AF666109

A World History of Neuroradiology

Daniel Birchall
Editor

President Wan-Yuo Guo

A World History of Neuroradiology

1990 to Present Day

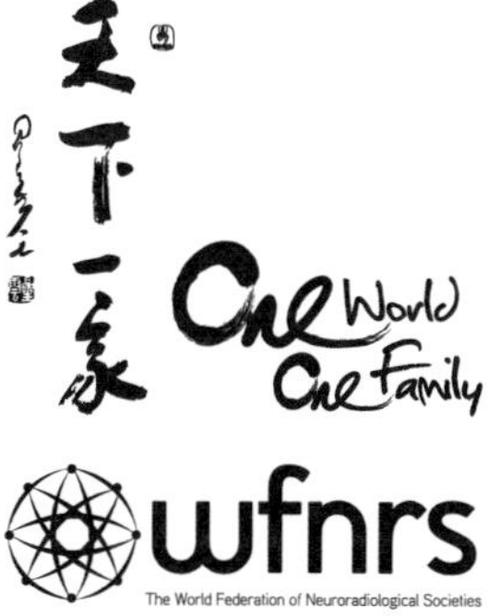

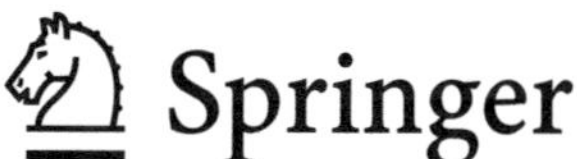

Editor
Daniel Birchall
Regional Neurosciences Centre
Royal Victoria Infirmary
Newcastle upon Tyne, UK

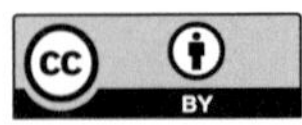

ISBN 978-3-032-16652-4 ISBN 978-3-032-16653-1 (eBook)
https://doi.org/10.1007/978-3-032-16653-1

The World Federation of Neuroradiological Societies

This Springer imprint is published by the registered company Springer Nature Switzerland AG
The registered company address is: Gewerbestrasse 11, 6330 Cham, Switzerland

Preface

The inspiration for the development of this project comes from the personal interactions that we have had with the very many inspirational Neuroradiologists from around the world. In our roles at the World Federation of Neuroradiological Societies, we are in a privileged position of being in contact with Neuroradiology Associations from all corners of the world and of being able to see and appreciate the inspirational stories and professional journeys of Neuroradiologists around the globe.

The last 30 years have seen extraordinary advances in Neuroradiology, and we are at an inflection point for our speciality where international collaboration, communication, and sharing of resources are becoming increasingly important, not only for better mutual understanding but also for the improvement of health outcomes across the world. This book seeks to enhance this common understanding and to help in strengthening the bridges between Neuroradiology Associations in all continents. It also aims to provide a record and a reflection of the extraordinary contributions already made.

This compilation represents the end result of a huge collaborative effort from individuals and Neuroradiology organizations from around the world. To all of these, we are enormously grateful. It remains a great privilege for us to have helped in some small way in shaping this book.

Oak Brook, IL, USA Wan-Yuo Guo
Newcastle, UK Daniel Birchall

WFNRS 2022–2026 ExCom

President:	Wan-Yuo Guo, MD, PhD	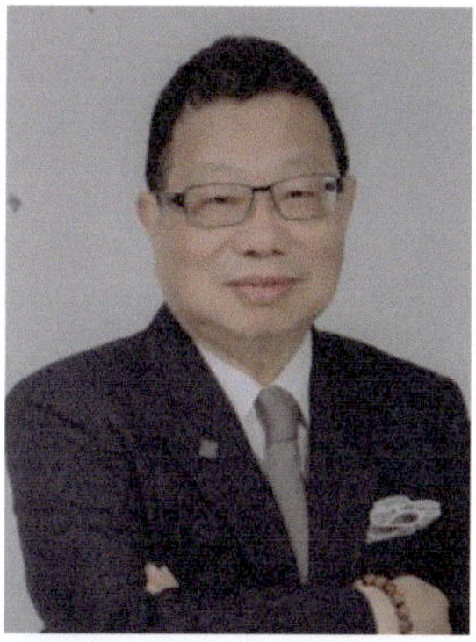
Vice-President/ President-Elect:	Daniel Birchall, MD, MBA	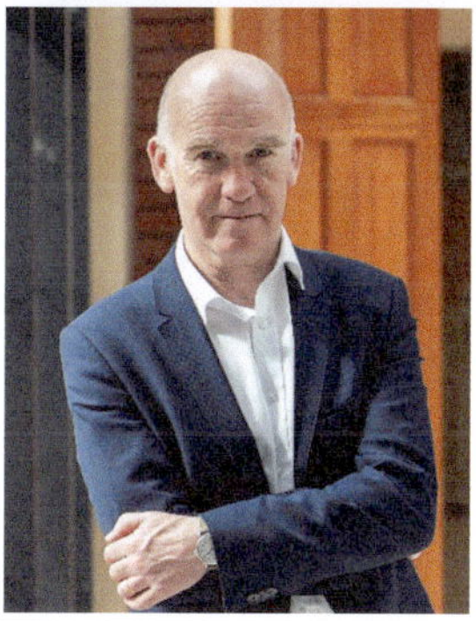

(continued)

Secretary General:	Pia Maly Sundgren, MD, PhD	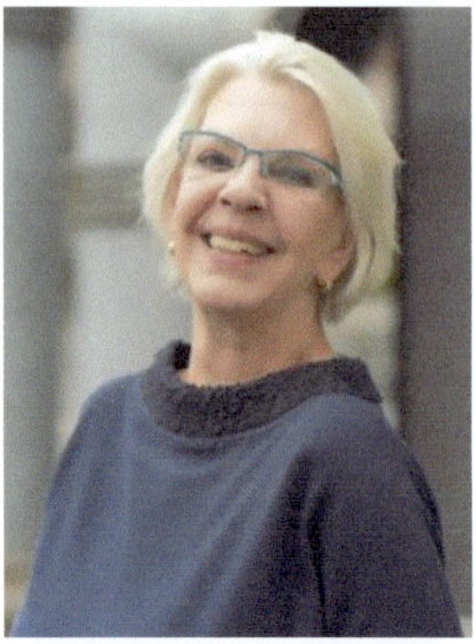
Treasurer:	Deborah Shatzkes, MD	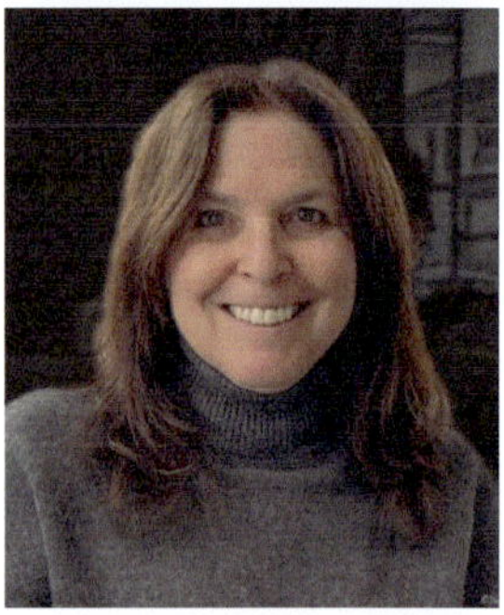
Member-at-Large:	Maria de Fatima Viana Vasco Aragao, MD, PhD	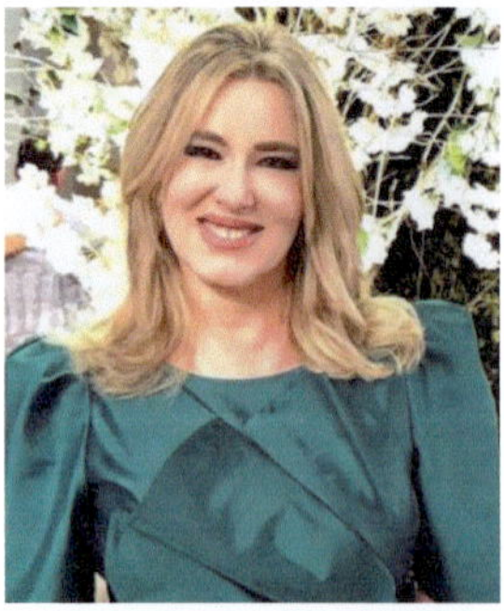
Member-at-Large:	Tracy Kilborn, MBChB, FRCR	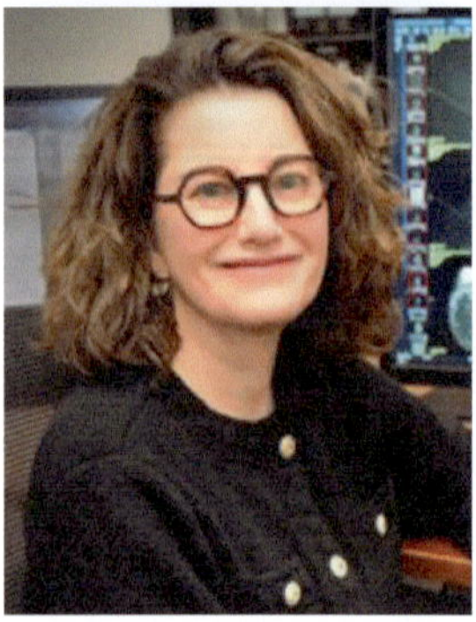

(continued)

Member-at-Large:	Paul Parizel, MD, PhD	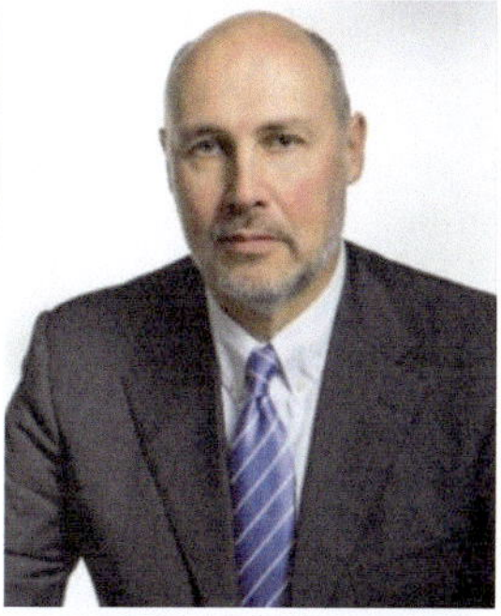
Immediate Past President, WFNRS:	E. Turgut Tali, MD	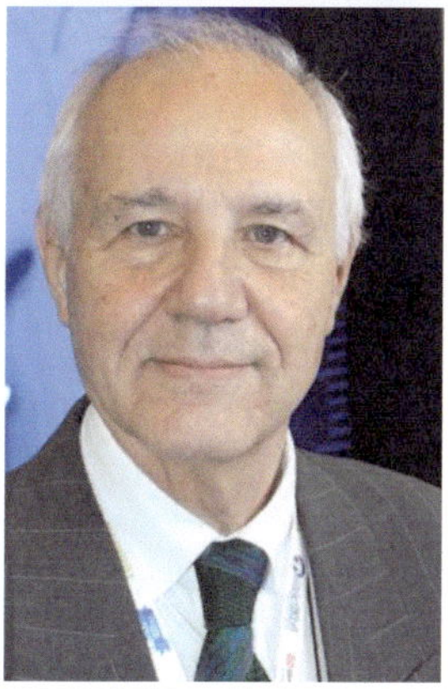
XXII SNR President:	Mauricio Castillo, MD, FACR	mauricio_castillo@med.unc.edu
XXIII SNR President:	Tarek Yousry, MD	t.yousry@ucl.ac.uk

Staff (Central Office)	Karen Lyp	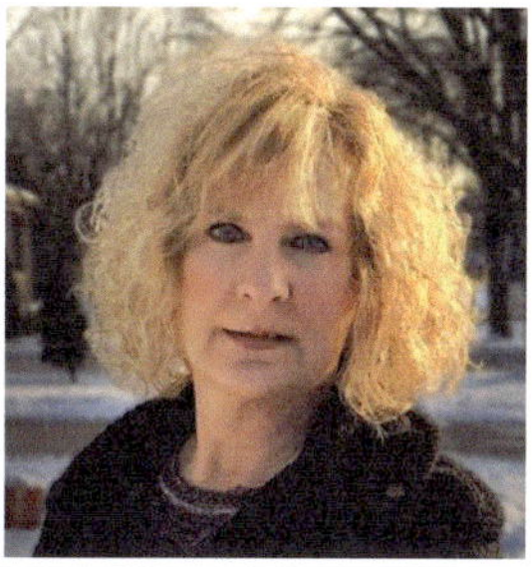
820 Jorie Blvd. Suite 300		
Oak Brook, IL 60523		
1-630-574-0220/Fax 1-630-572-0661		

(continued)

Staff (Taiwan Office) Rm 203, 2nd Floor, LiFu Educational Building, China Medical University No. 91, Hsueh-Shuh Rd., North District, Taichung City, 404, Taiwan Tel: +886-4-22053366 ext 7007	Hui-Yun Chen	twoffice@wfnrs.net

Acknowledgments

This book has taken several years to come to fruition, and we have benefited from the generosity, patience, expertise, and wisdom of many people.

I wish to thank Margaret Moore, Priyanka Dey, and the production team at Springer for their guidance and always thoughtful support in bringing the manuscript to completion.

I wish to express my gratitude to the Memorial Foundation of Ching-The Hsu for generous financial support for this project.

Recognition is due to Dr. Mat Elameer for his assistance, time, and editorial guidance, which were important in helping to shape this compilation.

Thanks are also due to Hui-Yun Chen and Karen Lyp for their administrative assistance and unfailing support throughout this process.

Above all, this book would not exist without the inspiration, energy, and vision of Professor Wan-Yuo Guo, the President of the World Federation. He has been a wise and constant captain of the ship, and this book is a fitting reflection of his constant warmth, openness, and kindness.

Daniel Birchall

The original version of the book has been revised. A correction to this book can be found at https://doi.org/10.1007/978-3-032-16653-1_27

Stories from Across the World of Neuroradiology

When you tell a story, you spark a connection. This is the power of storytelling.
–Jay O'Callaghan

The World Federation of Neuroradiological Societies (WFNRS) was established in 1994 by the great visionary Derek Harwood Nash to promote international collaboration and global development in our chosen field of Neuroradiology. This year marks the 30th anniversary of the founding of the Federation. As part of this anniversary, we are pleased to present a history of Neuroradiology over the last 30 years, as seen through the stories told by our member Societies and Associations.

The Federation is a dynamic network of nearly 50 Neuroradiology Societies and Associations from across the world, representing Africa, Asia, Europe, the Middle East, North America, Oceania, and South America. The Federation provides a platform on which our member Societies and Associations can share their experience and stories, and in doing so, the Federation aspires to promote mutual understanding and respect. The rapid development of digital communications over the last few years have revolutionized how we interact and engage internationally, and has made global connectivity a reality. Professor Nash can only have dreamed of the connectivity and connectedness that have become so central and ubiquitous to our personal and professional lives.

It is this ease of connection and our human drive to engage that has made partnerships and collaborations between geographically disparate places a day-to-day reality. The revolution in connectedness brings us together in a way that was unimaginable 30 years ago, and creates an extraordinary mix of inspiration and energy that makes the network such an exciting, catalytic "world city."

As part of the Federation's aspiration to continue to be as modern, impactful, and meaningful as possible, we see this compilation as an important part of the process of networking through deepening of mutual understanding across countries and continents.

This compilation of stories highlights and extols the extraordinary contributions made to International Neuroradiology by individual Neuroradiology Societies and Associations across the globe. Each Society has traveled its own path, and each has its own unique and special story to tell, with its own integral dynamism, energy, and direction. We are defined by our history and by our geography, and by bringing together the stories from our member Societies across the world, not only can we celebrate the past, but we can understand the present and plan for the future. The increasing dynamic toward collaboration across countries and continents can only be strengthened by such an understanding of each other's perspectives. This compilation is a celebration not only of what we share in common but also of what makes our individual journeys all so unique.

An important theme that becomes very apparent is the extraordinary contribution to progress, education, and training that has been provided by women in our speciality. It is fair to say that as the last 30 years have evolved women have taken the lead in the forward development of Neuroradiology across the world, with very many inspirational figures and stories. This compilation recognizes and reflects this, and we are proud to present additional chapters that highlight the pioneering roles played by women in Neuroradiology around thc world.

This compendium also includes a review of the keynote conference of the Federation, the Symposium Neuroradiologicum, the 4-yearly coming together of Neuroradiology Associations from around the world. This review of the previous Symposia is a remarkable record of aspiration, effort, and educational excellence, all for the benefit of International Neuroradiology, and is a testament to the tremendous contributions made by Neuroradiologists from around the world. This encapsulates the goals of the Federation in providing connectivity, excellence in education, and togetherness in our chosen field.

We are enormously indebted to our member Societies and Associations for their contributions to this compilation. Each chapter tells its own wonderful story, and brings a different color to the rainbow that is International Neuroradiology.

I also wish to commend to you Professor Wan-Yuo Guo, President of WFNRS. He has been the inspiration behind this book. Without his vision, enthusiasm, drive, and boundless energy, this compilation would not have come to fruition.

On behalf of Professor Wan-Yuo Guo and the WFNRS Executive Committee, I thank the individual authors for their time, commitment, and thoughtfulness in making this volume possible.

We hope that the stories that are contained within this volume will become an important step in strengthening the bridges between us.

> Individually, we are one drop. Together, we are an ocean. –Ryunosike Satoro

World Federation of Neuroradiological Societies
Oak Brook, IL, USA

Daniel Birchall

Contents

Part I A History of World Neuroradiology

1 A Brief History of the Symposium Neuroradiologicum 3
Paul M. Parizel
Acknowledgement of Bibliographic Sources 5
1939—The Ist SNR—Antwerp (Belgium)—Rudolph Thienpondt 5
1949—The IInd SNR—Rotterdam—Bernard George Ziedses des Plantes 6
1952—The IIIrd SNR—Stockholm (Sweden)—Erik Lindgren....... 7
1955—The IVth SNR—London (UK)—James William Douglas Bull . 8
1957—The Vth SNR—Brussels (BE)—Donald Lane McRae........ 9
1961—The VIth SNR—Rome (IT)—Giovanni Ruggiero 9
1964—The VIIth SNR—New York City/USA—Juan Manuel Taveras . 10
1967—The VIIIth SNR—Paris/FR—Hermann Fischgold........... 11
1970—The IXth SNR—Göteborg/SE—Ingmar Wickbom 12
1974—The Xth SNR—Punta del Este/UY—Néstor Azambuja....... 12
1978—The XIth SNR—Wiesbaden/DE—Sigurd Wende............ 13
1982—The XIIth SNR—Washington DC/US—Giovanni Di Chiro ... 14
1986—The XIIIth SNR—Stockholm/SE—Torgny Greitz........... 15
1990—The XIVth SNR—London—Edward Philip George Houssemayne du Boulay.......... 16
1994—The XVth SNR—Kumamoto/JP—Mutsumasa Takahashi 16
1998—The XVIth SNR—Philadelphia/PA, USA—Sadek Kamel Hilal 17
2002—The XVIIth SNR—Paris/FR—Luc Picard 18
2006—The XVIIIth SNR—Adelaide/AUS—Michael R. Sage 18
2010—The XIXth SNR—Bologna/ITA—Marco Leonardi 19
2014—The XXth SNR—Istanbul/TR—E. Turgut Tali.............. 20
2018—The XXIst SNR—Taipei/TWN—Wan-Yuo Guo 20
2022—The XXIInd SNR—New York City/NY, USA—Mauricio Castillo 21
2026—The XXIIIrd SNR—London—Tarek Yousry 22

2030—The XXIVth SNR—Sapporo—Prof. Kohsuke Kudo and Prof. Minako Azuma 22
Final Thoughts 23
Further Reading 25

2 Purpose-Driven Mission: A History of the American Society of Neuroradiology (ASNR): 1990–2024 29
Jonathan D. Clemente
Preamble: 1962 to 1990 29
ASNR Strategic Goals and Initiatives Since 1990 30
Practice/Advocacy 30
Education/Training 31
Governance 35
ASNR Physician Leadership 36
ASNR Executive Committee 36
ASNR Committee Structure 37
Evolution of the ASNR Constitution 38
Research 40
Conclusion 43
Appendix: Past Presidents of the American Society of Neuroradiology . . . 43
References 45

3 Asian-Oceanian Society of Neuroradiology and Head & Neck Radiology: The Early Years 49
Francis Hui and C. C. Tchoyoson Lim
Introduction 49
Founding of the AOSNHNR 49
World Wide Web Presence 52
The Future and Challenges Facing Neuroradiology and AOSNHNR . . . 57
Challenges in the Asian-Oceanian Context 58
References 59

4 Australian and New Zealand Society of Neuroradiology (ANZSNR) 1990 to Present Day 61
Makhan S. Khangure
Introduction 61
The Beginning 62
Post 1990 64
Training 65
Society Presidents 66
Current Status 68
Publications 68
Conclusion 69

5 Austrian Society of Neuroradiology (Österreichische Gesellschaft für Neuroradiologie—ÖGNR) 71
Elke R. Gizewski, Hannes Deutschmann, Gregor Kasprian, Julia Furtner, Michael Sonnberger, and Johannes Trenkler
Introduction 71
Organization 72
Annual Meetings 73
Current Situation of Neuroradiology in Austria 76
Training 76
Academia 77
References 77

6 Recent History of the Brazilian Society of Diagnostic and Therapeutic Neuroradiology 79
Carlos Clayton Macêdo de Freitas, Claudio C. V. Staut, Francisco Mont'Alverne, Felipe T. Pacheco, Carlos Batista Alves de Souza Filho, Carlos Michel A. Peres, Christiane M. S. Campos, Eric Homero Albuquerque Paschoal, Eduardo Floriani Raupp, Gelson Luis Koppe, José Guilherme Caldas, Maria de Fátima Viana Vasco Aragao, Michel Eli Frudit, Pedro S. C. Magalhães, Raquel Trovo Hidalgo, Ricardo Abkalaf, and Rogério Zenóbio Darwich
The Dawn of a New Society 80
The Recent History (2018 Until Now) 82
SBNR'S Partnership with Other Institutions 85
Advancements and Collaborations 87
Future Challenges for Interventional Neuroradiology in Brazil 88
References 89

7 A History of the British Neuroradiology from the Perspective of British Society of Neuroradiologists 91
Christopher Rowland-Hill and Dipayan Mitra
Early Days 91
1990s 92
Year 2000 Onwards 93
Academic Subcommittee 94
Standards Subcommittee 94
Training and Education Subcommittee (TESC) 95
BSNR Constitution 96
Online Presence 96
Conclusion 96

8 World History of Neuroradiology: Croatia 97
Dijana Zadravec, Mia Smoljan Basuga, and Matea Prenc

9 Neuroradiology in Germany 107
Peter Schramm, Ansgar Berlis, and Florian Schneider
Scope of Work: Diagnosis and Intervention 107
Organizational Structures 110
References. 111

10 History of the Israeli Society for Neuroradiology 1990–2024 113
Ayelet Eran and Eliel Ben-David

11 History of Italian Neuroradiology, 1990–2023 115
Giuseppe Scotti
AINR: Associazione Italiana di Neuroradiologia 117
Congresses, Meetings, and Courses 117
Hospital Departments 118
Neuroradiology Departments 2023. 119
Academic Positions, Teaching, and Research. 119
International Relationships 120
Italian Neuroradiologists Abroad 120
Lost Colleagues 1990–2023 121
The Future. 121
National Congresses (Before 1990) 122
National Congresses After 1990 123
Pediatric Section 123
Honorary Members and Gold Metal Awards 124
Presidents or Board Members of the International Societies of Neuroradiology. 125

12 Japanese Society of Neuroradiology (JSNR): 1990 to The Present . . . 127
Yukio Miki
Membership Composition. 127
Leadership. 127
Legal Status. 128
Standing Committees 128
Fiftieth Anniversary Commemorative Events. 128
Kato Prize 129
Website 129
Foreign Honorary Members 129
Hosting the Symposium Neuroradiologicum (SNR) 129
Official Journal 130
Logo 130
Future Prospects 130

13 A Brief History of Neuroradiology in South Korea: From a Small Beginning to an Ever-Growing Leading Role 131
Hye Jin Baek, Ji-hoon Kim, and Won-Jin Moon
Introduction. 131

History of Neuroradiology in South Korea Centered on the Korean Society of Neuroradiology (KSNR) 132
Conclusion 140
References. 140

14 Neuroradiology in Norway; The Last 25 Years 143
Per Hjalmar Nakstad
References. 145

15 A Brief History of Portuguese Neuroradiology: The Last 30 Years . . . 147
Rui Manaças, Luísa Biscoito, Inês Carreiro, and Ana Mafalda Reis

16 SILAN Society: History and International Impact 1988–2024. 157
Ramón E. Figueroa

17 History of South African Neuroradiology. 173
Clive Wyndham Sperryn, Sally Candy, Ebrahim Kader, Andre MacDonald, Duncan David Royston, Victor Mngomezulu, Coert de Vries, Shalendra Kumar Misser, Leon Janse van Rensburg, and Linda Tebogo Hlabangana
The Context. 174
The Early Years 175
Diagnostic Neuroradiology. 176
Paediatric Neuroradiology 181
Several South African Radiologists Have Made an International Name in Paediatric Neuroradiology 181
Neuro-intervention 182
Academic Support and Continuing Medical Education 185
The Future. 186
References. 188

18 The History of Swiss Neuroradiology 189
Karl-Olof Lövblad, Isabel Wanke, Luca Remonda, and Daniel Rüfenacht
The Swiss Society for Neuroradiology (SGNR/SSNR) 189
Before the Swiss Society of Neuroradiology 190
Neuroradiology in the Various Institutions and Cantons 191
The Swiss Title in Neuroradiology 193
Neuroradiology and Research. 194
References. 195

19 The Neuroradiological Society of Taiwan. 197
Chao-Bao Luo, Wan-Yuo Guo, and Michael Mu-Huo Teng
The Asian-Australasian Federation of Interventional and Therapeutic Neuroradiology (AAFITN 2008). 199
XXI SNR in Taiwan 199

20 **Neuroradiology in Türkiye** 203
E. Turgut Tali
References 214

21 **History of the Swedish Society of Neuroradiology and Swedish Neuroradiology 1990–2024** 215
Isabella M. Björkman-Burtscher, Ida Blystad, Tobias Granberg, and Pia Maly Sundgren
The Swedish Society of Neuroradiology, SSNR (Svensk Förening för Neuroradiologi, SFNR) 216
References 222

Part II Women in Neuroradiology

22 **Women in Neuroradiology in Africa** 227
Clive Wyndham Sperryn, Napo Kasirye-Mbugua, Sally E. Candy, Sahar Saleem, Amal Saleh Nour, Hafisatu Gbadamosi, Sheila Waa, Phyllis Mezue, Hamdi Mohamed Isse, Thandi Eunice Buthelezi, Gopolang Mndebele, Ugumba Mussa Kwikima, Valeria Nabossa, Rita Nassanga, and Sarah B. Nshimbi
Egypt 229
Ethiopia 232
Ghana 233
Kenya 238
Nigeria 240
Somalia 241
South Africa 241
Tanzania 249
Uganda 252
Zambia 257
Summary 261
References 264

23 **History of Women in Neuroradiology in Asia Oceania** 265
Kumiko Ando, Patrcia Desmond, Lou Xin, Christina Andica, Sri Andreani Utomo, Mohit Agarwal, Won-Jin Moon, Norlisah Mohd Ramli, Ling Ling Chan, Chao-Bao Luo, Nitaya Suwanwela, Laetitia de Villiers, Lee-Anne Slater, Lesley Cala, and Patricia Desmond
Introduction 265
Women in Neuroradiology and Neurointervention in Australia 267
Women in Neuroradiology and Neurointervention in China 272
Women in Neuroradiology in Indonesia 282
History of Women Neuroradiologists in India 285
History of Woman in Neuroradiology in Japan 286
Pioneers 287
Promising Talents 303

History of Women Neuroradiologists In Korea 314
Women in Radiology and Neuroradiology in Malaysia 327
Women In Radiology and Neuroradiology in Nepal 333
Women in Neuroradiology in Singapore 334
Women in Neuroradiology in Taiwan............................ 343
Women In Neuroradiology and Neurointervention in Thailand....... 345
References.. 354

24 Women's Contribution to the World History of Neuroradiology: Europa Chapter.. 357
María Isabel Vargas, Sofie Van Cauter, Zulejha Merhemic, Primarius Martina Špero, Jennifer Linn, Chiara Zini, Nicoletta Emanuela Anzalone, Anna Zimny, Marta Drake-Perez, Pia C. Sundgren, Kees J. Simon, Frans W. Zonneveld, Aysenur Cila, and Isil Saatci
Women in Neuroradiology: Belgium 358
Women in Neuroradiology: Bosnia and Herzegovina 362
Women in Neuroradiology: Croatia 365
Women in Neuroradiology: Germany........................... 370
Women in Neuroradiology: Italy 374
Women in Neuroradiology: Poland............................. 378
The Role of Women in Spanish Neuroradiology 387
Women in Neuroradiology: Sweden............................ 394
Women in Neuroradiology: Switzerland......................... 404
Women in Neuroradiology: The Netherlands..................... 406
Women in Neuroradiology: Turkey 413
Further Reading 415

25 The History of Women in Neuroradiology in Latin America 419
Maria de Fátima Viana Vasco Aragao, Carolina Tramontini, Katiuzka Casares, Jose Alejandro Bacalla, Carolina Mejias Soto, Carlos Rugilo, Eduardo Gonzalez, Carolina Servin, Janeth Bu, Valeria Schoenstedit, Maria Honrado, and Jorge Boschi
History of Women Neuroradiologists in Brazil 420
History of Women Neuroradiologists in Peru..................... 429
History of Women Neuroradiologists in Colombia 432
History of Women Neuroradiologists in Costa Rica................ 434
History of Women Neuroradiologists in Argentina................. 434
History of Women Neuroradiologists in Paraguay 439
History of Women Neuroradiologists in Mexico 441
History of Women Neuroradiologists in Honduras................. 442
History of Women Neuroradiologists in Chile 443
History of Women Neuroradiologists in the Dominican Republic..... 446
History of Women Neuroradiologists in Uruguay 446
Conclusion 447
References.. 447

26 The History of Women in Neuroradiology in North America from 1990 to the Present 449
Anne G. Osborn, Patricia Rhyner, Carolyn C. Meltzer, Pamela W. Schaefer, Laurie A. Loevner, Pina C. Sanelli, Tina Young Poussaint, Erin Simon Schwartz, Yvonne W. Lui, Yoshimi Anzai, Donatella Tampieri, Wendy Smoker, Vijay Rao, Michelle Michel, Deborah Shatzkes, Nancy Fischbein, Kristine Mosier, Christine Glastonbury, Jody Tanabe, Jill Hunter, Caroline Robson, Susan Palasis, V. Michelle Silvera, Judy Donovan Post, Alyssa Watanabe, Michelle Johnson, Lubdha Shah, Wende Gibbs, Mary E. Jensen, Raquel Z. del Carpio-O'Donovan, Rona Woldenberg, Tabassum Kennedy, Achala Vagal, Birgit Ertl-Wagner, Tammie Benzinger, Soonme Cha, and Patricia Ellen Grant
Introduction 452
Leadership 452
Clinical Innovation and Research 453
Education 455
Diversity, Equity and Inclusion, and Global Outreach 455
Biographical Sketches 456
Conclusion 495
References 495

Correction to: A World History of Neuroradiology C1
Daniel Birchall

Epilogue of the Book 497

Index 499

Contributors

Ricardo Abkalaf Interventional Neuroradiology Service, Hospital A.C. Camargo Cancer Center, São Paulo, Brazil

Mohit Agarwal Department of Radiology, Medical College of Wisconsin, Milwaukee, WI, USA

Christina Andica Faculty of Health Data Science, Juntendo University, Bunkyo, Tokyo, Japan

Department of Radiology, Juntendo University Graduate School of Medicine, Bunkyo, Tokyo, Japan

Kumiko Ando Department of Diagnostic Radiology, Kobe City Medical Center General Hospital, Kobe, Japan

Yoshimi Anzai University of Utah Hospital, Salt Lake City, UT, USA

Nicoletta Emanuela Anzalone Neuroradiology Department, IRCCS San Raffaele Scientific Institute, Milan, Italy

Vita-Salute San Raffaele University, Milan, Italy

Maria de Fátima Viana Vasco Aragao Universidade de Federal de Pernambuco, São Paulo, Brazil

Department of Radiology, Clinica Diagnostika Endoscopia e Radiologia, LTDA, Recife, Brazil

Department of Surgery and Postgraduate Department of Neuropsychiatry and Behavioral Sciences at UFPE, Centro de Ciencias Medicas da Universidade Federal de Pernambuco (UFPE), Recife, Brazil

Jose Alejandro Bacalla Department of Diagnostic Imaging, Instituto Nacional De Ciencias Neurologicas, Lima, Peru

Hye Jin Baek Department of Radiology, Pusan National University Yangsan Hospital, Pusan National University School of Medicine, Yangsan, Republic of Korea

Mia Smoljan Basuga Croatian Society of Neuroradiology, UHC Sestre Milosrdnice, University of Zagreb School of Dental Medicine, Zagreb, Croatia

Eliel Ben-David Department of Radiology, Shaare Zedek Medical Center, Jerusalem, Israel

Faculty of Medicine, The Hebrew University, Jerusalem, Israel

Tammie Benzinger Mallinckrodt Institute of Radiology, Neuroradiology Section, Washington University in Saint Louis, St. Louis, MO, USA

Ansgar Berlis University hospital Augsburg, Germany, Diagnostic and Interventional Neuroradiology, Augsburg, Germany

Luísa Biscoito Centro Hospitalar e Universitário de Lisboa Norte, Lisbon, Portugal

Isabella M. Björkman-Burtscher University of Gothenburg, Gothenburg, Sweden

Ida Blystad Linköping University, Linköping and President of SSNR, Linköping, Sweden

Jorge Boschi Department of Radiology, Medica Uruguaya, Montevideo, Uruguay

Janeth Bu Department of Radiology, hospital de especialidades instituto honduras, Comayagua, Honduras

Thandi Eunice Buthelezi Department of Diagnostic Radiology, Chris Hani Baragwanath Academic Hospital, Johannesburg, South Africa

University of the Witwatersrand, Johannesburg, South Africa

Lesley Cala Department of Radiology, Monash Health and School of Clinical Sciences Monash University, Clayton, VIC, Australia

José Guilherme Caldas Hospital of Clinics of University of São Paulo, São Paulo, Brazil

Christiane M.S. Campos Hospital da Beneficência Portuguesa de São Paulo, São Paulo, Brazil

Sally E. Candy Department of Diagnostic Radiology, Groote Schuur Hospital/ University of Cape Town, Cape Town, Western Cape, South Africa

Inês Carreiro Centro Hospitalar e Universitário de Coimbra, Coimbra, Portugal

Katiuzka Casares Department of Neuroimaging, National Institute of Neurology and Neurosurgery, Mexico City, Mexico

Ling Ling Chan Department of Neuroradiology, Division of Radiological Sciences, Singapore General Hospital, Singapore, Singapore

Duke-NUS Medical School, Singapore, Singapore

Soonme Cha Department of Radiology & Biomedical Imaging, University of California, San Francisco, San Francisco, CA, USA

Aysenur Cila Radiology Department, Medipol University, Istanbul, Turkey

Jonathan D. Clemente Charlotte Radiology, PA, Neuroradiology Section, Charlotte, NC, USA

Rogério Zenóbio Darwich Rede D'or Biocor, Belo Horizonte, Minas Gerais, Brazil

Carlos Clayton Macêdo de Freitas Neurosurgery and Interventional Neuroradiology, São Paulo State University, Botucatu, São Paulo, Brazil

Raquel Z. del Carpio-O'Donovan McGill University Health Center, Montreal, QC, Canada

Patricia Desmond Royal Melbourne Hospital, University of Melbourne, Melbourne, VIC, Australia

Carlos Batista Alves de Souza Filho Interventional Neuroradiology, Hospital Santa Casa, Belo Horizonte, Minas Gerais, Brazil

Hannes Deutschmann Division of Neuroradiology, Vascular and Interventional Radiology, Department of Radiology, Medical University of Graz, Graz, Austria

Laetitia de Villiers Department of Radiology, Monash Health and School of Clinical Sciences Monash University, Clayton, VIC, Australia

Department Neurointerventional Radiology, Gold Coast University Hospital, Southport, QLD, Australia

Qscan Radiology Clinics, Neutex Image Guided Surgical and Robotics Training Centre, Southport, QLD, Australia

Coert de Vries Scholtz and Partners, Midstream Mediclinic, Centurion, South Africa

Marta Drake-Perez Department of Radiology—Neuroradiology, Hospital Universitario Marqués de Valdecilla and IDIVAL, Santander, Spain

Ayelet Eran Department of Radiology, Rambam Health Care Campus, Haifa, Israel

Faculty of Medicine, Technion – Israel Institute of Technology, Haifa, Israel

Birgit Ertl-Wagner Department of Diagnostic & Interventional Radiology, The Hospital for Sick Children, Toronto, ON, USA

Department of Medical Imaging University of Toronto, Toronto, ON, USA

Ramón E. Figueroa Emeritus Professor of Neuroradiology, Medical College of Georgia at Augusta University, Augusta, GA, USA

Nancy Fischbein Department of Radiology, Center for Academic Medicine, Stanford University, Stanford, CA, USA

Michel Eli Frudit Department of Interventional Neuroradiology—INRAD/HCFMUSP and Department of Interventional Neuroradiology, Albert Einstein Hospital, São Paulo, Brazil

Julia Furtner Research Center for Medical Image Analysis and Artificial Intelligence, Danube Private University, Krems an der Donau, Austria

Hafisatu Gbadamosi Department of Radiology, Korle Bu Teaching Hospital, Accra, Ghana

Department of Radiology, University of Ghana Medical School, Accra, Ghana

Wende Gibbs Department of Neuroradiology, Barrow Neurological Institute, Phoenix, AZ, USA

Elke R. Gizewski Department of Radiology, Neuroimage Core Facility, Medical University Innsbruck, Innsbruck, Austria

Christine Glastonbury University of California, San Francisco, San Francisco, CA, USA

Eduardo Gonzalez Radiología-Radiology, Hospital Universitario CEMIC, CEMIC University Hospital, Caba, Argentina

Tobias Granberg Karolinska Institutet, Stockholm, Sweden

Patricia Ellen Grant Boston Children's Hospital, Harvard Medical School, Boston, MA, USA

Wan-Yuo Guo Department of Radiology, Taipei Veterans General Hospital, Taipei, Taiwan

Raquel Trovo Hidalgo Hospital de Base, São José do Rio Preto, São Paulo, Brazil

Linda Tebogo Hlabangana Diagnostic Radiology, University of Witwatersrand, Johannesburg, South Africa

Maria Honrado Department of Nueroradiology, CIMEN S.A.S, Santiago, Dominican Republic

Francis Hui Radiology, National University Hospital, Singapore, Singapore

Jill Hunter Baylor College of Medicine, Houston, TX, USA

Department of Pediatric Radiology, Texas Children's Hospital, Houston, TX, USA

Hamdi Mohamed Isse Department of Radiology, Sahan Diagnostic Center, Mogadishu, Banadir, Somalia

Leon Janse van Rensburg Division of Radiodiagnosis, Tygerberg Academic Radiology, Cape Town, South Africa

Mary E. Jensen Department of Radiology and Medical Imaging, University of Virginia Health, Charlottesville, VA, USA

Michelle Johnson Yale New Haven Hospital, New Haven, CT, USA

Ebrahim Kader General and Neuro Interventional Radiology, Morton and Partners Inc, Cape Town, South Africa

Napo Kasirye-Mbugua Department of Radiology, Foothills Medical Centre, Calgary, AB, Canada

Gregor Kasprian Department of Biomedical Imaging and Image-Guided Therapy, Medical University of Vienna, Vienna, Austria

Tabassum Kennedy University of Wisconsin School of Medicine and Public Health, Madison, WI, USA

Makhan S. Khangure Department of Diagnostic and Interventional Radiology, Royal Perth Hospital, Perth, WA, Australia

University of Western Australia, Perth, WA, Australia

Ji-hoon Kim Department of Radiology, Seoul National University Hospital, Seoul National University College of Medicine, Seoul, Republic of Korea

Gelson Luis Koppe Hospital Cajuru, São Paulo, Brazil

Ugumba Mussa Kwikima Department of Radiology, Lugalo Military Hospital & Muhimbili University of Health and Allied Sciences, Dar es Salaam, Tanzania

C.C. Tchoyoson Lim Department of Neuroradiology, National Neuroscience Institute, Singapore, Singapore

Duke-NUS Medical School, Radiological Sciences Academic Clinical Programme, SingHealth Duke-NUS Academic Medical Centre, Singapore, Singapore

Jennifer Linn Institute for Diagnostic and Interventional Neuroradiology, University Hospital Carl Gustav Carus, Dresden, Germany

Medical Faculty of the Technical University Dresden, Dresden, Germany

Laurie A. Loevner Division of Neuroradiology, University of Pennsylvania Health System, Philadelphia, PA, USA

Karl-Olof Lövblad Division of Neuroradiology, Dépmartement diagnostique, Hôpitaux Universitaires de Genève, Genève, Switzerland

Yvonne W. Lui Department of Radiology, NYU Langone Health/Grossman School of Medicine, New York, NY, USA

Chao-Bao Luo Department of Radiology, Taipei Veterans General Hospital, Taipei, Taiwan

Andre MacDonald SCP Radiology, Panorama, Cape Town, South Africa

Pedro S.C. Magalhães Neurology, Neurosurgery and Neuroradiology Services, HMSJ, Joinville, Santa Catarina, Brazil

Rui Manaças SPNR (Portuguese Society of Neuroradiology), Lisbon, Portugal

Carolyn C. Meltzer Keck School of Medicine of USC, Los Angeles, CA, USA

Zulejha Merhemic Faculty of Health Care and Pharmacology, University Travnik, Travnik, Bosnia and Herzegovina

Phyllis Mezue Everlight Radiology, London, UK

Michelle Michel Froedtert Hospital and Medical College of Wisconsin, Milwaukee, WI, USA

Yukio Miki Department of Diagnostic and Interventional Radiology, Graduate School of Medicine, Osaka Metropolitan University, Osaka, Japan

Shalendra Kumar Misser Radiology, Lake Smit and Partners, Durban, South Africa

Dipayan Mitra Royal Victoria Infirmary, Newcastle upon Tyne, UK

Gopolang Mndebele Department of Radiology, Nelson Mandela Children's Hospital, Johannesburg, South Africa

Victor Mngomezulu Diagnostic Radiology, Chris Hani Baragwanath Academic Hospital/University of Witwatersrand, Johannesburg, South Africa

Francisco Mont'Alverne Interventional Neuroradiology Department, Hospital Geral de Fortaleza, Fortaleza, Ceara, Brazil

Won-Jin Moon Department of Radiology, Konkuk University Medical Center, Konkuk University School of Medicine, Seoul, Republic of Korea

Kristine Mosier Department of Radiology, Section of Neuroradiology and Imaging Sciences, Indiana University School of Medicine, Indianapolis, IN, USA

Valeria Nabossa Department of Radiology, Uganda Cancer Institute and Makerere University College of Health Sciences, Kampala, Uganda

Per Hjalmar Nakstad Neuroradiology, Oslo University Hospital, Oslo, Norway

Rita Nassanga Department of Radiology, Uganda Cancer Institute and Makerere University College of Health Sciences, Kampala, Uganda

Amal Saleh Nour Department of Radiology, School of Medicine, College of Health Sciences, Addis Ababa University, Tikur Anbessa Specialized Hospital, Addis Ababa, Ethiopia

Sarah B. Nshimbi Department of Radiology, University Teaching Hospitals – Adult Hospital, Lusaka, Zambia

Anne G. Osborn University of Utah, Salt Lake City, UT, USA

Felipe T. Pacheco Health Sciences from Santa Casa de Misericórdia, São Paulo, Brazil

Susan Palasis Emory University School of Medicine, Atlanta, GA, USA

Children's Healthcare of Atlanta, Atlanta, GA, USA

Paul M. Parizel Royal Perth Hospital (RPH), Perth, WA, Australia

University of Western Australia (UWA), Perth, WA, Australia

National Imaging Facility (NIF), St Lucia, QLD, Australia

Royal Australian and New Zealand College of Radiologists (RANZCR), Sydney, NSW, Australia

University of Antwerp (UA), Antwerp, Belgium

Eric Homero Albuquerque Paschoal Instituto Amazonas, São Paulo, Brazil

Carlos Michel A. Peres Neurosurgery Department, Hospital Santa Julia, Manaus, Amazonas, Brazil

Judy Donovan Post Boston University Chobanian & Avedisian School of Medicine, Boston, MA, USA

University of Miami Miller School of Medicine, Miami, FL, USA

Tina Young Poussaint Boston Children's Hospital, Harvard Medical School, Boston, MA, USA

Matea Prenc Croatian Society of Neuroradiology, UHC Sestre Milosrdnice, University of Zagreb School of Dental medicine, Zagreb, Croatia

Norlisah Mohd Ramli University Malaya, Kuala Lumpur, Wilayah Persekutuan Kuala Lumpur, Malaysia

College of Radiology, Academy of Medicine of Malaysia and Malaysian Society of Radiologists, Kuala Lumpur, Wilayah Persekutuan Kuala Lumpur, Malaysia

Asian Oceanian Society of Radiology Akriti Baral, MD, Kuala Lumpur, Wilayah Persekutuan Kuala Lumpur, Malaysia

Vijay Rao Jefferson Health, Sidney Kimmel Medical College, Thomas Jefferson University, Philadelphia, PA, USA

Eduardo Floriani Raupp Santa Casa de Misericórdia Hospital, Porto Alegre, Brazil

Ana Mafalda Reis Unidade Local de Saúde de Matosinhos, Hospital de Pedro Hispano, Matosinhos, Portugal

Luca Remonda Division of Neuroradiology, Kantonsspital Aarau, Aarau, Switzerland

Patricia Rhyner Mayo Clinic, Jacksonville, FL, USA

Caroline Robson Department of Radiology, Department of Otolaryngology, Boston Children's Hospital, Boston, MA, USA

Christopher Rowland-Hill Hull Royal Infirmary, Kingston upon Hull, UK

Duncan David Royston Lake Smit and Partners Radiology, Entabeni Hospital, Cape Town, South Africa

Daniel Rüfenacht Swiss Neuro Institute, Zurich, Zurich, Switzerland

Carlos Rugilo Diagnostic Imaging, Hospital Garrahan, Buenos Aires, Argentina

Isil Saatci Private Koru Hospitals, Interventional Neuroradiology Department, Ankara, Turkey

Sahar Saleem Department of Radiology, Kasr Al Ainy Faculty of Medicine-Cairo University, Cairo, Egypt

Pina C. Sanelli Northwell Health, Manhasset, NY, USA

Pamela W. Schaefer Department of Radiology, Massachusetts General Hospital, Boston, MA, USA

Harvard Medical School, Boston, MA, USA

Florian Schneider Deutsche Gesellschaft für Neuroradiologie e.V., Berlin, Germany

Valeria Schoenstedit Department of Radiologia, Clínica Alemana De Santiago, Santiago, Chile

Peter Schramm Institut für Neuroradiologie, UKSH Universitätsklinikum Schleswig-Holstein Campus Lübeck, Universität zu Lübeck, Lübeck, Germany

Erin Simon Schwartz Division of Neuroradiology, Lurie Family Foundations' MEG Imaging Center, Philadelphia, PA, USA

Perelman School of Medicine, University of Pennsylvania, Philadelphia, PA, USA

Giuseppe Scotti Centro Diagnostico Italiano (CDI), Milan, Italy

Università Vita Salute e Ospedale San Raffaele, Milan, Italy

Carolina Servin Medical Imaging, Centro Medico La Costa, Asunción, Paraguay

Lubdha Shah University of Utah Hospital, Salt Lake City, UT, USA

Deborah Shatzkes Zucker School of Medicine at Hofstra/Northwell Health, New York, NY, USA

V. Michelle Silvera Mayo Clinic, Rochester, MN, USA

Kees J. Simon Historical Section of the Dutch Society of Radiology, Domus Medica, Utrecht, The Netherlands

Lee-Anne Slater Department of Radiology, Monash Health and School of Clinical Sciences Monash University, Clayton, VIC, Australia

Wendy Smoker University of Iowa Health Care, Iowa City, IA, USA

Michael Sonnberger Institute of Neuroradiology, Neuromed Campus, Kepler University Hospital Linz, Linz, Austria

Carolina Mejias Soto Centro Nacional de Imágenes Médicas, Caja Costarricense del Seguro Social, Alajuela, Costa Rica

Primarius Martina Špero Department of Radiology, Affidea, Zagreb, Croatia

Clive Wyndham Sperryn Neuroradiology, Morton and Partners, Cape Town, South Africa

Morton and Partners Inc., Vincent Pallotti Hospital, Cape Town, Western Cape, South Africa

Claudio C.V. Staut Hospital of Clinics of University of São Paulo, São Paulo, Brazil

Pia C. Sundgren Department of Radiology, Institution of Clinical Sciences/Lund, Lund University, Lund, Sweden

Pia Maly Sundgren Lund University, Lund, Sweden

Nitaya Suwanwela Department of Radiology, King Chulalongkorn Memorial Hospital and Chulalongkorn University Medical School, Bangkok, Thailand

E. Turgut Tali Department of Radiology, Lokman Hekim University Faculty of Medicine, Ankara, Turkey

Donatella Tampieri Queen's University Hospital, Kingston, ON, USA

Jody Tanabe University of Colorado Anschutz, Aurora, CO, USA

Michael Mu-Huo Teng Department of Radiology, Cheng-Hsin General Hospital, Taipei, Taiwan

Carolina Tramontini Radiologia Departmente, Clínica Universitaria Colombia, Clinicas Colsanitas, Bogota, Colombia

Johannes Trenkler Institute of Neuroradiology, Neuromed Campus, Kepler University Hospital Linz, Linz, Austria

Sri Andreani Utomo Department of Radiology, Dr. Soetomo General Hospital, Surabaya, Indonesia

Faculty of Medicine, Universitas Airlangga, Surabaya, Indonesia

Achala Vagal Department of Radiology, UC College of Medicine, Cincinnati, OH, USA

Center for Clinical and Translational Science and Training (CCTST), University of Cincinnati Medical Center, Cincinnati, OH, USA

Sofie Van Cauter Department of Medical Imaging, East-Limburg Hospital Genk, Genk, Belgium

María Isabel Vargas Clinique des Grangettes, Hirslanden, Chêne Bougeries, Geneva, Switzerland

Sheila Waa Department of Radiology, Aga Khan University Hospital, Nairobi, Kenya

Isabel Wanke Swiss Society of Neuroradiology, Swiss Neuro Institute, Zurich, Zurich, Switzerland

Alyssa Watanabe University of Southern California, Los Angeles, CA, USA

CureMetrix, San Diego, CA, USA

Rona Woldenberg Zucker School of Medicine at Hofstra/Northwell, Manhasset, NY, USA

Lou Xin Department of Radiology, Chinese People's Liberation Army General Hospital, Beijing, China

Dijana Zadravec Croatian Society of Neuroradiology, UHC Sestre Milosrdnice, University of Zagreb School of Dental medicine, Zagreb, Croatia

Anna Zimny Department of General and Interventional Radiology and Neuroradiology, Wroclaw Medical University, Wroclaw, Poland

Chiara Zini Department of Radiology, USL Toscana Centro, Firenze, Italy

Frans W. Zonneveld Historical Section of the Dutch Society of Radiology, Domus Medica, Utrecht, The Netherlands

Part I
A History of World Neuroradiology

Chapter 1
A Brief History of the Symposium Neuroradiologicum

Paul M. Parizel

There is a tide in the affairs of men,
Which taken with the flood,
Leads on to fortune …
We must take the current when it serves,
Or lose our ventures.

—Shakespeare, Julius Caesar IV, iii

Since their inception, SNR meetings have served as the rallying point for active researchers, innovators, and clinicians in neuroradiology from across the entire world, providing them with an international stage to compare the results of their investigations and openly exchange ideas and opinions in a positive and friendly atmosphere that encourages scientific inquiry. The Latin-sounding name, "*Symposium Neuroradiologicum,*" was coined to indicate that this scientific meeting, to be held once every 4 years, should have a different character as compared with the (annual) meetings of national and (supra)regional neuroradiological societies.

SNR meetings serve as an open-access platform for neuroradiologists with diverse backgrounds and wide-ranging areas of interest to present their research, freely exchange ideas and concepts, and engage in fruitful discussions with colleagues from across the world. As Dr. Erik Lindgren wrote in a comment to the publication of the proceedings in Acta Radiologica (1953, vol 40, pp. 85–87): *These meetings should be* ***symposia****, and not congresses, that is, that every speaker must have the time he/she desires at his/her disposal. The word 'symposium' may*

P. M. Parizel (✉)
Royal Perth Hospital (RPH), Perth, WA, Australia

University of Western Australia (UWA), Perth, WA, Australia

National Imaging Facility (NIF), St Lucia, QLD, Australia

Royal Australian and New Zealand College of Radiologists (RANZCR), Sydney, NSW, Australia

University of Antwerp (UA), Antwerp, Belgium

D. Birchall (ed.), *A World History of Neuroradiology*,
https://doi.org/10.1007/978-3-032-16653-1_1

also be taken to imply that each lecture will be delivered with the aim of stimulating exchanges of views, and therefore be regarded as an introduction to a discussion. Almost 40 years later, in 1992, in Stockholm, the presidents reconfirmed the vision that *The meeting should be wholly devoted to the presentation and full discussion of scientific matter. ... On the other hand, courses for trainees and didactic lectures do not form part of the essential central purpose of such a symposium. ... It should also be noted that good science is not confined to the more developed countries*.

Given the spectacular growth of neuroradiology, it has become increasingly difficult to comply with these noble goals. Progressively, SNR meetings have attracted greater numbers of neuroradiologists, from all over the world. Despite the ambition to keep the SNR a scientific meeting of neuroscientists, favouring "cutting-edge research," many younger neuroradiologists are also interested in teaching and education. In recent times, SNR meetings have aspired to serve as a platform to innovation and research, while at the same time offering high-level medical education.

Table 1.1 provides a chronological overview of the SNR, listing years, locations (host cities), and Roman numeral references, from 1939 until 2030.

Table 1.1 Chronological overview of the SNR

1939	Antwerp/BE	I
1949	Rotterdam/NL	II
1952	Stockholm/SE	III
1955	London/UK	IV
1957	Brussels/BE	V
1961	Rome/IT	VI
1964	New York City/US	VII
1967	Paris/FR	VIII
1970	Gothenburg/SE	IX
1974	Punta del Este/UY	X
1978	Wiesbaden/DE	XI
1982	Washington DC/US	XII
1986	Stockholm/SE	XIII
1990	London/GB	XIV
1994	Kumamoto/JP	XV
1998	Philadelphia/US	XVI
2002	Paris/FR	XVII
2006	Adelaide/AU	XVIII
2010	Bologna/IT	XIX
2014	Turkey/TR	XX
2018	Taipei/TW	XXI
2022	New York City/US	XXII
2026	London/UK	XXIII
2030	Sapporo/JP	XXIV

Acknowledgement of Bibliographic Sources

In the preparation of this text, I am indebted to several eminent neuroradiologists who have made significant contributions to the history of neuroradiology:

- In 1967 *A Short History of Neuroradiology* was published by **Profs. Herman Fischgold & James Bull**, on occasion of the VIIIth Symposium Neuroradiologicum which was held in Paris, in September 1967. Unfortunately, I never had access to this original source, but it is referred to by other authors.
- In 1989, **Prof. Emmanuel Alain Cabanis**, together with **Dr Marie-Thérèse Iba-Zizen Cabanis**, edited a seminal book with the bilingual title *Contribution à l'histoire de la Neuroradiologie Européenne/Contribution to the history of European Neuroradiology.* In 1989, Emmanuel Cabanis was the president of the XVIth Congress of the European Society of Neuroradiology in Paris, 2–6 July 1989; a printed copy of the book was offered to all delegates, as part of their registration. The book was published by Éditions Pradel (Paris, France, 1989) and contained photocopies of many original documents, papers, articles, interviews, etc.
- In 1994, a *second edition* of the book was produced and published by Éditions Vigot, Paris. The project was financially supported by Laboratoire Guerbet, the leading French manufacturer of contrast media. The subtitle of this book was "ESNR 1969–1994" and it was published to celebrate the 25th anniversary of the European Society of Neuroradiology (ESNR). The second edition was presented to the participants of the XXth Congress of the European Society of Neuroradiology in Nancy (France), 14–18 June 1994. As for the previous edition, the **editors** of the book were listed **Emmanuel Alain & Marie-Thérèse Cabanis**.
- In 2002, *A History of Neuroradiology (1895–2002)* was published on the occasion of the XVIIth Symposium Neuroradiologicum, which was held in Paris, France, August 18–24, 2002. This was essentially a 3rd edition of the previous works. The **editors** were: **Emmanuel Alain Cabanis, Marie-Thérèse Iba-Zizen Cabanis, and Luc Picard** (who was the president of the XVIIth SNR), and the copyright belonged to the Symposium Neuroradiologicum. For this book, I could find the following information: ISBN: 9782913628113, 2913628117; OCLC Number/Unique Identifier: 496562157; 368 pages; 30 cm format.

1939—The Ist SNR—Antwerp (Belgium)—Rudolph Thienpondt

The *first-ever* Symposium Neuroradiologicum was a 5-day meeting that took place in Antwerp, Belgium from Monday 24th to Friday 28th July 1939. In fact, this first meeting was called *Conférences et Travaux Pratiques de Radiologie Crânienne.* It was only during the second Symposium Neuroradiologicum in Rotterdam, in 1949, that the Antwerp meeting was retrospectively labelled as the first SNR.

This first meeting was organised by Dr. Rudolph Thienpondt, a Belgian oto-rhino-laryngologist and ophthalmologist, who had trained in Germany and England, and who had started practising in Antwerp in 1927. Dr. Thienpondt had established himself as an expert in radiology of the temporal bone. The co-chair of this first meeting was Dr. Clément Sylvain Chaussé, a famous otoradiologist from Paris who had invented the technique of stereo-radiography of the temporal bone. Dr. Chaussé could not arrange for the meeting to be held in Paris, so it was moved to Antwerp, Belgium. The event was announced in the journal *La Presse Médicale* on 26 April 1939.

The meeting took place in the **Prince Leopold Institute of Tropical Medicine (ITM)** in Antwerp, Belgium, which was founded in 1906 by King Leopold II as a School for Tropical Diseases. It quickly evolved into a global centre for research and education in tropical medicine. In 1933, it moved into a newly commissioned building in Art Deco style in Antwerp. This architecturally beautiful and visually striking edifice was very much a state-of-the art 'modern' venue at the time of the meeting in 1939.

The *Conférences et Travaux Pratiques de* ***Radiologie Crânienne*** meeting 24–28 July 1939, Antwerp was attended by roughly 50 delegates. The registration fee was 300 **Belgian Francs**, *for the morning lectures ("conférences")* and *for the afternoon workshops ("travaux pratiques")*. Sponsorship was obtained from two industry partners:

- *Société Gevaert (now part of Agfa)*
- *Compagnie Générale de Radiologie (CGR, now part of GE Healthcare)*

A group photograph was taken on the steps in front of the main building of the Institute of Tropical Medicine. The 21 lectures and the practical demonstrations were mainly devoted to otoradiology. Lectures were held during the morning sessions, while the practical demonstrations took place in the afternoons. Interestingly, the two organisers, Dr. Thienpondt and Dr. Chaussé, were oto-rhino-laryngologists. Of the 13 speakers, there were five radiologists: Bertolotti, Tieschendorf, Lysholm, Schüller, and Ziedses des Plantes. Of the 21 papers and demonstrations, only two were concerned with contrast radiology:

- *Ventriculography (by prof. Lysholm from Stockholm, Sweden)*
- *Cerebral arteriography (by prof. Dyes from Würzburg, Germany)*

Prof. Ziedses des Plantes discussed the principles of both tomography and subtraction.

Many of the participants would not survive the Second World War, which started shortly after the meeting.

1949—The IInd SNR—Rotterdam—Bernard George Ziedses des Plantes

In 1949, under the presidency of Prof. Dr. Bernard George Ziedses des Plantes, Rotterdam hosted the first SNR after the Second World War (WW2). Dutch-born Dr. Ziedses des Plantes (1902–1993) trained in Utrecht, the Netherlands, as a specialist in nervous system diseases, but his lifelong passion was to improve X-ray imaging of living tissues. He was a pioneer in the practical implementation of plain film tomography (1931), also known as planigraphy, in which the X-ray tube and the film moved together around the plane of interest. In 1934, he designed a subtraction (1934) method to improve image quality after injection of contrast agents. Eventually he essentially became a full-time radiologist. He had attended the 1939 meeting in Antwerp.

At this point, it is useful to provide some background information regarding the historical setting of this 'second' SNR, which took place 4 years later the end of WW2. The city of Rotterdam had been subjected to heavy aerial bombardment during the German invasion of the Netherlands, given its strategic location and the economic importance of its harbour. During the bombardment of 14 May 1940, the entire historic city centre had been destroyed, and after the end of the hostilities, the city needed to be completely rebuilt. Amidst the difficult early post-WW2 years, the SNR served as a beacon of scientific collaboration and intellectual exchange, fostering advancements in diagnostic imaging techniques. The first post-war SNR provided a platform for the dissemination of new discoveries, thereby reshaping the future direction of neuroradiology. In a spirit of camaraderie among participants, lasting professional connections and friendships were crafted. As the curtains closed on the symposium, its legacy endured, leaving an indelible mark on the landscape of neuroradiology.

At the Rotterdam meeting, Prof. Schüller was elected as honorary president (in absentia) of the second Symposium Neuroradiologicum. Prof. Schüller was a prolific writer and authored or co-authored more than 300 publications covering not only radiology of the skull but also various aspects of neurology, surgery, and psychiatry. Because of his Jewish background, at the age of 65, he had been forced to leave the Vienna University School of Medicine in 1938 and would spend the later years of his life in Melbourne, Australia, where he continued to work at St Vincent's Hospital.

1952—The IIIrd SNR—Stockholm (Sweden)—Erik Lindgren

The 1952 SNR took place under the presidency of Prof. Dr. Erik Lindgren, a pioneer in cerebral angiography, pneumoencephalography, and gas myelography. Erik Lindgren had been appointed as Professor of Roentgen Diagnostics with Neuroradiology at the Karolinska Institute. In 1949, he had succeeded his famous predecessor, Professor Erik Lysholm, who was a pioneering neuroradiologist in Sweden, serving as the head of the Department of Neuroradiology at the Seraphimer Hospital (Serafimerlasarettet) and the Karolinska Institute (Karolinska Universitetssjukhuset) during the 1930s and 1940s.

Stockholm proved to be an excellent venue for an international meeting in the early 1950s. As one of very few countries in Europe, Sweden had remained neutral throughout the Second World War, and the city of Stockholm was untouched. The country was undergoing a period of social and economic transformation, and the capital Stockholm was at the forefront of these changes. It was a vibrant and dynamic city, with a reputation for its thriving cultural activities, with theatres, galleries, and concert halls attracting both local and international talent.

Under the dynamic leadership of Prof. Lindgren, neuroradiology became recognised as a specialty. This heralded the beginning of a golden age for Swedish neuroradiology. Under Lindgren's guidance, Seraphimer Hospital became the "Mecca of Neuroradiology." The Seraphimer School of Neuroradiology was a world-leading radiologic institution and attracted talent from around the globe. Prof. Lindgren had a huge influence on neuroradiology, and he trained an entire generation of neuroradiologists. No fewer than 6 of his pupils were to become presidents of the SNR in the ensuing decades. They were Giovanni Ruggiero (SNR President in 1961), Ingmar Wickbom (SNR President in 1970), Néstor Azambuja (SNR President in 1974), Sigurd Wende (SNR President in 1978), Giovanni di Chiro (SNR President in 1982), and Torgny Greitz (SNR President in 1986). The disciples of the Swedish neuroradiology school would go on to lead and define the specialty in the coming decades.

1955—The IVth SNR—London (UK)—James William Douglas Bull

At the age of 44, Prof. Dr. James Bull became the president of the IVth SNR, which was held in London in 1955. It took place at the University of London, Mallett Street campus, London, W.C.1 from 13th to 17th September 1955. A scientific exhibition, open throughout the week to all members of the Symposium, was held in the Institute of Education at the University of London. Participants were informed that there was to be an exhibition of specialised X-ray apparatus and of surgical instruments, pharmaceutical preparations, photographic materials, and protective clothing.

Prof. Dr. James Bull specialised in radiology. Thanks to a Rockefeller travel fellowship, he had travelled to Sweden in 1938 to study the new techniques of neuroradiology under Prof. Erik Lysholm at the Seraphimer Hospital (Serafimerlasarettet) in Stockholm. Shortly after the Second World War broke out, he was posted to Singapore. With the fall of Singapore, he spent three and a half difficult, starving years as a prisoner of war (POW) in the Changi POW camp. Shortly after WW2, he returned to Stockholm where Prof. Erik Lindgren had meanwhile taken over as chair at the Karolinska Hospital, developing the techniques of percutaneous angiography and pneumoencephalography. After his return to the United Kingdom, in 1946, James Bull was appointed at the Atkinson Morley Hospital as a neuroradiologist. In 1947, he joined the National Hospital for Nervous Diseases, Queen Square. There, Prof. James Bull introduced technique of percutaneous angiography, which he brought back with him from Sweden. His energy, determination and ability in negotiation and persuasion were instrumental in the introduction of the advancement of neuroradiology.

Prof. James Bull served for many years as the Director of the Lysholm Department of Neuroradiology at the National Hospital for Neurology and Neurosurgery, Queen Square. The department was named in honour of Prof. Erik Lysholm, his friend and Swedish mentor. Prof. James Bull trained many neuroradiologists of the next generation; many of those who had spent time at Queen Square would rise to positions of prominence in North America.

1957—The Vth SNR—Brussels (BE)—Donald Lane McRae

The Vth Symposium Neuroradiologicum in Brussels in 1957 SNR was organised under the presidency of Prof. Donald L. McRae, a prominent Canadian neuroradiologist from the Montréal Neurological Institute who is considered the "father of Canadian neuroradiology." This Vth SNR in Brussels was most unusual for two reasons. Firstly, while all other symposium presidents before and ever since have chosen to hold the meeting in their country of origin, Prof. McRae opted to have the meeting in Belgium, jointly with the World Congress of Neurology. Secondly, throughout the 1950s and 1960s, the symposia were always held at three-year intervals. The 1957 symposium in Brussels, which followed that in London in 1955, was an exception to that rule.

Prof. Donald McRae had served as a radiologist in the Royal Canadian Navy during WW2, from 1942 to 1945. After the war, he was appointed radiologist-in-chief in Montréal at the children's Memorial Hospital, and the Montréal Neurological Institute. Towards the later part of his career, he served as Professor of Radiology at University of Toronto from 1967 to 1978. To this day, Donald McRae is affectionately considered as the "Dean" or the "Father of Neuroradiology" in Canada. He made great contributions in the study of pneumoencephalography, radionuclide brain scanning, as well in describing abnormalities of the cervical spine and craniocervical junction. To this day, we teach our trainees that the McRae line is a radiographic line drawn on a lateral view that connects the anterior and posterior margins of the foramen magnum (basion to opisthion). It is used to detect the presence of basilar invagination (atlantoaxial impaction) and to determine the position of the cerebellar tonsils relative to the foramen magnum.

1961—The VIth SNR—Rome (IT)—Giovanni Ruggiero

In 1961, Professor Giovanni Ruggiero received the honour to organise and chair the VIth SNR in Rome, Italy. The meeting was announced in the journal *Radiology*. The president, Prof. Ruggiero, genuinely embraced the idea of a united Europe. After having worked for some time in Stockholm, Sweden, he moved to Paris, France (where he was and still is considered one of the founders of French neuroradiology). Eventually, he would return to Italy, where he was appointed director of the Department of Neurosurgical Diagnosis at the Bellaria Hospital in Bologna, which included an inpatient ward.

Prof. Ruggiero was a visionary but demanding chief. He only accepted pupils with a documented neurological culture who were able to accept and treat their patients, while working within a team framework. Prof. Ruggiero was a man of contrasts: he was a great enthusiast, supportive of new ideas, but he was also known to be highly critical, and he could be very tough with his trainees. He has been the driving force and guide for Italian neuroradiologists (AJNR 17:721–730, Apr 1996 0195–6108/96/1704–0721).

In retrospect, the VIth SNR in Rome may well be considered the first truly modern international neuroradiology meeting with participants from all over the world. Neuroradiologists learned about the great progress in this specialty being made, especially in Europe, but also in North America. A plethora of papers were read by such illustrious neuroradiology giants as Chase, Leeds, Taveras, Potts, Pribram, LeMay, Hanafee, Newton, McRae, and Di Chiro. For all those who attended the symposium, it was obvious that a quantum leap had been made. The VIth SNR made it clear that neuroradiology needed to be considered a separate science, at the crossroads between radiology and neurology; this meeting marked the birth of modern neuroradiology in Italy.

1964—The VIIth SNR—New York City/USA—Juan Manuel Taveras

The presidency of the VIIth Symposium Neuroradiologicum, to be held in New York City, was awarded to Prof. Dr. Juan Manuel Taveras, who had been appointed following the previous SNR meeting in Rome. Prof. Taveras was a leading figure in neuroradiology, and at the time, he was the Director of Neuroradiology at the Neurological Institute of Columbia-Presbyterian Medical Center in New York City. The VIIth SNR was held at the Waldorf-Astoria Hotel in New York City, from 20 to 25 September 1964. This marked the first time the SNR was to be held in North America, a historic event, and a recognition of the rapidly growing role of the New World in neuroradiology.

Prof. Juan M. Taveras (1919–2002) is widely regarded as the father of neuroradiology. His stellar international reputation was linked to his role as a founder of the American Society of Neuroradiology (ASNR) where he served for several years as president. He also founded the American Journal of Neuroradiology (AJNR) of which he was the founding editor for many years. Based on their work at the Neurological Institute of New York City's Columbia Presbyterian Medical Center in 1960, Juan M. Taveras and Ernest Wood published an encyclopaedic 2-volume textbook, titled *Diagnostic Neuroradiology,* which was to remain the go-to reference for the next decades. The book focused on the emerging techniques in neuroradiology such as neuroangiography, pneumoencephalography, and myelography.

In the mid-1980s, when I served as a *Clinical Fellow in Neuroradiology* at the Massachusetts General Hospital and *Research Fellow* at Harvard Medical School, Boston, MA, I had the good fortune of getting to know Prof. Taveras personally. At that time, he was Radiologist-in-Chief at the Massachusetts General Hospital and Professor at Harvard Medical School. He took a very keen interest in the work of the neuroradiology fellows. Prof. Taveras and his wife invited me to his home, and I distinctly remember him asking me if I was aware that the very first SNR had been held in my hometown, Antwerp. I remember him as a great role model, and an exemplary leader for neuroradiology.

1967—The VIIIth SNR—Paris/FR—Hermann Fischgold

The VIIIth SNR was held in Paris at the UNESCO Building from 25 to 30 September 1967. The president was Prof. Herman Fischgold (1899–1982), who served as Professor of Neuroradiology at the CHU Hôpital Universitaire Pitié-Salpêtrière, from 1963 to 1969.

Prof. Fischgold was a prolific researcher and writer, and has been called the founder, thinker, and organiser of French neuroradiology. He had received his early medical training in Bucharest where he was awarded his medical degree in 1925. In the setting of a cultural exchange between France and Romania, he travelled to Paris. In 1946, he became "Assistant des Hôpitaux de Paris," in 1947 "Electroradiologiste des Hôpitaux" and finally, chief of the department of EEG and neuroradiology at La Pitié Hospital in 1956. In 1962, Prof. Fischgold became chairman of radiology; he retired in 1970.

His enthusiasm led him to organise courses, seminars, and congresses, to write books and monographs, and to serve as an editor of *Traité de Radiodiagnostic*, which is the materialisation of his knowledge in general radiology. He was also elected president of the International Symposium of Neuroradiology in Paris in 1967. His main scientific contributions to neuroradiology concern the base of the skull and the cervico-occipital region and their relationships with the cranial nerves, radio-anatomy, direct magnification, subtraction, radio-ophthalmology and otology, forensic radiology, and microradiography. On the occasion of the VIIIth SNR, a medallion was coined (reproduced in: *Lev MH, Gadde JA, Wiggins RH. A Brief History of Neuroradiology and the 60th Anniversary of the ASNR: "Through the Decades with ASNR." AJNR Am J Neuroradiol. 2022 Dec;43(12):E54–E59*). The obverse of the medallion shows individuals considered to be pivotal in the development of neuroradiology (Schüller, Dandy, Lysholm, Sicard, Moniz); the reverse lists the locations and dates of previous meetings (Anvers (sic) 1939; Rotterdam 1949; Stockholm 1952; Londres (sic) 1955; Bruxelles 1957; Rome 1961; New-York 1964; Paris 1967).

1970—The IXth SNR—Göteborg/SE—Ingmar Wickbom

Under the Presidency of Prof. Ingmar Wickbom, the IXth SNR returned to Sweden, in the city of Gothenborg (Göteborg), from 24 to 29 August 1970. The announcement published in Radiology (June 1969) indicated that the SNR would deal mainly with the following subjects: hydrocephalus, brain atrophy, and cerebral spinal fluid circulation; the central nervous system in the perinatal period (normal and developmental disturbances); advances in ultrasound and diagnostic isotope methods; cerebral angiography, physiologic and anatomic aspects; radiobiology of the nervous system; use of the proton beam in therapy of the brain; and radiological examinations of the spinal canal. Round table discussions would be arranged on the factors influencing the development of hydrocephalus and how to determine "brain death." Papers dealing with other subjects would also be accepted. There were to be scientific as well as technical exhibits in connection with the meeting.

Prof. Ingmar Wickbom served as the head of one of the two departments of general radiology at Shalgrens Hospital (Shalgrenska Sjukhuset), Gothenburg, Sweden. He had been a student of Prof. Erik Lindgren in Stockholm, and he was well prepared to meet the needs of the newly opened department of neurology and neurosurgery. Wickbom was a pioneer in the technique of electronic subtraction, most useful with angiography and now almost indispensable in interventional neuroradiology, which he developed in a collaboration with Henry Wallmann, an American-born professor of medical electronics at Chalmer's Technical Institute in Gothenburg. Wallman and Wickbom were the first to combine television technology with the image intensifier to allow roentgen screening in daylight. Wickbom became professor of general radiology in 1968. He resigned in 1973 and moved to the USA.

1974—The Xth SNR—Punta del Este/UY—Néstor Azambuja

For the Xth edition, in 1974, the SNR moved to Uruguay. It was the first SNR meeting in the Southern Hemisphere and only the second on the American continent. The Xth SNR in Punta del Este was organised and presided over by Dr. Néstor Azambuja. It was attended by 400 neuroradiologists from all around the world. The Presidency of the Xth SNR had been awarded to Dr. Néstor Azambuja, since he had been admitted in 1957 as a foreign resident at the Seraphimer Hospital in Stockholm, under the direction of Prof. Erik Lindgren. The choice of Punta del Este was an interesting albeit an audacious one. The 1970s were a politically turbulent period in Uruguay, characterised by social unrest and by the rise of leftist guerrilla movements and subsequent government crackdowns. However, Punta del Este, where the Xth SNR was held, was a haven of peace and prosperity: it was (and still is) an affluent resort on Uruguay's Atlantic coast with pristine beaches and a vibrant cultural life.

Dr. Néstor Azambuja had a background in neurosurgery and radiology. He was an alumnus of the Swedish School of Neuroradiology. Upon his return to Uruguay, he worked as a neuroradiologist at the Neurology Institute in Montevideo and the Hospital Británico (British Hospital), where the first Lysholm table in Montevideo was installed. He was affiliated with the University of Montevideo where he eventually held the Chair of Radiology. In Montevideo, Néstor Azambuja created one of the most important schools of neuroradiology in Latin America. He described "central ventriculography," as an important tool for the diagnosis of posterior fossa tumours in the pre-CT era. He advocated the use of small quantities of air, without removing CSF, a technique that became known as "fractional pneumoencephalography."

1978—The XIth SNR—Wiesbaden/DE—Sigurd Wende

The XIth SNR was organised in Wiesbaden by Prof. Sigurd Wende, from 4 to 10 June 1978. The Proceedings were published by Springer Verlag in 1978, as a 646-page document (ISBN-10: 3540087826; ISBN-13: 978-3540087823). Wiesbaden is a picturesque city nestled in the heart of Germany's Rhine-Main region, known for its stylish architecture, lush parks, and historic thermal baths. It has a reputation as an elegant spa town, attracting visitors seeking relaxation and rejuvenation. For international congress delegates, Wiesbaden was very easy to reach, thanks to its proximity to the international Frankfurt am Main Airport.

The president of the XIth SNR, Prof. Sigurd Wende graduated in medicine in 1952 from the Free University of Berlin. He became Medical Assistant at the Neurological and Psychiatric Hospital of the Free University of Berlin and was certified as a specialist in neurology and psychiatry in 1958. In 1959, he worked under the guidance of Professor Lindgren at the Seraphimer Hospital of Stockholm. In 1962, he was admitted as a University Lecturer in Berlin and travelled as the recipient of a Henry Ford Foundation stipend to spend a year in the United States of America, where he worked with Prof. Juan Taveras in Neuroradiology at the Neurological Institute of the Columbia Presbyterian University, New York; with Dr. Robins at the Department of Radiology of the Massachusetts General Hospital, Boston, and with Dr. Morgan at the Department of Radiology of Johns Hopkins Hospital, Baltimore. Between 1952 and 1989, Sigurd Wende published 192 papers on neuroradiological, general radiological, and neurological subjects and was the co-author of 12 books. His research on brain tumours was exemplary, and he worked generally as a member of a multidisciplinary team (neurologist, neurosurgeon, and neuropathologist).

When Prof. Sigurd Wende was elected to the Presidency of the XIth SNR, the decision was made in recognition of his original research and organisational abilities. The SNR in Wiesbaden in 1978 was *an outstandingly good meeting, memorable for the rigour of the method of blind selection of oral presentations, the beautiful opera house, the boat trip on the Rhine and a nightingale that sang daily in the sunshine beside one of the busy roads.*

1982—The XIIth SNR—Washington DC/US—Giovanni Di Chiro

The XIIth SNR took place in Washington, D.C., the capital of the United States of America. Italian-born Professor Giovanni Di Chiro (1926–1997) served as president, and Hillier L. Baker, Jr. as vice president of the XIIth SNR in Washington, D.C. It was the second of the symposia to be held in North America. The meeting occurred during the Reagan presidency, with the continuing arms race with the Soviet Union in the background, in the waning years of the Cold War. Geopolitically, the year 1982 was characterised by the short but fierce Falklands War, which had erupted between Argentina and the United Kingdom.

Prof. Giovanni Di Chiro had graduated as a medical doctor from the University of Naples but spent most of his professional life living and working abroad, first in Sweden, afterwards in the United States of America. Between 1949 and 1953, he had trained as a neuroradiologist in Stockholm in various hospitals such as the Serafimerlassarettet and Sodersjukhuset, which were affiliated with the Karolinska University. In 1953, he moved to the United States, working at Boston City Hospital on a 6-month Fullbright Fellowship. He returned to Italy, where he established the radiology departments of the Neurological Institute of the University of Naples and the St. Mary's Hospital in Aversa. In October 1957, he returned to the United States of America, to Washington, D.C. He was offered a staff position at the National Institute of Neurological Disorders and Stroke (NINDS), which is a part of the US National Institutes of Health (NIH). Very quickly after his appointment, he established what became known as the NINDS Neuroimaging Branch in 1958. In 1977, he founded the *Journal of Computer Assisted Tomography ("JCAT")*, one of the major scientific publications in cross-sectional imaging.

In 1982, the president, Giovanni Di Chiro, and the vice president, Hillier L. Baker, Jr., of the XIIth Symposium Neuroradiologicum established an important innovation, the Fellowship Awards, which would first be presented at the XIIIth Symposium in Stockholm, for *the best original work by a radiologist relating to the application of radiology and radiologic science to the study of the nervous system.* The XIIth SNR marked the first time that the neuroradiological community had been exposed to magnetic resonance images (MRI) of the brain; this technique would come to dominate diagnostic neuroradiology in future years. A selection of the abstracts that were presented during the XIIth Symposium Neuroradiologicum, October 10–16, 1982, in Washington, D.C., was published in Radiology in September 1982 (*Abstracts for presentation at XII symposium neuroradiologicum, October 10–16, 1982, Washington, D.C. Radiology 1982 144:4, 943–962*).

Prof. Giovanni Di Chiro was one of the true giants of neuroradiology. He was a talented and inquisitive researcher, best known for his groundbreaking contributions to diagnostic neuroradiology, computed tomography, and magnetic resonance imaging.

1986—The XIIIth SNR—Stockholm/SE—Torgny Greitz

Under the presidency of Prof. Torgny Greitz, the XIIIth SNR returned to Sweden for the third time, and to Stockholm for the second time, after 1952. Prof. Torgny Greitz, a graduate of the Stockholm School of Neuroradiology at the Seraphimer Hospital, quickly became a well-known neuroradiologist. In 1956, he spent a year at Washington University in St. Louis to practise and teach neuroradiology at the famous Mallinckrodt Institute of Radiology. He returned to Sweden and would later become the chief of the Department of Neuroradiology at the Karolinska Hospital. He was a leader in the development of clinical applications of computed tomography (CT) and positron-emission tomography (PET).

The XIIIth SNR was held in Stockholm, Sweden, from 23 to 28 *June* 1986. For me personally, it was the first SNR meeting I attended; I remember that the weather was beautiful, with long days and short nights. The meeting featured fascinating presentations, lectures, and workshops, covering a wide range of topics related to neuroradiology. Attendees had the opportunity to exchange ideas, share research findings, and collaborate on innovative approaches to diagnosing and treating neurological disorders. A new feature was the Fellowship Awards, which had been established in 1982 in Washington, D.C., by the president, Giovanni Di Chiro, and the vice president, Hillier L. Baker, Jr., of the XIIth SNR. The first awards were presented at the XIIIth Symposium in Stockholm, for *the best original work by a radiologist relating to application of radiology and radiologic science to the study of the nervous system.* The recipients of these first Fellowship Awards were:

- Isabelle Berry, University of Toulouse, France, and University of California, San Francisco
- Robert R. Edelman, Massachusetts General Hospital, Boston, Massachusetts
- Gerald O'Reilly, Beth Israel Hospital, Boston, Massachusetts

The award winners received a round-trip airfare to Stockholm, 3 days per diem, a cash prize, and a diploma. In addition, the contributions presented by Dr. T. Yamaguchi et al., and Drs J.B. Rubin and D.R. Enzman were selected for an honourable mention, receiving a cash award and a diploma. Yamaguchi.

The Proceedings of the XIIIth Symposium Neuroradiologicum were published as a voluminous 774-page supplement to Acta Radiologica (*XIII Symposium Neuroradiologicum. Stockholm, June 23–28, 1986. Acta Radiol Suppl. 1986; 369:1–774. PMID: 2908789*). This was in contradistinction to the previous, XIIth SNR, for which only a small selection (20 pages) of abstracts had been published in Radiology (*Abstracts for presentation at XII symposium neuroradiologicum, October 10–16, 1982, Washington, D.C. Radiology 1982 144:4, 943–962).* The XIIIth SNR played an important role in shaping the future direction of research and clinical practice in neuroradiology, leaving a lasting impact on everyone who attended the meeting.

1990—The XIVth SNR—London—Edward Philip George Houssemayne du Boulay

Professor George Houssemayne du Boulay was honoured by the prestigious invitation to be the president of the XIVth SNR, which took place in London from 17 to 23 June 1990. It was a testimony to the enormous personal respect in which he was held by the world's leading academic neuroscientists. It was the second time that the SNR visited London. The Proceedings of the XIVth SNR were published in a hardcover volume, edited by Profs. George du Boulay, Andrew Molyneux, and Ivan Moseley.

Prof. George du Boulay was one of Britain's leading neuroradiologists, and—interestingly—he was also a world-famous veterinary radiologist. During the Second World War years, he had been a medical student at King's College, London, and Charing Cross Hospital Medical School, qualifying in 1945. George du Boulay had a privileged professional relationship with Prof. James Bull, who was his senior, and who had served as the convenor for the IVth SNR in London in 1955. Despite their difference in age, they were close friends. When Prof. James Bull retired in 1975 from Queen Square, Prof. George du Boulay succeeded him as director. A year later was awarded the first academic chair in neuroradiology in Britain, at the Institute of Neurology. He served as the director of the famous Lysholm radiological department at the National Hospital for Neurology and Neurosurgery, Queen Square, London until his retirement in 1985. His department was a veritable incubator for talent and ideas; it catalysed the careers of an entire generation of neuroradiologists from all parts of the world.

Prof. George du Boulay also served as the editor-in-chief for Neuroradiology. When the four-yearly SNR was to be held in London in 1990, he was the obvious choice as president, even though this event arrived at a relatively late stage of his illustrious career.

1994—The XVth SNR—Kumamoto/JP—Mutsumasa Takahashi

Japanese neuroradiology received the great international honour of hosting the XVth SNR in Kumamoto from 25 September to 1 October 1994 under the Presidency of Prof. Mutsumasa Takahashi. It was the first such event to be held in Asia. More than 1200 delegates convened to discuss the most recent developments, including interventional neuroradiology, functional imaging, MRI contrast media, new techniques in MRI, iodinated contrast media, and other topics. The proceedings were published in a hardcover volume, edited by Profs. Mutsumasa Takahashi, Yukunori Korogi, and Ivan Moseley.

The XVth SNR was held in Kumamoto, a city on the southern Japanese island of Kyushu, rich in culture and history. Kyushu is known for its natural beauty, and offers spectacular vistas of mount Aso, one of the largest active volcanoes in the world. Though Kumamoto is a growing and modern city, it still retains its traditional charm and historical significance.

The president of the XVth SNR was Prof. Mutsumasa Takahashi. In 1960, he had graduated as a medical doctor from Kyushu University at Fukuoka. He became one of the founding board members of the Japanese Society of Neuroradiology, which had been formed in 1972, at Noguchi Hideyo Memorial Hall in Tokyo. In 1980, he was appointed as professor and chairman of radiology at Kumamoto University School of Medicine. He held this position until 2001 when he became professor emeritus.

Professor Takahashi was a prolific author and served as an editor-in-chief of Neuroradiology.

1998—The XVIth SNR—Philadelphia/PA, USA—Sadek Kamel Hilal

In 1998, the XVIth SNR convened in Philadelphia. Prof. Sadek K. Hilal served as president, while his colleague and good friend Prof. Stephen A. Kieffer acted as vice president.

The XVIth SNR was a special event for three reasons. To start with, it was the first SNR to be presented under the auspices of the recently established World Federation of Neuroradiological Societies (WFNRS), which had been founded in 1994 at the XVth SNR in Kumamoto, Japan thanks to the driving force of Prof. Derek Harwood Nash. Secondly, it was conceived and organised as a conjoint, back-to-back meeting between the XVIth SNR (Thursday 15th May to Sunday 17th May 1998) and the 36th Annual Meeting of the American Society of Neuroradiology (from Sunday 17th May to Thursday 21st May 1998), both held at the Pennsylvania Convention Center in Philadelphia, USA. Thirdly, it would be the third such event to be held in North America (after New York in 1964 and Washington D.C. in 1982), and the neuroradiological community saw it as a recognition of the great advances that had been made on their continent. The host city, Philadelphia, is one of the oldest cities in North America and has always enjoyed a special place in American history and culture. The Declaration of Independence was conceived, written, and signed in this city on fourth July 1776. The proceedings were published as a supplement to The Neuroradiology Journal (Volume 11 Issue 1_suppl, May 1998).

The President, Prof. Sadek K. Hilal was born in Cairo, Egypt, in 1930 and received his medical degree from the University of Cairo in 1955. He was an innovative thinker and developed many original research ideas. He was passionate about quantification of cerebral blood flow using diverse imaging techniques. In the early 1960s, he developed a technique for catheter cerebral angiography which led to his becoming one of the early pioneers in interventional neuroradiology. During his most academically productive years, he served as the Director of Neuroradiology at the Neurological Institute of Columbia Presbyterian Medical Center in New York.

2002—The XVIIth SNR—Paris/FR—Luc Picard

The XVIIth SNR was held in Paris, from 18–24 August 2002 under the presidency of Prof. Luc Picard. The meeting took place in the Palais des Congrès de Paris at the Porte Maillot, as a conjoint meeting with the European Society of Neuroradiology (ESNR). Several of the SNR's past-presidents were united in Paris: Giovanni Ruggiero, Nestor Azambuja, Torgny Greitz, George du Boulay, Mutsumasa Takahashi. The Proceedings of the XVIIth SNR were published as a two-volume supplement of Rivista di Neuroradiologia, allowing indexing in the scientific literature. At the occasion of the XVIIth SNR, a book entitled "L'histoire de la Neuroradiologie mondiale" ("The History of World Neuroradiology") was published and distributed among the participants.

The president, Prof. Luc Picard was a neurologist by training, a clinician at heart, and a pioneer of interventional neuroradiology. He had spent his entire professional career in Nancy, France, where he had created a strong school of neuroradiology, together with a closely knit team of loyal collaborators. Throughout his career, Prof. Picard laboured tirelessly to further the development of French neuroradiology and increase its scientific, medical, and political influence. He was one of the founders of the French Society of Neuroradiology in 1970. He was the editor-in-chief of the *Journal of Neuroradiology* for 24 years from 1977 to 2001. In 1990, he created the WFITN (*World Federation of Interventional Neuroradiology*) and served as its president and vice-president from 1991 to 1995. Luc Picard was an exceptional person and a role model for his many students and collaborators.

2006—The XVIIIth SNR—Adelaide/AUS—Michael R. Sage

In 2006, the XVIIIth SNR moved to Adelaide, the capital of South Australia, under the presidency of Prof. Michael R. Sage. The meeting was held from 19 to 24 March 2006 under the auspices of, and with financial support from, "The Australian and New Zealand Society of Neuroradiology" (ANZSNR). The ANZSNR logo was incorporated into the SNR logo.

The modern and versatile Adelaide Convention Centre was a perfect venue for the XVIIIth SNR and the meeting was attended by 743 delegates and 81 partners from around the world. An excellent scientific programme was created by a large national and international faculty of experts and consisted of several symposia covering cerebrovascular disease, subarachnoid haemorrhage, cerebral arteriovenous malformations, epilepsy, dementia, brain tumours, cerebrospinal fluid, spine and spinal cord, skull base, paediatric neuroradiology, paranasal sinuses, and head and neck tumours. However, the choice to organise the meeting in Adelaide had not been without risk. Though Adelaide is renowned for its elegant architecture, lush parklands, and vibrant cultural scene, the city is relatively remote and difficult to reach, with few direct flights from other parts of the world.

The convenor, Prof. Michael R. Sage, had served as the first president of "The Australian and New Zealand Society of Neuroradiology" (ANZSNR), which had been founded in 1993, and which held its first meeting at the Sydney Convention Centre at Darling Harbour on Thursday 21st October 1993, with 19 members in attendance. The next year, at the XVth SNR in in Kumamoto, ANZSNR was to become one of the founding members of the World Federation of Neuroradiological Societies (WFNRS). In September 1994, Prof. Sage was elected the first secretary-general of the WFNRS.

Professionally and scientifically, Michael Sage had been a well-known neuroradiologist since many years. He was chairman of the Department of Radiology at Flinders Medical Centre and held an academic appointment at the College of Medicine and Public Health at Flinders University. Professor Sage and his colleagues at Flinders University focused their research to contribute significantly to the understanding of the blood-brain barrier.

2010—The XIXth SNR—Bologna/ITA—Marco Leonardi

The XIXth SNR took place in Bologna, Italy, from 4 to 9 October 2010, under the presidency of Prof. Marco Leonardi, with Prof. Anton Valavanis acting as vice-president. However, it was not the original plan to organise the meeting in Bologna. When Marco Leonardi pitched his project to the WFNRS, the plan had been to organise the meeting in Venice, and this proposal was approved. Approximately 1 year before the scheduled start of the meeting, Prof. Marco Leonardi informed the community that (for 'important technical reasons') he had been obliged to move the Symposium site venue from Venice to Bologna, which also implied the dates of the meeting were changed to 4–9 October 2010. Prof. Leonardi stated that while *Bologna is not well known and of course lacks the charm of Venice, it is a very nice and interesting city too* and he confirmed that all the participants would like it. The meeting was held in the Palazzo della Cultura e dei Congressi, Bologna, under the banner of The World Congress of Diagnostic & Therapeutic Neuroradiology.

At the time of the XIXth SNR, Prof. Marco Leonardi held the Chair of Neuroradiology at the University of Bologna and was the director of the Servizio di Neuroradiologia in the Ospedale Bellaria. After he obtained his medical degree in Medicine and Surgery in 1967, he specialised in radiology in Padua. For a short term, he was a fellow of Prof. Giovanni Ruggiero, one of the founders of European Neuroradiology, but he left to be nominated as the Chief of Neuroradiology in at the University of Udine. After 13 years, he moved to the University of Milan where he was appointed as full professor of Neuroradiology. Eventually, he would move back to Bologna, to become chief at the Bellaria Hospital.

I remember Prof. Marco Leonardi as an innovator and an astute advocate of neuroradiology, in Italy and internationally. He held many positions of leadership in scientific organisations, and he was the founder and editor of "The Neuroradiology Journal" and "Interventional Neuroradiology."

2014—The XXth SNR—Istanbul/TR—E. Turgut Tali

The XXth SNR was held in Istanbul, from 7 to 12 September 2014 at the Lutfi Kirdar International Convention and Exhibition Center under the presidency of Professor Turgut Tali. While the WFNRS is the organisation that provides support and energy behind the Symposium, all the practical arrangements were very much the work of the Symposium President, Professor Turgut Tali who organised a remarkable meeting in Istanbul, the city where East meets West, and tradition embraces innovation. The XXth SNR was conceived as a celebration of the power of neuroradiology to bridge borders and transform lives, advancing scientific knowledge and improving patient outcomes worldwide.

The proceedings of the XXth SNR were published as a 476-page Supplement to Neuroradiology (*XXth Symposium Neuroradiologicum. Neuroradiology* ***56*** *(Suppl 1), 1–476 (2014). https://doi.org/10.1007/s00234-014-1405-4*), including abstracts from lectures and poster presentations covering stroke, head and neck, paediatric diagnostic neuroradiology, spine and interventional neuroradiology, adult diagnostic neuroradiology, intravascular interventional neuroradiology.

The XXth SNR President, Prof. Turgut Tali received a medical degree from The Hacettepe University. He has had a most distinguished career as prominent Turkish neuroradiologist, holding many national and international positions of leadership in Neuroradiology. In 2014, at the time of the XXth SNR, he was Director of the Division of Neuroradiology at The Gazi University School of Medicine. He currently serves as Professor and Chairman of the Department of Radiology at Lokman Hekim University in Ankara, Türkiye. Prof. Tali is a leading figure in his field, having held many distinguished functions as president of the European Society of Neuroradiology (ESNR), president of the Turkish Society of Neuroradiology (TSNR), president of the World Federation of Neuroradiological Societies (WFNRS), and Chief Examiner for the European Board of Neuroradiology. Dr. Tali's expertise and research interests include advanced imaging of the brain and spine. In 2025, he served as congress president of the first-ever Joint Congress of the Asian-Oceanian, European, and Turkish Societies of Neuroradiology, combining forces with European Society of Neuroradiology (ESNR), the Asian-Oceanian Society of Neuroradiology and Head and Neck Radiology (AOSNHNR) and the Turkish Society of Neuroradiology (TSNR).

2018—The XXIst SNR—Taipei/TWN—Wan-Yuo Guo

The XXIst SNR (The World Congress of Neuroradiology 2018) took place under the presidency of Prof. Wan-Yuo Guo and was held from 19 to 23 March at the Taipei International Congress and Exhibition Centre (TICC), Taipei, Taiwan. The meeting was hosted by the Neuroradiological Society of Taiwan (NRST). The meeting was held in combination with the 12th Asian-Oceanian Congress of Neuroradiology and Head & Neck Neuroradiology (AOCNHNR) .

Prof. Wan-Yuo Guo had been elected as the president of the XXIst SNR in 2010 during the XIXth SNR in Bologna, Italy. After 8 years of preparation, the XXIst SNR successfully united more than 1000 attendees from 50 countries over five continents and 39 industry sponsors. The 5-day meeting consisted of 74 sessions on 6 themes, including Brain, Head & Neck, Paediatric, Spine, Intervention, Highlights and special sessions such as "Master to Master" and "Junior Meets Junior." In addition to the comprehensive scientific programme, the XXIst SNR Organizing Committee unprecedentedly invited famous Taiwanese artists to join the Congress and exhibit their artworks, as well as hosted tea art performances throughout the Congress at the Congress Venue of TICC. It is the true form of realisation and unification of "The Art of Healing, the Healing of Art." And as for the attendees, the Organizing Committee hosted a "Photography Exhibition Competition" that allowed the attendees to submit their photography works and displayed them during the congress.

Professor Wan-Yuo Guo received the medical degree (MD) from China Medical College, Taichung, Taiwan. In 1993, he obtained a PhD degree from the Karolinska Institute, Stockholm, Sweden. He trained as a neuroradiologist at the Radiology Department, Taipei Veterans General Hospital, Taipei, Taiwan, between 1983 and 1989. He is currently Chief of the Division of Neuroradiology, Radiology Department, Taipei Veterans General Hospital, and Professor of radiology with National Yang-Ming University, Taipei. His research interests include foetal magnetic resonance (MR) images, MR perfusion images, gamma knife radiosurgery, MR diffusion tensor imaging, as well as artificial intelligence (AI) applications such as Federated Learning.

2022—The XXIInd SNR—New York City/NY, USA—Mauricio Castillo

The XXIInd SNR was held from 14 to 16 May 2022 at the New York City Hilton Hotel under the presidency of Prof. Mauricio Castillo. It was a joint meeting, followed back-to-back by the 60th anniversary Annual Meeting of the ASNR from 16 to 18 May 2022. Authors were encouraged to choose between four submission categories:

- Scientific oral presentation—to be included during ASNR only
- Electronic scientific poster—to be shown during both meetings
- Electronic educational exhibit—to be shown during both meetings
- Excerpta (oral presentations)—to be included during SNR only

Due to the Covid-19 pandemic, which had entered its third year, both events were offered as hybrid meetings (i.e. live/remote). Delegates had the option to attend in-person or virtually. Participants were given the option to transfer their registration to an alternative form of participation at no additional cost.

The president of the XXIInd SNR, Prof. Mauricio Castillo, was born in Guatemala. He graduated as a medical doctor from the University of San Carlos. His career in the USA started with 1½ years as a Research Fellow at MD Anderson Hospital in Houston. He went on to complete a residency in Diagnostic Radiology at the University of Miami, followed by a 2-year Neuroradiology Fellowship at Emory University in Atlanta. He returned to the University of Texas in Houston and, in 1992, was recruited to the University of North Carolina. Dr. Castillo served as Chief of the Neuroradiology Division for over 28 years. Prof. Castillo is one of the visionary leaders of our discipline. He has received many distinguished honours, including as president and Gold Medallist of American Society of Neuroradiology and of the American Roentgen Ray Society (ARRS). For many years, he served as the editor-in-chief of the American Journal of Neuroradiology. It is therefore not surprising that he was called to serve as President of the XXIInd Symposium Neuroradiologicum, the world's oldest neuroradiology meeting.

2026—The XXIIIrd SNR—London—Tarek Yousry

The XXIIIrd SNR will convene in London, United Kingdom, from 30th September to fourth October 2026, with Prof. Tarek A. Yousry serving as president. The XXIIIrd SNR will be held under the auspices of the WFNRS, and it will be held in conjunction with the 49th European Society of Neuroradiology (ESNR) Annual Meeting, and the meeting of the British Society of Neuroradiologists. The meeting motto is "MIND THE FUTURE—From innovation to impact," and the meeting symbol shows a lateral view of the human brain with a superimposed schematic transport map representing the coloured lines and stations of the London Underground.

Prof. Tarek Yousry is Professor of Neuroradiology and Head of the Division of Neuroradiology and Neurophysics at the University College London (UCL) Institute of Neurology, and he serves as Head of Lysholm Department of Neuroradiology, National Hospital for Neurology Neurosurgery, UCLH Foundation Trust. Prof. Yousry graduated as a medical doctor and obtained the Habilitation from the Ludwig-Maximillans-Universität in Munich. He received the Fellowship from the Royal College of Radiologists. His work focuses on the translation of research from the basic science level to clinical applications, using advanced MR imaging techniques to improve diagnosis and treatment of CNS disease, especially MS, movement disorders and intrinsic brain tumours.

2030—The XXIVth SNR—Sapporo—Prof. Kohsuke Kudo and Prof. Minako Azuma

The XXIVth SNR will be held in Sapporo, Hokkaido, Japan, under the presidency of the "Program Chairs," Professor Kosuke Kudo, (Department of Radiology, Graduate School of Medicine, Hokkaido University), and Professor Minako Azuma,

(Department of Radiology, Faculty of Medicine, Miyazaki University). It will be the first time in 36 years that the SNR will be held in Japan. The previous time was the XVth meeting of SNR (Kumamoto, 1994). The website of the Japan Convention Bureau announces the event as the 24th Symposium of the World Federation of Neuroradiological Sciences. The event will likely take place in June or July 2030, and the organisers expect approximately 1200 participants from different countries and regions around the world.

Final Thoughts

In researching and writing this chapter, I often thought about Mark Twain's famous dictum, which states that *History never repeats itself, but it does often rhyme.* This statement perfectly applies to the history of the Symposium Neuroradiologicum (SNR). The first part of the quote emphasises that every SNR meeting is unique, one of a kind, with its own distinct vibe and flavour, and the circumstances are never identical to a past event. The second part of the quote indicates that, even though all SNR meetings are different, their presidents share similar dreams and objectives, while facing comparable challenges and difficulties; this is the "rhyming" part of the statement.

At the end of his paper *A history of neuroradiology in Italy,* Marco Leonardi wrote (AJNR Am J Neuroradiol 1996; 17(4): 721–730): *That's the end of my story. There is no conclusion because (luckily) history is still in the making.* This holds true for the SNR: our history does not end at the time this chapter was written, but continues into the future. Our community looks forward with great anticipation to the next editions in London (SNR XXIII, 2026) and Sapporo (SNR XXIV, 2030) and we are confident that these meetings will unite neuroradiologists from across the globe.

It is, however, worthwhile to think how the rapidly evolving scientific landscape, including the transformative role of artificial intelligence, in combination with geopolitical and demographic fluctuations will change the scope of SNR meetings to come. The spectacular development of neuroradiology starting in the mid-twentieth century has been mainly driven by European-influenced schools. As shown in Table 1.2, SNR meetings have been held predominantly in the Northern Hemisphere. Of the 24 SNR editions up to and including 2030, 15 will have taken place in Europe (62.5%), 5 on the American continent (21%), 3 in Asia (12.5%), and 1 in Australia-Oceania (4%).

There have been only two meetings in the Southern Hemisphere (Punta del Este and Adelaide). The SNR has never been held on the African continent.

This distribution hardly reflects the scientific, economic, or demographic reality of our world in the twenty-first century. The 'Eurocentric' world view of neuroradiology prioritises European and North American perspectives, often to the detriment of non-Western schools of thought. The SNR needs to acknowledge other perspectives and foster inclusive dialogues with other medical and academic communities.

Table 1.2 Overview of the SNR meeting by continents, countries, host cities, years, and roman numeral identifiers

Asia ($n = 3$)	Japan	Kumamoto	1994	XV
		Sapporo	2030	XIV
	Taiwan	Taipei	2018	XXI
Australia—Oceania ($n = 1$)	Australia	Adelaide	2006	XVIII
Europe ($n = 15$)	Belgium	Antwerp	1939	I
		Brussels	1957	V
	France	Paris	1967	VIII
		Paris	2002	XVII
	Germany	Wiesbaden	1978	XI
	Italy	Rome	1961	VI
		Bologna	2010	XIX
	Netherlands	Rotterdam	1949	II
	Sweden	Stockholm	1952	III
		Gothenburg	1970	IX
		Stockholm	1986	XIII
	United Kingdom	London	1955	IV
		London	1990	XIV
		London	2026	XIII
	Turkey	Istanbul	2014	XX
North America ($n = 4$)	USA	New York City	1964	VII
		Washington DC	1982	XII
		Philadelphia	1998	XVI
		New York City	2022	XXII
South America ($n = 1$)	Uruguay	Punta del Este	1974	X

In Asia, Latin America, the Middle East, and Africa, neuroradiology is rapidly expanding, addressing different realities and healthcare issues which are influenced by social, economic, and environmental factors.

The WFNRS bears the solemn responsibility of choosing the host cities for the next SNR meetings, and needs address the consequences associated with those geopolitical decisions, which are of vital importance to ensure ongoing success. International air travel is expensive, complex, stressful, and time-consuming for delegates attending SNR meetings. Ideally, SNR host cities should have easy-to-reach major airport hubs, with scheduled direct flights offered by different airlines. This makes it more convenient, cheaper, and faster for attendees to fly in, limiting the number of flights and the time wasted in airport layovers. From past experiences, we have learned that SNR locations that were difficult to reach struggled to attract enough delegates to defray the costs of hosting the meeting. Complex, expensive, and time-consuming travel itineraries act as significant deterrents; they create barriers to participation and contribute to social exclusion, with particular impact on delegates from low- and middle-income countries. Similarly, preference must be given to inner-city SNR congress venues, which are reachable by a well-developed public transportation system, allowing delegates to access the meeting without the need for private cars, taxis, or buses.

All SNR presidents dream of creating a unique and memorable meeting, delivering impactful, lasting, and scientifically stimulating experiences to the participants. Yet all SNR presidents face similar financial and organisational challenges. History rhymes, even though it does not repeat itself. The organisation of a large international meeting is an increasingly complicated and costly endeavour. Rather than leveraging the experience, knowledge, and resources of their predecessors, SNR presidents must essentially start from scratch to address the organisational challenges in the chosen venue. This is in contradistinction to other large scientific societies (e.g. the Radiological Society of North America or the European Society of Radiology) which offer all-inclusive event management services that protect the president and other stakeholders from the financial liability, time commitment, stress, and complexity of planning and running a large conference. The WFNRS should consider developing a roadmap for future SNR meetings to improve efficiency, achieve objectives, and ensure alignment with the ongoing goals of the international neuroradiology communities. The development of such a directive requires financial and human resources, but it will provide invaluable assistance to the SNR president to plan the meeting, develop the programme, define clear objectives, and support WFNRS goals. An uninterrupted stream of thought linking past SNR meetings to present challenges and future strategic opportunities is vital to sustain the continuous growth of the SNR meetings. Future SNR presidents should be able to build upon the success of their predecessors, learn from past failures, avoid repeating mistakes, implement improvements and innovations to ensure the ongoing success of the SNR. Alignment with the WFNRS goals will become ever more important as the SNR family expands to embrace diverse neuroradiological communities in other continents, addressing complex societal and healthcare issues, and developing alternative diagnostic and therapeutic perspectives for a diverse and rapidly growing population.

For figures related to the contents, the readers are recommended to contact the chapter correspondent for further information.

Further Reading

1. de Morsier G. Le Symposium neuroradiologicum de Rotterdam [The Rotterdam symposium on neuroradiology]. Confin Neurol. 1951;11(1):5–9. PMID: 14831337.
2. Fischgold H. Introduction à la Neuroradiologie [Introduction to neuroradiology]. J Radiol Electrol Med Nucl. 1964;45:18–22. PMID: 14143085.
3. Bull JW. The history of neuroradiology. Proc R Soc Med. 1970;63(6):637–43. https://doi.org/10.1177/003591577006300640. PMID: 4916568; PMCID: PMC1811576.
4. Pendergrass HP. James William Douglas Bull, M. D. (1911–1987). Radiology. 1979;130(2):550. https://doi.org/10.1148/130.2.550. PMID: 366669.
5. Shapiro BJ. Donald Lane McRae, M.D.—1912–1982. Radiology. 1983;146(2):565. https://doi.org/10.1148/radiology.146.2.565-a.

6. XII Symposium Neuroradiologicum. Washington, DC, October 10–16, 1983. AJNR Am J Neuroradiol. 1983;4(3):219–882. PMID: 6410704; PMCID: PMC8334977.
7. XIII Symposium Neuroradiologicum. Stockholm, June 23–28, 1986. Acta Radiol Suppl. 1986;369:1–774. PMID: 2908789.
8. Greitz T. The Symposium Neuroradiologicum. Acta Radiol. 1987;28(6):657–8. PMID: 2962596.
9. du Boulay G. James William Douglas Bull, 1911–1987. AJNR Am J Neuroradiol. 1988;9(3):532.
10. du Boulay G. Professor Dr. med. Sigurd Wende. Neuroradiology. 1992;34:171–2. https://doi.org/10.1007/BF00596329.
11. Sage MR. The history of neuroradiology: an Australian perspective. AJNR Am J Neuroradiol. 1995;16(6):1295–302. PMID: 7677029; PMCID: PMC8337848.
12. Takahashi M. Pioneers and history of Japanese neuroradiology. AJNR Am J Neuroradiol. 1995;16(4):741–4. PMID: 7611031; PMCID: PMC8332308.
13. Houser OW. Neuroradiology: a historical perspective. Radiology. 1995;196(1):1–2. https://doi.org/10.1148/radiology.196.1.7784551. PMID: 7784551.
14. Greitz T. The history of Swedish neuroradiology. Acta Radiol. 1996;37(3 Pt 2):455–71. https://doi.org/10.1177/02841851960373P209. PMID: 8652312.
15. Leonardi M. A history of neuroradiology in Italy. AJNR Am J Neuroradiol. 1996;17(4):721–30. PMID: 8730193; PMCID: PMC8337264.
16. Huckman MS. Giovanni Di Chiro (1926–1997). AJNR Am J Neuroradiol. 1998;19(6):1007–10. PMID: 9672004; PMCID: PMC8338636.
17. Picard L. The XVII Paris symposium neuroradiologicum, August 18–24, 2002. J Neuroradiol. 2000;27(2):83–4. PMID: 10970956.
18. Huckman MS. Dinner at Keen's: the founding of the American Society of Neuroradiology. AJNR Am J Neuroradiol. 2001;22(9):1803–5. PMID: 11673184; PMCID: PMC7974432.
19. Huckman MS. Juan Manuel Taveras, 1919–2002. AJNR Am J Neuroradiol. 2002;23(7):1065–8. PMCID: PMC8185710.
20. Cabanis EA, Iba-Zizen Cabanis MT, Picard L. A history of neuroradiology: XVIIth symposium neuroradiologicum: Paris, France, August 18–24, 2002.
21. X Symposium Neuroradiologicum, Punta del Este, Uruguay, 1974. In: Cabanis EA, Iba-Zizen MT, editors. A history of neuroradiology (1895–2002), Toulouse, Europa Edition. 2002. p. 55.
22. Greitz T, Hindmarsh T. Erik Lindgren (1905–2005). AJNR Am J Neuroradiol. 2006;27(7):1396. PMID: 16927472; PMCID: PMC7977540.
23. Leonardi M. Invitation to attend the Symposium Neuroradiologicum. Neuroradiology. 2010;52:329–31.
24. Abstracts of the XIX Symposium Neuroradiologicum. The World Congress of Diagnostic & Therapeutic Neuroradiology—Bologna, Italy, 4–9 October 2010. Neuroradiol J. 2010;23(Suppl 1):1–488. Epub 2010 Sept 20. PMID: 24477266.
25. Sabattini L. To Professor Giovanni Ruggiero. Neuroradiology. 2010;52:655–6. https://doi.org/10.1007/s00234-010-0688-3.
26. van Gijn J, Gijselhart JP. Ziedses des Plantes: uitvinder van planigrafie en subtractie [Ziedses des Plantes: inventor of planigraphy and subtraction]. Ned Tijdschr Geneeskd. 2011;155:A2164. PMID: 21418697 (Dutch).
27. Hoeffner EG, Mukherji SK, Srinivasan A, Quint DJ. Neuroradiology back to the future: brain imaging. AJNR Am J Neuroradiol. 2012;33(1):5–11. https://doi.org/10.3174/ajnr.A2936. Epub 2011 Dec 8. PMID: 22158930; PMCID: PMC7966158.
28. Abstracts of the XXth Symposium Neuroradiologicum, September 7–12, 2014, Istanbul, Turkey. Neuroradiology. 2014;56(Suppl 1):1–476. https://doi.org/10.1007/s00234-014-1405-4. PMID: 25107432.
29. XXIst Symposium Neuroradiologicum. Neuroradiology. 2018;60(Suppl 1):1–406. https://doi.org/10.1007/s00234-018-1983-7. PMID: 29520428.

30. Hindmarsh T, Kaijser M. One hundred years of neuroradiology in *Acta Radiologica*: a Swedish perspective. Acta Radiol. 2021;62(11):1451–9. https://doi.org/10.1177/02841851211051027. Epub 2021 Nov 11. PMID: 34761691.
31. Lev MH, Gadde JA, Wiggins RH. A brief history of neuroradiology and the 60th anniversary of the ASNR: "through the decades with ASNR". AJNR Am J Neuroradiol. 2022;43(12):E54–9. https://doi.org/10.3174/ajnr.A7712. Epub 2022 Dec 1. PMID: 36456083.

Chapter 2
Purpose-Driven Mission: A History of the American Society of Neuroradiology (ASNR): 1990–2024

Jonathan D. Clemente

Preamble: 1962 to 1990

The American Society of Neuroradiology (ASNR) was established on April 19, 1962, in New York City under the leadership of Dr. Juan M. Taveras [1]. The 14 founding members created a professional society "(1) To develop and support standards for the training and practice of neuroradiology; (2) To foster independent research in neuroradiology; and (3) To promote a closer fellowship and exchange of ideas among neuroradiologists." [2]

During its first three decades, ASNR organized its activities around its original mission and focused on "creating an identity of neuroradiology as an autonomous discipline." The Society developed its governance and committee structure to meet the needs of its growing membership and annual meeting and to achieve other goals [3]. Advances in CT, MRI, and PET fueled growth in neuroimaging and interest in the field. In 1980, ASNR launched its official journal, the *American Journal of Neuroradiology* (AJNR). By 1990, the annual meeting, once a closed scientific meeting held in a single conference room, evolved into a multiday affair attracting a broad audience and covering a wide range of topics.

US policymakers and insurance carriers began to increasingly scrutinize rising healthcare expenditures and raised questions about the value of neuroradiology. Concerns over the proposed "healthcare reform" legislature in the early 1990s, along with diminishing funding for research, and an increasingly complex regulatory environment led ASNR to pursue a proactive role in shaping healthcare policy as a forceful advocate for neuroradiology.

During the last three decades, ASNR's strategic goals, organization, and governance structure have progressed to address the dynamic challenges and opportunities, although its core mission and vision remain the same. From focusing on

J. D. Clemente (✉)
Charlotte Radiology, PA, Neuroradiology Section, Charlotte, NC, USA

D. Birchall (ed.), *A World History of Neuroradiology*,
https://doi.org/10.1007/978-3-032-16653-1_2

education, practice and training standards, research, and public policy to adapting to technological advancements and enhancing diverse member engagement, ASNR's activities reflect a commitment to advancing neuroradiology and maximizing patient care.

ASNR Strategic Goals and Initiatives Since 1990

ASNR has driven its activities by strategic goalsetting and based on practice and advocacy, education and training, governance, and research. Before 1990, Society officers undertook planning with input from committee chairpersons. ASNR began a formal strategic planning process in the spring of 1994 under the leadership of its new Executive Director, James B. Gantenberg, and Dr. R. Nick Bryan [4]. Developed over a yearlong process, the 1994 strategic plan was shaped by internal factors (e.g., members' surveys on policy and future direction and needs assessment on programs and services) and external factors (e.g., emerging legislative and regulatory issues or turf battles). ASNR has updated its Strategic Plan every 3–5 years except in the early 2000s, when the focus temporarily shifted to needs assessment and developing educational programming [5]. While ASNR has updated strategic plans periodically, the core pillars undergirding them are unchanged since its founding.

Practice/Advocacy

ASNR has elevated neuroradiology by promoting high standards of practice and through advocacy work. The Society has sought to demonstrate its value to its members and establish neuroradiology's vital role in patient care.

Intersociety collaboration has been key to the development of "Practice Parameters and Technical Standards" for neuroradiology [6]. ASNR has worked effectively with the American College of Radiology (ACR), other radiology organizations, and neurological and neurosurgical societies to develop practice parameters and training, competency, and credentialing standards for neuroradiological procedures [7].

In September 1994, ASNR achieved a long-sought goal of subspecialty certification in neuroradiology by the American Board of Radiology, signifying neuroradiology as a distinct medical subspecialty [8]. Although controversial at the time, the Society later encouraged "Maintenance of Certification" [9] and provided members with resources to fulfill requirements [10]. No longer serving as the surrogate certifying body for neuroradiologists, ASNR could then focus on building a more inclusive society [11].

While ASNR has long aligned closely with ACR on political matters, it has been prepared to "go it alone," and lobby on its behalf [12]. In 1995, a "Clinical Practice Committee" (CPC), initially led by J. Arliss Pollock, MD, was created to focus on socioeconomic issues impacting neuroradiologists [13]. In 1996, ASNR gained a seat in the American Medical Association (AMA) House of Delegates and its influential Current Procedural Terminology Editorial Panel (CPT), and the Resource-based Relative Value System Update Committee (RUC) [14]. These committees play a major role in coding and reimbursement decisions in the United States, and ASNR's seat allowed member's voices to be heard.[1] In 2000, ASNR CPC helped achieve six new billing codes for common neuroradiological exams [15]. To strengthen its relationship with ACR, the CPC and its subcommittees aligned with ACR Neuroradiology Commission in 2011 [16]. Since 2012, ASNR has participated in over 100 support letters, tasks forces, and coalitions with other organizations on a range of issues related to health care policy, reimbursement, and practice standards [17].

ASNR has endeavored to be an inclusive society in recognition that international outreach and collaboration are vital to neuroradiology's future. In 1991, ASNR advocated for the creation of the World Federation of Neuroradiological Societies out of the Symposium Neuroradiologicum [18]. ASNR launched an International Imaging Symposia program in 2016. In 2017, the Society created the "Anne G. Osborn ASNR International Outreach Professor Program" to formalize the sponsorship of visiting professorships to developing nations [19].

Patient outreach has assumed greater importance for ASNR. In 2003, ASNR published three information pamphlets on stroke, AVM, and aneurysm for distribution to patients [20]. The Society created a "Patient-centered Ad Hoc Committee" in 2011 to promote the value-added role of neuroradiology [21].

Education/Training

ASNR fulfills its education mission through its annual meetings, publications, practice standards, guidelines, and curriculum development.

Annual Meeting

The Annual Meeting, held in major cities across North America in late spring, is a premier educational event.[2] A topical Symposium sponsored by the ASNR's Research Foundation precedes the main meeting. The Program Committee has

[1]The AMA stipulated that greater than 25% of a professional society's voting members also be AMA members to qualify for a seat in the House of Delegates. The ASNR almost lost its seat in 2011 by not reaching this threshold.

[2]The Society's 50th Annual Meeting took place in New York City in 2012. The COVID-19 Pandemic caused the 2020 and 2021 meetings to be held virtually. Over 4000 people attended the first virtual meeting. The 2022 and 2023 meetings here hybrid virtual/in-person. The 2024 meeting returned to an in-person format.

tailored meeting content to be "timely and relevant" to the membership, which is equally represented by academic and community practice radiologists. The Society has made significant efforts—particularly after the 2010 Strategic Plan—to enhance the meeting's value for the entire constituency, including research scientists, and members-in-training [16].

Concurrent neuroradiology subspecialty society programming by ASHNR, ASSR, ASTIN (later SNIS), and ASPNR began in 1996, and by ASFNR in 2005. At the 1999 meeting in San Diego, ASNR formalized the responsibility of subspecialty societies for planning their annual meeting content.

Multidisciplinary case-based reviews with partner organizations like the Society of Neuro-Oncology have been popular, as have advanced imaging seminars and interactive scientific poster sessions introduced in 2010. Joint programming with ISMRM began in 2010. The creation of ASNR Study Groups in 2014 strengthened the Society's ties with the broader neuroscience research community by uniting investigators with common interests, such as Vessel Wall Imaging and AI [22]. Corporate sponsorship for the meeting has varied over time depending on a range of factors such as federal regulations on funding for medical meetings. ASNR currently benefits from corporate support and vendor-sponsored programming.

ASNR has fostered international collaboration by hosting the Symposium Neuroradiologicum in 1998 and 2022 and by incorporating sessions led by the Sociedad Ibero Latino Americana de Neurorradiología Diagnóstica y Terapéutica (SILAN),[3] the European Society of Neuroradiology (ESNR), and the Asian-Oceanian Society of Neuroradiology and Head & Neck Radiology (AOSHNR).

ASNR introduced the "Audience Response System" in 2005 along with dedicated SAM and MOC sessions to help members earn credit toward recertification.[4] In 1998, ASNR introduced Informatics programming as the "Electronic Learning Center" (rebranded "Synaptic Junction" in 2010 and "Computer Science & Informatics" in 2013). At the 2015 Symposium, patients participated in sessions to discuss their experience dealing with disease. Other important non-interpretive programming introduced since 2010 include Young Professionals (2010), Evidence-based Medicine (2017), and Diversity and Inclusion (2021). The meeting format has also embraced a digital presence. By 2000, presenters submitted 99% of abstracts online. ASNR has made meeting content available through a variety of electronic media, such as CD-ROM, flash drive, and via mobile app (2012), with electronic exhibits available online for several months after the event [23].

[3] Iberolatinoamericana Society of Diagnostic and Therapeutic Neuroradiology.

[4] SAM Self-Assessment Module; MOC Maintenance of Certification.

Publications

ASNR's flagship publications are the AJNR and *Neurographics*, launched in 1980 and 2011, respectively. During its first decade of publication, the *American Journal of Roentgenology* co-published articles in the AJNR, reflecting the journal's co-ownership by the American Roentgen Ray Society (ARRS). On January 1, 1986, full ownership of the AJNR passed from the ARRS to ASNR [24].

AJNR has had seven editors-in-chief: Juan M. Taveras (1980–1989), Michael S. Huckman (1989–1997), Robert M. Quencer (1997–2005), Robert I. Grossman (Jan 2006–2007), Mauricio Castillo (2007–2015), Jeffrey Ross (2015–2023), and Max Wintermark (2023–present). Since the 1990s, AJNR has increased in size, article submissions, international authorship, and impact factor. AJNR has grown from 6 to 12 issues a year, began digital publication in September 2000, and launched a mobile app in 2010. In January 2025, AJNR transitioned its publication to an all-digital format. A major update to AJNR's website "WEB 2.0" in 2010 added "Case of the Week," "Classic Case," AJNR Blog, podcasts, and a Fellows' Club among other features [25]. Manuscript submissions have steadily increased since the 1990s, from 610 in 1998 to over 1700 in 2020 [26]. By 2007, over 50% of submissions to the journal came from outside the United States [27]. Between 2010 and 2023, AJNR's impact factor has ranged from 2.9–4.9. Since 2016, the ASNR has offered free or low-cost journal access to developing nations through the WHO HINARI program. Current Editor, Dr. Max Wintermark has introduced the AJNR Academy of Reviewers to elevate the quality of the peer review process, and AJNR "SCANtastic" to promote AJNR content via social media [28].

Neurographics is ASNR's peer-reviewed, quarterly, educational journal published online since June 2011, and bimonthly since 2015. *Neurographics* serves "to supplement the basic and clinical science research published in the AJNR with high-quality neuroradiology educational articles." [29] Since March 2013, Neurographics has offered Continuing Medical Education (CME) credits. Drs. Quencer and Castillo served as the initial editors and the journal consisted of educational exhibits selected from the annual meeting. Barton F. Branstetter IV MD, then Chair of the ASNR Education Committee, was the first editor-in-chief. He was succeeded as editor-in-chief by Joshua P. Nickerson, MD in June 2020. In early 2026, *Neurographics* was rebranded as AJNR *Clinical Practice*, focused on high-quality, peer-reviewed, practice-oriented clinical content.

The monthly AJNR Podcast reviewing journal highlights began with the November–December 2009 issue. There have been five podcast editors to date: C. Douglas Philips, MD (2009–2012) Yvonne W. Lui, MD (2013–2017), Wende Gibbs, MD (2017—2021), Courtney Tomblinson, MD (2021), and Keven Hiatt, MD (2021-Present). Mauricio Castillo started the AJNR Blog in January 2009 to provide space for book reviews, annotated bibliography of neuroradiological literature, and other important editorial news. By December 2009, the Blog received about 5000 visits per month [30].

Standards, Guidelines, and Curriculum Development

ASNR's educational, training, and curriculum development activities have advanced to meet the changing needs of neuroradiology professionals, embracing state-of-the-art technology, and ensuring the relevance of continuing education.

Initiatives are as follows: Introduction of the Core Curriculum Course in 1994, development of the Bracco-sponsored Neurocurriculum Live in 2014,[5] creation of the Neuroradiology Fellowship Curriculum in January 2021, and a Comprehensive Neuroradiology Course in September 2022 to supplement institutional curricular offerings. Currently, ASNR's Education Connection platform provides a library of on-demand webinars, podcasts, and other resources. Since its launch in September 2019, ASNR has hosted over 120 webinars and learners have earned over 84,000 CME hours [31].

The Society secured accreditation for neuroradiology fellowships by the Accreditation Council for Graduate Medical Education (ACGME) in 1992, with the objectives of addressing the subspecialty workforce crisis in the late 1990s and adapting training standards to innovative technologies and practice patterns. ASNR advocated for a "Neuroradiology Fellowship Match" in January 2001 which organized and streamlined the trainee selection process, improved fairness, and reduced no-show rates among fellows.

ASNR focused on recruiting and supporting future leaders through leadership development programs, targeted meeting features for fellows, and the establishment of the Young Professionals Committee in 2014. Free membership for "Members-in-Training" category, and the development of a Career Center arrived in March 2021.

ASNR has collaborated with other societies, such as SNIS and AANS[6] to define practice standards for neuroradiology, including guidelines for neurointerventional training and artificial intelligence standards.

ASNR Digital Presence and Social Media

ASNR has embraced digital presence and social media as crucial components of its strategy to engage members, disseminate knowledge, and foster community within neuroradiology. The journey began on December 20, 1996, with the launching of its website, marking the start of its online presence. Over the years, ASNR has matured its digital strategy, including major website redesigns in 2008 and in 2022 to improve user experience, searchability, and access to curated content, embracing social media platforms in April 2010 and launching a Facebook page in December 2012 [32].

[5] Neurocurriculum Live was rebranded "Neuroradiology Core Education Series" in 2022.

[6] Society of Neurointerventional Surgery and American Association of Neurological Surgeons.

Governance

ASNR Executive Leadership

During its early years, a small Executive Committee comprising elected officers conducted the Society's business. ASNR lacked physical headquarters or administrative staff. ASNR presidents relied on their personal staff and resources to fulfill their duties. The increasing complexity of the Annual Meeting in the 1970s, coupled with membership growth, led the Society to seek an experienced meeting planner and managerial support. ASNR approached the Radiological Society of North America (RSNA) for help. In 1983, ASNR hired George F. Schuyler, the RSNA's director of scientific meetings, to assist in planning its annual meeting and other activities. Schuyler was both a "Meeting Consultant" and a "Managing Director." In that capacity, he remained an RSNA employee and worked for the ASNR part-time [33].

Schuyler retired from RSNA in 1989 and was succeed by Patricia Grosshauser who had served as ASNR's assistant managing director since 1985. Grosshauser played an instrumental role in gaining ownership of AJNR [34]. In the Summer of 1990, ASNR achieved full independence from RSNA with its own office and administrative staff. After Grosshauser left, the ASNR began a search for a new Executive Director.

In 1993, ASNR hired James B. Gantenberg, FACHE to serve as Executive Director. Gantenberg brought a wealth of managerial experience, including 5 years as Executive Director of the American Society of Clinical Oncology. Gantenberg brought skills in strategic planning and implementation, organizational development, corporate relations, fundraising, and fiscal management to bear on the challenges facing the Society. He built ASNR's professional staff, from 5 to 17, bringing in experts in functional areas like finance, human resources, technology, and meeting planning.

Over the next two decades, Gantenberg and physician leaders oversaw the growth and evolution of ASNR from a radiology subspecialty society operating under the auspices of RSNA into an independent national organization with over 5500 members and strong international partners. With Gantenberg scheduled to retire at the end of 2016, ASNR conducted a national search and selected Mary Beth Hepp, MBA to succeed him. Hepp came to ASNR with over a decade of executive leadership experience, most recently as Executive Director and Foundation President of Helping Hand Center, a large social services organization [35]. In her role as ASNR Executive Director, Hepp oversees a staff of 17 and the work of ASNR's Board of Directors to ensure that the society remains dedicated to the fulfillment of its educational, research, and advocacy missions.

ASNR Physician Leadership

The ASNR physician leadership structure has changed in size, structure, and composition since its founding. ASNR chooses officers annually. Until the early 1990s, a "Nominating Committee" made recommendations on a slate of candidates, effectively *selected* the president without input from the members. Historically, ASNR leadership has come from major academic institutions on the east and west coasts of the United States and the Mayo Clinic. In 1992, in response to member feedback that elections were undemocratic, ASNR began soliciting its general membership for nominations for elected positions [12]. In 1995, Dr. Robert Lukin was the first president of the ASNR *elected* through this more inclusive member ballot process.

In its 61-year history, ASNR has made strides, particularly in the last decade, to improve the diversity of the senior leadership to reflect the changing membership, and the elevation of women, and community practitioners. To date, ten women have served as president. The first woman to serve as president was Anne G. Osborn, MD in 1988–89. Another 17 years would pass before a second woman, Patricia A. Rhyner, MD, was elected president in 2005. Since that time, eight other women have served as president, including Tina Young Poussaint, MD, FACR, and Past President Yvonne W. Lui, MD FACR [36]. In 2018, Robert M. Barr became the first private practice neuroradiologist to be elected ASNR president.[7]

ASNR Executive Committee

The ASNR Executive Committee (The "Ex Comm") had been the society's principal decision-making body since October 1962. The Ex Comm functioned like a traditional corporate board of directors empowered to conduct the society's business, controlled funds and "the safe keeping or sale of property." [37] For many years, the Ex Comm consisted of the president, president-elect, vice president, secretary, and treasurer. All standing committees of the ASNR reported up to the Ex-Comm. By the early 1990s, members raised concerns that the Ex Comm had become too insular, unresponsive to the needs of subspecialists and private practitioners, inadequately defended turf, and lacked participation in reimbursement policy decisions. In 1992, the ASNR revamped its governance structure to allow for greater member representation, greater authority, and expansion into new fields of public policy and practice standards [38].

By 1994, the Ex Comm had grown to include the senior elected officers, one member-at-large, the three most recent past presidents, the chair of the Rules Committee, and representatives of the Subspecialty Groups recognized by the Executive Committee [39]. That year, a small "Administrative Committee" was

[7] An appendix provides a full list of ASNR past presidents.

established.[8] The Ex Comm was empowered to carry out business between meetings of the *membership*. Whereas the Society empowered the Administrative Committee to conduct business between meetings of the *Executive Committee* [40].

Over the next decade, ASNR's Ex Comm expanded to incorporate representatives of preexisting standing committees and those of newly formed committees created over the years to address various issues such as health policy, research, and fellowship training. By 2014, the Ex Comm had 22 voting members and 11 non-voting members [41]. The Ex Comm became a valuable component of the ASNR leadership, fostering collaboration among various regional and subspecialty societies and including input from committee chairs, the ACR council, and other societies. It had also become unwieldy. ASNR needed a smaller, nimbler group to oversee management and functions and to improve the efficiency and focus of leadership [42].

In 2015, ASNR restructured its governance, rebranding the Administrative Committee as the "Board of Directors" (BOD). The new BOD consisted of the president, president-elect, vice-president, secretary, treasurer, first, second, and third president, executive director (ex-officio, non-voting), Chair of the Foundation of the ASNR Board of Trustees, editor-in-chief of the American Journal of Neuroradiology (AJNR), and up to three additional members chosen by the Board [43].

Four years later, in 2019, ASNR underwent another significant leadership reorganization, replacing the Ex Comm with the Board of Directors and a new Advisory Council ("AC"). The BOD retained its composition and fiduciary responsibilities, while the larger AC (comprising the elected officers and chairs of the standing committees) functions to advise the Board in meeting strategic goals and initiatives and has some specific authorities. ASNR redefined terms of service of its officers, and assigned the vice president as chair of the AC [44].

ASNR Committee Structure

ASNR's committees are necessary to promote the Society's mission and fulfill its vision. Hundreds of dedicated neuroradiology professionals have volunteered their time and energy to serve on various committees. Whereas the ASNR BOD steers the ship, the committees have provided the power to generate ideas, solve problems, implement programs, and serve as a training ground for the Society's future leaders. Headquarters administrative staff—who provide critical liaison services including facilitating planning, communications, advice on policy and procedures, and program implementation—have assisted ASNR committees.

[8] The Administrative Committee consisted of the president, president-elect, vice president, secretary, treasurer, first past president, and the executive director (ex-officio, non-voting).

The modern committee structure of ASNR has its origins in the early 1970s, which, broadly speaking, has consisted of standing, ad hoc, and annual meeting program-related committees reporting up through the Ex Comm [45] and, after 2019, through the BOD. The number of ASNR standing committees has risen steadily from 6 in 1962 (Executive, Auditors, Rules, Membership, Program, and Nominating) to 31 in 2015–2016. The Society has formed new committees to oversee increasingly complex daily business (e.g., Finance, Publications, and Commercial Relations committees) and through the strategic planning process (e.g., Fellowship Directors and Social Media committees).

In 2013–2014, ASNR underwent a major expansion of its standing committees, many of which existed for years. Committees were grouped into five broad categories: Core Missions (Health Policy, Research, and Education), Meeting-related (Program and Technical/IT), Social Engagement (Membership, Commercial Relations, ASNR Foundation, Publication, Infrastructure, and Intersociety Relations), Administrative (Admin and Ex Comm, Human Resources, Audit, Finance, Rules, Nominating), and Honorific (Honorary Membership, Outstanding Contributions in Research, and Gold Medal Award) [46]. The three long-standing Health Policy subcommittees on "Economics," "Quality Safety and Value," and "Standards and Guidelines" were all elevated to committee status reflecting the complexity of practice and payor issues. Among the new committees formed were "Computer Science and Informatics," "Website and Online CME," "Young Professionals," and "International Collaborations." [47]

Further restructuring and consolidation of committees occurred between 2017–2023, to align those with similar purposes such as "Website" with "Social Media" or to incorporate important committees like Health Policy and the Special/Regional Societies into the Advisory Committee. In 2020, ASNR BOD established a standing committee on "Diversity and Inclusion "to ensure that the 'increasingly diverse and complex' nature of the Society was incorporated into its many programs, functions and activities." [48] Most recently, in 2023, the AJNR editor-in-chief position was removed from the Board of Directors, to reflect best practice and consistency with other societies' practices. The editors-in-chief of all ASNR publications (currently AJNR and *Neurographics*) remain on the ASNR Advisory Council [49].

Evolution of the ASNR Constitution

The foundational governance document of ASNR is its "Constitution," first codified in April 1962 and updated on a near-annual basis. Over six decades, its basic structure has remained stable; defining the Society's objectives, roles, and terms of officers, membership criteria, and functions of major committees. Since the 1980s, ASNR's Constitution has become more detailed. These changes reflect a commitment to maintaining a dynamic and relevant professional organization and a continued evolution of the society's governance and operational procedures, aiming to provide transparency and flexibility, and to reflect current and best practices. ASNR has made some major changes to its constitution.

Elections In 1992, ASNR decided to increase its role in socioeconomic issues, public relations, interaction with government and private payers, and explore inter-society collaboration. The Society therefore undertook “extensive constitutional reform, to improve the operational efficiency of a larger society and democratization of the selection of [its] leadership.” [50] From that point, ASNR made an open call to its membership for nominees for officers [51].

Objectives Between 1969 and 1994, the ASNR constitution added four new objectives: (1) providing for an annual scientific and educational meeting, (2) promoting close cooperation with other related specialties, (3) establishing a channel to publish neuroradiology research, and (4) promoting understanding of neuroradiology among patients, the public, and other medical specialists [52].

Membership Before 1990, membership was by “invitation only” and for fellowship-trained neuroradiologists. As membership plateaued, the Society sought to attract new members from neuroradiology, the broader neuroscience research community, and from outside North America. Periodically, ASNR has amended its membership categories to be more inclusive and to streamline the application process. Achieving the milestone of subspecialty certification required the ASNR to compromise with organized radiology by allowing all qualified individuals actively engaged in the professional practice of neuroradiology to sit for the exam. In 1995, the ASNR constitution was amended to create a new route for “Junior” members to advance to “Senior” membership and also enabled any radiologist who had received a subspecialty certification in Neuroradiology from the ABR to be eligible for senior membership [53]. Since 1962, ASNR has admitted international physicians designating them “corresponding members” until 1999 when they were folded into the “Member” category. In 2014, the Society created a new member category called “International Outreach” to include individuals from developing countries with an annual per-person GDP of $10,000 or less [54]. As of 2024, there were seven member categories.[9]

Constitutional Crisis Changes to the ASNR Constitution have seldom generated controversy. In 2007, the ASNR Executive Committee’s proposal to include non-neuroradiologists as “Senior Members” caused great consternation among the Society’s members [55]. An earlier decision by ASNR to add a dues assessment of $1800 on top of regular member dues to fund the Society’s philanthropic foundation had the unintended consequence of a 5–10% attrition in membership. Some members chose not to renew, while others converted to a less expensive member category.

[9]These categories are Senior Member, Junior Member, Member-in-Training, International Outreach Member, Research Scientist Member, Emeritus Member, and Honorary Member.

ASNR leadership had strategized ways of increasing member ranks by removing financial and bureaucratic barriers and eliminating the perception of a “second class status” of non-senior members who lacked voting rights or the ability to chair committees. Societal growth helped introduce fresh ideas and new potential leaders, fostered collaboration with other specialties, and increased international participation at a time when over 50% of AJNR manuscripts came from outside the United States. A larger ASNR also meant greater influence within organized Medicine. David M. Yousem, MD, then president-elect of the ASNR, noted “This is not just about money. It is about expanding the sphere of influence of the ASNR, making it a broader more scientific, international, and far-reaching society.” [56]

Member sentiment was decidedly against the proposed changes, fearing that it would dilute the influence of neuroradiologists, devalue senior membership status, and open the Society up to domination by non-neuroradiologists. Furthermore, as written, ASNR would no longer require Senior Members to practice neuroradiology 50% of their time, be board-certified, or reside in North America [56]. ASNR quickly rescinded the dues increase and took other measures to control costs such as decreasing the length of the annual meeting and limiting spending on social events. The 2007 amendments did not pass and instead the Society later created “Member-in-Training” and “Research Scientist” member categories to encourage fellows and neuroscientists to join the Society [57].

Modernization In 2019, ASNR undertook a comprehensive review of its Constitution and made substantial changes to reflect current best practices, clarifying governance roles of the Executive Committee, and affirming its important advisory role. Extensive wordsmithing to the Constitution improved its clarity and consistency and introduced gender-neutrality. The Society created a new “ASNR Policy and Procedure Manual” to contain operational procedures and logistical details of committee structures that were previously in the Constitution. This change was meant to streamline the document and improve the flexibility of ASNR for growth and innovation.

Research

“Those who do the research, control the field.” [58] ASNR has long recognized the critical importance of research for the future of neuroradiology [59]. The Society has been proactive in supporting neuroradiological research through various initiatives starting with a Fellowship in Basic Science Research Award in 1986 to foster the scientific development of young researchers [60], the creation of a Research Committee in 1991 to oversee research activities, and the establishment of a philanthropic foundation in late 1994 to secure financial resources necessary to ensure research and educational opportunities for its members.

Expansion of the ASNR’s role in education and research and the need for aggressive fundraising to support research independent from members’ donations, other radiology organizations, government and corporate sources have been consistent with the Society's strategic plans. Around 2010, ASNR recognized that it had "lost the lead in neuroimaging research" and that the Society needed to grow its Foundation and develop a sustainable structure for research, including projects that benefited community-based neuroradiologists [61]. The 2018–2021 Strategic Plan highlighted the need to develop the governance and interoperability of the ASNR Board, its Foundation, and the ASNR Research Committee so that the research agenda was aligned with strategic initiatives, and that research priorities cascaded throughout the Society [62].

Foundation of the ASNR (FASNR)

The Foundation of the ASNR (FASNR) began operating as a tax-exempt, non-profit organization in 1995 [63]. The Foundation was governed by a small Board of Trustees that was expanded in 2002 to include more representation by community neuroradiologists [64]. From 1994 until 2014, the Foundation's Board had a single Chair: Burton P. Drayer, MD (1995–2001), A. James Barkovich, MD (2001–2007), Eric J. Russell, MD (2007–2010), and Howard A. Rowley, MD (2010–2014).

In 2014, the Foundation restructured its leadership into two branches with Co-Chairs for "Research and Grants" and "Funding and Development." This reorganization intended to facilitate the evaluation and administration of an increasing number of grants, develop a "more inspired approach to fundraising," [65] and a sustainable framework for ASNR-sponsored research [66]. Pina C. Sanelli, MD, MPH, FACR served as Co-Chair (Research and Grants) from 2014–2023 and was succeeded by Christopher P. Hess, MD, PhD in 2023. Laurie A. Loevner, MD has served as Co-Chair (Funding and Development) from 2014 to present. The Board of Trustees currently consists of two Co-Chairs, the ASNR President, the President-elect/Program Chair, two Members-at-Large, and the ASNR Executive Director. In 2020, the ASNR entered into a new financial and management agreement with the Foundation to simplify the contractual terms around use of the Society's staff and administrative resources [67].

Individual member donations, periodic financial support from growth in ASNR financial reserves, and corporate sponsorship have been the Foundation's principal funding sources. Historically, 7–10% of ASNR members have donated to it. During Fiscal Year 2022 alone, 214 individuals donated a total of $158,000 [68]. In 2018, the ASNR BOD began sponsoring a matching grant for first-time donors, yielding a 17% increase in such donors [69]. Corporate sponsors to the FASNR have included Target Therapeutics, Berlex Pharmaceuticals, and Bracco, among others. In 2023, the FASNR received a $four million charitable contribution to establish the Aldon Mark Berger Fund for Research and Education in Mental Health to develop competitive research grants and education related to mental health [70].

In 2019, the FASNR established three giving circles: the Leadership Circle, the Chairman's Society, and the Corporate Giving Circle. The goals of the giving circles include increasing Foundation giving (annual, major, and planned gifts), creating an organizational identity, and building camaraderie among philanthropists who consistently support the Foundation. Recently, the FASNR redesigned its website to highlight donors and grant recipients [71]. The ASNR and its Foundation remain financially strong, with over $11 million in reserve as of 2021 [72].

Since 1995, the FASNR has awarded over $8.83 million in grants; with 75% of funding awards made through the Boerger Research Fund for Alzheimer's Disease and Neurocognitive Disorders ($2.12 m), the Basic Science Award ($1.82 m), and Scholar Award in Neuroradiology Research ($1.75 m) [73]. More than 116 individual researchers have been funded since 1987. FASNR awards over $340,000 in grants annually [74].

As of 2024, the FASNR offers The Foundation Grant Program (for promising young researchers), the Alzheimer's' Association/Foundation of the ASNR Imaging Grant in Alzheimer's Disease and Neurodegenerative Diseases, the Trainee Research Grant in Neuroradiology, the Aldon Mark Berger Mental Health and Neuropsychiatry Imaging Research Grant, and the Women in Neuroradiology Leadership Award (funds attendance at the ACR's annual Radiology Leadership Institute Summit) [75]. The Foundation has also recently established an "Innovative Research Fund" to support research in AI, clinical data analytics, comparative effectiveness, novel neuroimaging techniques, and translational research.

The Foundation has a tripartite mission to support excellence in patient care, research, and education. The FASNR has funded some of the advocacy work of the Health Policy Committee, which has benefited all members, and educational activities such as *Neurographics*, eCME, Neurocurriculum Live, and the annual meeting Symposium [76]. In 2016, the Foundation provided $150,000 in support to the neuroradiology subspecialty societies to develop research programs. The FASNR has fostered relations with the NIH (2006, 2010), collaborated with ISMRM (2007), and co-sponsored grants with the RSNA (2013) and ARRS (2014). To keep members up-to-date on emerging neuroimaging techniques, such as fMRI and diffusion tensor imaging, the Foundation introduced "hands-on workshops" at the 2014 Annual Meeting.

ASNR Research Committee

The ASNR Research Committee, established in the early 1990s, is "responsible for fostering research in neuroradiology, for overseeing researchers and research activities funded by or through the Society." [77] The Committee evaluates applications for competitive grants, makes recommendations on grant recipients to the Foundation's Board of Trustees, and monitors the progress of research by funded individuals. The Research Committee has played a vital role in developing strategies to increase NIH funding and fostering intersociety collaboration with the RSNA, ISMRM, the Organization for Human Brain Mapping (OHBM), and the Society for Neurosciences (SfN).

ASNR-sponsored research has spanned from basic science to clinical applications, including morphologic and physiologic imaging, outcomes research, and the development of new diagnostic and therapeutic devices. Recent efforts have emphasized evidence-based medicine, comparative effectiveness research (CER) and artificial intelligence (AI) [78].

Conclusion

Since its inception in 1962, ASNR has evolved from a small, visionary group of founders to a major force in the field of neuroradiology. The Society has stayed true to its original mission while adapting to the vast changes in healthcare, technology, and the socioeconomic environment that have occurred since 1990. The society's strategic shifts toward inclusivity, advocacy, education, and research reflect its commitment to advancing neuroradiology and optimizing patient care. With continuous strategic planning, ASNR has not only navigated challenges but has also seized opportunities to promote excellence in practice, advocate for the specialty, foster international collaboration, and drive forward with innovation in research and education. The enduring legacy of ASNR is a testament to its members' dedication and the pivotal role neuroradiology plays in modern medicine.

Acknowledgments The author would like to acknowledge the following individuals who provided encouragement and invaluable support toward the completion of this endeavor: Mary Beth Hepp, Yvonne W. Lui, MD, James B. Gantenberg, FACHE, Karen Lyp, Robert M. Quencer, MD, Mauricio Castillo, MD, William P. Dillon, MD, Robert M. Barr, MD, Patrick A. Turski, MD, Eric J. Russell, MD, Robert I. Grossman, MD, Robert R. Lukin, MD, David M. Yousem, MD, Pina C. Sanelli, MD, Barton F. Branstetter IV, MD, Carolyn C. Meltzer, MD, and Erin Simon Schwartz, MD.

Appendix: Past Presidents of the American Society of Neuroradiology

2023–24 Yvonne W. Lui, MD, FACR
2022–23 Erin Simon Schwartz, MD, FACR
2021–22 Tina Young Poussaint, MD, FACR
2020–21 Joshua A. Hirsch, MD, FACR, FSIR, FSNIS
2019–20 Robert M. Barr MD, FACR
2018–19 Pina C. Sanelli, MD, MPH, FACR
2017–18 Jacqueline A. Bello, MD, FACR
2016–17 Howard A. Rowley, MD
2015–16 Laurie A. Loevner, MD
2014–15 Gordon K. Sze, MD, FACR
2013–14 Mauricio Castillo, MD, FACR

2012–13 Pamela W. Schaefer, MD
2011–12 David B. Hackney, MD, FACR
2010–11 Carolyn Cidis Meltzer, MD, FACR
2009–10 John R. Hesselink, MD, FACR
2008–09 Robert D. Zimmerman, MD, FACR*
2007–08 David M. Yousem, MD, MBA
2006–07 Robert I. Grossman, MD
2005–06 Patricia A. Rhyner, MD
2004–05 Victor M. Haughton, MD
2003–04 Charles M. Strother, MD
2002–03 Patrick A. Turski, MD, FACR
2001–02 William P. Dillon, MD
2000–01 William S. Ball, Jr., MD
1999–00 Eric J. Russell, MD, FACR
1998–99 A. James Barkovich, MD
1997–98 Richard E. Latchaw, MD
1996–97 Burton P. Drayer, MD
1995–96 Robert R. Lukin, MD
1994–95 Robert M. Quencer, MD
1993–94 Glenn S. Forbes, MD, FACR
1992–93 David Norman, MD
1991–92 R. Nick Bryan, MD, PhD
1990–91 Anton N. Hasso, MD, FACR*
1989–90 Joseph F. Sackett, MD
1988–89 Anne G. Osborn, MD
1987–88 Michael S. Huckman, MD*
1986–87 Derek C. Harwood-Nash, MD*
1985–86 R. Thomas Bergeron, MD
1984–85 Samuel M. Wolpert, MD*
1983–84 O. Wayne Houser, MD*
1982–83 Arthur E. Rosenbaum, MD
1981–82 Gabriel H. Wilson, MD*
1980–81 George Wortzman, MD
1979–80 David O. Davis, MD*
1978–79 Stephen A. Kieffer, MD*
1977–78 Sadek K. Hilal, MD*
1976–77 Norman E. Leeds, MD*
1975–76 Irvin I. Kricheff, MD*
1974–75 Hillier L. Baker, Jr., MD*
1973–74 T. Hans Newton, MD*
1972–73 Fred J. Hodges, III, MD*
1971–72 Norman E. Chase, MD*
1970–71 D. Gordon Potts, MD*
1969–70 Giovanni Di Chiro, MD*
1968–69 Colin B. Holman, MD*

1967–68 Harold O. Peterson, MD*
1966–67 Ernest H. Wood, MD*
1965–66 Donald L. McRae, MD*
1964–65 Mannie M. Schechter, MD*
1962–64 Juan M. Taveras, MD*

Founding Members

Norman E. Chase, MD*
Giovanni Di Chiro, MD*
William N. Hanafee, MD*
Fred J. Hodges, III, MD*
Colin B. Holman, MD*
Norman E. Leeds, MD*
Eugene V. Leslie, MD*
Donald L. McRae, MD*
Thomas H. Newton, MD*
Harold O. Peterson, MD*
D. Gordon Potts, MD*
Mannie M. Schechter, MD*
Juan M. Taveras, MD*
Ernest H. Wood, MD*
*Deceased

References

1. Huckman MS. Dinner at Keen's: the founding of the American Society of Neuroradiology. AJNR Am J Neuroradiol. 2001;22(9):1803–5.
2. Kieffer SA. ASNR recollections: a brief history of the American Society of Neuroradiology, 1988, Glenn S. Forbes Collection, ASNR digital archive.
3. *Ibid*, Kieffer, pg. 7.
4. ASNR Strategic Plan, May 1995. Bryan had served as ASNR President from 1991–92.
5. James B. Gantenberg and Patrick A. Turski, MD FACR, Personal Communication.
6. Jordan JE, Norbash A. A call to improve the visibility and access of the American College of Radiology Practice Parameters in neuroradiology: a powerful value stream enhancer for both neuroradiologists and patients. AJNR Am J Neuroradiol. 2019;40(2):213–6.
7. See for example, Connors JJ 3rd, Sacks D, Furlan AJ, Selman WR, Russell EJ, Stieg PE, Hadley MN; NeuroVascular Coalition Writing Group. Training, competency, and credentialing standards for diagnostic cervicocerebral angiography, carotid stenting, and cerebrovascular intervention. AJNR Am J Neuroradiol 2004;25(10):1732–1741.
8. Sackett JF. The ultimate recognition for neuroradiology. AJNR Am J Neuroradiol. 1992;13(3):833.
9. Lukin RR, Forbes GS. Why I should take my CAQ recertification examination. AJNR Am J Neuroradiol. 2004;25(5):668–9. The ABR now calls MOC Continuing Certification."
10. John H. ASNR President and Yousem D, 2nd Past President, President's Message: Don't Mock the MOC! Thursday, April 15, 2010, www.asnr.org (via Internet Archive, web.archive.org).

11. ASNR Strategic Plan, 1999–2000.
12. Bryan RN. 1992 ASNR presidential address. AJNR Am J Neuroradiol. 1992;13(6):1652–4.
13. ASNR strategic plan, strategic issue #3, socioeconomics, May 1995. ASNR renamed the clinical practice committee as the "Health Policy Committee" in April 2012.
14. Pollack A, Turski P. Representation of the ASNR in the AMA house of delegates at risk. AJNR Am J Neuroradiol. 2006;27(2):239–40.
15. Donovan WD. The resource-based relative value scale and neuroradiology: ASNR'S history at the RUC. Neuroimaging Clin N Am. 2012;22(3):421–36.
16. ASNR 2010 Strategic Plan.
17. Minutes, ASNR 2023 Annual business meeting, Tuesday, May 2, 2023, ASNR Advocacy Activities, https://www.asnr.org/asnr-advocacy-activities/. Accessed 10 Mar 2024.
18. Harwood-Nash DC. The world federation of neuroradiological societies: a proposal. AJNR Am J Neuroradiol. 1991;12(5):845–7.
19. ASNR International Imaging Series, https://www.asnr.org/international-education-collaborations/. Accessed 3 Mar 2024.
20. ASNR Offers Patient Information Pamphlets on Stroke, AVM and Aneurysm, Posted August 14, 2003, www.asnr.org, (via Internet Archive, web.archive.org).
21. Meltzer CC. American Society of Neuroradiology President's Report, "Planning for Our Future in a Changing Health Care Environment," ASNR 2011 Annual meeting, Seattle.
22. The ASNR "Study Groups" include CSF flow/hydrocephalus (2012), Vessel Wall imaging (2014), Tumor genomics (2014), fMRI/DTI (2014), Alzheimer's disease/ARIA (2019), and PET neuro-oncology (2024).
23. Proceedings from past ASNR meetings., https://www.asnr.org/meeting-proceedings/. Accessed 5 Mar 2024.
24. Taveras JM. Editor's comments on the 10th anniversary of AJNR. AJNR Am J Neuroradiol. 1989;10(1):1–2.
25. Castillo M. Editor-in-chief, midterm report. AJNR Am J Neuroradiol. 2011;32(6):977–8.
26. Minutes, ASNR 2021 Annual business meeting (Virtual), 2021., www.asnr.org
27. Grossman RI. Last words. AJNR Am J Neuroradiol. 2007;28(8):1426.
28. Wintermark M. Introducing AJNR SCANtastic and the AJNR academy of reviewers. AJNR Am J Neuroradiol. 2023;44(12):1357.
29. Branstetter IV, Barton F. Neurographics. 2011;1(1):1. https://doi.org/10.3174/ng.1110007.
30. AJNR Blog reaches 50,000 visits! https://www.ajnrblog.org/2009/12/09/ajnrblog-reaches-50000-visits/. Accessed 8 Mar 2024.
31. Op. Cit, ASNR 2021 Annual Business Meeting Minutes.
32. ASNR Shared its first post on X (formerly Twitter) in April 2010. As social media began to grow and become an integral part of organizations' communication strategies, a presence on Facebook, LinkedIn, and Instagram followed. Annually, the society shares more than 1,600 posts per year across its social platforms and receives more than 94,000 visitors to its website. ASNR remains committed to digital strategies to ensure timely flow of information to members and the neuroradiology community.
33. Zylak CJ, Hasso AN. RSNA and ASNR: a decade of collaboration. Radiology. 1991;179(2):578.
34. Schuyler G. In memory Patricia Grosshauser, 1937–1994. AJNR Am J Neuroradiol. 1995;16(4):786.
35. ASNR News Release, Mary Beth Hepp Named New, Executive Director for the American Society of Neuroradiology (ASNR), Posted on: September 9, 2016, www.asnr.org, (via Internet Archive, web.archive.org).
36. Meltzer CC, Sanelli PC, Hepp MB, Bello JA. Women rising to the top: the tipping point for the ASNR. AJNR Am J Neuroradiol. 2019;40(1):2–4.
37. ASNR Constitution. January 1986 rev., Glenn Forbes Collection, ASNR Digital Archive.
38. *Ibid*, Bryan.
39. In 1994, Recognized subspecialty groups were: the American Society of Head and Neck Radiology (ASHNR), the American Society of Interventional and Therapeutic Neuroradiology

(ASITN, now called the Society for Neurointerventional Surgery), the American Society of Pediatric Neuroradiology (ASPNR), and the American Society of Spine Radiology (ASSR). The American Society of Functional Neuroradiology (ASFNR) was established in June 2004.
40. ASNR Constitution, Revised May 1994.
41. The Ex Comm voting members included the elected officers, chairpersons of major standing committees, and representatives of the five subspecialty societies. ASNR Constitution, Revised August 14, 2014.
42. Barr RM. Personal communication.
43. ASNR Constitution, Revised February 9, 2015.
44. ASNR Constitution, Revised December 2023, Robert M. Barr, MD FACR, Personal Communication,
45. *Ibid*, Kieffer, pg. 8.
46. ASNR 2013 Strategic Plan (Issue 5), Subcommittee Report on Developing ASNR Leadership.
47. ASNR Constitution, Revised August 14, 2014.
48. Jordan JE. ASNR e-news: diversity and inclusion and the ASNR, Posted on: March 16, 2020, www.asnr.org
49. ASNR Constitution, Revised December 2023.
50. Drayer BP. Secretary's report 1991–1992. AJNR Am J Neuroradiol. 1992;13(6):1655.
51. Lui YW. Personal Communication.
52. ASNR Constitution, Revised May 1994; Revised December 2023.
53. Quencer RM. 1995 ASNR presidential address. AJNR Am J Neuroradiol. 1995;16(10):2136–7.
54. ASNR Constitution, Revised August 2024.
55. Hunter GJ. Rules Committee Chair, Letter to ASNR Senior Members on Proposed Constitutional Amendments, April 2007.
56. Letter to ASNR Members from David M. Yousem, MD, President-Elect, ASNR on proposed changes to the ASNR Constitution and Frequently Asked Questions, 28 September 2007, www.asnr.org
57. ASNR Constitution, Revised 20 July 2010.
58. ASNR 1995 Strategic Plan, Strategic issue #6, Neuroscience Research, May 1995.
59. Latchaw RE. The American Society of Neuroradiology. Neuroradiology research: the opportunities and the challenges. Radiology. 1998;209(1):3–7.
60. Bergeron RT. ASNR fellowship in basic science research sponsored by Berlex Imaging, 16 December 1985, Glenn S. Forbes Collection, ASNR Digital Archive.
61. ASNR Strategic Plan 2010, Strategic issue 3, ASNR's role in supporting research.
62. ASNR Strategic plan, goals and objectives, 2018–2021., www.asnr.org. Accessed 10 Mar 2024.
63. In 2002, the foundation of the ASNR was rebranded as the "Neuroradiology Education and Research Foundation" (NERF). NERF reverted to its original name "Foundation of the ASNR" in 2011. New for 2011—Rebranding of the Foundation, Monday, February 28, 2011, www.asnr.org
64. Dillon WP. 2002 Presidential Address. AJNR Am J Neuroradiol. 2002;23(8):1433–5.
65. ASNR E-News, ASNR President's review of 2014, Gordon Sze, MD, Posted on: March 2, 2015., www.asnr.org
66. ASNR 2013 Strategic plan implementation grid, Strategic issue #3, Role in Sponsoring Research.
67. Barr RM. ASNR 2020 Presidential Address.
68. Op Cit., Dillon, 2002 Presidential Address; ASNR President's Report 2013–2014, Mauricio Castillo, MD FACR. ASNR's reserves exceeded $13m in 2021. (ASNR 2021 Annual Business Meeting (Virtual) Wednesday, May 26, 2021).
69. 2018 Annual Report of the Foundation of the ASNR, foundation.asnr.org. Accessed 10 Mar 2024.
70. Foundation of the ASNR to Establish New Mental Health Research and Education Initiative, https://foundation.asnr.org/page/our-impact/bergerfund/. Accessed 10 Mar 2024.
71. Foundation of the ASNR, 2024 First Quarter Newsletter, foundation.asnr.org

72. Minutes, ASNR 2023 Annual business meeting, Tuesday, May 2, 2023.
73. Information provided by ASNR Executive Director, Mary Beth Hepp.
74. FASNR Impact, https://foundation.asnr.org/page/our-impact/. Accessed 10 Mar 2024.
75. Other FASNR grants and awards include: the outstanding contributions award, the comparative effectiveness research award, the research scientist award, the ASNR/RSNA Research Scholar Grant, the Anne G. Osborn ASNR International Outreach Professor Program, the Neuroradiology Research Grant in Artificial Intelligence, and the David M. Yousem Research Fellow Award. Some research grants have been sunset over the years based on need and relevance.
76. Letter from the President—Search for New Leaders of the Foundation of the ASNR, Gordon Sze, M.D., FACR Chair, Search Committee for Chair of the FASNR President, ASNR, posted January 27, 2015, www.asnr.org
77. ASNR Research Committee. https://www.asnr.org/about-us/committees/research-committee/. Accessed 10 Mar 2024. ASNR recently renamed Neurocurriculum Live as "ASNR Neuroradiology Core Education."
78. The ASNR established an Evidence Based Medicine Committee in 2017 to promote "the application of sound clinical research methods in neuroradiology by offering educational sessions and hands-on assistance to prospective investigators." (ASNR EBM Committee, https://www.asnr.org/about-us/committees/evidence-based-medicine-committee/, Accessed 10 Mar 2024) Since 2019, the ASNR and RSNA have co-sponsored AI challenges on intracranial hemorrhage, brain tumors, and lumbar degenerative disc disease.

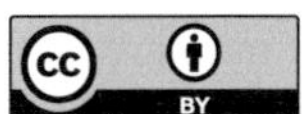

Chapter 3
Asian-Oceanian Society of Neuroradiology and Head & Neck Radiology: The Early Years

Francis Hui and C. C. Tchoyoson Lim

Introduction

The Asian and Oceanian Society of Neuroradiology and Head & Neck Radiology (AOSNHNR) is a federation of Neuroradiological Societies comprising neuroradiologists and head and neck radiologists, dedicated to the science and the arts of diagnostic and interventional radiology within the region of Asia and Oceania [1]. This chapter chronicles the founding and development of the Society to the present day, focusing especially on our Congresses. The AOSNHNR works closely with international partners in Europe, the Americas and also with general radiology Societies and those of our allied health professionals. Many individual members have made important contributions, and individual Asian and Oceanian national societies have written other chapters in this book; which readers are encouraged to peruse.

Founding of the AOSNHNR

In the early 1990s, the need for a society in the Asian and Oceanian countries to promote neuroradiology and head and neck radiology was growing. The impending establishment of the World Federation of the Neuroradiological Societies (WFNRS)

F. Hui
Radiology, National University Hospital, Singapore, Singapore

C. C. T. Lim (✉)
Department of Neuroradiology, National Neuroscience Institute, Singapore, Singapore

Duke-NUS Medical School, Radiological Sciences Academic Clinical Programme, SingHealth Duke-NUS Academic Medical Centre, Singapore, Singapore
e-mail: tchoyoson@duke-nus.edu.sg

D. Birchall (ed.), *A World History of Neuroradiology*,
https://doi.org/10.1007/978-3-032-16653-1_3

at the same time, gave new impetus to our radiologists to form a society to provide representation from the Asian and Oceanian regions [2].

Through the initiative of Prof. Mutsumasa Takahashi, a meeting was arranged in January 1994 among interested participants attending the 18th International Congress of Radiology in Singapore in 1993. At this first organizational meeting of the AOSNHNR, the representatives of the countries and regions of Asia and Oceania met and discussed the organization of the Society and its Constitution [3]. Prof. Takahashi was designated President-Elect and asked to organize the first scientific meeting to coincide with the XV Symposium Neuroradiologicum scheduled to be held in Kumamoto in September 1994. The Constitution of the Society was carefully discussed by the representatives and finally adopted through mail ballots.

First Congress and XV Symposium Neuroradiologicum: Kumamoto 1994

The final organizational meeting of the society was held at the Hotel New Otani, Kumamoto, Japan on September 25, 1994 [4]. More than 30 representatives from Asia and Oceania region founded the society. The office of the society was located at the Department of Radiology, Kumamoto University School of Medicine, Japan. The Constitution of the society was adopted officially and the office bearers were elected by representative National Delegates.

The very first Officers of the AOSNHNR Council were duly elected as follows:

President: Mutsumasa Takahashi (Japan)
Vice-President: Tsuen Chang (Taiwan)
Treasurer: Michael Mu-Huo Teng (Taiwan)
Secretary: Mutsumasa Takahashi (Japan)

National and Regional Delegates:	Mark Soo	(Australia)
	Elizabeth Thompson	(Australia)
	Rajesh Kapur	(India)
	Hayao Shiga	(Japan)
	Shinpei Tada	(Japan)
	Kee Hyun Chang	(Korea)
	Kyu Ho Choi	(Korea)
	Jung-Ho Suh	(Korea)
	Francis Hui	(Singapore)
	Jackson C. T. Lin	(Taiwan)
	Chau-Chin Lee	(Taiwan)
	Nitaya Suwanwela	(Thailand)
	Hon-Shing Lam	(Hong Kong)
	Jian-Ping Dai	(China)

It was decided at the council meeting that the AOSNHNR would join the WFNRS as well as the International Congress of Head and Neck Radiology. The delegate to the WFNRS would be Nitaya Suwanwela of Thailand and the delegate to the ICHNR would be S. Tada of Japan. It was also agreed that in the following years, the meeting would be held every 3 or 4 years in various cities of the Asian and Oceanian countries.

Following the organizational meeting and a brief opening ceremony, with an address by Prof. Takahashi, 9 proffered papers were presented with stimulating discussions. A special lecture, "Spinal Cord Injury: MR Imaging and Evolving Concepts in Treatment" by Dr. R. M. Quencer (USA) was also included in the program.

Following the inaugural meeting, the secretariat lost no time in reaching out and collating the list of national delegates among potential member countries.

Second Congress: Taipei 1997

The second Congress of the AOSNHNR, held in Taipei, Taiwan from March 23 to 27, 1997 under the Presidency of Dr. Tsuen Chang, proved to be a successful meeting which attracted 228 delegates; Secretary General was Michael Mu Huo Teng, and Scientific Committee Chairman was Professor Wan-Yuo Guo. During the Council meeting, important amendments to the Constitution of the Society were also passed. New National Delegates were admitted into the council. They were Benny Huwae, Benjamin D Adapon, Adel Shannan, Umair Rashid Chaudhry and Jehad Al Watban. Dr. Tsuen Chang was elected as President, Prof. Michael Sage as Vice-President and Prof. Michael Teng as Secretary General/Treasurer.

Third Congress: Adelaide 1999

The third AOCNHNR Congress was held in Adelaide, Australia from June 18 to 211,999. At the Council meeting, Prof. Michael Sage was elected President, Prof Kee-Hyun Chang as Vice-President and Prof. Brian Tress as Secretary General/ Treasurer. Prof. Sage, reported that over 70 posters were submitted [5].

Fourth Congress: Seoul 2001

The fourth AOCNHNR Congress took place very soon after the 9–11 tragedy when international air travel was still severely impacted. Nevertheless, the organizing committee led by the chairman, Kee-Hyun Chang bravely soldiered on and worked hard to put together a very fruitful meeting with a detailed scientific program for the

385 attendees from 23 countries [6]. The program featured refresher courses, symposia, special lectures, and 144 scientific paper presentations, with more than 90% of oral presenters using the new computer-linked presentations.

At the Council meeting, Prof. Kee-Hyun Chang was elected as President, Jian-Ping Dai as Vice-President and Prof. Dong Ik Kim as Secretary General/Treasurer.

World Wide Web Presence

In July 2003, the official website of the Society at http://www.aosnhnr.org was set up thanks to the hard work of the Korean Society of Neuroradiology and Head & Neck Radiology to enhance visibility of the organization and promote easy broadcasting of news and future events of interest to all members [1]. It also served to encourage interaction among member countries.

Fifth Congress: Shanghai 2004

The fifth AOCNHNR Congress was held in Shanghai, China; Chairman of the organizational committee, Dr. Xiaoyuan Feng, reported that the number of registrants totaled 337, of which 117 were from overseas and 220 were local. The scientific program consisted of 37 refresher course lectures, 70 oral presentations and 53 scientific poster exhibitions. At the council meeting of the AOSNHNR, Jian-Ping Dai was elected as President, Francis Hui as Vice-President and Xiaoyuan Feng as Secretary General/Treasurer [7].

Sixth Congress: Singapore 2007

The sixth AOCNHNR Congress was held in Singapore from February 2–52,007. Dr. Francis Hui reported that the number of registrants totaled 456, of which 113 were local and 343 were from 29 other countries [8]. The keynote presentation of the Congress was named the Takahashi Lecture, in honor of Mutsumasa Takahashi, the Founding President of the Society. Prof Pierre Lasjaunias was the distinguished speaker for the inaugural Takahashi Lecture and he delivered a stirring oration on the "Anatomy and Development of the Cerebral Venous System." The scientific program included 12 plenary lectures, 39 topical lectures and 13 concurrent symposiums.

At the Council meeting, Francis Hui was elected President, Benny Huwae as Vice-President, Vincent Chong as Secretary General and Tchoyoson Lim as Treasurer. During the meeting, a proposal was made to shorten the name for future congresses to Asian & Oceanian Congress of Neuroradiology (AOCNR).

The management of the official AOSNHNR website was handed over from the Korean society to the Singapore society in March 2008. This was after a long process of passing over the ownership of the website and transfer of data contained in the website and finding a company to manage the website.

In July 2008, the AOSNHNR community was left in shock at the sudden passing of Prof Pierre Lasjaunias of Paris, France. Prof Lasjaunias was a dear friend and a strong supporter of neuroradiology education and research in this region. It was indeed a very great loss for many of us.

Seventh Congress: Bali 2009

The seventh AOCNR was held in Bali, Indonesia from July 9–11, 2009. Benny Huwae, the organizing chairman reported a total number of 620 participants: 180 overseas participants and 440 local participants [9]. The Takahashi Lecture was delivered by Prof Anne Osborn.

At the Council meeting, Benny Huwae was elected President, Nitaya Suwanwela as Vice-President, Sri Andreani Utomo as Secretary General and Cindy Sadikin as Treasurer. There were changes to the list of national representatives: Myanmar and Sri Lanka were welcomed as new members of the society. Their national representatives are Lim Tun and Nirmala Wijesinha, respectively. New national representatives of current member countries included Wong Yiu Chung of Hong Kong; Yukunori Korogi, Kazuhiro Katada and Shinichi Kan of Japan; Woo Suk Choi of Korea; David Perry of New Zealand and Suthisak Suthipongchai and Sirintara Pongpech of Thailand.

Eighth Congress: Bangkok 2012

The eighth AOCNR was originally scheduled to be held in Bangkok, Thailand on October 26–28, 2011 but a serious flood situation forced the event to be postponed to August 1–3, 2013. In spite of the change, Nitaya Suwanwela, the organizing chairman reported a successful meeting with a total number of 498 participants registered. There were 150 overseas participants and 348 local participants. The scientific program included the Takahashi Honorable Lecture and the Pierre Lasjaunias Honorable Lecture. There were 9 symposia, 21 lectures, 8 interactive sessions and 3 luncheon symposia. The social program included a Presidential Dinner cruise on the Chaophrya River. At the Council meeting, Nitaya Suwanwela was elected President, Henry Adapon as Vice-President and Anchalee Churojana as Treasurer.

Ninth Congress: Cebu 2014

The ninth AOCNR was originally planned to be held in Cebu in the autumn of 2013 but the Philippines was hit by a strong earthquake and a supertyphoon, requiring a postponement of the Congress to February 12–14, 2014. At the council meeting, the organizing chairman, Henry Adapon shared the challenges of holding the meeting and showed gratitude to the Council members who helped out with the scientific program. At this meeting, Henry Adapon was elected President, Yukunori Korogi as Vice-President and Anchalee Churojana as Treasurer.

September 16, 2013 was a sad day for the Society when news of the passing of the Society's Founding President, Prof Mutsumasa Tahahashi filtered through the community in Asia and Oceania. Prof Takahashi was a kind figure to all who knew him but at the same time also a giant in teaching and research in Neuroradiology and Head & Neck Radiology. We had indeed lost a dear friend and pioneer.

Tenth Congress: Fukuoka 2015

The tenth AOCNR was held in Fukuoka, Japan from November 5–7, 2015. The organizing chairman, Yukunori Korogi reported on the meeting's success as a genuine regional meeting in Asia and Oceania. There were invited lecturers from the United States and France, namely, Mauricio Castillo, Christophe Cognard and Suresh K. Mukherji. Together with a faculty of 79 Asian lecturers comprising 43 from Japan and 36 from other countries in the Asian Oceanian region. There were 49 oral presentations and 121 poster presentations. A Takahashi Memorial Travel Fund was established for overseas attendants to support their travel fee to the congress. There was also a Fukuoka City Award for both domestic and overseas participants for excellence in the papers presented. The congress attracted 467 participants of which 177 were from overseas and 290 were local [10].

Eleventh Congress: Beijing 2017

The 11th AOCNR was held in Beijing, China from August 18–21, 2017. At the council meeting, the organizing chairman, Lin Ai, detailed that the number of participants registered was 222 from 8 countries/regions. The scientific program included a faculty of 7 international speakers and 35 speakers from the Asian-Oceanian regions. There were 50 special sessions, 9 sponsored seminars,16 oral and 16 poster presentations. Among the items on the agenda was the issue of the AOSNHNR trophy which generated a vigorous exchange of opinions among the member countries.

As the next AOCNR meeting would be very close to the current meeting, it was proposed that the President of the Society will be Lin Ai of China until August 2019 and Sandy Cheng-Yu Chen of Taiwan after that date. Members agreed to the proposal.

Twelfth Congress & XXI Symposium Neuroradiologicum: Taipei 2018

The 12th AOCNR was held in Taipei, Taiwan from March 19–21, 2018 in conjunction with the XXI Symposium Neuroradiologicum: the first 3 days were for the AOCNR and the following 3 days were for the SNR, with some overlapping programs. There were 457 registrants from 54 countries with 110 taking part in the AOCNR only. The faculty included 122 speakers and moderators [11].

Thirteenth Congress: Seoul Online 2021

The 13th AOCNR was scheduled to be held in Seoul, Korea in April 2021, a beautiful time in Korea with spring flowers in bloom for all to wonder at. Unfortunately, 2020 saw the devastating impact of the Covid-19 virus across the world. Humankind was held captive and world travel was paralyzed by a miniscule virus. This presented the organizers with a great problem. By the end of 2020, the infections had not abated and it was clear that an in-person congress would not be able to proceed as originally planned. Cancelling the congress would have repercussions on the future planning of the congresses. Postponing the meeting was also tricky since at that point in time, there was still no indication if or when the infections would be under control. Crucially, no one knew for sure when air travel would return to normal.

It was the second time the Korean organizers had been hampered by severely impacted air travel. But like their previous compatriots, they met the challenges head on and the 2021 organizing committee with Sang Hoon Cha at the helm, worked tirelessly to introduce critical changes to adapt to those adverse conditions. They basically changed the format of the entire Congress to make it possible for participants to join the virtual AOCNR online. Their hard work and indomitable spirit paid off with a successful pioneering online Congress, and set an example for us to follow, especially if there are future pandemics or disasters. Despite being held online, the AOCNR 2021 conference maintained an exceptional level of quantity and quality. A total of 662 participants from 24 countries and regions registered. The scientific program featured 11 international and 31 Asian-Oceanian speakers. The agenda included one Takahashi lecture, four plenary lectures, 19 scientific sessions with 72 lectures, five sponsored symposia with seven lectures, five oral presentation sessions with 44 presentations, and 95 e-poster presentations.

Fourteenth Congress: Singapore 2023

The 14th AOCNR was held in Singapore from August 18–20, 2023. Despite the post-pandemic uncertainties, financial challenges and difficulties, the organizing chairman, Prof Tchoyoson Lim reported great response and support from our region, with over 800 participants (425 overseas), over 200 invited speakers (76 overseas from 21 countries) in diagnostic neuroradiology, interventional neuroradiology and head and neck parallel sessions. Prof. Paul Parizel gave the Takahashi Lecture, Prof. Timo Krings and Dr. Daniel Birchall were Plenary speakers. There were 231 accepted abstracts (21 oral presentations and 210 posters), demonstrating that in-person meetings are still welcomed by our members, and that the social and human connections are very important [12]. At the council meeting, there was an interesting discussion on the payment of membership fees to the AOSNHNR and WFNRS.

The Story of the AOSNHNR Trophy

Made for the second AOSNHNR congress in 1997 by an expert craftsman in Taiwan, the trophy was meant to be a symbol of the society to be prominently displayed at every Congress organized by the Society [13]. Since then, it has also been a tradition for the outgoing President to hand over the trophy to the current Congress chairman as a symbolic transfer of stewardship to the person who will become the next President of the Society.

The trophy is made of two components, the first is a beautiful blue glass sculpture with a map of the Asian Oceanian region which is attached to the second piece, a rectangular wooden base with a front panel inscribed with the sites of the previous Congresses. However, over the years and after several expeditions across Asia and Australia, it began to show signs of structural fatigue. That it was very heavy and very fragile, making it all the more susceptible to the knocks and vibrations inherent in air transportation.

When it was deemed too risky to be transported to the next congress, Dr. Korogi, who was custodian of the trophy at that time, informed the council at the 2017 AOSNHNR council meeting in Beijing. The council discussed what would be the most appropriate replacement for the trophy as the Society's next emblem and suggestions of a medal, chain, trophy and crown were raised. Dr. Korogi found out that the artist of the trophy was still in Taipei and so he brought the trophy over to him to repair. The artist was also able to fabricate a custom-made box for the trophy so that it could be safely transported to the following meetings.

The Future and Challenges Facing Neuroradiology and AOSNHNR

Information Overload: Workload and Manpower Shortages

Since 2021, neurological diseases have become the leading cause of overall disease burden in the world: stroke, neonatal encephalopathy, migraine, dementias, are on the top 10 list of highest age-standardized causes of disability-adjusted life years [14]. Although patient demand and clinical needs are increasing exponentially, the number of qualified diagnostic neuroradiologists is increasing very slowly, resulting in a worldwide shortage of radiologists [15, 16]. With an overwhelming diagnostic and therapeutic workload, risks of diagnostic errors, radiologist burnout and patient safety become particularly acute, and international collaborative efforts to address them are becoming necessary [17, 18]. Post-graduate radiological education (and possibly subspecialty neuroradiology accreditation) will increase in importance; senior leaders will need to engage the next-generation of Residents and Medical Students to attract them to practice Neuroradiology.

Artificial Intelligence and Technical Advances

Modern neuroimaging technologies generate vast quantities of data: the challenge is how to present, visualize and consume the data, how to integrate this information into the patient's record, and communicate to other healthcare workers in a way that neuroradiologists are not overwhelmed [19]. Artificial intelligence has been advocated as a panacea for all problems, but despite the change in perception from AI as a threat to AI as a desired assistant, neuroradiology has not yet successfully incorporated it at scale into daily clinical use, let alone into our academic teaching and research missions [20]. These challenges are particularly urgent in light of above-mentioned workload and manpower problems facing us, and neuroradiologists should think about big-picture financial life cycles and systems engineering, in order to understand and work with hospital leadership and government funders. Other, non-AI technological advances in ultralow field MRI, PET and non-traditional imaging sources also have the potential to disrupt and improve our mission to provide safer, faster and more accessible patient care.

Challenges in the Asian-Oceanian Context

Diversity in Local Disease Patterns and Healthcare Systems

Asian patients exhibit a higher prevalence of intracranial atherosclerosis and intracranial hemorrhage, necessitating a tailored approach to acute endovascular stroke interventions [21]. The diversity in socioeconomic conditions and demographics results in healthcare system variations: the political, financial landscape and healthcare systems vary significantly across Asian countries, presenting challenges in standardizing stroke care and other neuroradiological practices. Furthermore, ageing societies (first in Japan, Singapore, Korea, then China and others), political instability and underinvestment in healthcare in several South-East Asian nations such as Myanmar have resulted in significant setbacks in the past decades; Central and West Asian nations are not well-represented in our Society, and more can be done to engage nascent neuroradiology groups in these regions. Nevertheless, the diverse and varied health systems can be a strength, and intra-regional collaborative learning and exchange of ideas has great potential for the future.

Financial Viability and Secretariat

Although rapid economic growth, improving healthcare infrastructure investment and access to modern imaging technologies have in the past decades provided neuroradiologists with the tools they need for accurate diagnosis and treatment, more can be done to improve our patients' lives. Through the untiring efforts of Secretary/Treasurer Prof Kei Yamada, the AOSNHNR has established a professional Secretariat based in Japan that interfaces with National Delegates, engages with other Societies, and also maintains our website. It is an important but uncompleted task to improve the processes and communications within the AOSNHNR to ensure its long-term financial and professional viability.

Working Together

In spite of the challenges we face, there are opportunities for standardizing best practices across different countries to ensure consistent and high-quality patient care [20]. Regular AOCNR Congresses are necessary conditions to promote and connect neuroradiologists and groups, but we can do more to promote neuroradiology and assure the diffusion of knowledge throughout Asia and Oceania. We can enhance training programs and continuing education opportunities within Asia and Oceania to support training and attachment: to this end, regional diploma certification may be an idea whose time has come. AOSNHNR can also promote research and collaboration, particularly in diseases such as nasopharyngeal cancer and intracranial atherosclerosis to address region-specific challenges.

Multidisciplinary interaction has always been a strength of neuroradiology: we have worked well with neurology, neuropathology, neurosurgery, neuro-oncology, and psychiatry to develop new paradigms and tools to integrate complex information (from molecular data to behaviors) into health systems, via caring for individual patients. Working within Asia-Oceania and with our colleagues in the American and European Societies of Neuroradiology and the WFNRS, we can go from strength to strength, and look forward to the future.

Acknowledgments The authors thank Professors Sang Hoon Cha, Kei Yamada, Wan-Yuo Guo, Michael Mu Huo Teng, Sandy Chen and Umair Chaudhry for their photographs and suggestions.

References

1. Asian-Oceanian Society of Neuroradiology and Head & Neck Radiology Aims [Internet]. [cited 2024 May]. Available from https://www.aosnhnr.org/whats_about.html.
2. Harwood-Nash DC. The World Federation of Neuroradiological Societies: a proposal. AJNR Am J Neuroradiol. 1991;12(5):845–7.
3. Asian-Oceanian Society of Neuroradiology and Head & Neck Radiology Founding [Internet]. [cited 2024 May]. Available from https://www.aosnhnr.org/about.html.
4. Asian-Oceanian Society of Neuroradiology and Head & Neck Radiology 1st Kumamoto Congress [Internet]. 1994 [cited 2024 May]. Available from https://www.aosnhnr.org/pdf/1stAOCNHNR_1994.pdf.
5. Asian-Oceanian Society of Neuroradiology and Head & Neck Radiology 3rd Adelaide Congress [Internet]. 1999 [cited 2024 May]. Available from https://www.aosnhnr.org/pdf/3rdAOCNHNR_1999.pdf.
6. Kim JH, Chang KH. The fourth Asian-Oceanian Congress of Neuroradiology and Head & Neck Radiology. AJNR Am J Neuroradiol. 2002;23(3):499.
7. Asian-Oceanian Society of Neuroradiology and Head & Neck Radiology 5th Shanghai Congress [Internet]. 2004 [cited 2024 May]. Available from https://www.aosnhnr.org/pdf/5thAOCNHNR_2004.pdf.
8. Asian-Oceanian Society of Neuroradiology and Head & Neck Radiology 6th Singapore Congress [Internet]. 2007 [cited 2024 May]. Available from https://www.aosnhnr.org/pdf/6thAOCNHNR_2007.pdf.
9. Asian-Oceanian Society of Neuroradiology and Head & Neck Radiology 7th Bali Congress[Internet]. 2009 [cited 2024 May]. Available from https://www.aosnhnr.org/pdf/7thAOCNHNR_2009.pdf.
10. Asian-Oceanian Society of Neuroradiology and Head & Neck Radiology 10th Fukuoka Congress [Internet]. 2015 [cited 2024 May]. Available from https://www.aosnhnr.org/pdf/10thAOCNHNR_2015.pdf.
11. Asian-Oceanian Society of Neuroradiology and Head & Neck Radiology 12th Taipei Congress [Internet]. 2018 [cited 2024 May]. Available from https://www.aosnhnr.org/pdf/12thAOCNHNR_2018.pdf.
12. Asian-Oceanian Society of Neuroradiology and Head & Neck Radiology 14th Singapore Congress [Internet]. 2023 [cited 2024 May]. Available from https://www.aosnhnr.org/pdf/AOCNR-Programme-list-Aug-2023.pdf.
13. Asian-Oceanian Society of Neuroradiology and Head & Neck Radiology Trophy [Internet]. [cited 2024 May]. Available from https://www.aosnhnr.org/about-history.html.

14. GBD 2021 Nervous System Disorders Collaborators. Global, regional, and national burden of disorders affecting the nervous system, 1990–2021: a systematic analysis for the Global Burden of Disease Study 2021 [published correction appears in Lancet Neurol. 2024;23(5):e9]. Lancet Neurol. 2024;23(4):344–81. https://doi.org/10.1016/S1474-4422(24)00038-3.
15. Yamada K. What has caused the shortage of radiologists? Features exclusive to Japan. Korean J Radiol. 2023;24(10):933–5. https://doi.org/10.3348/kjr.2023.0815.
16. Meng F, Zhan L, Liu S, Zhang H. The growing problem of radiologist shortage: China's perspective. Korean J Radiol. 2023;24(11):1046–8. https://doi.org/10.3348/kjr.2023.0839.
17. Nakajima Y, Yamada K, Imamura K, Kobayashi K. Radiologist supply and workload: international comparison—working group of Japanese College of Radiology. Radiat Med. 2008;26(8):455–65. https://doi.org/10.1007/s11604-008-0259-2.
18. Wintermark M, Gupta V, Hess C, et al. Realistic productivity in academic neuroradiology: a national survey of neuroradiology division chiefs. AJNR Am J Neuroradiol. 2023;44(7):759–61. https://doi.org/10.3174/ajnr.A7912.
19. Lui YW, Chang PD, Zaharchuk G, et al. Artificial intelligence in neuroradiology: current status and future directions. AJNR Am J Neuroradiol. 2020;41(8):E52–9. https://doi.org/10.3174/ajnr.A6681.
20. Wintermark M, Yamada K, Lim T, Riascos R, Torres C, Yousry T. Striking a balance: global perspectives on neuroradiology workload and quality of service. AJNR Am J Neuroradiol. 2024;45(2):127. https://doi.org/10.3174/ajnr.A8125.
21. Ng JC, Churojana A, Pongpech S, et al. Current state of acute stroke care in southeast Asian countries. Interv Neuroradiol. 2019;25(3):291–6. https://doi.org/10.1177/1591019918811804.

Chapter 4
Australian and New Zealand Society of Neuroradiology (ANZSNR) 1990 to Present Day

Makhan S. Khangure

Introduction

In the 1980s, diagnostic neuroradiology was practised mainly by general radiologists with an interest in neuroradiology. There were only a few trained dedicated neuroradiologists. Cerebral angiography, myelography, discography, and pneumoencephalography were the predominant invasive procedures. Computed Tomography was the non-invasive tool, whilst Doppler ultrasound was the mainstay of evaluation of the cervical neck vessels.

Interventional procedures for head and neck tumours and vascular malformations were performed at Royal Perth Hospital (RPH) in Perth, Royal North Shore Hospital and Royal Prince Alfred Hospital in Sydney, and Royal Melbourne and Monash Hospitals in Melbourne. The first intracranial intervention was performed by Drs H T ApSimon and M S Khangure at RPH in 1979, a successful occlusion of a traumatic carotico-cavernous fistula using the Debrun detachable balloon system. Further developments in this field subsequently followed a few years later at RPH.

With the installations of MRI scanners in Australia and New Zealand in the late 1980s the need for trained dedicated neuroradiologists rapidly became apparent. Many newly qualified radiologists commenced fellowship training in neuroimaging and later in Interventional Neuroradiology. The impetus to form a Society of Neuroradiology was self-evident. The Royal Australian and New Zealand College of Radiology (RANZCR) and ANZSNR have worked closely with a shared vision

M. S. Khangure (✉)
Department of Diagnostic and Interventional Radiology, Royal Perth Hospital, Perth, WA, Australia

University of Western Australia, Perth, WA, Australia

D. Birchall (ed.), *A World History of Neuroradiology*,
https://doi.org/10.1007/978-3-032-16653-1_4

of the need for an appropriate level of training and for its fellows to provide expert patient care. Prior to the formation of ANZSNR several INR courses were organised by the RANZCR. Many INR presentations were part of the RANZCR annual scientific meetings and many presentations were also made at the Interventional Radiology Society of Australasia (IRSA) meetings.

The Beginning

The inaugural meeting to establish the Society was held in Queensland in October 1992 and attended by approximately 30 Fellows and Education Affiliates of RANZCR. The meeting was chaired by Prof. Michael Sage who was subsequently elected as the founding President. Guidelines were established and agreed unanimously. The first Annual General Meeting (AGM) of the Society was held in Sydney in October 1993. It was agreed that the Society letterhead would indicate that the Society incorporated neuroradiology, INR, and head and neck/ENT radiology. A proposed constitution was endorsed. Membership was initially open to all Fellows and Education Affiliates with a nominal membership fee. At that time, only a handful of RANZCR Fellows were trained as dedicated neuroradiologists. Prof. Sage was generous in offering the services of his secretaries (Helen Sainsbury and Sue Edwards) to administer the affairs of the Society which they diligently carried out from 1992 to 2011.

The first Committee of ANZSNR was elected at the second AGM to serve for a period of 3 years from January 1 and consisted of: President; Secretary/Treasurer; Representatives of the State Branches: New South Wales, Victoria, Queensland, Western Australia, South Australia, New Zealand, and Tasmania; and Representatives from the following: RANZCR, MRI, Interventional Radiology, World Federation of Neuroradiological Societies (WFNRS), and the Academic Convenors for the next 3 years. Prof. Sage asked the members to design a logo for the Society.

The second Committee consisted of: President, Immediate-Past President, Secretary-General, Councillors (one from each state and NZ), and the following Representatives: RANZCA, IRSA, WFITN, World Federation of Head & Neck Radiology (WFHNR), Asian Oceanic Society of Neuroradiology & Head & Neck Radiology (AOSNHNR).

The third Committee was elected to occupy office from January 2000 and its tenure was to expire on 30 June 2003. This adjustment was required to align the financial report with the national taxation requirements. All committees after 2003 were elected to office from July 1 to June 30.

The composition of the subsequent committees remains similar but include representatives of The American Society of Neuroradiology (ASNR) and The European Society of Neuroradiology (ESNR). The Society members and representatives for the organisations listed above informed the Society regarding developments and other issues of common interest. WFITN representatives had a seat at the WFITN council in its earlier years. At the 2023 AGM, it was ratified that the composition of council officially included a Head & Neck/ENT representative and a Paediatric Neuroradiology representative.

All office bearers are eligible for re-election for a second 3-year term. Most have exercised this option and have been re-elected.

The first ASM of the Society, convened by Prof. Brian Tress, was held in Melbourne in April 1994 and was attended by 56 delegates with both luminary international speakers and local faculty. Since the first meeting, the Society has held an AGM and ASM (some combined with international meetings), other than in 2021 when there were no meetings due to COVID.

At the second International Conference in Magnetic Resonance Imaging 5–9 April 1995, held in Melbourne, the neurological section of the MRI meeting, with input from Prof. Tress and Dr. William Sorbey, was identified with ANZSNR, in effect the second ASM of the Society.

The third ASM, under the banner of ANZSNR, and with Prof. Sage as convenor, was held at the Adelaide Convention Centre South Australia and attended by 267 delegates. This was in fact a conference on radiologic-pathologic correlation. An excellent scientific programme was organised providing an overview of neuropathology as relevant to imaging. Prof. Anne Osborn was supported by six leading Australian Pathologists and Society members.

It was decided that most future Society ASMs would be small gatherings to foster local members to present their research, imaging, and INR experience. This philosophy was adopted and has paid dividends in developing local expertise, in-depth knowledge, and clinical/scientific presentations.

The ASM is held in a different state each year, convened by local members of the Society. A family friendly venue is always chosen. The learning is supplemented by social gathering including a gala dinner. The ASM has expanded in both scope and content each time, from an initial one-and-half days' meeting with no parallel sessions to a two-and-half days' meeting with parallel sessions, covering neurointervention and neuro imaging, including spine and head and neck, with some joint plenary sessions. An international and very able local faculty present an outstanding learning experience for both "the experts" and the trainees. The attendance at the last few meetings is a marker of the quality and friendly nature of the meetings. In 2020, there were 163 delegates. In 2022, the attendance was 123 in person with 48 virtual attendees. In 2023, there were 170 delegates. Trainee participation in oral and poster presentations are of a high quality and improve with each ASM. Industry support has been greatly appreciated and each year there are many "hands on" interactive displays for participation by the delegates.

Cerebral angiography via femoral artery catheterisation was well established in the 1980s. External carotid artery territory vascular malformation, fistulae, and tumours were being embolised at several centres as was the treatment of CC fistulae using the Debrun detachable balloon system. In 1982, Dr. Trevor ApSimon assembled a dedicated team of radiographers, nurses, and with Dr. Mark Khangure established the first INR team in Australia/New Zealand. The team performed its first cyanoacrylate (super glue) brain AVM embolisation, using the Kerber calibrated leak balloon microcatheter in 1983. In the following years, Mr. David Hartley, senior radiographer and member of the team, engineered "in house" latex micro balloons and valve sealing detachable balloons, removing the need to tie the balloons to the catheter. The latter were subsequently commercially manufactured by Cook Australia. Detachable balloons filled only with iodine-based contrast were unstable as the contrast either leaked or leeched out of the balloon. Prof. Khangure developed a formulation of iodine-based contrast and soluble monomer 2-Hydroxyethyl Methacrylate (HEMA) with added ferrous ammonium sulphate as the "contrast" to opacify and position the balloon. Addition of hydrogen peroxide to the solution polymerised the HEMA to a solid insoluble polymer over about 2 min, allowing minor repositioning of the balloon. This overcame the issue of balloon deflation. The team also developed safer ways of delivering superglue to a specific location using additional nondetachable balloon catheters to arrest flow, divert flow, and protect a major vessel with collateral connections to a vessel being embolised. These techniques were also adopted at other centres, predominantly for dural vascular malformation and fistulae.

Post 1990

In 1991, the Federal Department of Health Australia (DOHA) recognised Royal Perth Hospital as a Centre of Excellence and funded the INR unit to treat interstate patients and train others to provide INR service in all states. Joint Centre of Excellence status was granted to Royal North Shore Hospital and Royal Prince Alfred Hospitals in Sydney with a single team of neuroradiologists. By the time of Dr. ApSimon's retirement in 1995, upwards of 200 brain, spine, and dural vascular malformations were treated with superglue including the first vein of Galen malformation in a neonate in 1994. The first aneurysm to be treated by the Gugliemi detachable coil (GDC) was in 1994.

The RPH unit participated in the International Subarachnoid Haemorrhage Trial (ISAT) as the only centre from Australasia. RPH was the first centre to commence a fellowship programme, initially for INR and in later years for diagnostic neuroradiology and INR. (Prof. Tress established a fellowship programme soon after at Royal Melbourne Hospital). Workshops were held at RPH to demonstrate and teach interstate neuroradiologists the scope of INR. By the time the findings of ISAT were made available, in October 2002, INR teams were operating at multiple centres. All had at least one fellowship trained operator and all were well skilled and competent. Many fellows acquired their training and skills in the USA, Canada, and quite a few in Perth and some in the UK. Carotid artery angioplasty and stenting was being performed at many centres in patients with an elevated risk for surgical intervention.

Training

The RANZCR registrar training programme runs over 5 years, covering all aspects of radiology. In the final year, the registrars can request to devote at least 6 months in a given subspeciality. For diagnostic neuroradiology, this provides a good foundation. In 1996, a subcommittee of the Society was established, chaired by Prof. Khangure to consider the training requirements for neuroradiology, in particular INR. The committee considered a minimum of a year (preferably 2 years) of dedicated fellowship, after the final year of training, and at an appropriate centre, was desirable for diagnostic neuroradiology. For INR, a minimum of 2 years at a centre providing a comprehensive INR service was deemed appropriate. The fellows were to document their training. The recommendations of the committees were endorsed at the 1998 AGM.

Advancements in CTA, MRA, and Doppler ultrasound reduced the need for catheter angiography to very few clinical indications. The Society was concerned regarding maintenance of skills by radiologists who would only perform the procedure a few times a year. Prof. M Khangure and Dr. W Chong, serving as RANZCR councillors, raised their concerns regarding this issue and the potential for patient harm. At Council meetings, they were tasked with obtaining a broad opinion from all stakeholders the minimum numbers of cerebral angiographic studies that a RANZCR fellow required over a 2-year period to maintain adequate skills. The number suggested, after much debate by the Society and RANZCR Council, was 20! Following the publication of ISAT, in the early 2000s, there was subspecialisation of neurosurgery; centralisation with smaller numbers of vascular neurosurgeons and a smaller number of vascular neurosurgical units, in order for practitioners to maintain skills. This, coupled with INR units, removed the need for catheter angiography outside these centres, further improving patient safety.

From 2000 onwards to 2007, Prof Khangure organised a half-day meeting before the ASM of the Society for INR members as mortality and morbidity (M&M) coupled with "difficult cases discussion" as a learning experience for all. This session was well attended and continues to the present time.

From 2009 onwards (15thmeeting in August 2024), Dr. Jason Wenderoth (NSW) and Dr. Hal Rice (now Assoc. Prof. Qld) organised an annual meeting, named Neuro Exchange, for the expanding INR group over one and half days, discussing difficult cases, M&M, new and evolving technologies, and often with industry experts on site and presenting. These meetings, like the ANZSNR ASMs, were and are held in different states in Australia and in New Zealand.

By 2010, INR units were performing mechanical thrombectomy for acute stroke. The need to again expand the INR workforce was urgent. In addition to ANZSNR members taking on this additional work and increases in fellowship training positions, locally and overseas, other craft groups were attracted. Prof. Alan Coulthard, along with Prof. Khangure and Dr. Wenderoth as ANZSNR members, invited representatives of the Neurosurgical Society of Australasia (NSA) and Australia and New Zealand Association of Neurologists (ANZAN) to a joint meeting, convened at the

RANZCR premises, to discuss national training standards in INR. After a number of meetings held over several months, chaired by a member of each group, agreement was reached as to the required training and a "Conjoint Committee for Recognition of Training in INR(CCINR) was established." Those already in INR practice with a proven record were grandfathered, and those in training were to produce the documents supporting their training. This was a great achievement in providing patient safety; all practitioners requiring certification of INR by this tripartite committee. Many health institutions in Australia quickly adopted the CCINR certification as a credentialing requirement for INR practice. The role of CCINR was further endorsed under Prof. Mitchell as president with requirement that practitioners be CCINR certified to provide mechanical thrombectomy on the Medical Benefits Schedule.

Several Society members have been part of the local faculty at many RANZCR ASMs delivering both diagnostic and INR presentations. Several members have organised didactic neuro imaging courses outside of the Society's ASM on a broad range of topics, ranging from anatomy, pathology, routine clinical imaging to more challenging MRI techniques. These have been well attended by both trainees and consultants. Several members have presented and have been on the faculty of Asian and Oceanic conferences, including AOSNHNR, JSNR, and KSNR.

Society Presidents

There have been six previous presidents and a seventh incumbent. They are:

Prof. Michael Sage, Prof. Brian Tress (3-year term each), Prof. Makhan (Mark) Khangure, Dr. Winston Chong (now Professor), Prof. Alan Coulthard (two 3-year terms each), and Dr. Peter Mitchell (now Assoc. Professor). The incumbent Dr. Constantine (Con) Phatouros is serving his successive second 3-year term. The first three presidents are recipients of the Gold Medal of the Society presented to all 3 at the 2019 ASM in Adelaide. Prof. Coulthard will be presented the Gold Medal at the 2025 ASM.

All presidents and their elected councils have incrementally advanced the standing of the Society. They have advocated for patient safety and well-being, which includes developing and mandating the minimum training standards for neuroradiology. They have worked tirelessly with RANZCR councils and boards to lobby governments for funding (Profs. Sage and Khangure were RANZCR presidents and Profs. Coulthard and Chong long-term councillors of RANZCR and ANZSNR). Prof. Khangure was an Australian Medical Association (AMA) councillor for 10 years, enlisting the help of the AMA to engage with the Federal Department of Health in pursuit of the recognition of the importance of radiology and INR in patient management. They have worked with and collaboratively negotiated with other stakeholders on issues relating to scope of practice. The expansion of the ASMs, content and duration are self-evident of the improvement, as is the expansion of the membership numbers. The Society's financial position has also improved from the larger number of delegates and industry sponsorship. The annual subscription for membership was maintained according to the national consumer price index (CPI) and ASM registration kept as low as possible. In the early years, there was an annual newsletter sent out with the Society's agenda papers. This was increased to two newsletters. Currently there are quarterly newsletters which follow each meeting of council. The importance of collegial contact and friendship with other neuroradiology societies in North America, Europe, and the Asia-Pacific region was recognised and is a primary goal of the Society. Many international invited speakers to the society ASMs became long-lasting friends.

In 2010, the Society provided a grant of $25,000 to Prof. Coulthard for a pilot project in establishing a "Collaborative Research Network" using the ANZSNR framework to improve neurological practice and research throughout Australasia. Prof. Coulthard also took on the task of developing a web page for the society, maintaining and improving it.

The Society's constitution was updated twice in the early years. Prof. Peter Mitchell, as President, commenced an in-house review of the constitution and the committee's proposals, including guidelines for awarding the Gold Medal. These were approved at the 2018 AGM. The current council, under the leadership of Dr. Phatouros, has reviewed and revised the constitution further with a legal expert review to align it with contemporary requirements. Dr. Phatouros, with input from several Society members, working with RANZCR, has led an ANZSNR delegation over 2 years, in collaboration with IRSA and RANZCR, to advocate for the recognition of INR as a speciality within radiology. RANZCR has lodged the submission with the Australian Medical Council (AMC) for Interventional Neuroradiology and Interventional Radiology to be recognised as specialities. This recognition will provide significant patient benefit and enable Radiology trainees to undergo subspecialisation into INR or IR at an earlier stage of training.

The secretarial support to the Society, provided by Prof. Sage, ended in 2011. Dr. Mitchell, as incumbent secretary-general, assumed this task for a short period before RANZCR agreed to provide some part time secretarial support. With an increasing complexity in the Society's activities, including managing the video-recorded ASM, the need for full-time administration support became urgent. RANZCR was unable to provide this. Dr. Phatouros, as current president, sought and appointed an excellent full-time administration support group for the society in November 2019, wholly under the management of ANZSNR executive and fully funded by the Society.

In 1999, the third AOCNHNR was convened in Adelaide under the auspices of the ANZSNR with Prof. Sage as convenor. The format was similar to the very successful CME meeting held at the same venue. There were 350 delegates.

Prof. Tress requested the Society to support the nomination of Prof. Sage to the Symposium Neuroradiologicum Nominating Committee to organise the Symposium in 2006 under the auspices of ANZSNR. This nomination was fully supported and was successful. The Society provided the seed money for the very successful Symposium held in Adelaide in March. There were 743 delegates from all around the world.

A joint ninth AAFITN/ 19th ANZSNR meeting, convened by Drs Chong and Trost, was held in Melbourne in April 2010, attended by 620 delegates. There were more than 40 invited speakers for both meetings from 15 neighbouring countries in the Asia-Pacific region. This was the first time these two societies had jointly participated in a meeting in Australasia. Dr. Chong was appointed president of AAFITN in 2012.

A large group of Australasian Interventional Neuroradiologists attended the 2011 WFITN meeting in Cape Town, South Africa. Drs Hal Rice and Laetitia de Villiers presented a bid to host the 2015 meeting under the auspices of ANZSNR at the Gold Coast, Queensland. They were supported by Dr. Chong as current ANZSNR President and Prof. Khangure as ex-President. Despite presentations from other nations, the delegates voted for the Gold Coast, Australia as the next venue. Dr. Chong was nominated as the meeting President by the WFITN executive with Prof. Khangure as Honorary President. Prof. Coulthard as the ANZSNR President in 2015 hosted the meeting. A highly successful meeting was held in November, attended by 1200 delegates from all parts of the world who enjoyed the scientific programme and an excellent social programme.

Current Status

There are 215 ANZSNR members, including student members. There are 164 fully trained neuroradiologists and 46 in-training members.

There are eight diagnostic neuro fellows and eight INR fellows in Australian departments and one diagnostic and an INR fellow in Auckland.

There are academic neuro radiology positions in Victoria, Queensland, and Western Australia, including Professor Paul Parizel in Western Australia and Professor Meng Law in Victoria. Both are widely recognised in the international community for their research and teaching. National active researchers include Prof. Trish Desmond, Assoc. Prof. Sandeep Bhuta, Prof. Peter Mitchell, Prof. Alan Coulthard, and many other members with clinical publications in INR (collaborative material) and diagnostic neuroradiology. Prof. Mitchell has been very active in the field of stroke research and the first to perform in human brain-computer interface implantation. Dr. Geoff Parker (NSW) has made important contributions in intracranial venous stenting.

Publications

An extensive literature search for peer-reviewed publications, (Endnote Library Compression File) for named society members yielded 1073 entries for the period 1990 to 2024. Over 30 publications a year from a small society membership is pleasing.

The Society established a Research Committee in 2021 and has awarded its first research grant to a fellow in 2023 investigating the role of diffusion tensor imaging in assessment of cervical nerve roots in patients with cervical radiculopathy. Several applications for research grants in 2024 are currently in progress.

In 2021, the society was successfully registered with the Australian Charities and Not-for-profits Commission, allowing it to receive charitable donations.

Current Objectives of the Society as per the 2024 Constitution

1. To advance, promote, and develop education and training in neuroradiology
2. To advance, promote, and develop standards for the practice of neuroradiology
3. To advance, promote, and support research in neuroradiology
4. To be the reference body for training and practice in diagnostic neuroradiology, interventional neuroradiology, and head and neck radiology in Australia and New Zealand
5. To promote fellowship and the exchange of ideas among neuroradiologists
6. To provide a forum for the presentation of papers and the dissemination of knowledge in relation to diagnostic neuroradiology, interventional neuroradiology, and head and neck radiology
7. To promote close cooperation between neuroradiology and other branches of medicine and the allied sciences
8. To promote close association with other neuroradiological groups such as ESNR, ASNR, WFITN, AOSNHNR and WFNRS
9. To cultivate and maintain the highest principles of practice and ethics in respect of diagnostic neuroradiology, interventional neuroradiology, and head and neck radiology
10. To establish, administer, and contribute to any charitable or benevolent fund in connection with or for the benefit of deserving persons engaged in the pursuit or practice of diagnostic neuroradiology, interventional neuroradiology, and head and neck radiology
11. To confer, co-operate, or correspond with any association, societies, bodies, or individuals, whether incorporated or not, in relation to any of the objects of the Association, or on any other matter of interest to the Association or its members

Conclusion

The ANZSNR has performed a vital role in the development of the field of neuroradiology in Australia and New Zealand over the past four decades. It has fostered the subspecialisation of radiologists into the subspeciality areas of diagnostic neuroradiology, interventional neuroradiology, head & neck/ENT radiology, and spine radiology. It has provided an indispensable forum for national alliance and education. This has further extended across international borders to symbiotic affiliations with international societies. The society has promoted and advanced research and teaching and functioned as an advocate to government and health institutions in advancing the practice of neuroradiology and maintaining high clinical and professional standards that serve the patient interest. All members of the council and executive have performed their duties in an honorary capacity without remuneration, motivated primarily by the betterment of the profession. It is anticipated the Society will flourish well into the future assisting our venerable subspeciality adapt to an ever-changing clinical landscape whilst promoting collaboration, collegiality, and clinical excellence.

Acknowledgments I gratefully acknowledge Dr. Constantine (Con) Phatouros for his contribution to this chapter.

Chapter 5
Austrian Society of Neuroradiology (Österreichische Gesellschaft für Neuroradiologie—ÖGNR)

Elke R. Gizewski, Hannes Deutschmann, Gregor Kasprian, Julia Furtner, Michael Sonnberger, and Johannes Trenkler

Introduction

Strictly speaking, Neuroradiology started in the Austria of Emperor Franz Joseph with the work of Arthur Schüller. The radiologist Arthur Schüller received his doctorate and habilitation at the Faculty of Medicine of the University of Vienna with the habilitation thesis: "X-ray diagnostics of diseases of the head" [1]. Schüller coined the term "Neuro-Röntgenologie" for the first time [2] and is now regarded internationally as the "Father of Neuroradiology" [2].

E. R. Gizewski (✉)
Department of Radiology, Neuroimage Core Facility, Medical University Innsbruck, Innsbruck, Austria
e-mail: elke.gizewski@i-med.ac.at

H. Deutschmann
Division of Neuroradiology, Vascular and Interventional Radiology, Department of Radiology, Medical University of Graz, Graz, Austria
e-mail: hannes.deutschmann@medunigraz.at

G. Kasprian
Department of Biomedical Imaging and Image-Guided Therapy, Medical University of Vienna, Vienna, Austria
e-mail: gregor.kasprian@meduniwien.ac.at

J. Furtner
Research Center for Medical Image Analysis and Artificial Intelligence, Danube Private University, Krems an der Donau, Austria
e-mail: Julia.furtner@dp-uni.ac.at

M. Sonnberger · J. Trenkler
Institute of Neuroradiology, Neuromed Campus, Kepler University Hospital Linz, Linz, Austria
e-mail: michael.sonnberger@kepleruniklinikum.at; johannes@trenkler.at

D. Birchall (ed.), *A World History of Neuroradiology*,
https://doi.org/10.1007/978-3-032-16653-1_5

In today's Austria after 1945, neuroradiological examinations have been carried out by neurosurgeons, neurologists and less so by radiologists. First tendencies toward an independent neuroradiology started in major neurological-neurosurgical hospitals by departments in Linz (Benno Hammer) and Salzburg (Hermann Mösl) since 1969.

An important step was the foundation of a computed tomography (CT) study group within the scope of the Austrian Society of Radiology by B. Hammer in 1978. In the mid-1980s, magnetic resonance imaging (MRI) was included as well.

Jean-Paul Braun (at that time president of the European Society of Neuroradiology; ESNR) initiated at the Symposium Neuroradiologicum 1986 in Stockholm a round table of neuroradiologists from Switzerland and Austria, resulting in organizing joint-meetings of Swiss and Austrian neuroradiologists that took place in Salzburg, Zurich and Udine 1986/87.

The Austrian Society of Neuroradiology (ÖGNR) was founded on May 5th, 1990.

Essential steps were the establishment of Neuroradiological divisions in the General Hospital of Vienna/Medical University of Vienna in 1991, in the University Hospital of Graz in 2003, University Hospital of Innsbruck in 2007 and the University Hospitals of Tulln and St. Pölten since 2014. With the foundation of University Hospitals in Linz and Salzburg, independent Institutes of Neuroradiology were established (2016 and 2019, respectively).

There are ongoing efforts to establish a subspecialty in Neuroradiology, which is supported by the Austrian Society of Radiology.

Organization

The ÖGNR is a non-profit scientific association aiming to promote diagnostic and interventional neuroradiology in clinical practice, teaching and research in collaboration with radiology, neurosurgery, neurology, psychiatry, otorhinolaryngology, cranio-maxillofacial surgery, orthopedics, ophthalmology and pediatrics as well as in collaboration with neurosciences. The society also intends a close collaboration with the ESNR and with neuroradiological societies of countries surrounding Austria.

The executive committee with the leading president is responsible for the management of the society (Table 5.1). It consists of the president, the vice-president, the past president, the secretary and the treasurer. It is also possible to co-opt

Table 5.1 List of presidents of the Austrian Society of Neuroradiology

Presidents of the Austrian Society of Neuroradiology	
1990–2000	Erwin Schindler
2000–2002	Mario Grobovschek
2002–2008	Erich Klein
2008–2016	Johannes Trenkler
2016–2020	Hannes Deutschmann
2020–2024	Elke Gizewski

Table 5.2 List of honorary members of the Austrian Society of Neuroradiology

Honorary members of the Austrian Society of Neuroradiology		
	Names	City, Country
	Prof. Dr. Jean Paul Braun†	Colmar, France
	Prof. Dr. Benno Hammer†	Linz, Austria
	Prim. Dr. Hermann Mösl†	Salzburg, Austria
	Prof. Dr. Peter Huber†	Bern, Switzerland
	Dr. Hildegard Böhm-Jurkovic	Linz, Austria
	Prof. Dr. Pierre Rabischong	Montpellier, France
2008	Prof. Dr. Erich Klein	Graz, Austria
2013	Prof. Dr. Gerhard Schroth	Bern, Switzerland
2018	Prof. Dr. Georges Rodesch	Paris, France
2019	PD Dr. Mark McCoy	Salzburg, Austria
2019	Dr. Johannes Trenkler	Linz, Austria
2021	Prof. Dr. Anton Valavanis†	Zürich, Switzerland
2022	Prof. Dr. Daniela Prayer	Wien, Austria

† has died

members in the executive committee, typical functionaries to the interest of the society (e.g., national delegates of the ESNR, World Federation of Neuroradiological Societies (WFNRS), etc.). Within recent years, the structure was further developed in order to account for recent developments in digitalization and in regard to promote young radiologists. Therefore, a co-opted member for Internet and web-based teaching was established as well as a group of young neuroradiologists.

The function period of the ÖGNR executive committee lasts 4 years. The membership is structured in full members, associate members and honorary members (Table 5.2). The general assembly is to be held once a year.

The Austrian Society of Neuroradiology holds institutional memberships to the ESNR and to the WFNRS and is part of Clinical Neuroradiology as associated Journal of ÖGNR, German Society of Neuroradiology (DGNR) and Swiss Society of Neuroradiology (SGNR).

The society currently has 120 members (2024).

Annual Meetings

One of the main activities of the society is the organization of annual meetings (Table 5.3).

The founding conference on the occasion of an honorary symposium for Prof. Hammer (25 Years of Neuroradiology in Upper Austria) took place in May 1990 in Linz, the first annual meeting was held in May 1991 in Vienna.

From the beginning, the ÖGNR was a society with high interest in networking across the borders. In 1994, the annual meeting was held jointly with the Hungarian Society of Neuroradiology in Balatonfüred, Hungary.

Table 5.3 List of annual meetings of the Austrian Society of Neuroradiology

Annual meetings of the Austrian Society for Neuroradiology				
Date of Meeting Start	Date of meeting end	Name of Meeting	Location	Congress President
05.05.1990		Founding conference on the occasion of an honorary symposium for Prof. Hammer (25 Years of Neuroradiology in Upper Austria)	Linz	Jurkovic
25.05.1991		1st Annual Meeting	Vienna	Schindler
23.05.1992		2nd Annual Meeting	Graz	Ebner
15.05.1993		3rd Annual Meeting	Salzburg	Grobovschek
26.05.1994	28.05.1994	4th Annual Meeting together with the 5th Annual Meeting of the Hungarian Society of Neuroradiology	Balatonfüred, HU	Schindler/ Miklos
07.09.1995	09.09.1997	30th Annual Meeting DGNR/7th Annual Meeting SGNR/5th Annual Meeting ÖGNR	Würzburg, DE	Nadjmi/ Valavanis/ Schindler
11.05.1996		6th Annual Meeting	Innsbruck	Schindler
23.05.1997	24.05.1997	7th Annual Meeting	Linz	Jurkovic
05.06.1998	06.06.1998	8th Annual Meeting	Graz	Klein
07.09.1999	11.09.1999	XXV. ESNR Congress (no annual meeting ÖGNR)	Vienna	Schindler
26.05.2000	27.05.2000	9th Annual Meeting	Velden	Haselbach
18.05.2001	19.05.2001	10th Annual Meeting	Salzburg	Grobovschek
30.05.2002	31.05.2002	11th Annual Meeting	Innsbruck	Waldenberger
06.06.2003	07.06.2003	12th Annual Meeting	Graz	Klein
14.05.2004	15.05.2004	13th Annual Meeting	Vienna	Prayer
02.06.2005	04.06.2004	14th Annual Meeting	Linz	Trenkler
19.05.2006	20.05.2006	15th Annual Meeting	Salzburg	Grobovschek
2007		no Annual Meeting		
02.10.2008	04.10.2008	16th Annual Meeting/5thGrazer INR-Kurs	Graz	Klein
29.10.2009	31.10.2009	17th Annual Meeting/6th Erich-Klein-Kurs INR	Linz	Trenkler
18.11.2010	20.11.2010	18th Annual Meeting/7thErich-Klein-Kurs INR	Innsbruck	Schocke
17.11.2011	19.11.2011	19th Annual Meeting/8th Erich-Klein-Kurs INR	Klosterneuburg	Nasel
22.11.2012	24.11.2012	20th Annual Meeting/9th Erich-Klein-Kurs	Graz	Deutschmann
10.10.2013	12.10.2013	neuroRad 2013, 21st Annual Meeting ÖGNR, 48th Annual Meeting DGNR	Köln, DE	Trenkler/ Dörfler
20.11.2014	22.11.2014	22nd Annual Meeting/10th Erich Klein Kurs INR	Salzburg	McCoy

(continued)

Table 5.3 (continued)

Annual meetings of the Austrian Society for Neuroradiology				
19.11.2015	21.11.2015	23. Annual Meeting/11. Erich-Klein-Kurs	Klagenfurt	Hausegger
05.10.2016	08.10.2016	neuroRad 2016, 24. Annual Meeting ÖGNR, 51. Annual Meeting DGNR	Köln, DE	Gizewski/Berlis
16.10.2017	18.10.2017	25. Annual Meeting/12. Erich-Klein-Kurs INR	Graz	Deutschmann
15.11.2018	17.11.2018	26. Annual Meeting/13. Erich-Klein-Kurs INR	Vienna	Prayer/ Kasprian
09.10.2019	12.10.2019	neuroRad 2019, 27. Annual Meeting ÖGNR, 54. Annual Meeting DGNR	Frankfurt, DE	Trenkler/ Zimmer
2020		cancelled (Corona)	Salzburg	McCoy
18.11.2021	20.11.2021	28. Annual Meeting/14. Erich-Klein-Kurs INR	Klagenfurt	Hausegger
03.11.2022	05.11.2022	29. Annual Meeting/15. Erich-Klein-Kurs INR	Innsbruck	Gizewski
04.10.2023	06.10.2023	neuroRad 2023, 30. Annual Meeting ÖGNR, 58. Annual Meeting DGNR	Kassel, DE	Pfaff/Hattingen
07.11.2024	09.11.2024	31. Annual Meeting/16. Erich-Klein-Kurs INR	Graz	Deutschmann

In 1995, on the occasion of the 100th anniversary of the discovery of X-rays by Conrad Wilhelm Röntgen in Würzburg, a common meeting was organized by Prof. Nadjmi for the DGNR, Prof. Schindler for the ÖGNR and Prof. Valavanis for the SGNR.

In 1999, Prof. Schindler, the then president of the ÖGNR, succeeded to organize the XXVth ESNR Congress in the Vienna Imperial Palace—strongly supported by the ÖGNR.

Due to the rapid development of Interventional Neuroradiology (INR), a popular course in INR was integrated into the national annual meetings since 2008 as the "Erich Klein Course in Interventional Neuroradiology," named after Prof. Klein, an Austrian pioneer of Interventional Neuroradiology.

In 2012, the DGNR and the ÖGNR under the presidencies of Prof. Olav Jansen and Prim. Johannes Trenkler agreed to a common annual meeting every 3 years known as the "neuroRad." The first joint meeting took place in 2013 in Cologne (Germany) organized by Prof. Arnd Dörfler and Prim. Trenkler. Since then, this successful joint meeting was held in 2016 in Cologne, 2019 in Frankfurt and 2023 in Kassel. For 2025, the next joint meeting is planned to take place in Salzburg for the first time in Austria.

Current Situation of Neuroradiology in Austria

As mentioned above, at the moment, there is no subspecialty for neuroradiology in Austria. However, within the curriculum of radiology, a dedicated neuroradiology module is established.

Today, diagnostic neuroradiology and most neurointerventional procedures are provided by radiologists and, to a lesser extent, by neurosurgeons. Dedicated departments or centers of neuroradiology in university hospitals are established as follows:

Clinical divisions in Vienna, Graz and Innsbruck as part of the Departments of Radiology of the University Clinics.
University Institute of Neuroradiology in Salzburg
Neuroradiology in University Hospitals St. Pölten and Tulln
Institute of Neuroradiology at Kepler University Hospital, Neuromed Campus Linz here one location is missing: Professorship for Neuroradiology at Medical University Innsbruck as part of Department of Radiology, Innsbruck

Neuroradiology is a focus specialty in General Hospitals with neurological—neurosurgical or neurological services. To date, there are no independent or private practices with a pure neuroradiological focus.

Training

The training structure is according to the European training curriculum radiology:

Level 1 (Years 1–3) is finalized with an exam. Level 2 (Years 4–5) allows a specialization in neuroradiology as radiologist.

The Level 3 subspecialization neuroradiology is still to be established. As there is no subspecialization in neuroradiology in Austria at the moment, the ESNR and European Society of Minimally Invasive Neurological Therapy (ESMINT) courses are attended by neuroradiological-interested fellows, they are encouraged and financially supported to aim for appropriate diplomas provided by ESNR or ESMINT.

Based on the German concept and in cooperation with the corresponding German societies, the Austrian Society of Interventional Radiology (ÖGIR) and the ÖGNR implemented a modular gradual approach to train and certify individuals and centers in neurovascular therapy. To ensure quality assurance, the participation, in a dedicated quality-assurance software, is provided.

Further practical training for radiologists with a main focus in neuroradiology is possible in well-equipped institutions (mostly universities) that run, for instance, 1.5–3 T MR-units, biplane angiography and technical high-end CT scanners.

Academia

There are well-established research programs for young radiologists who are interested in neuroradiology at all university clinics/hospitals in Austria. This research is based on a tight collaboration with neurology and neurosurgery as well, as there is a broad interdisciplinary cooperation with other neurosciences (e.g., neuropathology, psychiatry, psychology, neurophysiology, cognitive and basic neurosciences, etc.)—which have been recently organized in centers of shared academic clinical and scientific interests.

Furthermore, dedicated lectures in neuroradiology are offered as part of the graduate medical school curriculum as well as postgraduate PhD programs. According to the subspecializations within the field neuroradiology (diagnostic, interventional, pediatric, functional, etc.), there are different scientific and clinical focuses amongst Austrian neuroradiological academic institutions—which regularly attract international visiting fellows to broaden their experience in the field. The ÖGNR encourages all those who are interested in neuroradiology to attend the ESNR-courses for neuroradiology. After completion of the whole ESNR course circle—including all mandatory examinations—the ÖGNR officially recognizes the subspecialization.

All universities run masters and doctoral thesis as well as PhD programs, which include clinical neuroradiological topics.

Scientific publishing is encouraged by the scientific Arthur Schüller Award, provided and sponsored by the ÖGNR annually.

References

1. Schindler E. Arthur Schüller: pioneer of neuroradiology. AJNR Am J Neuroradiol. 1997;18:1297–302.
2. Schüller A. Röntgenologie in ihren Beziehungen zur Neurologie. Dtsch Z Nervenheilkd. 1914;50:188–207.

Chapter 6
Recent History of the Brazilian Society of Diagnostic and Therapeutic Neuroradiology

Carlos Clayton Macêdo de Freitas, Claudio C. V. Staut, Francisco Mont'Alverne, Felipe T. Pacheco, Carlos Batista Alves de Souza Filho, Carlos Michel A. Peres, Christiane M. S. Campos, Eric Homero Albuquerque Paschoal, Eduardo Floriani Raupp, Gelson Luis Koppe, José Guilherme Caldas, Maria de Fátima Viana Vasco Aragao, Michel Eli Frudit, Pedro S. C. Magalhães, Raquel Trovo Hidalgo, Ricardo Abkalaf, and Rogério Zenóbio Darwich

C. C. M. de Freitas (✉)
Neurosurgery and Interventional Neuroradiology, São Paulo State University, Botucatu, São Paulo, Brazil
e-mail: c.freitas@unesp.br

C. C. V. Staut
Hospital of Clinics of University of São Paulo, São Paulo, Brazil

F. Mont'Alverne
Interventional Neuroradiology Department, Hospital Geral de Fortaleza, Fortaleza, Ceara, Brazil

F. T. Pacheco
Health Sciences from Santa Casa de Misericórdia, São Paulo, Brazil

C. B. A. de Souza Filho
Interventional Neuroradiology, Hospital Santa Casa, Belo Horizonte, Minas Gerais, Brazil

C. M. A. Peres
Neurosurgery Department, Hospital Santa Julia, Manaus, Amazonas, Brazil

C. M. S. Campos
Hospital da Beneficência Portuguesa de São Paulo, São Paulo, Brazil

E. H. A. Paschoal
Instituto Amazonas, São Paulo, Brazil

M. de. F. V. V. Aragao
Universidade de Federal de Pernambuco, São Paulo, Brazil

G. L. Koppe
Hospital Cajuru, São Paulo, Brazil

D. Birchall (ed.), *A World History of Neuroradiology*,
https://doi.org/10.1007/978-3-032-16653-1_6

Some Words

The dawn of a new society marks a transformative period in which fresh ideas, values, and structures begin to take shape. It represents the merging of diverse perspectives, fostering innovation and collaboration. This new society wishes to advance technology and social practices, reshaping how individuals interact and thrive. As challenges arise, the resilience and adaptability of the community play a crucial role in defining its future. The birth of a society is not just about survival; it's about the development of identity, community, and a shared narrative that continues to influence subsequent generations.

Carlos Clayton Macedo de Freitas

The Dawn of a New Society

Neuroradiology began with ventriculography in 1918, pneumoencephalography in 1919, and arteriography in 1927. Initially, air studies were common but were replaced by angiography in the 1950s and 1960s. Until the mid-twentieth century, neurosurgeons, neurologists, and general radiologists performed these examinations. In 1952, Dr. Juan M. Taveras became the head of the Radiology department at the Neurological Institute of Columbia Presbyterian Medical Center in New York, training specialists dedicated to Neuroradiology. This field has progressively developed in nearly all countries. Today, with advancements in CT, MRI, and PET, specialists carry out neuroradiology due to the increasing complexity of neuroscience and the need for dedicated professionals in endovascular treatments [1].

In Brazil, neuroradiology began with the pioneering efforts of Professor José Záclis, who established the first center at the Hospital das Clínicas da Faculdade de

E. F. Raupp
Santa Casa de Misericórdia Hospital, Porto Alegre, Brazil

J. G. Caldas
Hospital of Clinics of University of São Paulo, São Paulo, Brazil
e-mail: jose.caldas@hc.fm.usp.br

M. E. Frudit
Department of Interventional Neuroradiology—INRAD/HCFMUSP and Department of Interventional Neuroradiology, Albert Einstein Hospital, São Paulo, Brazil

P. S. C. Magalhães
Neurology, Neurosurgery and Neuroradiology Services, HMSJ, Joinville, Santa Catarina, Brazil

R. T. Hidalgo
Hospital de Base, São José do Rio Preto, São Paulo, Brazil

R. Abkalaf
Interventional Neuroradiology Service, Hospital A.C. Camargo Cancer Center, São Paulo, Brazil

R. Z. Darwich
Rede D'or Biocor, Belo Horizonte, Minas Gerais, Brazil

Medicina da Universidade de São Paulo in 1947. In 1964, he lectured on Pan-Cerebral Angiography at the V Symposium neuroradiologicum during the First Congress of Neurologic Sciences in Brussels, Belgium. This innovative technique significantly advanced neuroradiology by allowing comprehensive visualization of intracranial blood vessels. In 1976, the first computed tomography (CT) scans were implemented in clinical practice at Beneficência Portuguesa Hospital in São Paulo, with the active participation of Professor Nélio Garcia de Barros and Professor José Záclis, marking the beginning of a new era in the diagnosis and treatment of neurological diseases [2, 3].

During the 1960s, several notable figures emerged in the field of neuroradiology. Dr. Wilson Eliseu Sezana founded the Center for Neuroradiology at the Hospital de Base in Brasília. Dr. Glerystane R. B. de Holanda established the Neuroradiology department in Recife, Pernambuco. Dr. Sérgio Santos Lima, who trained in the United States, returned with valuable skills, including the technique for crafting handmade catheters using either a flame or warm water. At the same time, Prof. Sérgio Raupp in Porto Alegre, Rio Grande do Sul, conducted and published research on "Myelography with Liposoluble Positive Contrast." These individuals made remarkable contributions to the field during the 1960s, 1970s, and 1980s [4, 5]. Prof. Sérgio Raupp, the second president of SBNRDT, is a tireless personality who continues to participate in meetings, congresses, and every grand round at the Santa Casa de Porto Alegre Hospital with fellows.

The subsequent period of the SBNR was characterized by the strong influence of the French School (1990s timeline), which profoundly impacted Brazilian history. Distinguished mentors, including Professor Pierre Lasjaunias, Professor Luc Picard, Professor Jean Jacques Merland, and Professor Jacques Moret, were instrumental in cultivating expertise within this domain. Prominent Brazilian pioneers, such as Dr. Ronie Piske, Dr. José Maria Modenese Freitas, Dr. Márcio Sampaio, Dr. Carlos Abath, Dr. Paulo Passos, Dr. Claudio Staut, Prof. José Guilherme Pereira Caldas, Dr. Eduardo Ernesto, among others, received training from French professors at a different time. They successfully established the INR in their respective regions.

The SBNR holds Professor Pedro Lylyk in high regard as a prominent figure in South American interventional neuroradiology. His significant contributions to the field have trained numerous Brazilian neuroradiologists and fostered the development of innovative techniques, greatly enhancing the treatment of complex neurological diseases. As a leader in endovascular interventions, his work has been crucial in improving the management of strokes and cerebral artery diseases. His extensive academic and professional accomplishments highlight his considerable influence in the neurosurgical field, positioning him as a key player in advancing medical practices and education throughout Latin America.

During the "French period," these professionals have significantly advanced the treatment of cerebrovascular diseases in Brazil by incorporating innovative techniques learned abroad. Their efforts have improved considerably the care for brain and spine conditions. However, they face considerable challenges, such as needing more essential equipment, devices, and adequately trained personnel. Despite these obstacles, their dedication continues to drive progress in the field, ensuring better patient outcomes and laying the groundwork for future advancements in medical treatment across the country.

In 1997, a group of neuroradiologists established the Brazilian Society of Diagnostic and Therapeutic Neuroradiology (SBNRDT). However, it was not officially registered until September 2, 1998, during the II Congress of SBNRDT, held alongside the XVIII Congress of Neurology in São Paulo (see *timeline design*). Exclude the 3 words before (see timeline design) among parenthesis. Immediately above, the official register with all SBNRDT first members.

The Recent History (2018 Until Now)

The SBNR has grown in recent years, reaching almost 400 members, and it has worked with other sister societies in national and international collective actions in Brazil and South America. However, managing a country like Brazil means facing many challenges, such as vast geography and population distribution, historically concentrated training centers in the southeastern and southern regions, regional disparities in professional availability and quality, and different Human Development Indices. In response, a task group of over 30 experts developed a standardized curriculum based on competency education for Neuroradiology, which was approved as a medical residency program in 2018.

The Competency-Based Curriculum and the competency matrix opened a new era in Brazilian Neuroradiology. New training centers were established in underserved regions, promoting equity, and the number of fellows increased to nearly 50 per year, which is a clear indicator of the SBNR's commitment to enhancing professional practice in the country. Competency-based medical education (CBME) and entrustable professional activities (EPAs) are innovative approaches that have transformed the landscape of medical education and assessment. These frameworks focus on developing specific competencies and ensuring that medical trainees are entrusted with responsibilities that reflect their readiness and ability to perform key tasks in clinical practice.

CBME emphasizes the importance of outcomes and the mastery of skills, knowledge, and behaviors necessary for effective patient care. It encourages a more individualized and learner-centered approach to training, allowing for a tailored educational experience that caters to each student's needs.

Similarly, EPAs serve as concrete units of professional practice, defining what trainees should be able to do upon completion of their education. They provide a clear structure for assessing readiness for unsupervised practice and enhance the consistency of evaluations across different educational settings.

These advancements in medical education are part of a broader movement that spans various international societies. Collaborations are seen among the Brazilian Society of Neuroradiology (SBNR), the French Society of Neuroradiology (SFNR), the European Society of Neuroradiology (ESNR), and the Portuguese Society of

Neuroradiology (SPNR). Such collaborative efforts aim to unify standards and ensure the quality and relevance of medical education on a global scale.

In Latin America, several countries are working toward a unified educational framework, particularly in the medical field. Institutions such as the Colégio Argentino de Radiologia (CANI), Sociedad Ibero Latino Americana de Neuroradiology, Sociedad Chilena of Neuroradiology, Sociedad Peruviana of Neuroradiology, Sociedad Colombiana de Neurocirurgia, and the Sociedade Brasileira de Neurorradiologia (SBNR) began working on a homogeneous platform for education before 2020, emphasizing the value of a competence-based curriculum. This approach establishes standardized educational development in Knowledge, Skills, and Attitude, focused on Interventional Neuroradiology. By promoting collaboration and consistency across borders, these efforts seek to improve the quality and accessibility of medical education, ultimately benefiting healthcare outcomes in the region.

The Period of COVID-19. It Was a Dark Moment in Human Beings' History

It's impossible to describe recent human history without considering the COVID-19 pandemic, which has profoundly impacted global health systems and revealed significant vulnerabilities. Hospitals faced unprecedented challenges, including financial strain due to increased demand for medical supplies and equipment and the postponement of elective procedures. The economic crisis exacerbated these issues, leading to a rise in uninsured individuals as unemployment soared. Health systems struggled to maintain access to care, highlighting the need for robust pandemic preparedness and resilient healthcare financing.

All regions of Brazil have been affected, leading to new challenges to ensure adequate care for suspected or confirmed cases of COVID-19 and the safety of health professionals and other patients, reducing their exposure to the risk of infection and safeguarding the care of other potential life-threatening condition, like Acute ischemic stroke and Subarachnoid Hemorrhage. To provide an organization framework for acute stroke patients' healthcare and those who require urgent neurointerventional procedures in the COVID-19 pandemic setting of the Scientific Department on Cerebrovascular Diseases of the Brazilian Academy of Neurology, the Brazilian Society of Cerebrovascular Diseases and the Brazilian Society of Diagnostic and Therapeutic Neuroradiology created an expert joint consensus. It published a guideline in 2020 [6] (Mont'Alverne F et al. Arq Neuropsiquiatr. 2020;78(7):440–449). This was expanded, updated, and used in a review of recommendations published by the World Federation of Interventional Neuroradiology (Interv Neuroradiol. 2021;27(1_suppl):24–29) [6].

Despite the terrible coexistence of disease, suffering, and death, the primary instinct of human beings has also emerged: survival. In our profession, barriers have been broken, whether of knowledge, courage, challenge, or truths that turn into lies and vice versa. But at the same time, we have learned that the current stage of Internet technology allows us to remain connected and united and, better yet, continue to exchange experiences and knowledge. In this new scenario, where distances have been shortened with technology, the SBNR launched two main projects.

The first was a remote education platform for the Acute Management of Stroke disease associated with COVID-19 in the same case. It was coordinated by Dr. Francisco Jose Mont'Alvene, Prof. Marcos Lange (President of the Brazilian Society of Cerebrovascular Diseases), Prof. Carlos Clayton Macedo, Prof. Joao Jose Carvalho (Former President of the Brazilian Society of Cerebrovascular Diseases), Dr. Fabricio Oliveira Lima (Brazilian Society of Cerebrovascular Diseases) and Prof. Jose Batista Cysne (Educational coordinator). This course was addressed to Interventional Neuroradiology and Neurology fellows and based on an active pedagogy, addressing the specific learning objectives of each module: (1) Initial patient management; (2) neuroimaging; (3) decision-making process for reperfusion therapies; (4) patient management in Stroke Unit. Using distance learning pedagogy and Internet tools, it was possible to bring training centers closer by sharing their experiences in teaching the learning objectives and standardizing and improving care protocols, adding significant value to the resident's training to maintain the training of professionals. It's evolved with more than 100 participants from all over Brazil.

The second project was the CONNECTA BRASIL and SIG-CONNECTA Neuro, which proposed a rapprochement between Brazilian Neuroradiologists so that we could fraternally get to know each other better and exchange experiences through virtual meetings. Many meetings were held every 2 weeks or months in a virtual environment, each lasting 2 h, with a list of attendance and identification of all participants. This project took place in 2020 and 2021, coordinated by Dr. Elias Rabahi, Dr. Wilson Novais, and Prof. Carlos Clayton M de Freitas for therapeutic meetings and Dr. Felipe Pacheco from São Paulo, Dr. Pablo Coimbra from Ceará, Dr. Leonardo Macedo from Minas Gerais, and Dra. Nina Ventura from Rio de Janeiro for diagnostic meeting.

During this period of isolation, a fascinating association between Brazil and other countries in South America created the most prominent online meeting that we have ever seen on our continent, the GSANIT/CONNECTOR BRASIL. Many colleagues were founders of GSANIT, such as Prof. Luiz Lemme, Dr. Ronie Piske, Dr. Javier Echevarrieta, Prof. Orlando Dias, Dra. Azucena Davila Malaga, Dr. Luiz Portela, Dr. German Abdo, Dr. Gelson Koppe, Dr. Eduardo Raupp, Dr. Eduardo Bravo, Dr. Boris Pabon, Dr. Rodrigo Rivera Miranda, and others. Their initiatives include organizing academic meetings and events, such as the annual meeting in different South American countries, to discuss advancements and strategies in neuro intervention in a free ambiance. They also offer a robust library online (PNVS) with many case discussions and lectures, a vital tool for education.

The Old Became New

Despite the isolation and lockdown, the SBNR has found ways to stay connected, share knowledge, and support each other. The COVID-19 pandemic has been challenging for all of us, but it has also shown our resilience and ability to adapt. As we continue to navigate these difficult times, we must remember the strength and unity we have demonstrated as a global community.

The Interventional Neuroradiology (INR) simulation started before 2016, but only a few centers were used for training. Our first contact with the Mentice simulator was on May 27, 2019, during the SBNR certification. After that, the SBNR began to use the simulators in a hands-on course and certification.

We applied simulator-based learning with remote online teaching, adapting to the lockdown moment and allowing professors and fellows to continue developing their skills. The initiative aimed to maintain high standards of medical education and ensure that professionals remained proficient in advanced techniques, thereby supporting the society's mission to improve neuroradiology training in Brazil. In 2021, we successfully launched a turnaround initiative across 21 training centers spread across the country, providing a comprehensive 1-week course to all participants. This approach exemplifies the resilience and adaptability of medical education in challenging times.

The International Symposium of Neuroradiology embraces the lessons learned during lockdown by offering attendees a unique and immersive experience. Participants will engage in hands-on sessions focused on diagnostic neuroradiology, allowing for in-depth discussions of challenging cases with experts in the field. This interactive format enhances learning and fosters a sense of community among professionals, ensuring a valuable experience for all involved.

SBNR'S Partnership with Other Institutions

In recent years, SBNR has strengthened its relationship with SOBRICE, SBN, ABNc, SBDCV, SILAN, AMB, and CBR. This collaboration has facilitated numerous educational initiatives and support efforts focused on cerebrovascular disease in Brazil. Together, they aim to address the profound effects of stroke and related conditions.

SILAN BRAZIL 2004, an unforgettable meeting occurred in Costa do Sauípe, organized by SILAN and SBNR. This event was marked by high-level case discussions, showcasing cutting-edge technology and featuring esteemed international guests. The atmosphere was professional and friendly, fostering an environment conducive to learning and networking. Participants left with new insights and connections, making it a memorable experience for all involved.

By pooling resources and expertise, the SBNR strives to improve patient outcomes through innovative treatment strategies and comprehensive care models. Their work focuses on news images and technologies, and the recent neurointervention approach emphasizes pre-hospital care, treatment, rehabilitation, and long-term support for stroke survivors. The Resilient Trial was a national research network that resulted from this collaborative effort focused on stroke treatment. The trial aims to assess the efficacy of new treatment modalities and interventions for stroke patients, and its success depends on the active participation and support of multiple societies and organizations. This collective action reflects the commitment of the medical community to continuously enhance the quality of care and treatment options for individuals affected by stroke. This trial was approved and funded from the Brazilian Federal Government. The Hospital Geral of Fortaleza (HGF) national reference in Stroke care was the leading institution contributing to the Resilient Trial and Basic trial.

The first neuroradiology coding manual was created in 2019, establishing national parameters for charging professional fees. Last but not least, the societies involved have been developing guidelines to ensure that the best available scientific evidence is used to service patients with cerebrovascular disease [8].

Numerous impactful activities have occurred, such as meetings, congresses, symposiums, and online case discussions focused on political and educational objectives. It is worth highlighting the session at the national congress with deputies to discuss the planning for implementing thrombectomy financing in the country's SUS network.

In Memory of Professors Pierre Lasjaunias, Luc Picard, and Ronie Leo Piske

Professor Pierre Lasjaunias, who passed away in 2008, was a renowned figure in anatomy and neuroanatomy. He was a prolific author and dedicated educator, sharing his expertise in neuroradiology with students worldwide. Known for his strong personality, Lasjaunias made significant contributions to interventional neuroradiology, particularly in treating vein of Galen malformations. His sudden death profoundly impacted the medical community, underscoring the loss of a brilliant mind and compassionate clinician who transformed patient care with his innovative techniques.

Professor Luc Picard, a pioneer in interventional neuroradiology, passed away in 2021, leaving a profound legacy. His groundbreaking contributions to the field and his heartfelt commitment to curriculum development and ethical standards defined the WFITN approach's humanitarian spirit. Picard was deeply passionate about interventional neuroradiology, demonstrating unwavering care for his patients and a genuine concern for his student's growth. His contributions have left an indelible mark on the medical community, ensuring his influence will be felt for generations.

Dr. Ronie Leo Piske was a luminary in interventional neuroradiology whose contributions have left an indelible mark on the medical community. Born in São Paulo, Brazil, and of French descent, Dr. Piske was a pioneer in neurointervention, a field that combines radiology and neurology to treat complex brain and spinal conditions using minimally invasive techniques.

His career was largely centered at the Hospital da Beneficência Portuguesa in São Paulo, where he served as professor and mentor to many aspiring neuroradiologists. Dr. Piske's dedication to education and training helped shape the next generation of specialists, ensuring that his innovative techniques and compassionate approach to patient care continued to influence the field long after his passing.

Dr. Piske was a skilled clinician and prolific researcher. His work was widely published and frequently cited by peers, underscoring his role as a thought leader in interventional neuroradiology. His research contributions have been instrumental in advancing the understanding and treatment of neurological disorders, making complex procedures safer and more effective.

During his career, Dr. Piske consistently collaborated with other prominent figures in the field, including Jacques Moret and Laurent Spelle. These alliances encouraged a culture of innovation and excellence, reinforcing his status as a world leader in neurointervention.

Dr. Piske's legacy is reflected in his professional achievements and the respect and admiration he garnered from colleagues and patients alike. His commitment to patient care, combined with his pioneering spirit, made him a beloved figure in the medical community.

We honor Dr. Ronie Leo Piske, a devoted advocate for advancing medical science and enhancing patient outcomes. His work has laid the groundwork for future advancements in neuroradiology, and his impact will resonate for generations.

Advancements and Collaborations

The Brazilian Society of Diagnostic and Therapeutic Neuroradiology (SBNR) has made significant strides in advancing neuroradiology in Brazil. This progress is marked by the development of a comprehensive new curriculum, the establishment of new training centers, and the breaking of traditional paradigms. These efforts aim to enhance the quality and scope of neuroradiological practice in the country.

The new centers serve as hubs for education and research, fostering an environment of continuous learning and innovation. By expanding training facilities, the SBNR is addressing the growing demand for specialized neuroradiologists and ensuring practitioners have access to state-of-the-art resources and technology.

Since 2019, the Brazilian Society of Diagnostic and Therapeutic Neuroradiology has organized the International Symposium of Neuroradiology (ISN), a pivotal event in South America. The symposium covers cutting-edge topics such as high technology, hands-on training, innovation, case discussions, and online surgery. In 2022, the SBNR introduced a women's group for Neurointerventionists, highlighting their commitment to diversity and inclusion. This annual event provides a unique platform for professionals to engage in immersive learning experiences, fostering advancements in neuroradiology.

The hands-on course, which began in 2021 with online monitoring, is now offered by SBNR presence as a part of the curriculum and is available to fellows twice a year.

Collaboration and advocacy are pivotal to SBNR's strategy. By partnering with national and international institutions, the society shares knowledge and best practices, fostering advancements in global neuroradiology. Their commitment to diversity is evident through the Women's Group for Neurointerventionists. Engaging with the federal government, SBNR advocates for public health improvements, aiming to enhance the accessibility and quality of neuroradiological services in Brazil. These efforts underscore the society's dedication to advancing the field and improving healthcare outcomes.

In conclusion, the Brazilian Society of Diagnostic and Therapeutic Neuroradiology has committed to advancing the field through education, collaboration, and advocacy. By developing a new curriculum, establishing training centers, and engaging with other societies and the government, the SBNR plays a pivotal role in shaping the future of neuroradiology in Brazil. These efforts not only improve the standards of practice but also contribute to the overall improvement of public health systems in the country.

Future Challenges for Interventional Neuroradiology in Brazil

The future holds many uncertainties, yet we need to strategize in alignment with our objectives. The executive committee of SBNR is prepared for the new and excited challengers as:

1. *Geographic distribution and access*: Despite efforts to expand training centers, significant challenges may still exist in equitably distributing fused professionals nationwide. The historical concentration of training centers in the Southeast and South has caused many physicians to emigrate from their home regions, exacerbating inequities in the availability of specialists. The objective is to enhance professional training while collaborating with government entities to invest in public institutions. We can foster a more effective and impactful educational environment by improving research, assistance, and teaching through high technology and resources.
2. *Curriculum standardization*: Although a standardized curriculum has been developed and planned, uniform implementation across all training centers may continue to be challenging. Ensuring that all centers strictly follow the standardized curriculum is crucial to maintaining the quality of training.
3. *Integration of new technologies*: The rapid evolution of medical technologies requires that training programs continually adapt to incorporate new techniques and equipment. Keeping up with technological innovations and integrating effective forms into the curriculum may be an ongoing challenge. The cost and sustainability of high-complexity medicine are challenges not only to income countries but worldwide.

4. *International collaboration*: Although there are fellowship and exchange programs with other societies worldwide, maintaining and expanding these collaborations to ensure that Brazilian professionals can access international best practices can be challenging.
5. *Continuing professional development*: In addition to initial training, professionals must have access to ongoing professional development opportunities to update their skills and knowledge throughout their careers.

We conclude with the photo taken during the 17th Congress of WFITN in New York, USA. This photo symbolizes a nation ready to welcome the international community at the World Congress 2028.

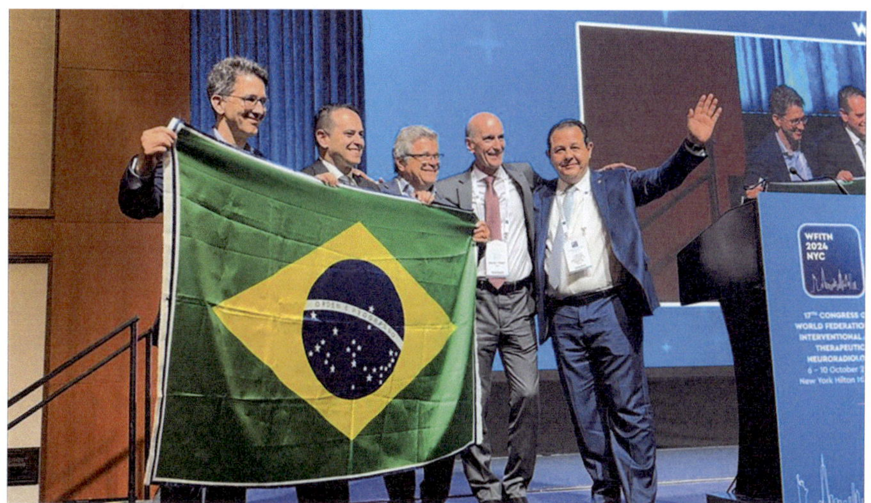

Readers are suggested to contact the corresponding author for figures if needed.

References

1. Bull JWD. Section of the history of medicine. Proc R Soc Med. 1970;63:637–43.
2. Manual do residente do Hospital das Clinicas da USP de Sao Paulo. https://doi.org/10.1590/S0004-282X1984000100017.
3. Zaclis J. Cerebral pan-angiography is the name we suggest for the visualization of all intracranial blood vessels after injection of contrast medium in one of the carotid arteries. Arq Neuropsiquiatr. 1959;17(1):1–22.
4. Sezana WE. Academia de Medicina de Brasilia. https://www.ameb.org.br/index.php/academicos/membros/33-emeritos/138-wilson-eliseu-sesana.
5. Raupp SF. Radiculografia com contraste hidro-solúvel. Porto Alegre: Universidade Federal do Rio Grande do Sul; 1960.

6. Mont'Alverne F, et al. Management of acute stroke and urgent neuro-interventional procedures during COVID-19 pandemic: recommendations on the Scientific Department on cerebrovascular diseases of the Brazilian Academy of Neurology, Brazilian Society of Cerebrovascular Diseases and Brazilian Society of Diagnostic and Therapeutic Neuroradiology. Arq Neuropsiquiatr. 2020;78(7):440–9.
7. Barros NG. https://inrad.hc.fm.usp.br/residencia-medica-em-radiologia-e-diagnostico-por-imagem/.
8. Pontes-Neto OM, et al. Brazilian guidelines for endovascular treatment of patients with acute ischemic stroke. Arq Neuropsiquiatr. 2017;75(1):50–6.

Chapter 7
A History of the British Neuroradiology from the Perspective of British Society of Neuroradiologists

Christopher Rowland-Hill and Dipayan Mitra

Early Days

The British Society of Neuroradiologists was conceived in the late 1960s and after preliminary gatherings, the first official meeting of the Society took place in London in May 1970. Membership comprised consultant neuroradiologists from neuroscience centres throughout the UK. At the time it was typical for these centres to only have 1 or 2 full-time neuroradiologists, and membership was less than 40. Throughout the 1970s the main business of the Society was to organise a 1-day annual scientific meeting (ASM), sometimes as a joint meeting with other societies, including the ESNR in 1972 and the Society of British Neurological Surgeons (SBNS) in 1973. Meetings were hosted by neuroscience centres within the UK on a rotational basis. Probably the most important and influential presentation at a BSNR meeting was given by Dr. Jamie Ambrose in Glasgow in 1972, describing his experience of the world's first CT scanner at Atkinson Morley's Hospital, London. The Society also set up small working groups to deal with standards, manpower and training and published reports covering these issues.

At the dawn of the 1980s, the Society was still exclusively male, welcoming the first female member in 1982. Whereas the 1970s had been the decade of CT, 1980 heralded the arrival of MRI with a presentation from Nottingham on NMR (as it was then known) at the 1980 ASM. In 1981, the ASM extended to two days and included a half-day Registrars Course with didactic teaching. With the emergence of

C. Rowland-Hill
Hull Royal Infirmary, Kingston upon Hull, UK
e-mail: chris.rowland-hill@nhs.net

D. Mitra (✉)
Royal Victoria Infirmary, Newcastle upon Tyne, UK
e-mail: d.mitra@nhs.net

D. Birchall (ed.), *A World History of Neuroradiology*,
https://doi.org/10.1007/978-3-032-16653-1_7

Interventional Neuroradiology as a major advance in treatment of neurovascular conditions, an Interventional Neuroradiology Working Party was formed after discussion at the 1983 meeting in Leeds.

1990s

The Annual Scientific Meeting of the BSNR was by now firmly established as a 2-day event, including a half day of didactic lectures, held in early October. This continued during the decade with the exception of 1997, when the ESNR was held in Oxford.

In 1990, the United Kingdom Neurointerventional Group (UKNG) was formed, open to all practising neurointerventionists, meeting twice per year to discuss scientific, clinical and technical developments and to present cases of interest. The meetings were generously sponsored by industry and, at most meetings, a leading international neurointerventionist was invited to speak.

There were concerns that the formation of the UKNG might split the BSNR and negatively impact on sponsorship for BSNR events. The Diagnostic Neuroradiology Forum (DNF) was set up as a separate group of diagnostic neuroradiologists but many felt that the BSNR already fulfilled this function. The DNF failed to establish itself in sufficient numbers and was disbanded after a small number of meetings.

The 1995 BSNR ASM included the introduction of an eponymous lecture in honour of Dr. James Bull, a key figure in the development of neuroradiology as a speciality in the UK and who was a founder member and the first President of the BSNR. The inaugural lecture was delivered by Professor Michael Sage from Adelaide on the topic of the Blood Brain Barrier. The James Bull Lecture is delivered every year at the ASM by a distinguished national or international speaker in the field of clinical or sometimes non-clinical neuroscience.

In 1996, the Society published the first edition of Effective Neuroradiology. This was a comprehensive 36-page guideline produced by a subcommittee chaired by Professor Ian Isherwood, intended as a reference document for the provision of neuroradiology services in the UK. The guideline encompassed facilities, staffing, training, provision of neurointervention and integration with other clinical neurosciences. An appendix provides a snapshot of UK neuroradiology manpower in the mid-1990s. There were 107 consultant neuroradiologists, averaging 2.6 per department and 8 training posts, of which 4 were based in London. There have been major revisions of this document in 2003 and 2012; the 2012 version was titled Safe Neuroradiology.

During the mid-late 1990s, there were discussions on whether or not a UK-based higher qualification in neuroradiology along the lines of the American Certificate of Added Qualification (CAQ), was required or desirable. Opinion was divided with some strongly in favour. It was recognised that setting up such a qualification would require considerable resource plus the support of the RCR, and ultimately, a UK CAQ equivalent never came to fruition.

In 1998, the BSNR's ASM was held overseas for the first time, in Kinsale, Ireland. At this time, the Irish Society of Neuroradiology was yet to exist. Further overseas meetings occurred in Amsterdam (2003) hosted by the late Dr. Gareth Davies and in Dublin (2017), the latter being a joint meeting with the Irish Society of Neuroradiology.

Up until the late 1990s, Officers of the BSNR had been nominated by the Committee with appointments ratified at the Annual Business Meeting held during the Annual Scientific Meeting. Feedback from neuroradiology trainees at the Kinsale meeting revealed that juniors felt the Society was undemocratic and out of touch. At the 1999 Annual Business Meeting (ABM) it was agreed that thenceforth candidates for the post of president and other Society Officers could be proposed and seconded by any full member of the Society, followed by an election with all full members entitled to vote. A Committee post of Junior Member was also established and the post of Educational Advisor was formalised.

Year 2000 Onwards

In the 1990s, Dr. Andrew Molyneux in Oxford had conceived the International Subarachnoid Aneurysm Trial (ISAT), a randomised, multicentre trial to compare the safety and efficacy of endovascular coiling with standard neurosurgical clipping for such aneurysms judged to be suitable for both treatments. The trial was stopped after 2143 patients had been enrolled. The results, published in the Lancet in 2002, showed conclusively that outcomes at 1 year post treatment were better in the endovascular group. This had major implications for neuroradiology in the UK. Although the endovascular treatment of aneurysms had risen steadily through the 1990s, the new high-level evidence-based need to provide coiling services on a 7- or at least 6-day basis was a major challenge for individuals, departments and national bodies, including the UKNG and BSNR.

Radiology training in the UK at the time was, and still is, based on three years of core training followed by two years of specialist higher training. Ideally, the Fellowship of the Royal College of Radiologists (FRCR) is passed, by written and viva examination, at the end of the third year of training or soon after. At the time, two years of higher training was available for neuroradiology whether just diagnostic or diagnostic plus intervention. The feeling among several interventionists was that two years was insufficient time to train adequately in both branches of neuroradiology. The BSNR's push for three years of higher training for neurointerventionists was initially met with resistance by the RCR and GMC. Fortunately, our colleagues in Interventional Radiology (non-neuro) were pursuing the same aim and eventually Interventional Neuroradiology and Interventional Radiology were incorporated into a 3-year higher training curriculum. The stage was set for expansion of training in neurointervention to meet the demand for the clinical service.

The business and meetings of the Society continued along the same lines during the decade. Having had exclusively male presidents, in 2003, the Society elected its first female president, Dr. Margaret Hourihan (President 2004–2006), who had also been one of the first female full members. Dr. Hourihan introduced the President's Medal, awarded at the discretion of the President at the end of their term of office to a member of the Society for outstanding achievement. Further diversity was achieved when, in 2009, the Society elected its first president from an ethnic minority, Dr. Anil Gholkar OBE (President 2010–2012).

Dr. Robin Sellar (President 2008–2010) observed that other clinical neuroscience bodies in the UK were significantly more structured than BSNR and introduced three new subcommittees—Academic, Standards and Training and Education. After the initial appointment of Chairs by the President, there was a very enthusiastic response from members to be involved. The chief benefits of the subcommittees were twofold. Firstly it provided the BSNR with considerably more manpower resource to contribute to all manner of issues facing the provision and development of neuroradiology as a speciality. Secondly, it provided opportunity for more members of the Society to become actively involved. Since formation, the activities of the subcommittees have included:

Academic Subcommittee

Establishment of the Du Boulay Professorship, in honour of Professor George du Boulay (President 1982–1984). The incumbent or incumbents (on occasions this has been a joint appointment) visit several training schemes in the UK during their two years of tenure, giving lectures and providing advice and guidance on how to pursue a career in neuroradiology.

The Isherwood Prize, in honour of Professor Ian Isherwood (President 1994–1996), was introduced as a pump priming grant, awarded on the basis of submission of a research proposal and subsequent interview.

The Academic Subcommittee also administers a series of Travelling Scholarships, providing funding for trainees to visit other neuroscience centres for a specific purpose.

Standards Subcommittee

Review and revision of the Safe Neuroradiology document, which has helped several departments with planning for staffing levels and equipment upgrades.

Neuroradiology input to the Royal College of Radiologists' iRefer resource, now electronic, which has had a significant impact on improving the appropriateness of referrals for neuroimaging.

Contribution to the development of numerous reports and guidelines, including the 2013 NCEPOD report on Subarachnoid Haemorrhage, Standards for safe Thrombectomy provision, National Clinical Guideline for Stroke and Guidance for Revalidation in Diagnostic and Interventional Neuroradiology.

Training and Education Subcommittee (TESC)

From the outset, the TESC has been involved in developing and improving the content of the curriculum for neuroradiology training, in conjunction with the curriculum committee of the RCR. Due to the limitations imposed on curriculum content by the General Medical Council (GMC), the TESC also developed curriculum support tools, providing detail to supplement the RCR curriculum and the opportunity for trainees to provide feedback to the BSNR.

BSNR stand-alone Trainee Days were established in 2015, expanding to two days in 2018. The unwelcome arrival of Covid-19 in 2020 resulted in cancellation of the 2020 event but opened the door to the establishment of more remote teaching online. This proved to be extremely successful. The audience for the BSNR training grew from what had been 30–40 physical attendees to around 200 trainees and consultants from around the world. The online training programme was formalised in Autumn 2020 with completion of the first 2-year cycle in July 2021 by which time there had been over 14,000 virtual attendances.

A virtual Grand Round was introduced in the summer of 2020. Initially UK-based, this has expanded to presentations from around the world, including Canada, Brazil, Hong King and the UAE as well as a number of European centres.

In 2020, an annual Christmas lecture was introduced, followed by an Easter lecture in 2021. Topics have ranged from the psychology of perception through clinical negligence to paleoradiology. In 2022, an Easter Quiz was introduced.

From the early years of the BSNR, a requirement of becoming a Full Member had been to have presented a scientific paper at the ASM. By 2015, it was felt this rule was anachronistic and out of keeping with other societies. Subsequently, it was decided that all consultant neuroradiologists would be eligible for full membership.

The 2016 ASM in York, hosted by the Leeds neuroradiology team, marked the introduction of a second eponymous lecture, in honour of Brian Kendall, a titan of British neuroradiology who had contributed so much to the field of adult and paediatric neuroradiology as well as pioneering work in neurointervention. The inaugural Brian Kendall lecture was delivered by Dr. David Fiorella.

A manpower survey in 2016 showed there were 230.5 WTE neuroradiologists in the UK, of whom 79 were interventionists. There were 24 vacancies in neurointervention. It was estimated that 140 neurointerventionists would be required to deliver a 24/7 mechanical thrombectomy service.

BSNR Constitution

The Society's constitution underwent three major revisions during the 2010s to accommodate the new subcommittees, adopt changes in membership requirements, update fiscal arrangements and responsibilities and, lastly, to become a registered charity.

Online Presence

A BSNR website was first established in the early 2000s during Dr. John Straiton's tenure as Secretary. For many years, this was a little-used resource with few hits, but more recently, this has been transformed to a comprehensive site with a great deal of information about the Society and its meetings, teaching events and other activities.

Conclusion

Since 1990, British Society of Neuroradiologist (BSNR) has developed from a relatively small, male-dominated group of interested Neuroradiologists to a highly structured, diverse and democratic organisation with a strong online presence and an academic programme which has been complimented and emulated by similar societies. Looking forward, BSNR wants to continue developing its educational and research activities as well as its global footprint while continuing its role in setting and reviewing standards in Neuroradiology.

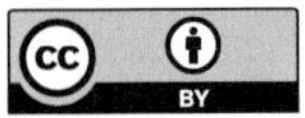

Chapter 8
World History of Neuroradiology: Croatia

Dijana Zadravec, Mia Smoljan Basuga, and Matea Prenc

Croatia is a country situated at the crossroads of Central and Southeast Europe. After the country's independence from the former Yugoslavia in the early 1990s, the healthcare system in Croatia has undergone various reforms.

Croatia's healthcare system is comparable to those in other European countries in terms of coverage and access to services. It is characterized by a combination of public and private services, delivered through a network of public hospitals, health centers, and specialized institutions, providing universal health coverage to its citizens.

Neuroradiology subspecialization is among three possible radiological subspecializations (ultrasound and interventional radiology being the other two) radiologists can choose from in Croatia.

There are currently 72 neuroradiologists in Croatia, practicing mainly in the University hospital centers. The majority work in the two University hospital centers in the capital of Zagreb. The second largest group of neuroradiologists works in the second largest Croatian city—Split. The neuroradiologists in University hospital centers mostly practice neuroradiology in their daily practice, with none or little general radiology, while in smaller regional hospitals, which usually have only a few neuroradiologists, neuroradiology is practiced only part-time.

Neuroradiology subspecialization is divided in two phases. The first phase (6 months) is dedicated to the clinical aspect and includes familiarizing the candidate with the fundamentals of clinical neuroradiology, neuropathology, and neurosurgery. In the second phase (16 months) of subspecialization, the candidate trains and works in an institution with a well-established neuroradiology department. In addition to work duties, lectures, colloquiums, and a final exam are included in the

D. Zadravec · M. S. Basuga (✉) · M. Prenc
Croatian Society of Neuroradiology, UHC Sestre Milosrdnice, University of Zagreb School of Dental medicine, Zagreb, Croatia
e-mail: zadravec@sfzg.hr; msmoljan@sfzg.hr; mprenc@sfzg.hr

D. Birchall (ed.), *A World History of Neuroradiology*,
https://doi.org/10.1007/978-3-032-16653-1_8

second phase of the subspecialization. A total of 256 hours of classes are foreseen in the form of seminars, lectures, and setting of diagnostic problems with independent participation of candidates.

During the second, radiological part of the program, neuroradiology candidates rotate through different neuroradiology subunits—neuroradiological emergencies, cerebrovascular diseases, inflammatory and parasitic diseases, degenerative diseases, neuro oncology, neuromuscular diseases, epilepsy, forensic neuroradiology, neuroradiologic methods in psychiatry, pediatric neuroradiology, and stereotaxy.

An important milestone for Croatian neuroradiology was the establishment of the Croatian network of interventional neuroradiology in 2023. It includes Primary centers organized in 18 hospitals throughout Croatia and Secondary centers organized in five university hospital centers where the neuroterventional procedures take place. The neuroradiological imaging and clinical data for mechanical thrombectomy or aneurysmatic embolization candidates are transferred from Primary centers to the Secondary centers via telemedicine and, if treatable, promptly transported to the nearest Secondary center. Therefore, the network shows its full potential in the early (the earliest possible) arrival of patients with the first symptoms of stroke and enables better treatment and recovery of patients.

The Croatian Society of Radiology (*Hrvatsko društvo radiologa*—HDR) was founded and named at the Founding Assembly held on April 22,1992, and the Section of Neuroradiology was the first section to be founded in 1993, in the very beginning of Croatia's independence. The first president of the Section was prof Nada Bešenski. Other notable neuroradiologists from that time are professors Zvonimir Sučić, Stipan Janković, Jurica Papa, and Ante Buća.

Prof Nada Bešenski, prof Stipan Janković and prof Ante Buča and their associates wrote two neuroradiology university textbooks in Croatian—*Klinička neuroradiologija mozga* (Clinical brain neuroradiology) and *Klinička neuroradiologija kralježnice* (Clinical spine neuroradiology), published in 2011 and 2013. The textbooks were reviewed by prof Zvonimir Sučić, Croatia's first neuroradiologist.

Section of Neuroradiology acted as a part of the HDR for years, but with the evolving neuroradiological modern techniques and developments, an aspiration among neuroradiologists within the HDR to form a separate society has emerged, a society devoted only to neuroradiology, head and neck radiology, and dental radiology, similar to Neuroradiological societies of other countries that have already been assembled.

The Croatian Neuroradiological Society (*Hrvatsko neuroradiološko društvo*, HNRD) of the Croatian Medical Association (*Hrvatski liječnički zbor*, HLZ) was founded at the end of 2017 at the Department for Diagnostic and Interventional Radiology at University Hospital Centre Sestre milosrdnice (UHC Sisters of Mercy) in Zagreb with the aim of gathering experts in the field of neuroradiology, head and neck radiology, and neurointervention, in order to make all important plans and decisions in the field of neuroradiology and neurointervention in the Republic of Croatia. The initiative was started by professor Dijana Zadravec (Fig. 8.1).

Meeting of the initiative committee for the establishment of HNRD was held on December 14, 2017, and on December 19, 2017, the decision of the Main Board of

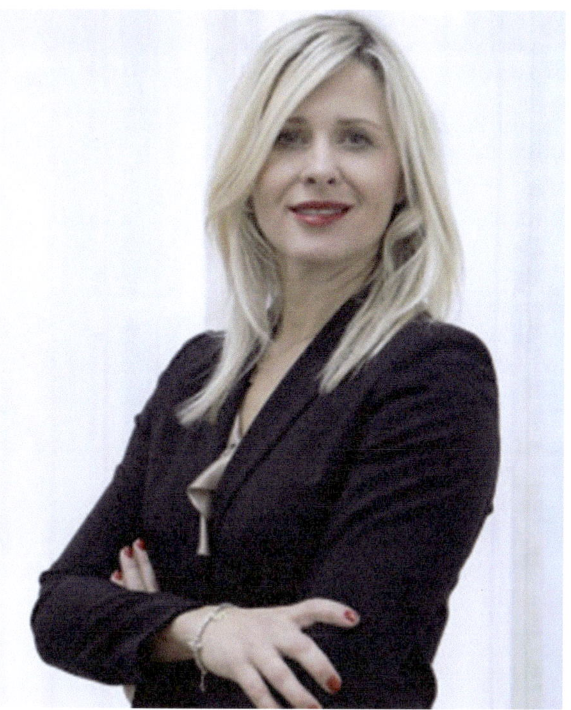
Fig. 8.1 Prof. Dijana-Zadravec—President of the Croatian Society of Neuroradiology

Croatian Medical Association to establish HNRD was made. Founding assembly was held on February 22, 2018, and the latest electoral assembly on March 22, 2022. prof Dijana Zadravec has been elected the president of the Society both times. The vice-president of HNRD is prof Zvonimir Sučić, and the Executive Commitee members are neuroradiologists Dr. Mia Smoljan Basuga, Dr. Tamara Rihtar, Dr. Ivana Župetić, Prim Stanko Belina, neurologist prof Iris Zavoreo, dental medicine doctor prof Tomislav Badel, and the secretary is Dr. Matea Prenc (Fig. 8.2).

The society is inclusive in nature, and, apart from neuroradiologists and radiologists and radiology residents showing a particular interest in neuroradiology, all other health care actors whose professional, scientific, or teaching interest is focused or connected to the field of neuroradiology, neuroscience, neurointervention, ophthalmology, otorhinolaryngology, dental medicine, and other related medical branches, as well as in prevention of neurological and head and neck diseases, are welcome. Therefore, members of the Executive committee as mentioned before, are not only neuroradiologists but also from other medical specialties. The goals of HNRD are based on a multidisciplinary approach to patient health, central nervous system, and head and neck disease prevention, enabling the most modern neuroradiological diagnostics and neurointerventional treatment, as well as increasing their accessibility to as many patients as possible evenly within Croatia. Being a relatively young society, Croatian Society of Neuroradiology wanted a modern and distinctive logo containing symbols and colors representing neuroradiology and the

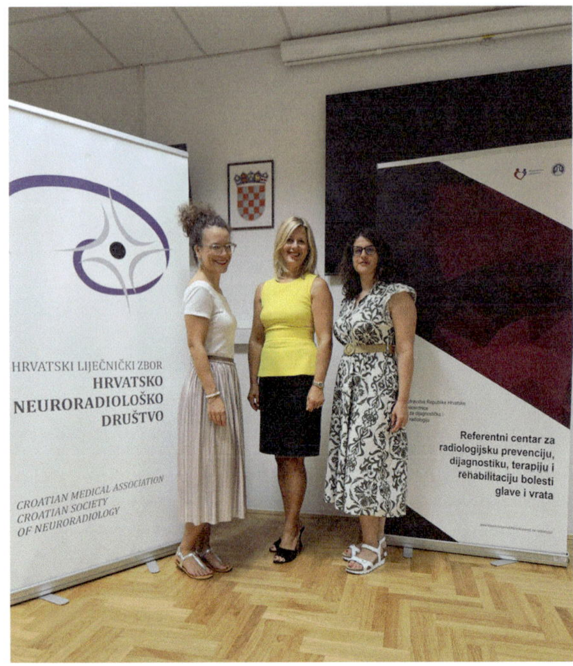

Fig. 8.2 Members of Croatian Society of Neuroradiology Executive committee Dr. Mia Smoljan Basuga, prof. Dijana Zadravec and Dr. Tamara Rihtar

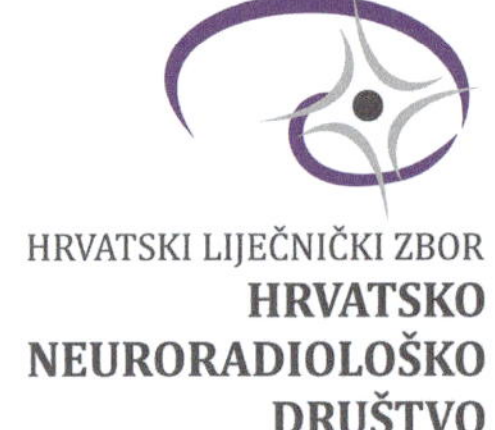

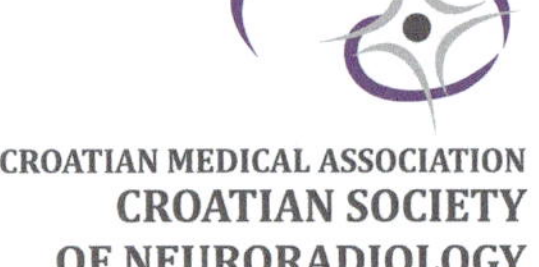

Fig. 8.3 A logo of the Croatian Society of Neuroradiology

Society itself. The grey color was chosen because of the grey matter and purple is the color of Croatian Society of Neuroradiology. Therefore, a stylized image of brain in purple, encompassing a grey neuron was picked for a logo of the Croatian Society of Neuroradiology (Fig. 8.3).

The special goals of the Society are the progress of the neuroradiology profession and neuroscience in the Republic of Croatia, representation of Croatian neuroradiology in the world, development of professional guidelines for the diagnostics and treatment of diseases of the central nervous system and head and neck in close cooperation with other relevant experts, as well as proposal of scientific projects concerning neuroradiology to European funds and the Ministries of the Republic of Croatia for development and modernization of scientific activity in the field of neuroradiology.

HNRD is focused on the permanent professional and scientific training of HNRD members through the organization of professional and scientific meetings, congresses, seminars, lectures, and courses, that is, all forms of permanent medical training, which is a particularly important part of the Society's program. HNRD has no membership fee. In just one year since the assembly, the Society doubled the number of members. Currently there are 97 HNRD members.

HNRD is engaged in the further development of neuroradiology in Croatia and in the organization of interesting, useful, and high-quality meetings and workshops.

So far, the following professional events have taken place:

1. Symposium Emergency Clinical Radiology with international participation

   November 17–18, 2017, Zagreb, Croatia

2. Radiology Academy 2018

   International Course in Head & Neck Radiology, Diagnostic and Interventional Neuroradiology and Dental Radiology
   May 21–23, 2018, Dubrovnik, Croatia

3. Interdisciplinary Expert Meeting—October 2018

   Dedicated to the World Stroke Day
   October 24, 2018, Zagreb, Croatia

4. Second Symposium Emergency Clinical Radiology with International

   Participation
   December 6–7, 2018, Zagreb, Croatia

5. Mechanical thrombectomy – a new era in ischemic stroke treatment

   Course in Diagnostic and Interventional Neuroradiology
   December 8, 2018, Zagreb, Croatia

6. Interdisciplinary Expert Meeting—March 2019

   Dedicated to Pediatric Neuropathology
   March 28, 2019, Zagreb, Croatia

7. Interdisciplinary Expert Meeting—July 2019

   Dedicated to Hydrocephalus
   July 3, 2019, Zagreb, Croatia

8. Interdisciplinary Expert Meeting—September 2019

   Dedicated to Epilepsy
   September 24, 2019, Zagreb, Croatia

9. Interdisciplinary Expert Meeting—November 2019

   Dedicated to Orbital Pathology
   November 12, 2019, Zagreb, Croatia

10. Third Symposium Emergency Clinical Radiology

    November 29, 2019, Zagreb, Croatia

11. Fourth Symposium Emergency Clinical Radiology with International

    Participation ONLINE
    December 11, 2020

12. First Croatian Neuroradiological Congress with International

    Participation ONLINE
    April 22–24, 2021, Rovinj, Croatia

13. Interdisciplinary Expert Meeting—December 2021

    Dedicated to AI
    December 16, 2021, Zagreb, Croatia

Radiology Academy has been a very well-appreciated first organizational venture of the Society, held in beautiful history-rich Dubrovnik. Faculty consisted of 17 international lecturers (Croatia, Belgium, the Netherlands, Italy, Finland, Slovenia, Turkey, the USA), who gave very interesting lectures from predominantly head and neck radiology, but also dental radiology, neuroradiology, and neurointervention.

HNRD has held four Emergency Clinical Radiology Symposia, always taking place at the end of the year, in Zagreb, the capital of Croatia. The meetings were multidisciplinary, hosting both clinicians (neurologists, internal medicine doctors, emergency medicine doctors, surgeons, otorhinolaryngologists) and radiologists as well as neuroradiologists from Croatia but also from abroad (Turkey, USA, Hungary, Canada, Belgium, Brazil) giving not only radiologists' but also clinicians' perspectives. The symposia were focused not only on neuroradiology but on emergency radiology in general.

The first Symposium was followed by a Course in Diagnostic and Interventional Neuroradiology—Mechanical thrombectomy—a new era in ischemia stroke treatment, where clinicians, neuroradiologists, and neurointerventional radiologists shared their view and knowledge on stroke treatment and mechanical thrombectomy with the participants. The course consisted of a lecture part, followed by a workshop.

The first Croatian Neuroradiological Congress with international participation took place during the COVID pandemic, so it was therefore a hybrid congress, held online for participants, with a part of the faculty giving lectures from the beautiful city of Rovinj in Croatia's biggest peninsula, Istria. The program included lecturers from North and South America, Australia, and Europe. HNRD was very proud that five eminent world-known neuroradiology experts gave plenary lectures on the first day of the congress—prof Anne Osborn, prof James Barkovich, prof Suresh K. Mukherji, prof Jan Casselman, and prof Meng Law. The second day of the congress was dedicated to neuroradiology of CNS tumors, stroke cerebrovascular diseases, and neurointervention, followed by issues in neuroimaging of infectious demyelinating and neurodegenerative diseases, as well as subjects pertaining to pediatric neuroradiology. Furthermore, topics such as neurologic manifestations and neuroradiological presentation of Covid-19 and use of artificial intelligence in neuroradiology were also discussed. The last day of the congress was devoted to approaches in imaging of neurotrauma pituitary region and skull base pathology and non-neoplastic lesions, with a separate section related to technological advances in neuroradiology.

The 2nd Croatian Neuroradiological Congress with international participation was organized in April 2025, where numerous eminent neuroradiologists from 17 countries actively participated and shared the newest professional and scientific achievements in their areas of expertise. Several interdisciplinary expert meetings have been organized so far, hosting clinicians from different fields related to neuroradiology or head and neck radiology, each time with a focus on a different topic. The first one was dedicated to the World Stroke Day, held at the end of October 2018, where a Croatian academic, neurologist Vida Demarin, gave an excellent lecture on stroke prevention. Croatian neuroradiologists and neurointerventional radiologists also gave lectures on the topic of stroke. The second interdisciplinary expert meeting was dedicated to pediatric neuropathology, hosting a neuropediatrician, neuroradiologist, and a pediatric neurosurgeon. The third meeting was on the topic of hydrocephalus, with lectures given by a neuroscientist with a scientific expertise in CSF dynamics, a neuroradiologist, and a neurosurgeon. The fourth meeting was focused on epilepsy, from a neurologist, neurosurgeon, and neuroradiologist's perspective. The fifth meeting was focused on orbits, therefore the discussions and the lectures were held by an ophthalmologist and a neuroradiologist. The sixth meeting was international and focused on artificial intelligence.

In 2019, professor Zadravec and associates were involved in the EU project Optimization and improvement of radiological diagnostics efficacy in the health care system of the Republic of Croatia—Radiological educational center (*Optimizacija i poboljšanje učinkovitosti radiološke dijagnostike u sustavu zdravstva Republike Hrvatske—Radiološki edukacijski centar*) (UP.02.2.1.05.0001). The project value was 4.3 million eu. The project lasted for four years and ended in December 2023. Numerous lectures and workshops about the MRI were provided and organized for three groups of medical professionals—the general practitioners, doctors specialized in non-radiological branches, and radiology technicians. The final goal of the project was the shortening of waiting lists for radiological exams in Croatia by raising the knowledge about radiological imaging possibilities and indications. The MR 3 T machine was obtained and a book, *MR Alphabet of Neuroradiology* (*MR abeceda neuroradiologije*), with many pictorial examples of neuroradiological pathologies has been published as a part of the project.

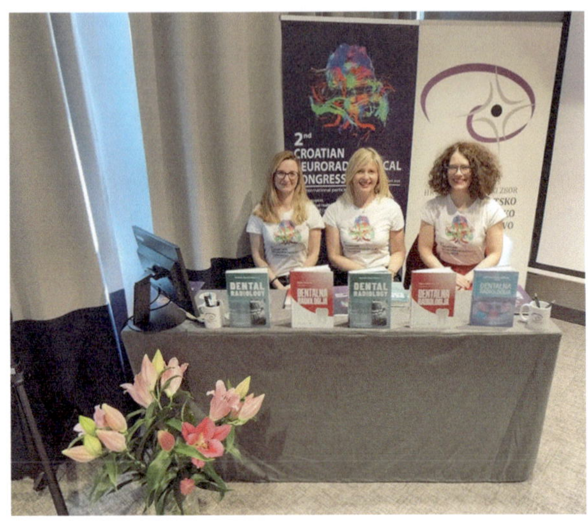

Fig. 8.4 Dr. Matea Prenc, prof. Dijana Zadravec and Dr. Mia Smoljan Basuga (from left to right) at the 2nd Croatian Neuroradiological Congress with international participation, presenting Dental radiology university textbook, 2nd edition

Prof Dijana Zadravec and associates also wrote and published *Dentalna radiologija* university textbook in Croatian in 2016 and also Dental Radiology in English in 2020. The second edition of *Dentalna radiologija* university textbook was published in 2023 (Fig. 8.4).

HNRD President prof Zadravec and Executive committee member Dr. Mia Smoljan Basuga are holders of the European Diploma in Neuroradiology (EDiNR), being among several other neuroradiologists in Croatia who have passed the EDiNR exam.

Prof Zadravec has been a deputy director of University hospital center Sestre milosrdnice since 2016 to 2020 and has been head of the department for diagnostic and interventional radiology from 2016 to 2021. She is head of Clinical unit for Neuroradiology at the University hospital center Sestre milosrdnice in Zagreb since 2016 and is the founder and head of the Referral center for radiological prevention, diagnostics, therapy, and rehabilitation of head and neck diseases of the Ministry of health, Republic of Croatia since 2015.

Prof Zadravec is Head of the General and Dental Radiology department at the University of Zagreb, School of Dental medicine. Two members of the HNRD Executive Committee are also involved at the University of Zagreb, Dr. Mia Smoljan Basuga, a postdoctoral teaching assistant, and Dr. Matea Prenc, a teaching assistant.

The Croatian Neuroradiological Society can be followed on its web page (www.neuroradiologija.org) where society professional activities are listed along with their programs and photos.

The Croatian Neuroradiological Society is a member of the World Federation of Neuroradiological Societies (WFNRS) since 2018 and the European Society of Neuroradiology (ESNR) since 2022. prof Dijana Zadravec is Croatian national delegate. Croatian Society of Neuroradiology will continue further development of Neuroradiology in Croatia and abroad.

Readers are suggested to contact the corresponding author for figures, if needed.

Chapter 9
Neuroradiology in Germany

Peter Schramm, Ansgar Berlis, and Florian Schneider

Scope of Work: Diagnosis and Intervention

Statistics

Neuroradiology in Germany is a focal subject of radiology. This means: The specialized training in neuroradiology builds on the specialist radiology training. The training period has been 24 months since the introduction of the model training regulations in 2018. Neuroradiological content is already part of the training for the specialist in Diagnostic and Interventional Radiology. According to statistics from the German Medical Association as of 12/22, 717 radiologists with a specialization/training in neuroradiology practised in Germany, 483 of them in in-patient care [1, 2].

P. Schramm
Institut für Neuroradiologie, UKSH Universitätsklinikum Schleswig-Holstein Campus Lübeck, Universität zu Lübeck, Lübeck, Germany
e-mail: Peter.Schramm@uksh.de

A. Berlis
University hospital Augsburg, Germany, Diagnostic and Interventional Neuroradiology, Augsburg, Germany
e-mail: ansgar.berlis@uk-augsburg.de

F. Schneider (✉)
Deutsche Gesellschaft für Neuroradiologie e.V., Berlin, Germany
e-mail: schneider@drg.de; dgnr@neuroradiologie.de; http://www.dgnr.org/

D. Birchall (ed.), *A World History of Neuroradiology*,
https://doi.org/10.1007/978-3-032-16653-1_9

Stroke Treatment

Ischemic stroke is one of the most common diseases in Germany, with about 270,000 cases annually, and the third leading cause of death. Since the mid-2010s, several international multicenter studies have proven the high efficacy of endovascular therapy developed primarily in neuroradiology. In this minimally invasive method, the blood clot is removed using a catheter system under angiographic image control (Mechanical Thrombectomy MT). MT has since become a cornerstone in the treatment of ischemic stroke. In 2023, almost 18,000 procedures were documented in the Intervention Register of the German Society for Interventional Radiology (DeGIR) and the German Society for Neuroradiology e.V. (DGNR), which means 8% of all ischemic strokes. In view of the voluntary documentation in the register, this is a high number (cf. Fig. 9.1). Neuroradiologists and radiologists with additional qualification from the professional societies (see below) are involved in the Stroke Unit certification of the German Stroke Society e.V. (DSG), which currently (2023) counts 349 certified Stroke Units in Germany, ensuring nationwide care for acute ischemic stroke [3, 4].

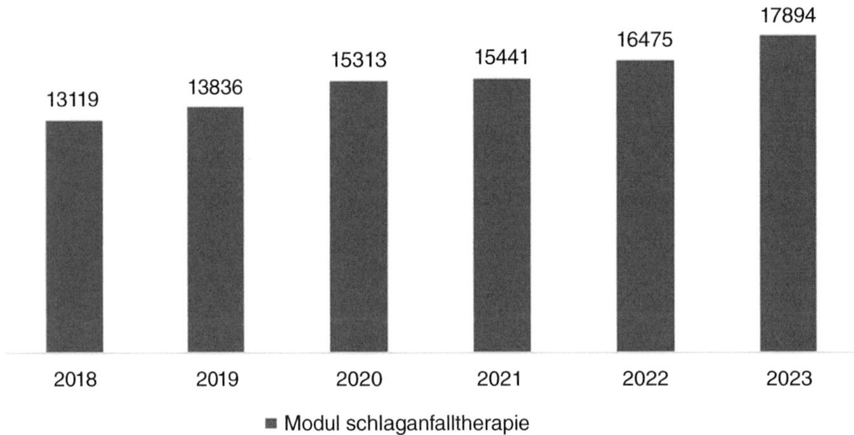

Fig. 9.1 Rising number of mechanical thrombectomy procedures for acute ischemic stroke in Germany from 2018 to 2023, as documented in the national DeGIR/DGNR intervention registry. The data reflect a significant increase in the application of this neuroradiological technique, underlining its pivotal role in modern stroke care. In the DeGIR/DGNR intervention register, the interventions of around 300 entering clinics are documented with regard to outcome, radiation exposure, treatment duration, etc. [5]. (Credits: DGNR)

Certification

Since 2012, the German Society for Neuroradiology e.V., in cooperation with the German Society for Interventional Radiology and Minimally Invasive Therapy (DeGIR), has been offering certificates for neuro-interventional procedures. "Module E," named after the ongoing series of interventional radiology treatment fields, includes all revascularization measures both outside and inside the skull (extra- and intracranial). These measures also include mechanical thrombectomy. One hundred procedures must be documented for module acquisition, including at least 30 intracranial and at least 10 extracranial interventions, preferably at a clinic with the appropriate structure with a Stroke Unit, and at least one cooperatively accessible neurosurgery. The prerequisite is a specialist in radiology. "Module F" certifies neurovascular embolization treatments (embolization and comparable procedures for intracranial aneurysms, embolization of intracranial and spinal vascular malformations, other intracranial embolizations). The prerequisite is the specialized designation in neuroradiology. In 2023, 502 colleagues had acquired Module E, and 287 had acquired Module F [6] (cf. Figs. 9.2 and 9.3).

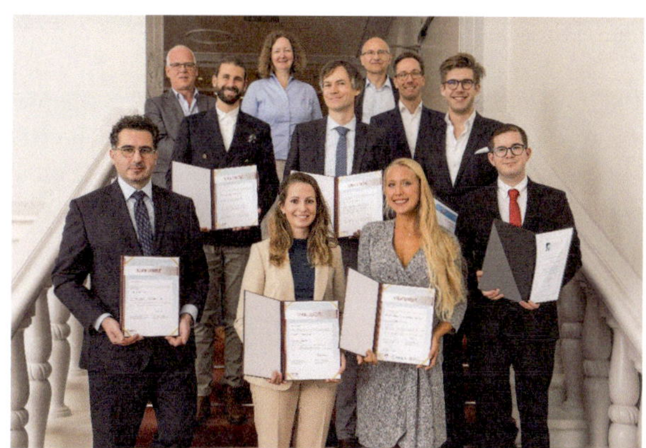

Fig. 9.2 Every year, the German Society of Neuroradiology awards specialist society prizes for outstanding scientific achievements in the field of diagnostic and interventional neuroradiology. Our photo shows the 2023 award winners. (All Rights Reserved by DGNR; Credits: DGNR)

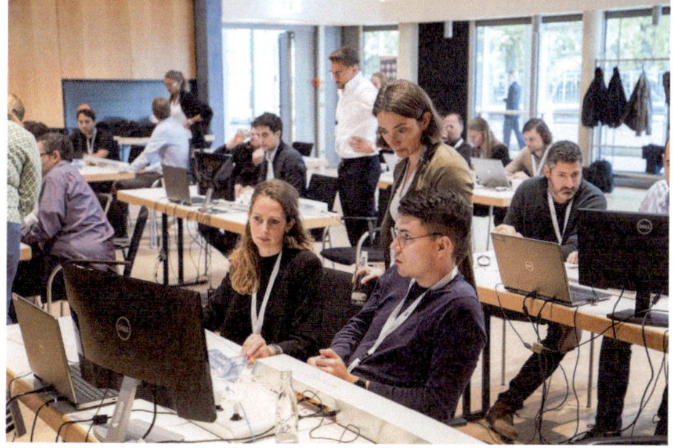

Fig. 9.3 The DGNR's innovative training formats also include simulator courses that simulate interventions such as thrombectomies as part of the German Stroke School at the DGNR's annual conference. (All Rights Reserved by DGNR; Credits: DGNR)

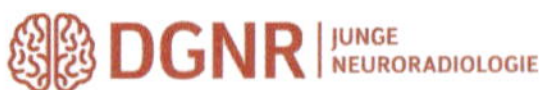

Fig. 9.4 Logo of "Young Neuroradiology" (JUNRAD), the junior organization of the German Society for Neuroradiology, founded in 2020 to represent the next generation of neuroradiologists. (All Rights Reserved by DGNR; Credits: DGNR)

Organizational Structures

German Neuroradiology is represented by two organizations. The German Society for Neuroradiology e.V., founded in 1967 in Mainz, currently has 1900 members, specialists with or without a specialized designation, and doctors in training in radiology or specialized training in neuroradiology. The DGNR offers a variety of continuing education activities, from the annual neurorad with about 1000 attendees to certification webinars and network events. Since 2020, the DGNR has had a Young Neuroradiology organization (cf. Fig. 9.4), offering many opportunities for the next generation of the field. The photo of the 2023 award winners highlights one such occasion (cf. Fig. 9.2). The DGNR maintains a close cooperation with the parent company, the German Radiological Society e.V. The current president is Prof. Dr. med. Peter Schramm www.dgnr.org.

The Professional Association of German Neuroradiologists e.V., founded in 1982 in Hamburg, currently has 150 members. Membership is statutorily linked to the specialized designation in neuroradiology. The BDNR is a full member of the Leading Association of Specialists in Germany (SpiFa e.V.). The current president is Prof. Dr. med. Bernd Turowski (Düsseldorf) www.bdnr.de.

Young Neuroradiology-Junge Neuroradiologie (JUNRAD)

In 2020, Young Neuroradiology was founded as a junior organization within the specialist society. The aim is to represent the interests of the next generation of neuroradiologists and to build a network. With many innovative training formats, its own program at the annual neurorad conference and digital offerings, Young Neuroradiology provides valuable impetus for the entire field. JUNRAD currently has 270 members.

A Look into the Future

How will the field develop? It is already foreseeable today that the diagnostic work of neuroradiology will change considerably as a result of artificial intelligence. Tumor detection and staging will become the work of AI, as will the monitoring and diagnosis of multiple sclerosis. At the same time, however, neurodegenerative diseases will increase in industrialized nations and the monitoring of success in the pharmacological treatment of dementia, for example, will bring additional diagnostic challenges—both qualitative and quantitative. Developments in the field of interventional neuroradiology will also remain extremely dynamic. Many indications for interventional therapy are associated with age, first and foremost strokes, but also intracranial aneurysms. The example of aneurysms is also a very good illustration of technical developments. The introduction of the flow diverter for the treatment of broad-based aneurysms has clearly shifted the treatment practice of these complex vascular diseases towards interventional radiology. Chronic subdural hematomas will also increase with age. With the embolization of the middle meningeal artery, a further field of treatment for neuroradiology is also developing here. German neuroradiology is well positioned to meet these challenges.

References

1. https://www.bundesaerztekammer.de/themen/aerzte/aus-fort-und-weiterbildung/aerztliche-weiterbildung/muster-weiterbildungsordnung
2. https://www.bundesaerztekammer.de/fileadmin/user_upload/BAEK/Ueber_uns/Statistik/AErztestatistik_2022_09062023.pdf
3. https://www.dgnr.org/de-DE/457/pressemitteilung-zum-tag-gegen-den-schlaganfall-10-05-2023
4. https://www.dsg-info.de/stroke-units-neurovaskulaere-netzwerke/
5. https://degir.de/qualitaet/degir-qs-register/
6. https://degir.de/zertifizierung/zertifizierung-personen/

Chapter 10
History of the Israeli Society for Neuroradiology 1990–2024

Ayelet Eran and Eliel Ben-David

During the 1990s, there were a small number of MRI machines in Israel, limited to large medical centers. The main focus of neuroradiology was based on CT, fluoroscopy, and diagnostic angiography. MRI exams were performed for specific indications. During these years, the Israeli Society for Neuroradiology joined as a recognized group within the Israeli Radiological Association (ISRA), with Dr. Dorith Goldsher as the first chairperson.

At the beginning of the new millennium, the society's activities included internal meetings every few months. Two international conferences were held in cooperation with the ESNR.

At the same time, more radiologists travelled for neuroradiology fellowships in accredited programs abroad, and a neuroradiology community began to develop, accompanied by broad neuroradiology education.

During the second decade of the 2000s, coinciding with an increase in the number of MRI machines and institutes, Prof. Chen Hofman (ISNR chair) and Prof. Jaacob Sosna (ISRA chair) acted to open a neuroradiology fellowship program with the support of the Ministry of Health. The first fellow was Dr. Nina Borisovsky from Bnei Zion Hospital, who trained at Rambam Hospital in Haifa. Since the commencement of the program, which is partially supported by the Ministry of Health, dozens of doctors have trained in the program.

A. Eran (✉)
Department of Radiology, Rambam Health Care Campus, Haifa, Israel

Faculty of Medicine, Technion – Israel Institute of Technology, Haifa, Israel
e-mail: a_eran@rambam.health.gov.il

E. Ben-David
Department of Radiology, Shaare Zedek Medical Center, Jerusalem, Israel

Faculty of Medicine, the Hebrew University, Jerusalem, Israel
e-mail: elib@szmc.org

D. Birchall (ed.), *A World History of Neuroradiology*,
https://doi.org/10.1007/978-3-032-16653-1_10

Before the outbreak of COVID, Prof. Ilan Shelef was appointed chairman of ISNR. During the years of the pandemic, online meetings were held every few months, and they continue to this day.

Today, the chairperson and secretary of the society are Dr. Ayelet Eran and Dr. Eli Ben-David, respectively. Dozens of Israeli society members are also members of different societies in Europe and North America.

Chapter 11
History of Italian Neuroradiology, 1990–2023

Giuseppe Scotti

The strength of today's Italian neuroradiology has its roots and foundations in the vision, determination, intelligence, and knowledge of the pioneers who promoted its birth and growth in the twentieth century.

The names of Lombardi, Passerini, Ruggiero, Calabrò, Galligioni, Smaltino, Benati, Nori, Bernasconi, Dettori, and Sicuro—just to mention a few, will remain forever as pioneers and leaders of the first generation who built the solid foundations of our discipline.

After this first wave, which characterized the modern development of the discipline from 1945 to 1970, a second wave appeared from the 1970s and beyond. The list is very long, but to mention a few: Raffaele Elefante, Giuseppe Scialfa, Ugo Salvolini, Luigi Bozzao, Mario Savoiardo, Marco Leonardi, Sossio Cirillo, Giancarlo dal Pozzo, Cesare Colosimo, Dodi Boccardi, Massimo Gallucci, Vincenzo Branca, Alberto Beltramello, Carla Carollo, Antonietta Vaghi, Tortori Donati, Boris Bradac, Frieda Valsecchi, Giorgio Belloni, Giuseppe Bonaldi. The names of the third wave of brilliant and determined leaders of the present generation, those representing Italian neuroradiology in 2023 and beyond, will be found in the following paragraphs dealing with academic careers, hospital departments, organization of meetings, congresses, refresher courses, research projects, and scientific papers.

The history of Italian neuroradiology and that of its relevant personalities before 1990 may be found in the dedicated chapters of the following books:

Before 1990: A Short Summary of the "Past".

G. Scotti (✉)
Centro Diagnostico Italiano (CDI), Milan, Italy

Università Vita Salute e Ospedale San Raffaele, Milan, Italy

D. Birchall (ed.), *A World History of Neuroradiology*,
https://doi.org/10.1007/978-3-032-16653-1_11

1. *Contribution à l'histoire de la Neuroradiologie Européenne*—éditions Pradel, Paris, 1989
2. *Contribution to the History of European Neuroradiology*—E.A. and M.T. Cabanis, Paris, 1994
3. *A History of Neuroradiology (1895– 2002)*—Europa editions—Toulouse, 2002

Marco Leonardi is the author of the last extensive history of Italian neuroradiology. Since his work is, in a way, preliminary to ours, it is worth reporting how Marco Leonardi had subdivided our history in the past century and envisaged its development in the twenty-first century.

The history of neuroradiology in Italy falls into four periods.

The first period was the dawning interest of different neurologists and radiologists in neuroradiology at the turn of the century until the early years of the First World War. It soon became apparent that not only did radiologists require neurological training, but above all neurologists required training in radiology. The radiology-neurology binomial symbolizes the meeting point between two complementary disciplines. The third discipline, neurosurgery, was still missing at this time and its subsequent development was to become the driving force behind neuroradiology.

The second period, a relatively short one, covered the Forties and Fifties and was characterized by the training of Italian neuroradiologists abroad, first in Sweden and later in France. In Sweden they learned to appreciate the role of the neuroradiologist as a separate figure, fully responsible for the risks entailed in invasive neuroradiological investigation, and thus responsible for the indications for examination. Di Chiro and Ruggiero are the leading exponents of the period…. This period of growing awareness and pinpointing targets ended in 1969 when new legislation reforming public hospitals included neuroradiology among the list of hospital specialties entitled to independent departments…..

The third period lasted from 1969 to date and was characterized by the growth of newly established hospital departments…. Unfortunately, this period also saw the development of a major conflict with radiology. Over the past thirty years the divide between professional approach of neuroradiologists and radiologists has widened in Italy. While neuroradiologists are "organ" radiologists in the true sense, radiologists bear the imprint of their technical specialty and include angiographers, computed tomographers, ultrasonographers etc…..While radiologists believed they were defending the integrity of the great mother figure of radiology, they provoked a serious split with neuroradiologists….Only recently has Radiology begun to change its attitude, system specialists now work alongside organ specialists: pediatricians, gastroenterologists etc. Within this framework, the chances of reaching an understanding with neuroradiologists are much greater, there is a plan to set up a joint specialization school, there is hope for future cooperation…

The fourth period is that of university acknowledgement of the neuroradiology discipline. It was only at the end of the Eighties that Italian universities finally recognized the importance of neuroradiology including the discipline in the Degree Course in Medicine. Initially confined to postgraduate specialization, neuroradiology teaching has now been extended to general medicine undergraduates. This important step forward should mark an increase in the number of teaching posts….in 1995 an agreement was reached with the radiologists to amend the Specialization in Radiology to offer two specialty courses: 1) Diagnostic and Therapeutic Radiology and 2) Neuroradiology. The courses started in 1996–1997.

Some have considered the neuroradiology specialty in the school of radiology as limiting, mainly due to the relatively scant clinical curriculum compared with the large number of radiology topics. However, this achievement does signify a clear-cut acknowledgement crowning the efforts of three generations of neuroradiologists. A point of arrival, but also a point of departure: future improvements will then be possible and will depend on our future work and on the work of our successors.

This optimistic scenario outlined in the conclusion of Marco Leonardi's report lasted for a short period, and a clear-cut university program that would have led to a specialty in neuroradiology has not yet been achieved. A proposed parliamentary-specific law, presented by a neuroradiologist member of the Parliament, Dorina Bianchi (16 October 2013), was never approved. The possibility of defining a certified Neuroradiology path within the Radiodiagnosis specialty course is currently being discussed.

In the following chapters, we will see the progress of neuroradiology in Italy from 1990 up to now. We will first have an overview of the growth of the number and of the quality of physicians practicing neuroradiology, spread of hospital departments, academic positions, and society membership. We will then approach the risks and the opportunities, for the next decades, that will require a clear vision and a strong determination not only to grow further but also not to lose the positions and recognitions acquired up to now.

AINR: Associazione Italiana di Neuroradiologia

In 2023, the members of the Italian Association of Neuroradiology (AINR), founded in 1961, were 722, of whom 290 were females and 432 males. The growth has been impressive: in 1990, the members of the society were less than 200.

The AINR is structured on a regional basis, with twelve representatives for the 20 regions (some regions are associated and have a single representative).

The members pay a regular annual fee; the board meets on a regular basis, and the minutes of the meetings may be found by the members on the web page at the following address: *https://ainr.it*

The AINR organizes a National Congress every 2 years, a Pediatric National Congress every 2 years, and educational courses, pediatric and interventional meetings that will be outlined in the following chapter.

The association has a strict relationship and cooperation with the Collegio dei Professori di Neuroradiologia, composed of the University Professors of Neuroradiology.

Italian neuroradiologists may also be members of the association of radiologists (SIRM—Società Italiana di Radiologia Medica), which has a specific section of neuroradiology. The current President of the Section is Alessandra Splendiani, Professor of Neuroradiology at the University of L'Aquila. Neuroradiology is also associated with neurologists and neurosurgeons in SNO (Scienze Neurologiche Ospedaliere).

Congresses, Meetings, and Courses

Until 2009, the AINR organized a National Congress on a yearly basis; subsequently, the national congress has taken place every other year. There is no fixed location and the congress is assigned by the executive committee on the basis of proposed candidatures by the members.

During the COVID-19 pandemic, the annual meeting was postponed by a few months but not discontinued.

Besides the National Congress, AINR organizes a congress of pediatric neuroradiology every other year; this takes place during the year when the National Congress does not take place. The general assembly of members takes place every year, either during the National Congress or the Paediatric Neuroradiology Congress. Also, a yearly interventional meeting, as well as a range of other courses and meetings, are organized.

Furthermore, since 2019, educational courses that lead to a master in Interventional Neuroradiology are promoted by the Collegio dei Professori Universitari in cooperation with several Italian universities, as well as, since 2021, a similar initiative that leads to a master in Diagnostic Neuroradiology. The registered participants just for the diagnostic master's 2024 are 120.

The pediatric section has about 100 members; since 1992, the section organizes a National Congress every 2 years.

Itinerant courses are organized every 6 months (1 for Northern Italy, 1 for Southern Italy), with the aim of basic training.

This report would not be complete without mentioning an original periodic event, a gathering of neuroradiologists that goes under the name of "Club Neuroradiologico Primavera". Starting in March 1990, Professor Giovanni Ruggiero promoted an original formula, a mixture of scientific meeting, social and literary entertainment of neuroradiologists for 1 week, usually in a location in the mountains, with skiing breaks, or at the seaside. From 1990 to 2010, when the Club was discontinued, a total of 19 reunions have contributed to strengthening friendly and professional relationships among Italian neuroradiologists, somewhat selected and invited by the founder of the "club," Professor Giovanni Ruggiero (1922–2009).

Hospital Departments

The number of Hospital Departments of Neuroradiology has significantly increased since 1990. Neuroradiology is practiced in hospital structures of different complexity, denominated according to the internal organization of Italian hospitals as Complex or Simple Operative Units. The complex units have complete autonomy and are chaired by a Director (Primario) who is fully responsible. The simple units may be part of a larger radiological department whose director, usually a radiologist, is ultimately responsible for the department and the neuroradiologist has a less complete responsibility for the unit.

The last official survey done by the AINR concerning the number and distribution of Services/sections of neuroradiology in Italy dates back to 1991 (*La Neuroradiologia in Italia, Censimento dei Servizi/Sezioni, Anno 1991. Editrice Omicron—I quaderni del Radiologo—n. 3/1992*).

This is the published table summarizing the results in 1991.

	North	Center	South	Total
A—Autonomous NRD service	17	13	13	43
B—Aggregated NRD Service	5	2	4	11
Total	**22**	**15**	**17**	**54**

A personal updated non-official survey allows us to witness a significant growth of the hospital departments, and can be summarized as such:

Neuroradiology Departments 2023

	North	Center	South	Total
Total	**37**	**30**	**30**	**97**

Notably, the size, workload, and number of doctors and technicians of the departments has significantly changed with the development of complex modern technical equipment and growth of the interventional activity.

Neuroradiology is practiced not only in Hospital Departments or University hospitals, but also in private clinics or diagnostic centers.

There is a large network of such facilities, usually well-equipped and highly qualified. In these clinics, neuroradiology is practiced both by retired neuroradiologists, full-time staff members and by part-time consultant neuroradiologists working also in public hospitals.

The private centers usually receive both private patients and patients covered by private insurances, as well as patients covered by the National Health Service.

Academic Positions, Teaching, and Research

The academic career in neuroradiology is regulated by national rules: "idoneità" and "concorsi," that is, first evaluation and promotion on the basis of scientific productivity, clinical involvement, and teaching activity and then appointment to the chair.

There are three levels of academic seniority:

1. Ricercatore (R)
2. Associate Professor (PA)
3. Full Professor (PO)

The number of academic positions has grown significantly since the early first chairs, in line with the growth and expansion of the discipline.

From the first appointment of a university professor in Naples in 1976, the number of university professors has grown to:

15 in 1990 (4 PO, 11 PA), to reach
39 in 2020 (11 PO, 22 PA, 6 R) up to the number of
54 in 2023 (20 PO, 18 PA, 16 R) of whom 25% are female.

All the University Professors are committed to teaching and research activities of their universities. Scientific research, however, is performed not only in university departments but also in the majority of hospital centers. The quality of Italian research in Neuroradiology is demonstrated by numerous prizes received by Italian neuroradiologists, national and European grants obtained, and the high Impact Factor of papers published in Italian and international journals.

The University Professors have their official organization and representation in the Collegio dei Professori di Neuroradiologia, whose current President is Alessandro Bozzao.

International Relationships

From 1990 until now, Italy has hosted and organized, besides national congresses and courses, a significant number of international meetings.

The presence of international guests as speakers has contributed to the strengthening of relationships with the most relevant and outstanding international colleagues in the field of neuroradiology, both in Europe and in the rest of the world.

Some of them were, or have become, good personal friends of many Italian neuroradiologists.

Just to mention a few, these include the late Derek Harwood Nash, Anne Osborn, Tom Naidich, the late Michael Huckman, Danielle Balériaux, the late Luc Picard, the late Pierre Lasjaunias, Claude Manelfe, Jordi Ruscalleda, Pia Sundgren, Tarek Yousry, Rolf Jaeger, Karell Terbrugge, Olaf Flodmark, and Majda Turner.

Italian Neuroradiologists Abroad

The names of Giovanni Di Chiro and Domenico Dilenge, as neuroradiologists of Italian origin and European culture and professional formation, who have become prominent figures of North American neuroradiology in the last century, are well known.

The role of Giovanni Ruggiero in promoting French neuroradiology in the 1960s is also notable.

More recently, we must mention Guido Guglielmi, who moved from Italy to Los Angeles, where he developed his world-renowned "Guglielmi detachable coils" method to treat intracranial aneurysms.

Among other figures of Italian neuroradiologists who have reached outstanding positions in hospital departments and universities outside Italy, we should mention:

Donatella Tampieri, Professor of Radiology, Lead of the Section of Neuroradiology at Queen's University, Kingston, Canada

Alessandra Biondi, Professor of Radiology and Director of the Department of Neuroradiology and Vascular Radiology. Besancon University Hospital, Besancon, France

Alessandro Cianfoni, Head of Neuroradiology, Neurocentro della Svizzera Italiana, Lugano

Felice D'Arco, Paediatric Neuroradiology Consultant at Great Ormond Street Hospital for Children in London

Francesco Carletti, full-time consultant in Diagnostic Neuroradiology at the National Hospital, Queen Square, London

Moreover, a large number of young Italian neuroradiologists have trained for periods of varying duration, from months to years, in the most important European or North American centers of diagnostic and interventional neuroradiology in the period from 1990 to 2023.

Lost Colleagues 1990–2023

From 1990 to 2023, we have lost, among others, the following outstanding colleagues and leaders in neuroradiology:

Angelo Passerini (1925–2004), Giovanni Ruggiero (1924–2009); Vincenzo Branca (1957–2010), Aristide Carella (1940–2011); Mario Savoiardo (1939–2014); Francesco Galligioni (1930–2015); Massimo Gallucci (1960–2015); Vittorio Bernasconi (1921–2016); Marco Leonardi (1944–2017); Maria Antonietta Vaghi (1930–2018); Giuseppe Scialfa (1942–2022); and Francesco Smaltino (1929–2022).

The Future

The task for the neuroradiologists of this decade, those who are now the actors and directors of this "story," is to complete *the long march* toward the specialty board certification and also to be leaders in the practice and teaching of diagnostic and interventional neuroradiology and in research in the field of neurosciences.

The scenario in which they are asked to act, however, is changing at a spectacular and unexpected speed.

From 1895, the year of the discovery of X-rays by Wilhelm Conrad Roentgen, the major steps of our disciplines in the past century have been in the 1920s, the introduction of contrast studies, followed by the advent of CT in 1972 and of MRI in the early eighties. We are now, almost 40 years later, probably facing a new revolution or significant step forward with the pervasive advent of AI and radiomics.

The "explosion" of artificial intelligence (AI) and its generative side will dramatically change not only the medical practice, especially in its diagnostic aspect, but also the modality of training future doctors and, in particular, specialists in neuroimaging, that is, the neuroradiologist.

Nobody has a crystal ball to look into the future, so we cannot know whether the prophecy of Jacques Attali that envisages that medicine in 2050 will mainly be "auto diagnosis" will come true. We definitely know that the gloomy prediction of Geoffrey Hinton, who back in 2016 stated that "*artificial intelligence will do better than radiologists and for this reason we should stop forming radiologists now,*" was wrong. We prefer to quote Curtis Langlotz, Professor of Radiology and Biomedical Informatics, who has said: "*Will AI ever replace radiologists? No, but radiologists who use AI will replace radiologists who don't.*"

The role of the neuroradiologist will, however, definitely change and we must be ready to be leaders in the field and continue to value our role as physicians who not only do not lose contact with the patient but also increase our role of being an inevitable interface between diagnostic data, their interpretation, and use, to give the best advice and help to the patients. We must also be in a strict relationship with biomedical engineers, neuroscientists, and clinicians.

The inevitable progress and increase in complexity of the interactions in the field of neurosciences will probably lead and determine the relationship with the radiological family and be a further factor, together with the growth of neuro intervention, to push toward the definitive recognition of neuroradiology as a medical specialty.

Acknowledgements I thank the following people for their help in revising and completing this report:

Nicoletta Anzalone, Alessandro Bozzao, Sandra Bracco, Ferdinando Caranci, Nadia Colombo, Andrea Falini, Simonetta Gerevini, Marcello Longo, Lillo Politi, Andrea Rossi, Alessandra Splendiani, Donatella Tampieri, Fabio Triulzi.

National Congresses (Before 1990)

I—Florence, 1980—President: A. Nori
II—Milan, 1982—P: A. Passerini
III—Bari, 1983—P: A. Carella
IV—Alghero, 1985—P: P.Dettori
V—Milan, 1986—P: G.Scialfa
VI—Bologna, 1987—P: G.Cristi
VII—Positano, 1988—P: R. Elefante
VIII—Padova, 1989—P: K: Pardatscher

National Congresses After 1990

9°—12-14 June 1991, Genova—P: Marco L. Rosa
10°—7-10 october 1992, Milano—P: G. Scotti
11°—10-12 June 1993, Ancona—P: U. Salvolini
12°—19-21 October 1994, Taormina—P: G. Pero
13°—19-21 October 1995, Roma—P: L. Bozzao
14°—16-18 October 1997, Cosenza—P: G. Santoro
15°—9-12 December 1998, Firenze—P: G. Dal Pozzo
16°—12-15 December 1999, Napoli—P: R. Elefante
17°—14-17 December 2000, Genova—P: P. Tortori Donati
18°—13-16 December 2001, Bologna—P: M. Leonardi
19°—15-18 May 2003, Verona—P: A. Beltramello
20°—22-25 September 2004, Milano—P: G. Scotti
21°—22-25 June 2005, Salerno—P: G. Sirabella
22°—4-6 October 2006, Milano—P: F. Triulzi
23°—20-23 June 2007, Bergamo—P: G. Bonaldi
24°—1-3 October 2008, Rome—P: L. M. Fantozzi
25°—9-12 December 2009, Firenze—P: G. Pellicanò
26°—19-22 October 2011, Padova—P: C. Carollo
27°—18-21 September 2013, Coppito (AQ)—P: M. Gallucci
28°—16-18 September 2015, Napoli—P: M. Muto
29°—27-30 September 2017, Milano—P: M.G Bruzzone, E. Ciceri
30°—2-5 October, 2019—Siracusa—P: C. Cristaudo, M. Longo, MP Pappalardo
31°—8–11 June 2022—Roma—P: A. Bozzao
32°—18–21 October 2023—Bergamo—P: S. Gerevini
33°—2025-Reggio Calabria—P: A. Armentano

Pediatric Section

I—1992, Padova—President: Carla Carollo
II—1994, Milano—7–9 April P: Fabio Triulzi
III 1996, Genova—P: Paolo Tortori Donati
IV—1998, L'Aquila—P: Massimo Gallucci
V—2000, Florence—11–12 May—P: Claudio Fonda
VI—2002, Bologna—22–24 November—P: Bruno Bernardi
VII—2004, Padova -15–17 April—P: Carla Carollo
VIII—2006, Ferrara—4–6 May—P: Ferdinando Calzolari
IX—2008, Catania—12–14 June—P: Giuseppe Pero
X—2010, Genova—10–12 December—P:Andrea Rossi
XI—2012, Ancona—28–30 June, P: Ugo Salvolini
XII—2014, Milano—2–4 October—P: Cristina Baldoli

XIII—2016, Rome—6–8 October—Ps: Bruno Bernardi and Andrea Rossi
XIV—2018, Brescia—11–13 October—P: R. Gasparotti
XV—2020, online—30 Nov-4 December (in conjunction with the Functional Neuroradiology Section)—Pres: Massimo Caulo, Cecilia Parazzini, Alessandra D'Amico
XVI—2023, Salerno—26–28 January, P: Alessandra D'Amico

The following list comprises the international meetings and courses organized in Italy:

1961—Rome, 18–22 September. VI SNR Symposium Neuroradiologicum. President: G. Ruggiero
1990—Milano, 4–8 September, European Course in Neuroradiology—Third Cycle, First Course. Intracranial Nervous System. Organizer G: Scotti
1996—Milano, 17–21 September XXII Congress of the European Society of Neuroradiology, ESNR. President G. Scotti
1996—Milano, September 18th: 6th Advanced Course of the ESNR—Functional Neuroanatomy of Motion and Vision—Course Directors Giuseppe Scotti and Denis Le Bihan
1998—Bologna, 22–27 May Fifth Cycle, Third Course—European Course in Neuroradiology—Spine and spinal cord—President Marco Leonardi—Course Director Cosma Andreula
2001—Ancona, 13–16 September 2001. 11th advanced Course and XXVII Congress of the European Society of Neuroradiology, President Ugo Salvolini
2010—Bologna, 4–9 October. XIX SNR. Symposium Neuroradiologicum Pres. M. Leonardi
2019—Naples, 21–24 October: 15th Congress of the World Federation of Interventional and Therapeutic Neuroradiology (WFITN)—President Mario Muto and Alessandra Biondi

Honorary Members and Gold Metal Awards

ESNR—European Society of Neuroradiology

Antonio Sicuro, 1995
Guido Guglielmi, 2006
Giuseppe Scotti, 2012
Massimo Gallucci, 2015
Marco Leonardi, 2016
Mario Muto, 2023

ASNR—American Society of Neuroradiology

Marco Leonardi 2000
Mario Muto 2021

ASPNR American Society of Pediatric Neuroradiology

Paolo Tortori Donati—2016
Andrea Rossi—2023

ESPR—European Society of Pediatric Radiology

Paolo Tortori Donati 1998
Andrea Rossi 2024

Presidents or Board Members of the International Societies of Neuroradiology

European Society for Neuroradiology

ESNR—Marco Leonardi—President 2008–2010
ESNR—Andrea Rossi—Vice President 2022; former Secretary General 2014–2022

Luigi Manfré Secretary General 2023—in office

Antonella Castellano and Nicoletta Anzalone Director of first Level Course of ESNR

WFNRS

Giuseppe Scotti has been a “member at large” of the board of the WFNRS

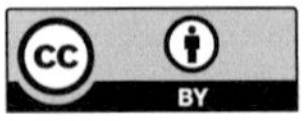

Chapter 12
Japanese Society of Neuroradiology (JSNR): 1990 to The Present

Yukio Miki

The Japanese Society of Neuroradiology (JSNR) boasts a history spanning over 60 years. Its origins trace back to the establishment of the Neuro-Radiological Association of Japan in 1960 by Dr. Toshio Kato and his colleagues. Although this association was briefly dissolved in 1969, it was reconstituted in 1971 as the Japanese Neuroradiological Society (later renamed to its current name). The first conference of the re-established society took place in 1972. The JSNR meeting held in 2024 marked the 53rd in the society's history. This chapter will focus on the society's history since 1990.

Membership Composition

In 2024, the society had 816 active members, distributed across various specialties: 539 radiologists (66%), 217 neurosurgeons (27%), 38 neurologists (5%), 7 pediatricians (1%), and 15 other specialties (2%). The JSNR's diverse membership is probably one of the very unique features of Japan, but we believe this facilitates robust interdisciplinary exchange.

Leadership

The JSNR presidents typically serve terms of 5–8 years, ensuring continuity and long-term strategic development. These are the presidents since 1990: Yutaka Kuru (1979–1994), Hayao Shiga (1994–1999), Tadayuki Maehara (2000–2007), Kazuhiro

Y. Miki (✉)
Department of Diagnostic and Interventional Radiology, Graduate School of Medicine, Osaka Metropolitan University, Osaka, Japan

D. Birchall (ed.), *A World History of Neuroradiology*,
https://doi.org/10.1007/978-3-032-16653-1_12

Katada (2007–2013), Yukunori Korogi (2013–2020), and Yukio Miki (2020–present).

Legal Status

In the past, the JSNR operated as an unincorporated association. However, in February 2022, the society transitioned into a general incorporated association. This shift provided the organization with a firm legal foundation, implementing the Articles of Incorporation and the Code of Ethics. The current Board of Directors consists of nine directors, two auditors, and five specially appointed directors (committee chairs).

Standing Committees

Prior to 2017, the JSNR relied on its presidents and the president's faculty members and secretaries for its operations. However, with the society's growth, it established standing committees in 2018, as suggested by Prof. Yukunori Korogi, then president. The initial committees included the Strategic Vision Committee, Social Media and Website Committee, Research and Education Committee, International Exchange Committee, and Public Relations Committee. Since then, additional committees–Diversity and Inclusion Committee, Finance Committee, Conflict of Interest Committee, Ethics Committee, Editorial Committee, and Rules and Regulations Committee, and Guideline Committee–have been added, resulting in 12 standing committees currently overseeing society operations.

Fiftieth Anniversary Commemorative Events

In 2021, the JSNR celebrated its 50th annual meeting at Osaka City Central Public Hall. Due to the COVID-19 pandemic, the event adopted a hybrid format, accommodating both in-person and online attendance. In celebration of its 50th anniversary, the society hosted special commemorative lectures and exhibitions. A commemorative publication was also released the following year to honor the milestone.

Kato Prize

The Kato Prize, established in 1979, honors Dr. Toshio Kato, one of the society's founders. It recognizes the JSNR member who produces the most outstanding paper in the field of neuroradiology each year. The award is the highest accolade in the field within Japan and serves as a benchmark for researchers. Award-winning papers historically focused on CT, but since around 1990, MRI research has become predominant. Among the awarded papers since 1990, the majority have been published in *Radiology* (11 papers), followed by the *American Journal of Neuroradiology* (AJNR) (9 papers), *European Radiology* (5 papers), and *Neuroradiology* (2 papers). Past winners and award-winning papers are listed on the website: https://neurorad.jp/english-page/kato-prize/

Website

The JSNR's website offers enhanced content, including information on board and committee members, rules, past and future conferences, research grants, Kato Prize submissions, and neuroradiology-related news. Webcasting of educational lectures from annual meetings began in 2023. An English version of the website was launched in 2023. https://neurorad.jp/english-page/

Foreign Honorary Members

The JSNR recently reinstated the appointment of Foreign Honorary Members in 2023. The new selection criteria include not only achievements in the field of neuroradiology, but also significant contributions to society and neuroradiology in Japan, such as accepting significant numbers of Japanese visiting researchers. Four neuroradiologists were selected as Foreign Honorary Members in 2023 and 2024, respectively.

https://neurorad.jp/english-page/organization/jsnr-honorary-members/

Hosting the Symposium Neuroradiologicum (SNR)

In 1994, SNR XV was hosted in Kumamoto, Japan, under the presidency of Prof. Mutsumasa Takahashi. In 2030, the JSNR will host SNR XXIV in Sapporo, marking its second time hosting the event. Prof. Kohsuke Kudo and Prof. Minako Azuma will serve as presidents for the conference. Sapporo is an attractive place that is popular among tourists, and we are aiming to make the conference a fulfilling one.

Official Journal

The JSNR's official journal, *Neuroradiology*, published by Springer, has published abstracts from the JSNR's annual meetings since 1981.

https://neurorad.jp/english-page/annual-meetings/

Logo

In 2021, the JSNR held a design contest among its members to select a new logo. The winning design features stylized Chinese characters for "neuro," morphing into the brain and spinal cord.

Future Prospects

Neuroradiology's progress aligns with advancements in diagnostic imaging technologies such as MRI and CT. The additional application of artificial intelligence shows promise. The JSNR aspires to foster global advancement in neuroradiology through strengthened international cooperation and collaboration. The society anticipates welcoming many neuroradiologists to SNR XXIV in Sapporo in 2030.

Readers are suggested to contact the corresponding author for figures if needed.

Acknowledgements DeepL and ChatGPT were used for Japanese-English translation and English editing.

Chapter 13
A Brief History of Neuroradiology in South Korea: From a Small Beginning to an Ever-Growing Leading Role

Hye Jin Baek, Ji-hoon Kim, and Won-Jin Moon

Introduction

The history of neuroradiology began to evolve with the invention of X-ray, as did the history of radiology. Therefore, the history of neuroradiology itself reflects the developmental history of radiology. Radiology was born on November 8, 1895, when Wilhelm Conrad Röntgen discovered X-rays, a new type of radiation with high penetrating capacity, and his achievement led to revolutionary development in the field of medicine [1, 2]. Then, Röntgen unveiled his discovery, "On a New Kind of Rays," by presenting it at a session of the Würzburg Physico-Medical Society, and it was subsequently published in the journal *Science* [3]. Owing to this pioneering discovery, X-rays promptly became a new tool in physics research, providing diverse opportunities to visualize and analyze the internal structures of the human body more systematically in medicine [1, 2]. Since then, Röntgen's discovery has been applied to imaging the skull and nervous system using a fast clip, and neuroradiology has established academic independence in radiology. Neuroradiology was further expanded by the subsequent launch of head and neck radiology as an early subspecialty in the early 1900s [2, 4, 5]. Additional innovations related to the

H. J. Baek
Department of Radiology, Pusan National University Yangsan Hospital, Pusan National University School of Medicine, Yangsan, Republic of Korea
e-mail: sartre81@pnuyh.co.kr

J.-h. Kim (✉)
Department of Radiology, Seoul National University Hospital, Seoul National University College of Medicine, Seoul, Republic of Korea
e-mail: jihnkim@snu.ac.kr

W.-J. Moon
Department of Radiology, Konkuk University Medical Center, Konkuk University School of Medicine, Seoul, Republic of Korea
e-mail: mdmoonwj@kuh.ac.kr

D. Birchall (ed.), *A World History of Neuroradiology*,
https://doi.org/10.1007/978-3-032-16653-1_13

widespread use of contrast agents, myelography, CT scanning, and MR imaging have become cornerstones in the development of neuroradiology. In addition, the adoption of cerebral angiography enabled neuroradiology to expand its field from diagnosis to neurotherapeutics as interventional neuroradiology [2, 6–9].

In South Korea, neuroradiology began to evolve as a subspecialty of radiology when the first CT scanner was installed at the Kyung Hee University Hospital in 1977. Since then, neuroradiology in South Korea has continued to develop in line with these changes and development trends by providing scientific evidence in daily clinical practice, advancing research, and establishing more systematic training programs. Over the decades, the efforts and passion of the early pioneers and all our members have been the basis for the remarkable development of the Korean Society of Neuroradiology (KSNR). Sometimes, the time filled with our history flows faster than the wind. However, we believe the eyes that were never extinguished within them were passed on to the next generation of Korean neuroradiologists. In this regard, we would like to begin this article by considering it an infinite honor to be able to perform meaningful work of looking back at and organizing the history of the KSNR.

History of Neuroradiology in South Korea Centered on the Korean Society of Neuroradiology (KSNR)

KSNR: The Period of Birth (1980–1990)

In the early stages, Korean neuroradiology also passed through a similar series of steps as the world's neuroradiology, with the need for clinical practice in the field of radiology based on radiological science and technical advances, and being stimulated by the trends of specialization in the departments of neurology and neurosurgery. This worldwide shift has steered the emergence of neuroradiology as one of the subspecialties in radiology in South Korea.

In South Korea, the introduction of CT scanners in the late 1970s has played a crucial role in the academic development of neuroradiology. The first CT scanner was installed at the Kyung Hee University Hospital in Seoul, South Korea, in 1977. Since other university hospitals adopted CT scanners in 1978, a few radiologists have recognized the need to initiate monthly meetings to discuss clinical cases of the brain obtained using CT scanners and exchange their clinical experiences. Thus, five pioneering neuroradiologists initiated an informal monthly study group in 1980, which became the KSNR forerunner. This played a pivotal role in learning about the new imaging modality and teaching other radiologists and trainees needing CT access. In 1983, the KSNR was formally organized as a subspecialty society of the Korean Society of Radiology (KSR) by a handful of radiologists who pioneered neuroradiology in South Korea, the same members as the informal monthly study group: Dr. Jung-Ho Suh (Yonsei University Severance Hospital), Dr.

Kee-Hyun Chang (Seoul National University Hospital), Dr. Chang-Gok Ham (Hanyang University Hospital), Dr. Soo-Jee Suh (Keimyung University Dongsan Hospital), and Dr. Choong-Ki Eun (Kyung Hee University Hospital) (Table 13.1). Dr. Jung-Ho Suh was elected as the first president, and Dr. Kee-Hyun Chang was the Secretary General of the KSNR. In 1995, Dr. Kee-Hyun Chang succeeded Dr. Suh as the president. In recent years, the strong leadership of these radiologists has become a major driving force in the development of neuroradiology in South Korea.

Ten years after the first CT scanner was installed in South Korea, the first domestically constructed clinical MR scanner was successfully developed by Zang Hee Cho, Ph.D., in collaboration with many scientists, radiologists, and industrialists. This 2.0 Tesla superconducting unit (Gold Star Electronics, South Korea) was installed at Seoul National University Hospital and Keimyung University Dongsan Hospital in Daegu. The impact of MRI on Korean neuroradiology is enormous, as it was in other countries, owing to its groundbreaking trialability in clinical practice by promising higher soft-tissue contrast and high resolution of anatomic detail in the body without radiation hazards compared to CT images.

Based on these technical advances, including the adoption of cross-sectional imaging such as CT and MRI, clinical practice and research in neuroradiology became

Table 13.1 The roster of KSNR presidents (1983–Present) and Founders

KSNR Presidents	
1980–1995 Jung-Ho Suh, MD, Yonsei University	2011–2013 Sang Joon Kim, MD, Ulsan University
1995–1999 Kee-Hyun Chang, MD, Seoul National University	2013–2015 Gyung Ho Chung, MD, Jeonbuk National University
1999–2001 KyuHo Choi, MD, Catholic University of Korea	2015–2017 Hyung-Jin Kim, MD, Sungkyunkwan University
2001–2003 Choong-Ki Eun, MD, Inje University	2017–2019 Kook-Jin Ahn, MD, Catholic University of Korea
2003–2005 Dong Ik Kim, MD, Yonsei University	2019–2021 Sang-Hoon Cha, MD, Chungbuk National University
2005–2007 Sun Yong Kim, MD, Ajou Univeristy	2021–2023 Chul-Ho Sohn, MD, Seoul National University
2007–2009 Woo Suk Choi, MD, Kyung Hee University	2023–2025 Ji-hoon Kim, MD, Seoul National University
2009–2011 Tae-Sub Chung, MD, Yonsei University	2025-present Chang-Woo Ryu, MD, Kyung Hee University
KSNR Founders	
Jung-Ho Suh, MD, Yonsei University Kee-Hyun Chang, MD, Seoul National University Chang-Gok Ham, MD, Hanyang University Soo-Jee Suh, MD, Keimyung University Choong-Ki Eun, MD, Kyung Hee University	

more active, and the area of interest in Korean neuroradiology began to expand further to neurotherapeutics by performing endovascular procedures with highly motivated neuroradiologists at the center. In 1984, Dr. Jung-Ho Suh of Yonsei University Severance Hospital and Dr. Kee-Hyun Chang of Seoul National University Hospital first treated carotid-cavernous fistulas with a detachable balloon in South Korea. In 1987, Dr. Dong Ik Kim of the Yonsei University Severance Hospital first treated a brain arteriovenous malformation with glue embolization. In 1990, the first official annual meeting of KSNR was held at Seoul National University Hospital.

KSNR: The Period of Growth (1991–2000)

Starting with a small, informal, monthly study group of only five pioneering radiologists in 1980, the KSNR developed rapidly as its membership grew to 36 in 1991, 76 in 1995, and 103 in 2000. As the number of members increased, academic activities also began to increase. A monthly neuroradiology meeting was held in the metropolitan area on the third Friday of every month. It consisted of exciting case discussions, lectures, and joint readings of the latest articles. An annual national meeting of the KSNR has been held since 1990. An annual national meeting was held twice a year, in spring and autumn, between 1994 and 1996. They are open to both member and non-member physicians, including radiology residents. The committee members decided the format of each meeting, which usually consisted of scientific presentations with free topics, special lectures, panel discussions, and quizzes on neuroradiology. In addition, the KSNR invited prominent foreign neuroradiologists to give lectures at annual national meetings (Fig. 13.1). In addition, casebooks of the KSNR were published from 1994 to 2002, and neuroradiological cases with high academic and clinical value were organized to satisfy the academic interests of our members. Identification reports and interchanges among members began with the publication of Newsletters from 1997 to 1999, and the KSNR website was opened in 1998 to establish a system for managing members and cases, as

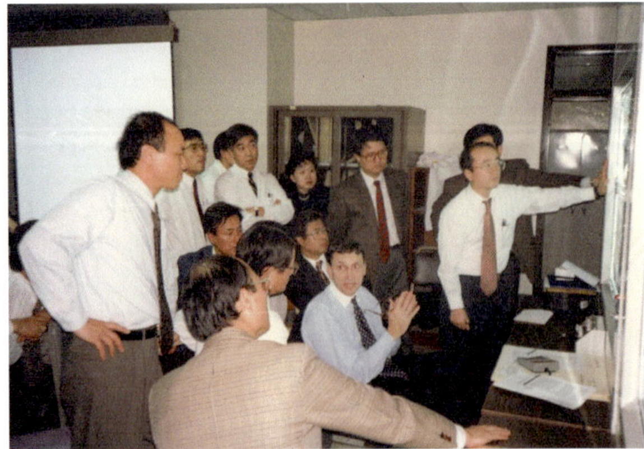

Fig. 13.1 Case discussion commemorating the invitation of Professor Robert I. Grossman, an editor-in-chief in AJNR and a section chief of neuroradiology at the University of Pennsylvania, in 1993

well as for sharing data. Furthermore, a monthly quiz for educational purposes of radiology residents began to operate on the website of the KSNR, and excellent residents were awarded at an imaging conference every year.

As the KSNR increased, standards for membership were required. However, there was a practical problem in discussing detailed regulations on fellowship training during this period. Only 30% of the members were fully dedicated to neuroradiology, and the others practiced neuroradiology as part of their work. Therefore, to be accepted as a member of the KSNR, the KSNR applied more relaxed regulations as follows: (1) the individual must be a physician certified (or eligible for certification) by the Korean Board of Radiology. The Korean Board Certification System has been adopted in North America. To become board-eligible, one must complete 5 years of postgraduate training: 1 year of internship and 4 years of radiology residency. The actual Board certificate in Radiology is given to those who pass a state-authorized test conducted after the radiology residency; (2) The individual must be interested in neuroradiology, but no other specific neuroradiological requirement is asked of the candidate.

In addition, interventional neuroradiology was considered an area of neuroradiology until the early 1990s because radiologists with neuroimaging backgrounds initiated and performed all procedures. During this period, most of these neuroradiologists took 1-year or 2-year training fellowships in interventional neuroradiology at leading overseas centers outside of South Korea, mainly in the United States or France. In 1994, eight neuroradiologists interested in interventional neuroradiology created an informal study group and began to hold a monthly meeting for clinical case discussions: Dr. Dong Ik Kim (Yonsei University Severance Hospital), Dr. Sun Yong Kim (Ajou University Hospital), Dr. Hong Sik Byun (SamSung Medical Center), Dr. Dae Chul Suh (Asan Medical Center), Dr. Hae Young Seol (Guro Korea University Hospital), Dr. Gil Woo Lee (Hallym University Kangdong Sacred Heart Hospital), Dr. Nam Joon Lee (Korea University Hospital), and Dr. Moon Hee Han (Seoul National University Hospital). In 1996, the Korean Society of Interventional Neuroradiology (KSIN) was formally organized into 25 members as a subsociety of neuroradiology. Dr. Hae Young Seol of Guro Korea University Hospital was elected as the first president of KSIN, and Dr. Hong Sik Byun of the Samsung Medical Center was the membership secretary of KSIN. In the same year, Dr. Dong Ik Kim (Yonsei University Severance Hospital) and Dr. Moon Hee Han (Seoul National University Hospital) respectively treated cerebral aneurysms with GDC coil embolization. After that, endovascular treatment for cerebrovascular disease began to take its place in South Korea.

KSNR: The Period of Dynamicity (2001–2010)

Over the past 30 years, the KSNR membership has steadily increased annually, reaching approximately 160 members (Fig. 13.2). During this period, the KSNR, along with its affiliated associations, made continuous efforts to provide clinical guidelines for diagnostic imaging and interactive management required by the daily

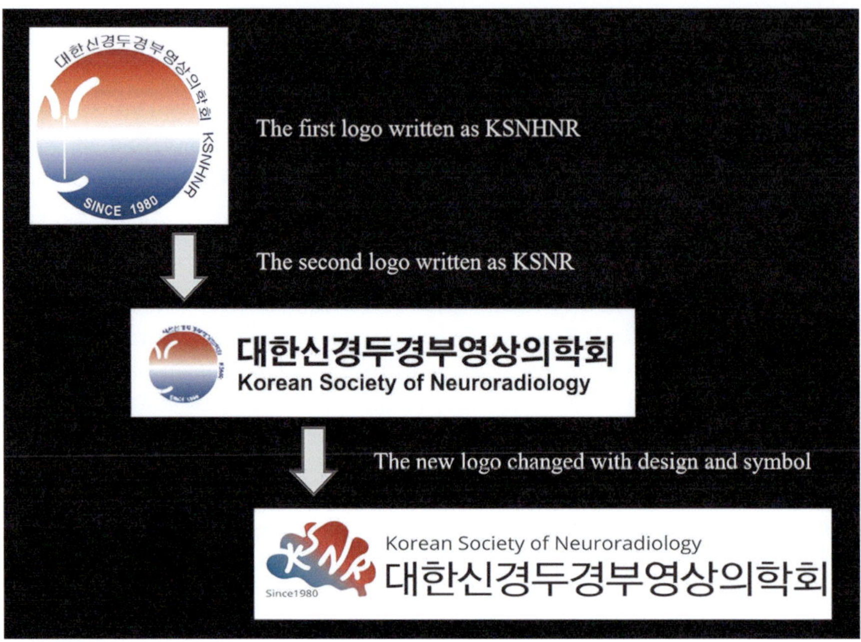

Fig. 13.2 A Changing History of the KSNR's Logo. The second logo was applied to the name of the English Literature Society, which changed from KSNHNR to KSNR in 2015. The KSNR uses a new logo that has changed with design and symbol in 2019

practice of neuroradiology, update information for its members according to changes in the domestic medical environment, support research activities, and develop training standards and educational programs for young radiologists, including radiology residents. The KSNR has begun training education courses for radiology residents since 2005; this systematic education for radiology residents is a 3-year training program that covers one topic each year: neuroanatomy, imaging findings for neurological diseases, and imaging findings for head and neck diseases. To strengthen case-based education for radiology residents, the KSNR works with the KSIN to hold two imaging conferences every spring and winter. Also, the KSNR published a textbook, "Thyroid Gland: Imaging and Interventional Procedures," in 2008 to strengthen education for radiology residents, board-certified radiologists, and medical students. Since the early 2000s, the KSNR has been systematically subdivided into several research committees and subsidiary societies officially established under the KSNR, as follows: Head and Neck Radiology Study Group (Dr. Ki Joon Sung, Wonju Severance Christian Hospital) in 2001, Stroke Study Group (Dr. Jae Hyoung Kim of Seoul National University Bundang Hospital) in 2004, Thyroid Radiology Study Group (Dr. Dong Gyu Na, Seoul National University Hospital) in 2005, and Brain Function Study Group (Dr. Sang Joon Kim of Asan Medical Center) in 2006. The Korean Society of Thyroid Radiology (KSThR), which originated from the Thyroid Radiology Study Group under the KSNR, was founded as an affiliated subspecialty of the KSR in 2009. These systematic changes and the expansion of the KSNR have laid the foundation for sustainable academic development through more in-depth interchanges between clinical cases and research. It also plays a vital role in effectively updating and sharing the subspecialized knowledge of neuroradiology.

Additionally, the KSNR has actively participated in international neuroradiology societies in Asia and elsewhere over the last 20 years. In particular, the KSNR has initiated international interchanges with neuroradiology societies in Asian countries such as Japan and Taiwan since the 2000s. In September 2001, the fourth Asian and Oceanian Congress of Neuroradiology and Head and Neck Radiology (AOCNHNR) was successfully held in Seoul, South Korea, hosted by the KSNR, through the efforts of Dr. Jung-Ho Suh (Yonsei University Severance Hospital) and Dr. Kee-Hyun Chang (Seoul National University Hospital), who led the organization committee. At that time, the number of registered participants was 385, including 160 international participants from 23 countries. The meeting was praised by participants as the most significant and highest-ranking neuroradiology conference ever held in the Asia-Pacific region. In parallel with the AOCNHNR, the KSIN hosted the 6th Congress of the World Federation of Interventional and Therapeutic Neuroradiology (WFITN) and completed a meeting with 426 registered participants from 31 countries.

KSNR: The Period of Diversity (2011–Present)

During this period, the KSNR membership steadily increased, reaching over 200. In particular, the number of female members steadily increased during the KSNR growth period, with the proportion of female members increasing significantly from 8.3% in the early 1990s to 57% of the total membership by 2020 (Fig. 13.3).

Since 2011, the KSNR has held a neuroimaging day to exchange and discuss the latest knowledge at the expert level, separate from the education for radiology residents. Also, in 2015, the KSNR published another textbook, "Head and Neck Imaging," to strengthen education for radiology residents, board-certified radiologists, and medical students. In 2017, an additional research committee was established as an aging and neurodegenerative imaging group (Dr. Won-Jin Moon, Konkuk University Medical Center).

Through changes over the past few years, the KSNR has become an ever-developing scientific society in South Korea that is academically progressive, fair, and open to all members and leads globally. For example, the KSNR is continuously making efforts to improve Korea's national healthcare system as an academic and professional community. For example, the KSNR produced guidelines for the legitimacy of diagnostic imaging studies jointly with the Korean Centers for Disease Control and Prevention and the KSR from 2015 to 2020, and also compiled guidelines for head and neck imaging in 2019. In addition, the KSNR carried out the tasks regarding clinical practice guidelines conducted by KSR, including "Expert

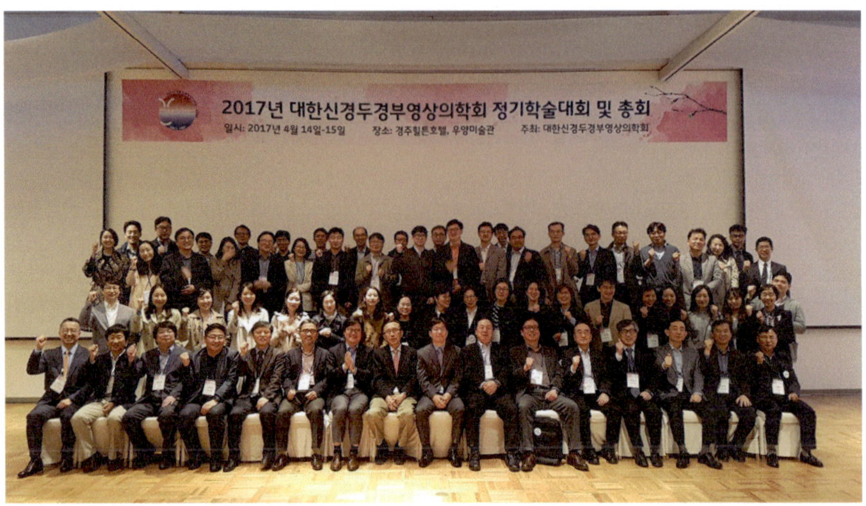

Fig. 13.3 KSNR's Annual Academic Conference and General Assembly in 2017

opinions and recommendations for the clinical use of quantitative analysis software for MRI-based brain volumetry" in 2017 and "Recommendations for the appropriateness of the clinical use of diagnostic imaging modalities in patients with tinnitus" in 2020.

Regarding international academic activities, the KSNR joined the international exchange program for the neuroradiology fellows with neuroradiology societies in Taiwan and Japan in 2012. Thus, two neuroradiology fellows in each country are exchanged for educational purposes every year. The Neuroradiology Forum was held over 2 days in Incheon, South Korea, in April 2014 and was co-hosted by neuroradiology societies in South Korea, Taiwan, and Japan. In addition, the 13th Asian Oceanian Congress of Neuroradiology (AOCNR) was held in Seoul, South Korea, in April 2021, hosted by the KSNR. This meeting, which has been held again in South Korea over the past 20 years, invited approximately 70 excellent speakers from domestic and abroad, including Asia, Oceania, North America, and Europe, to achieve exciting and beneficial academic venues by providing the latest knowledge and critical reviews in each field of neuroradiology (Fig. 13.4). We received 170 abstracts from 13 countries and 662 registered participants, including 343 international participants from 25 countries. Although the meeting was held virtually because of the COVID-19 social distancing, it was very successful. Hosting the 13th AOCNR in South Korea during the COVID-19 era was meaningful because it became an essential cornerstone for the KSNR to build a new platform for online domestic and international meetings without regional and time constraints. Beyond Asia, the KSNR joined the World Federation of Neuroradiological Societies (WFNRS). Our members have also actively participated and presented papers at many scientific meetings in North America and Europe, such as the Radiological Society of North America (RSNA), the American Society of Neuroradiology

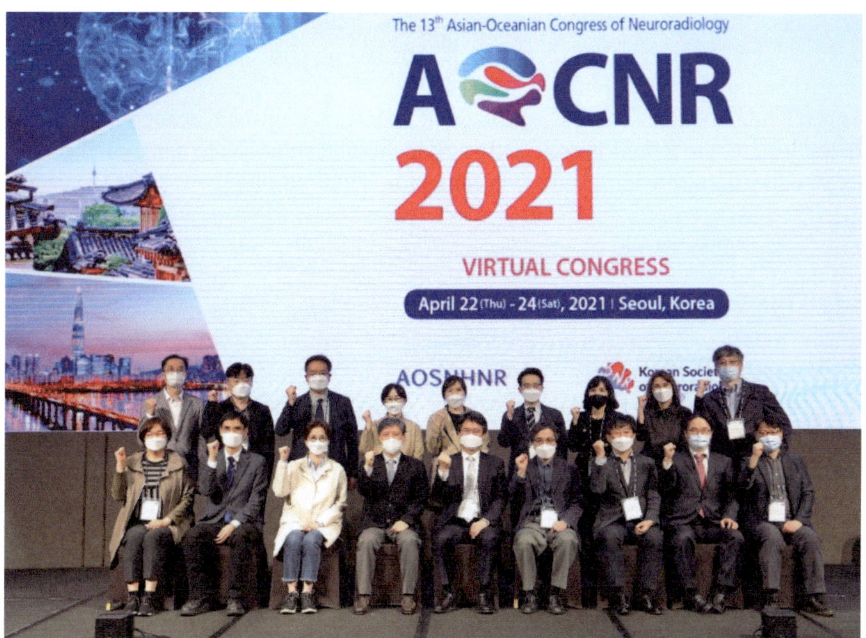

Fig. 13.4 The 13th Asian Oceanian Congress of Neuroradiology (AOCNR) as Virtual Meeting, Seoul, South Korea in 2021

(ASNR), the European Society of Neuroradiology (ESNR), the Symposium Neuroradiologicum (SNR), the American Society of Head and Neck Radiology (ASHNR), the European Society of Head and Neck Radiology (ESHNR), etc. Furthermore, the pursuit of diversity, equity, and inclusion has been recognized and evolved from an admirable ideal to an essential element of institutional excellence in international academia. To keep pace with this change, the KSNR has made steady efforts over the past decade to promote these values in neuroradiology as part of the medical workforce, which can be crucial in opening opportunities to minorities currently underrepresented in our field, reducing disparities, improving patient outcomes, expanding research protocols, and enhancing the quality of education.

Recently, artificial intelligence (AI) has been considered a key technology in medical advancement. As shown by a wide range of AI-based applications, such as machine learning algorithms and expert systems, AI's technological advancements and capabilities in radiology are expected to continuously transform various aspects of healthcare, such as diagnostics and personalized treatment planning [10]. Combined with this rapidly changing trend and Korea's strength as an IT powerhouse, our members' research results on AI and neuroradiology began to be published at the KSNR's annual academic conference in 2017. Since then, AI has gradually expanded into a new research area in Korean neuroradiology, and the active collaboration between neuroradiology and industry has opened new horizons for research.

To date, Korean neuroradiology, led by the KSNR, has continued to develop with technological advances. However, the KSNR has now faced difficulties with radiologist burnout, which is increasing globally owing to the increasing work burden. This phenomenon has caused a shortage of neuroradiologists in academic faculties. In this regard, the KSNR is constantly striving to find solutions to maintain the quality of education, research, and advancement in neuroradiology.

Conclusion

Looking back at the history of neuroradiology in South Korea, the KSNR in 2024 has grown to nearly 360 from an intimate, small study meeting of only five neuroradiologists in a metropolitan area in 1978. At present, the KSNR has continued to uphold its mission by playing a leading role in clinical practice and research for a systematic network of the KSNR and its sub-societies. This is achieved by holding an annual national meeting, providing clinical guidelines or standards for daily practice, conducting regular training education courses for radiology residents and young neuroradiologists, supporting the research efforts of our members, and maintaining close relationships with national and international organizations. Within the history of radiology in South Korea, the KSNR has reached its current standing by leading the adoption and application of new imaging technologies to daily clinical practice and by conducting a wide range of studies since the early period, including CT scanning in the late 1970s and MR in the 1980s and 1990s. Through decades of adversity and challenges experienced in making neuroradiology take root in South Korea, we look forward to continued growth domestically and playing a leading role in international societies of neuroradiology while adapting to the rapid changes of the times with new values.

References

1. Kornienko VN, Pronin IN. Neuroradiology: history and new research technologies. In: Diagnostic neuroradiology. Berlin, Heidelberg: Springer Berlin Heidelberg; 2009. p. 1–27.
2. Lev M, Gadde J, Wiggins R. A brief history of neuroradiology and the 60th anniversary of the ASNR: "Through the Decades with ASNR". Am J Neuroradiol. 2022;43(12):E54–E9.
3. Röntgen WC. On a new kind of rays. Science. 1896;3(59):227–31.
4. Leeds NE, Kieffer SA. Evolution of diagnostic neuroradiology from 1904 to 1999. Radiology. 2000;217(2):309–18.
5. Taveras JM. Diamond Jubilee lecture. Neuroradiology: past, present, future. Radiology. 1990;175(3):593–602.
6. Dandy WE. Roentgenography of the brain after the injection of air into the spinal canal. Ann Surg. 1919;70(4):397.
7. Sicard J, Forestier J. Methode radiographique d'exploration de la cavite epidurale par le lipiodol. Rev Neurol. 1921;37:1264–6.

8. Di Chiro G, Schellinger D. Computed tomography of spinal cord after lumbar intrathecal introduction of metrizamide (computer-assisted myelography). Radiology. 1976;120(1):101–4.
9. Ozdoba C, Gralla J, Rieke A, Binggeli R, Schroth G. Myelography in the age of MRI: why we do it, and how we do it. Radiol Res Pract. 2011;2011:329017.
10. Hamet P, Tremblay J. Artificial intelligence in medicine. Metabolism. 2017;69:S36–40.

Chapter 14
Neuroradiology in Norway; The Last 25 Years

Per Hjalmar Nakstad

Neuroradiology was already incorporated into the clinical work-up of neurological and neurosurgical patients in Norway from 1947. The so-called "Oslo School of Cerebral Angiography" attracted several colleagues from Europe and the USA. CT (1975) and MR technologies (1986) had spread rapidly around the country, contributing further to the development of neuroradiology. These technologies initiated a further need for neuroradiological departments, in addition to the departments established at Oslo University, The National Hospital, Rikshospitalet in 1962, and Oslo City Hospital, Ullevål Hospital, in 1964. These two university hospitals were merged in 2009 and called Oslo University Hospital (OUS). During the last 30 years, sections of Neuroradiology were established at Haukeland University Hospital, Bergen; University Hospital of North Norway, Tromsø; and St. Olavs Hospital, Trondheim University Hospital.

Due to the keen interest in angiographical interventional procedure at OUS, embolization of cerebral and dural arteriovenous malformations was started in 1988 and became a daily routine from 1992. The help from our American colleague, Professor Charles M. Strother, Madison, USA, was important. In addition to being an experienced neuroradiological interventionalist, he was a keen cross-country skier, combining interventional work with skiing in Oslo for 1 year in 1992/1993. At the same time, OUS was included as one of 12 European institutions in the international treatment strategy of using Guglielmi detachable coils in treating aneurysms. After that, interventional neuroradiology therapy slowly increased, despite a somewhat reluctant attitude of neurologists, but with important support from the neurosurgeons (Helge Nornes and Bjørn Magnæs) [1–3]. The first embolization of an aneurysm was performed at OUS (Rikshospitalet) in 1992. Embolizations of aneurysms were for many years exclusively performed at Oslo University Hospital.

P. H. Nakstad (✉)
Neuroradiology, Oslo University Hospital, Oslo, Norway
e-mail: p-h-na@online.no

D. Birchall (ed.), *A World History of Neuroradiology*,
https://doi.org/10.1007/978-3-032-16653-1_14

It was our opinion then that a one-center practice in our small country with excellent patient transportation facilities by air and land seemed justified [4]. Following the extensive development in techniques, equipment, and therefore the increased number of possible treatments, it seemed justified that other centers as well incorporated interventional neuroradiological treatment in their routine. In the beginning, Prof. P. Nakstad (PN) performed procedures for many years in the other university hospitals in Norway, as well as occasionally in Finland (Oulo University Hospital), Sweden (Karolinska University Hospital/University of Uppsala), and Iceland (Borgarspitalin). The engagement in Iceland lasted from 2000 to 2009 and was particularly challenging, since all instruments had to be carried along on the acute flight to Iceland. During the last 10–15 years, interventional neuroradiological procedures were implemented in four other university hospitals in Norway (Bergen, Tromsø, Trondheim, and Stavanger).

Since the scientific activity connected to the development of radiologic contrast media during the 1970s and 1980s resulted in the worldwide success of non-ionic contrast media (Amipaque/Omnipaque, Nycomed AS, later Amersham and General Electric), scientific work consequently continued with CT and MR with a special focus on contrast media. A PhD (doctoral thesis) has a high standing in Norway and may serve as a measure of scientific activity. The basis for the PhD thesis was, in addition to contrast media research, tumor diagnostic [5, 6], stroke [7], and interventional procedures [8]. MRI has had a great impact on the neuroradiological scientific work in Norway [9], and presently almost every hospital has installed MR as a routine acute service.

The European Society of Neuroradiology (ESNR) was founded in 1969, and the fifth ESNR congress was arranged in Norway (Geilo) in 1975 (president Per Amundsen). The next ESNR congress in Norway took place in Oslo in 2000 (president Per Nakstad) and then again in Oslo in 2020 (president Paulina Due-Tønnessen). The Norwegian National Society of Neuroradiology was established in 1985 during the ESNR congress in Amsterdam. Today, the National Society has 115 members.

The contribution in other important societies, such as The World Federation of Interventional and Therapeutic Neuroradiology and World Federation of Neuroradiological Societies (WFNRS) was established from the beginning as a founding member and member of the board (Per Nakstad). The activity in these societies is kept up to date by the Presidents of the National Society (Paulina Due-Tønnessen and Erik M. Berntsen).

Neuroradiology has maintained its status as a separately organized professional subspecialty despite the attempts to incorporate it more tightly with general radiology. Neuroradiologists are active at every university hospital and larger hospitals, and interventional neuroradiology is performed at all five university hospitals. The number of arteriovenous malformations and aneurysms in our population of merely five million inhabitants seemed earlier too low to maintain interventional treatment at five university hospitals [9]. However, the considerable increase in patients treated for strokes by transcatheter thrombectomy, in addition to other vascular diseases, has given the neuroradiologist the quantity necessary to maintain their skills and necessary continuous training at all five locations.

Most importantly, the health authorities have now given neuroradiology considerable economic support, enabling neuroradiology to prosper.

Readers are suggested to contact the corresponding author for figures if needed.

References

1. Nakstad P, Bakke SJ, Hald JK. Embolization of intracranial arteriovenous malformations and fistulas with polyvinyl alcohol particles and platinum fiber coils. Neuroradiology. 1992;34:248–51.
2. Nakstad P, Nornes H. Superselective angiography and surgery in treatment of cerebral arteriovenous malformations of the brain. Neuroradiology. 1994;36:410–3.
3. Nakstad P. Interventional neuroradiology. Review article. Acta Radiol. 1999;40:344–9.
4. Nakstad PH. Vascular interventional neuroradiology in a country with a small and scattered population. Twenty years of experience in Norway. Interv Neuroradiol. 2008;14:5–8.
5. Server A. Advanced neuroimaging in brain tumors: diffusion, spectroscopy, perfusion and permeability for the evaluation of tumor characterization and surgical treatment planning. Doctoral Thesis; 1997.
6. Server A, Kulle B, Mæhlen J, Josefsen R, Schellhorn T, Kumar T, Langberg CW, Nakstad PH. Quantitative apparent diffusion coefficients in the characterization of brain tumors and associated peritumoral edema. Acta Radiol. 2010;50:682–9.
7. Schellhorn T. Brain MRI findings associated with cognitive impairment before and after stroke. Doctoral Thesis; 2022.
8. Nome T, Bakke SJ, Nakstad PH. MR angiography in the follow-up of coiled cerebral aneurysms after treatment with Guglielmi detachable coils. Acta Radiol. 2002;22:10–4.
9. Berntsen EM. Preoperative planning and functional Neuronavigation. Doctoral thesis; 2009.

Chapter 15
A Brief History of Portuguese Neuroradiology: The Last 30 Years

Rui Manaças, Luísa Biscoito, Inês Carreiro, and Ana Mafalda Reis

The history of Portuguese neuroradiology over the last 30 years has been shaped by the dedication of pioneers whose enthusiasm and contributions have succeeded in establishing neuroradiology as a medical specialty in Portugal. Their efforts led to the definitive recognition of the several imaging techniques such as fluoroscopy, ultrasound, CT, and MRI techniques as indispensable tools in daily practice, along with the progressive acceptance of therapeutic techniques, namely endovascular (as safe methods for treating aneurysms, AVMs, AVFs, and acute ischemic stroke) and minimally invasive percutaneous spine procedures (such as vertebroplasty/kyphoplasty, facet joint radiofrequency, nucleolysis/ozonotheraphy, and percutaneous devices- spacers, screws…..).

In the preceding 70 years, this development was not an uninterrupted continuum but divided into two distinct phases, as described in the Portuguese chapter of *A History of Neuroradiology* (1895–2002) by Paulo Saraiva and Augusto Goulão (pages 377–388), presented at the XVII Symposium Neuroradiologicum, 2002, edited by E.A. Cabanis and M.T. Iba-Zizen.

The first phase began with the discovery of cerebral angiography in 1927 by Egas Moniz, leading to the creation of the Portuguese School of Angiography and the application of this technique to other organs and systems.

The second phase involved strengthening the field, with the establishment of a 5-year autonomous specialty in the late 1970s across three centers:

R. Manaças (✉)
SPNR (Portuguese Society of Neuroradiology), Lisbon, Portugal

L. Biscoito
Centro Hospitalar e Universitário de Lisboa Norte, Lisbon, Portugal

I. Carreiro
Centro Hospitalar e Universitário de Coimbra, Coimbra, Portugal

A. M. Reis
Unidade Local de Saúde de Matosinhos, Hospital de Pedro Hispano, Matosinhos, Portugal

D. Birchall (ed.), *A World History of Neuroradiology*,
https://doi.org/10.1007/978-3-032-16653-1_15

Lisbon—Hospital de Egas Moniz (Cruz Maurício), Coimbra—Centro Hospitalar de Coimbra (Faria Pais), and Porto—Hospital de Santo António (Paulo Mendo and Almeida Pinto). This significant leap contributed to the growing activity in hospitals, and the teaching of neuroradiology began in Central Hospitals. By 1982, there were three centers in Lisbon, two in Coimbra, and two in Porto, all with fully staffed neuroradiology departments comprising Heads of Service, Senior Consultants, Hospital Assistants, and Specialty Fellows.

Between these two phases, the neuroradiologic techniques available at the time using fluoroscopy—namely angiography, pneumoencephalography, ventriculography, and myelography—were performed in Portuguese hospitals primarily by neurosurgeons (neurologists also in Oporto).

In the 1990s, neuroradiology services or units expanded to five more hospitals in the National Health Care System: one in the north (Braga—led by Jaime Rocha), two on the outskirts of Porto (V.N. de Gaia—led by José Rocha Melo (1996) and later (1997) Matosinhos—led by José Rocha Melo) and two on the outskirts of Lisbon (Almada—led by Augusto Goulão, a former President of SPNR, and Amadora/Sintra—led by Rui Manaças, also a former President of SPNR).

The 1990s also saw the widespread adoption of MRI in diagnosing neurological and neurosurgical diseases. It is noteworthy that, as with CT in the 1980s, it was private initiatives by medical enterprises that facilitated patients' access to this then-revolutionary imaging technology. The dedication of many professionals led to the pioneering establishment of RM Caselas in Lisbon (Cruz Maurício, Eduardo Medina, Augusto Goulão, among others), SMIC in Porto (Almeida Pinto, Moreira Maia, Romeu Cruz, among others), and IMACENTRO and DIATOM in Coimbra (Faria Pais, Sousa Fernandes, among others). At the turn of the millennium, the Portuguese neuroradiology community had about 100 specialists; today, that number has grown to more than 250.

The first decade of this millennium saw the consolidation of Neuroradiology, with expanded diagnostic capabilities (most large centers now have two MRI machines and three CT scanners) and a growing focus on Interventional Neuroradiology.

In the North, four major hospitals have closely followed the growth of Neurology and Neurosurgery: two in Porto (the University Hospital Center of Porto, including the historic Hospital de Santo António, and the University Hospital Center of São João), one in Braga (also a University Hospital), and another in Vila Nova de Gaia.

In Porto's neuroradiology history, the key institutions are Hospital de Santo António and Hospital de São João. The former is considered the cradle of Portuguese Neuroradiology, where in the 1960s Paulo Mendo, one of the first Portuguese neuroradiologists, who started as Dr. Corino de Andrade's neurology fellow, was oriented by him to create the Neuroradiology Laboratory—the foundation of the first neuroradiology department in a public hospital in Portugal. Subsequent department heads in Santo António included José de Almeida Pinto, Romeu Cruz, and currently, João Xavier. In 2007, this hospital became part of the Porto Hospital and University Centre, incorporating the Maria Pia Paediatric Hospital and the Júlio Dinis Maternity

Hospital, followed by the Joaquim Urbano Psychiatric Hospital and the Dr. Jacinto Magalhães Medical Genetics Center in 2011.

Several key milestones in neuroradiology in northern Portugal are attributed to this group at Santo António: the installation of the first public hospital CT scanner in 1983, the first digital subtraction angiography (DSA) in 1994, the first cerebral aneurysm treated with GDC coils in 1995, the first intra-arterial thrombolysis in acute stroke in 1996, and the first mechanical thrombectomy in 2008. The 50th anniversary of the Neuroradiology Service at Hospital de Santo António was marked in 2016 with an international symposium, the "Oporto Neuroradiology 50th Anniversary International Symposium," and the publication of a commemorative book, *50 years—50 cases... and a few more from our friends*. In 2018, the service published another book, *Diagnostic and Therapeutic Neuroradiology: A Case-Based Guide to Good Practice* (João Xavier, Cristina Vasconcelos, Cristina Ramos, editors, Springer International Publishing AG, Cham, Switzerland, 2018).

At São João Hospital, neuroradiology began in the late 1960s under Joaquim Cruz as part of the neurosurgery service. By the early 1980s, with the advent of CT scanning, neuroradiology was separated from Neurosurgery and integrated into the Imaging Service. After Joaquim Cruz's retirement, the department was led by António Salgado and is currently directed by José Fonseca.

Pedro Hispano Hospital in Matosinhos also deserves recognition for its innovative model that directly integrates primary care services with the main hospital—the first in Portugal. Established in 1997, the neuroradiology department, initially led by José Rocha Melo, later by Pedro Moniz, and now by Ana Mafalda Reis, has advanced medical care, namely with pioneering minimally invasive spine interventions. Pedro Hispano Hospital also hosted the European Course on Spine Radiology, 2nd Cycle Module 1, in Porto from March 23–26, 2022, and since then, it annually hosts an International Spine Interventional Course (INSIC) also endorsed by the European Society of Neuroradiology (ESNR) (Fig. 15.1).

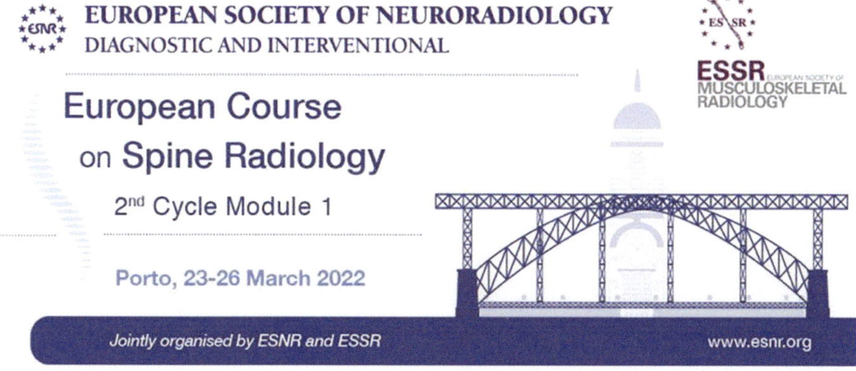

Fig. 15.1 European Course on Spine Radiology, 2nd Cycle Module 1, Porto March 23–26, 2022

In the central region, the University Hospital in Coimbra, formed from the merger of the University Hospital of Coimbra (HUC) and Coimbra Hospital Centre (CHC), also has a rich history in Neuroradiology. Key figures in the 1970s and 1980s included José de Sousa Fernandes (HUC) and Francisco Faria Pais (CHC), both of whom were founders of the Portuguese Nucleus of Neuroradiology, the precursor to the SPNR. Successive heads of neuroradiology have included Francisco Martins, Teresa Garcia, Cristina Moura, and currently, Egídio Machado. This hospital was the first in Portugal to offer an emergency rota of interventional neuroradiologists for Mechanical Thrombectomy, effective January 2, 2015—just one day after the scientific evidence for its efficacy was published.

In Lisbon, three major hospitals have been central to the practice and teaching of neuroradiology for decades. The Western Lisbon University and Hospital Center comprises Egas Moniz Hospital, Francisco Xavier Hospital, and Santa Cruz Hospital. Established in 2005, it coordinates clinical activities across a broad area of Lisbon. The Neuroscience Department, including Neuroradiology, primarily operates within Egas Moniz Hospital, which has a storied history. Founded in 1902 as Hospital Colonial de Lisboa, it initially served overseas military personnel, focusing on infectious diseases. After expansions, it was renamed Hospital do Ultramar in 1957, and following the 1974 revolution, it became Hospital de Egas Moniz.

The public hospital has played a foundational role in Portuguese Neuroradiology, establishing one of the first national departments. Professor Jaime Cruz Maurício, the founder and first head of the neuroradiology department, was also one of the founders of the "Núcleo Português de Neurorradiologia," the precursor to the SPNR. Successive department heads included Constança Jordão, Gabriel Branco, Pedro Soares, and currently, Pedro Vilela, a former SPNR President and President of the 44th ESNR Congress. The department has been at the forefront of innovations such as endovascular neuroradiology and the introduction of CT, training many of the country's leading neuroradiologists. Special mention goes to Professor Augusto Goulão, the department's first fellow, ESNR honorary member, and former SPNR President.

Today, the Neuroscience Department at WL-ULS (HEM) is known for its excellence in clinical and research activities, housing national reference centers in Interventional Neuroradiology, epilepsy surgery, and related areas such as cochlear implantation (Fig. 15.2).

Secondly, it is worth highlighting the role of HCL—Civilian Hospitals of Lisbon (as it was known at the time), where neuroradiology began formally in 1980, although informal practices date back earlier. Initially, it was conducted by neurosurgeons and neurologists who developed an affinity for the angiography room (used for angiography and pneumoencephalography) and the operating room with an X-ray machine (used for ventriculographies). These practitioners, led by Fernando Costa Reis, later dedicated themselves full-time to Neuroradiology, with Costa Reis recognized as the founder of the specialty in these hospitals.

At that time, these hospitals included Capuchos Hospital and São José Hospital, where the Neurology and Neurosurgery Services were based, alongside Curry Cabral Hospital (infectious diseases), Dona Estefânia Hospital (Pediatrics), and Santa Marta Hospital (Cardiovascular). Notably, it was at Santa Marta Hospital

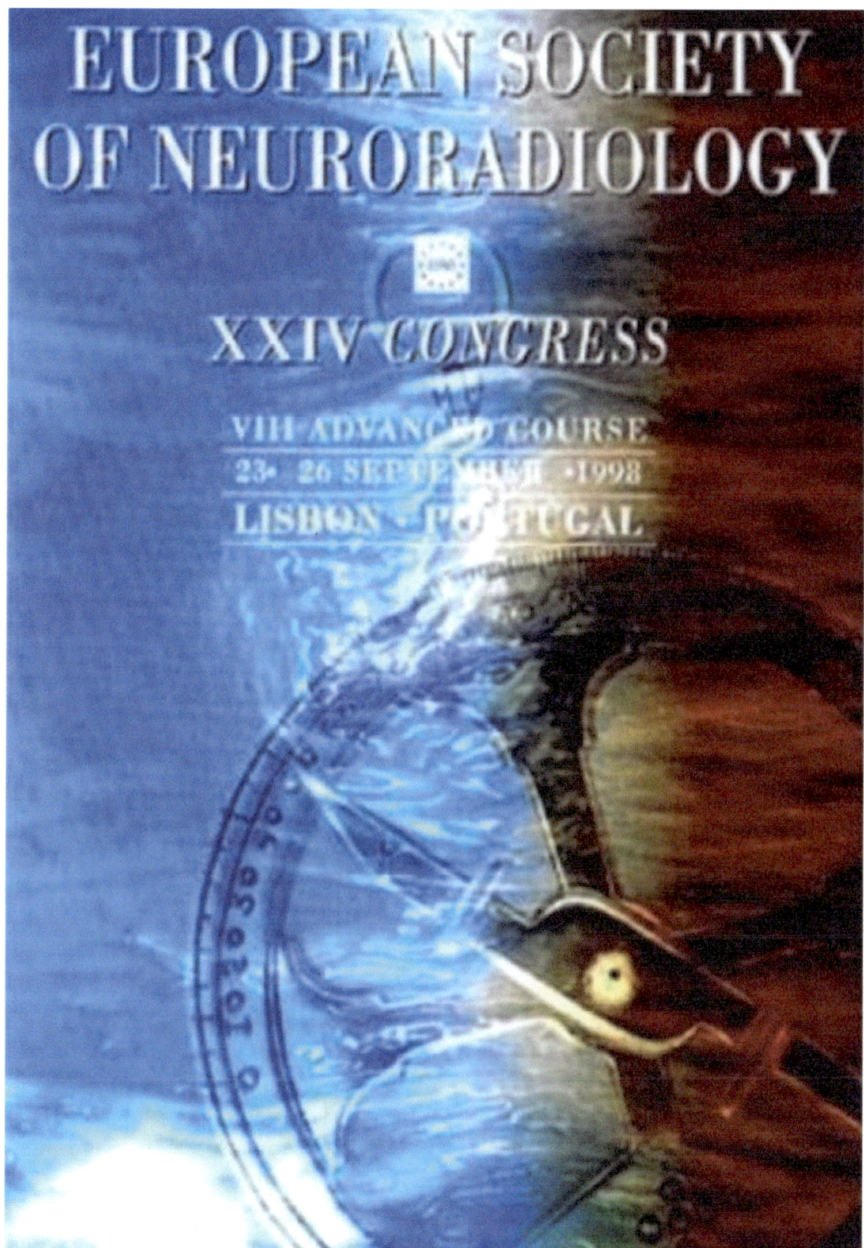

Fig. 15.2 XXIV ESNR Congress, Lisbon 1998

where Egas Moniz performed the first angiography in 1927. These institutions are historic, some originating as old monasteries, and one even predates the devastating earthquake and fire that struck Lisbon in 1755 (Fig. 15.3).

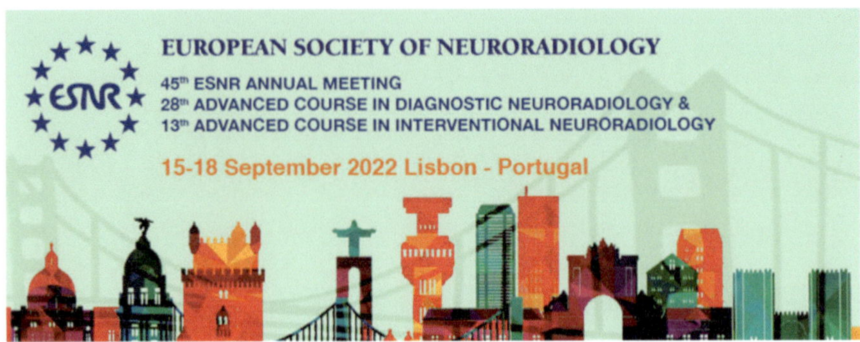

Fig. 15.3 45th ESNR Annual Meeting, Lisbon 2022

The Neuroradiology Unit was formally established in 1980, with the first fellows, João Reis and Rui Manaças, beginning their specialization in 1982. Both would later become Service Directors and prominent leaders of the specialty in Portugal in the following decades. During the 1990s, these hospitals split services: São José Hospital retained diagnostic neuroradiology (initially with only CT scans) and launched interventional neuroradiology, under João Reis as director of service, while Capuchos Hospital focused solely on diagnostics, bolstered in 1998 by one of the first MRI installations in Lisbon's public hospitals.

São José Hospital quickly became a pioneer in several vascular intervention techniques and spinal procedures. The first stroke treatment took place in 1999 using mechanical thrombolysis with a Sentry microballoon in a 20-year-old patient. In 1999 and 2000, the first stroke treatments using intra-arterial streptokinase were performed in the middle, anterior, and posterior cerebral arteries, both in proximal and distal segments. Additionally, in 2000, the first intracranial stent in Portugal was placed, and the first vertebroplasty was also performed. Over the subsequent years, the hospital was at the forefront of adopting new devices for stroke treatment, including the Stentriever Merci in 2003 and the TREVO and Solitaire devices in 2005.

In spinal care, São José Hospital also demonstrated a pioneering spirit. Besides the first vertebroplasty in 2000, the hospital introduced the first treatment for herniated discs using gelled alcohol in 2009, followed by the first intradiscal ozone therapy in 2012. Over the past 25 years, a remarkable generation of Interventional Neuroradiologists—around 14 in total—have passed through São José Hospital, many of whom now working in Central and Northern Portugal.

Today, at the Centro Hospitalar e Universitário de Lisboa Central (its current name), the neuroradiology department is led by João Reis and stands as the leading service in the country in terms of the number of specialists, fellows, and neuroradiological activities, both diagnostic and therapeutic.

In the third and largest hospital in Lisbon, Hospital de Santa Maria—now known as Centro Hospitalar Universitário de Lisboa Norte, formed by the merger of Hospital Santa Maria and Hospital Pulido Valente (the latter significant in early twentieth-century tuberculosis treatment)—there has also been a significant history in Neurosciences. Built in 1954, Santa Maria has a long tradition in this field, with its first Neurology Department established by Almeida Lima in 1954, later led by prominent figures such as neurologist José Ferro, known for his research in cerebral venous thrombosis, and neurosurgeon João Lobo Antunes, a former President of the European Society of Neurosurgery and a leading figure in Medical Neurosciences in Portugal and Europe. The Neurosciences Department even houses the Museum of Egas Moniz.

Much of the impetus for neuroradiology at this hospital was the result of the close collaboration with the neurology and neurosurgery departments, who helped to promote interventional neuroradiology as the future key choice for many neurovascular diseases. Neuroradiology began a bit later at Santa Maria, in the mid-1980s, with the arrival of Jorge Guedes de Campos. Although the neuroradiology fellowship only started in 2000, this did not prevent the hospital from becoming a center of excellence and a reference point for clinical practice, research, and teaching in neuroradiology in Portugal.

Jorge Guedes de Campos pioneered several interventional techniques in Portugal, including the first aneurysm treatment with GDC coils in 1993, performed in collaboration with Pedro Lylyk. The hospital was also the first in Portugal to use liquid embolic agents to treat AVMs and AVFs. More recently, with contributions from other team members, it introduced techniques such as balloon remodeling for aneurysm treatment and was the first to use flow diverters for brain aneurysms in the country. The department, currently headed by Graça Sá, hosts a large number of specialists and fellows and remains a pillar of teaching, research, and clinical care in Lisbon, its surroundings, and the southern region of Portugal. The department is recognized as a national reference center in Interventional Neuroradiology.

Jorge Campos also played a crucial role in organizing the 1999 WFITN congress in Portugal, held in Vilamoura, Algarve. He was a founding member of SILAN (Ibero-Latin American Society of Neuroradiology) in 1989, alongside pioneers like Fernando Vinuela and Juan Taveras, among others from Spain and Latin America. The first SILAN Congress was held in La Coruña in June 1989, followed by the second in Cascais, Portugal, in June 1990, with Jorge Campos serving as President. He also served as SILAN President from 1993 to 1995.

Several SILAN Congresses have been organized in Portugal, including one in June 1998 in Porto, with Joaquim Cruz as President, another in June 2003 in Estoril, with Carlos Morgado as President, one in October 2011 in Cascais, with Luísa Biscoito as President, and one in September 2019 in Porto, with Cláudia Pereira as President. Luísa Biscoito also served as SILAN President from 2017 to 2019 (Figs. 15.4 and 15.5).

One of the areas that has seen the most significant development in the past 7 years is the treatment of acute stroke, particularly following the establishment of Metropolitan Emergency Units in Porto and Lisbon in 2017. This initiative institutionalized reference centers for interventional neuroradiology in several locations: Braga, three hospitals in Porto/Vila Nova de Gaia, a central hospital in Coimbra,

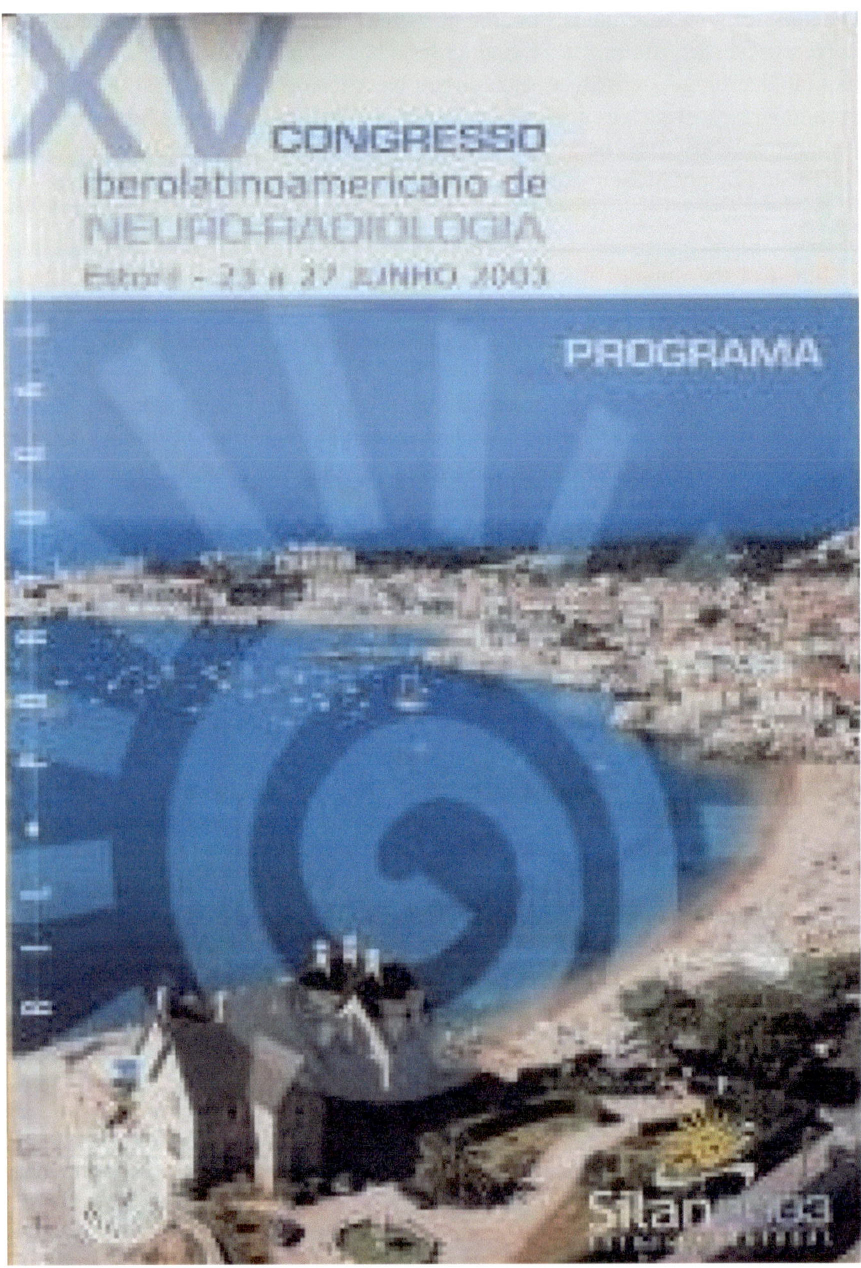

Fig. 15.4 XV Congress of SILAN, 2003, Estoril

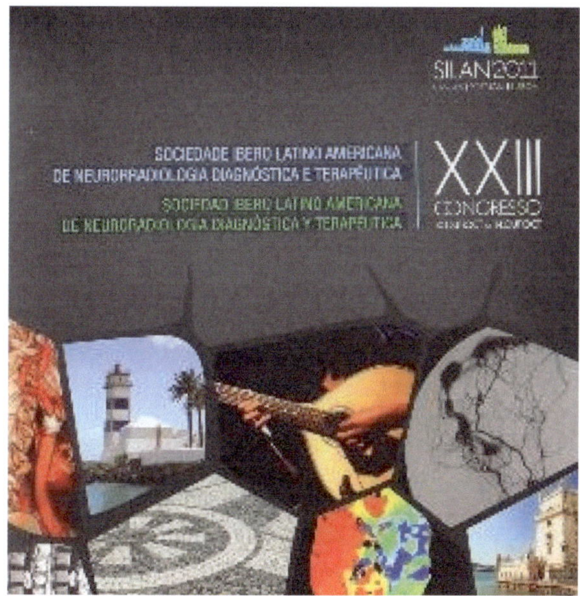

Fig. 15.5 XXIII Congress of SILAN, 2011, Cascais

and four hospitals in Greater Lisbon (three in Lisbon and Garcia de Orta Hospital in Almada). According to recent data, Portugal ranks among the top European countries in terms of the number of thrombectomies performed annually.

Two other hospitals in the Lisbon area also deserve to be mentioned, where neuroradiology departments were established by former neuroradiology fellows from the renowned Egas Moniz and Capuchos Hospitals. Garcia de Orta Hospital (founded in 1992 by Augusto Goulão) is a national reference center for Interventional Neuroradiology, co-chaired with Egas Moniz Hospital. The department has since been led by Maria Júlia Duarte and is currently headed by Cristina Rios. Another notable institution is Fernando Fonseca Hospital (founded in 1995 by Rui Manaças), which serves a large population in the western outskirts of Lisbon. This hospital has active Neurology, Ophthalmology, and Otolaryngology departments. In the late 1990s, the first digital subtraction dacryocystography was performed here, and several stents were implanted to treat nasolacrimal duct obstructions (led by Luisa Biscoito).

As previously mentioned, Portuguese neuroradiology currently has more than 250 doctors, distributed across approximately eleven hospitals from Braga to Faro. The specialty is supported by two scientific societies and is bolstered by a new generation of well-prepared professionals, ready to meet the significant challenges ahead. These challenges include the internationalization of the specialty, the free movement of professionals within the European space, and the growth of subspecialties such as interventional neuroradiology, head and neck imaging, and pediatric neuroradiology.

Much of the current success of Portuguese neuroradiology as an Autonomous Medical Specialty is due to the path, let's say original, of how training in neuroradiology is done in Portugal: since the 1980s, when it was created as a Hospital Specialty, which has been autonomous since its inception and not as in most countries, from which it derives from Radiology (with a common trunk of at least 3 years).

To conclude, quoting José Almeida Pinto, one of the founding fathers of Portuguese Neuroradiology, (October, 2020):

> *It is my pleasure to note that: (a) there is a progressive continuum between the beginning and the now; (b) the seed that the elders sowed more than 50 years ago has germinated and blossomed into the specialty we have today—indisputably beautiful, cultured, and now respected, which it wasn't always".*

Acknowledgment Special thanks are extended to Jaime Pamplona, João Xavier, Egídio Machado, and Pedro Vilela for their contributions to the preparation of this text.

Chapter 16
SILAN Society: History and International Impact 1988–2024

Ramón E. Figueroa

The Sociedad Ibero Latino Americana de Neurorradiología Diagnóstica y Terapéutica (also known as "SILAN") is an international professional nonprofit society constituted by 560 registered Spanish and/or Portuguese-speaking members from all countries in America, plus Spain and Portugal. From its inception in 1988 to the present, its main goal has been to advance the field of diagnostic and interventional neuroradiology in all its member countries through educational seminars, annual scientific meetings, and the sponsorship of international training scholarships in both diagnostic and interventional neuroradiology for young graduating residents from Radiology, Neurology, and Neurosurgery programs.

The origins of SILAN are traced to November 13, 1988, when a group of 24 Latin-American, Spanish, and Portuguese internationally recognized leaders coordinated by Dr. Fernando Viñuela (at the time the chief of Endovascular Therapy at UCLA) met at the XXIII Latin American Congress of Neurological Surgery in Acapulco, Mexico. The idea of advancing neuroradiology in Latin America through the creation of a Spanish and Portuguese-speaking neuroradiological society coalesced at this meeting. The initial Executive Committee was constituted by the elected President Dr. Juan M. Taveras (originally from Dominican Republic, who at the time was Chairman Emeritus of Radiology at Harvard's Massachusetts General Hospital); Dr. Jesús Rodriguez Carvajal as Vice President (who was the chief of neuroradiology at the National Institute of Neurosurgery and Neurology in Mexico City); Dr. Jorge Guedes Campos as Secretary (who was chief of neuroradiology at Hospital Santa Maria in Lisbon, Portugal); and Dr. Fernando Viñuela as Treasurer (originally from Uruguay, then chief of interventional neuroradiology at UCLA, Los Angeles, USA). The logo of SILAN was created at this time (Fig. 16.1), under the inspiration and guidance of Dr. Juan M. Taveras, the first president of

R. E. Figueroa (✉)
Emeritus Professor of Neuroradiology, Medical College of Georgia at Augusta University, Augusta, GA, USA

D. Birchall (ed.), *A World History of Neuroradiology*,
https://doi.org/10.1007/978-3-032-16653-1_16

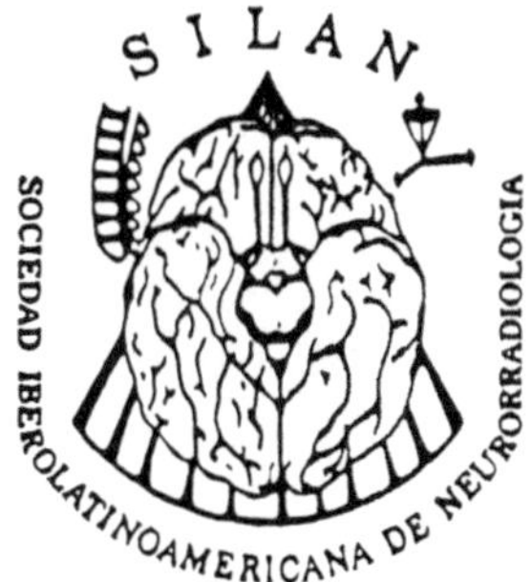

Fig. 16.1 The SILAN logo shows a base view of the brain overlying a CT x-ray fan beam, with a multidetector CT array on the left side and the symbol of a spinning proton referencing Magnetic Resonance Imaging on the right side of the brain. The name of the society outlines the lateral and inferior margins

SILAN. In addition, four Members of the Board were also selected to increase the membership representation and assist the elected officers in their functions: Drs. Jorge Vázquez Rebollar (Galicia, Spain), Bernardo Boleaga Durán (Mexico, DF), Genaro Herrera García (Lima, Perú) and Enrique Palacios Mayorga (Chicago, USA). (Fig. 16.2b).

The main goals for the establishment of SILAN were to bring together all Spanish- and Portuguese-speaking radiologists, neurologists, and neurosurgeons devoted to the practice of the different fields within neuroradiology, to establish a professional society that could represent our particular identity and needs, and to support the professional development of its members. From the outset, there was a unanimous decision to have annual scientific meetings in different countries, alternating between Spain and Portugal 1 year, followed by three sequential annual meetings in different countries in Latin America. At the time, only the United States had a formally established national neuroradiological society (American Society of Neuroradiology, founded by Dr. Taveras and 23 additional founding members in New York City in 1964). It was the first specific goal of SILAN to use the annual scientific meetings to foster the creation and to strengthen national neuroradiological societies in each one of the individual member countries. The second specific goal of SILAN was to bring state-of-the-art neuroradiological education to the member countries, presented preferentially in Spanish or Portuguese, the official languages of the society. This was an imperative for the development of local societies since language barriers made it difficult for the audiences to absorb difficult imaging or therapeutic concepts in those days. Our meetings are still conducted in Spanish and Portuguese, with the non-member guest speakers usually presenting in English, with available simultaneous translation for the participants who may need it. The third specific goal of SILAN was to develop centers of excellence in different countries where SILAN could sponsor young radiologists, neurologists, and neurosurgeons who would compete for training scholarships in both diagnostic and interventional neuroradiology, and then return to their countries of origin after completion

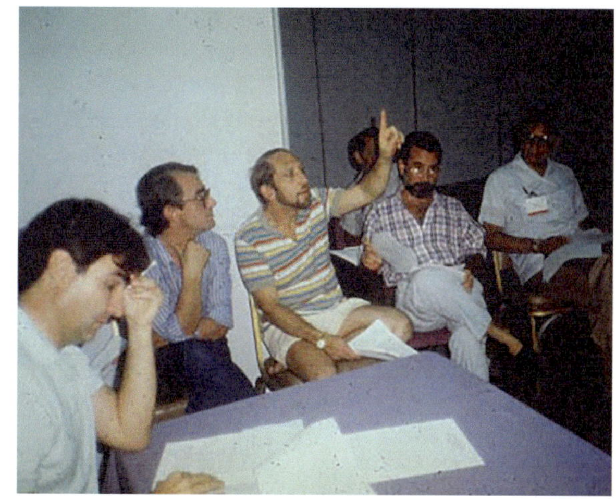

Fig. 16.2 Founding meeting of SILAN, Acapulco, Mexico, November 1988: Planning sessions with Founding members from left to right Fernando Viñuela, Eduardo García Cervigón, Alex Berenstein, Jorge Vázquez Rebollar, and Jesús Rodriguez Carvajal

of their training, thus improving the availability and expertise of neuroradiology practitioners across our member countries.

SILAN was registered as a nonprofit organization in Mexico City on June 22, 1989. Since its inception, SILAN has continued to grow each year, with Spanish or Portuguese-speaking members in both the diagnostic and therapeutic neuroradiology categories, representing Spain, Portugal, Brazil, and most other countries in North, Central, and South America.

The 24 founding members of SILAN were Dr. Alejandro Berenstein (USA), Dr. Bernardo Boleaga Durán (México), Dr. Francisco Correa-Paz (USA), Dr. Roque H. Ferreiro Irigoyen (México), Dr. Eduardo Floriani Raupp (Brazil), Dr. Eduardo García Cervigón (Spain), Dr. Jorge Guedes Campos (Portugal), Dr. Genaro Herrera García (Perú), Dr. José Luis Jiménez (México), Dr. Luis A. Lemme Plaghos (Argentina), Dr. Pedro Lylyk (Argentina), Dr. Marco A. H. Modesto (Brazil), Dr. Ernesto Mena (Guatemala), Dr. Carlos Muñoz Rivera (México), Dr. Enrique Palacios Mayorga (USA), Dr. Leopoldo José de Paula Assis (Canada), Dr. Ramón Peña Álvarez (México), Dr. Jesús Rodríguez Carvajal (México), Dr. Jordi Ruscalleda (Spain), Dr. José Antonio Santoyo Vázquez (México), Dr. Juan M. Taveras (USA), Dr. Jorge Vázquez Rebollar (Spain), Dr. Fernando Viñuela (USA), and Dr. Marco A. Zenteno (México).

The past presidents of SILAN since the establishment of the society in 1988 follow, in chronological order: Dr. Juan M. Taveras (USA, 1988–1991), Dr. Jesús Rodríguez Carvajal (México, 1991–1993), Dr. Jorge Guedes Campos (Portugal, 1993–1995), Dr. Fernando Viñuela (USA, 1995–1997), Dr. Jordi Ruscalleda (Spain, 1997–1999), Dr. Pedro Lylyk (Argentina, 1999–2001), Dr. Ramón E. Figueroa (USA, 2001–2003), Dr. Claudio Cesar Vilela Staut (Brazil, 2003–2005), Dr. Fernando Gómez Villafañe (Colombia, 2005–2007), Dr. Eduardo González Toledo (Argentina, 2007–2009), Dr. Teresa Sola Martínez (Spain, 2009–2011), Dr. Alejandro Berenstein (USA, 2011–2013), Dr. Rafael Rojas Jasso (USA, 2013–2015),

Dr. Orlando Diaz Daza (USA, 2015–2017), Dr. Luisa Biscoito (Portugal, 2017–2019), Dr. José Manuel Pumar (Spain, 2019–2022), Dr. Carlos Torres (Canada, 2022–2024), Dr. Roy Riascos (USA, 2024–2026).

Since its establishment as a professional society, SILAN has sponsored 33 annual meetings, only missing years 2020 and 2021 due to the COVID-19 global pandemic, when we sponsored web-based seminars instead. There are already two additional meetings scheduled for 2024 and 2025. The previous and future annual meetings are as follows:

SILAN I in La Coruña, Spain (June 1989). Fig. 16.3b.
SILAN II in Cascais, Portugal (June 1990).
SILAN III in Guadalajara, México (October 1991). Fig. 16.4b.
SILAN IV in Santo Domingo, Dominican Republic (December 1992).
SILAN V in Florianopolis, Brazil (October 1993).
SILAN VI in Madrid, Spain (June 1994). Fig. 16.5c.
SILAN VII in Buenos Aires, Argentina (October 1995).
SILAN VIII in Caracas, Venezuela (October 1996).
SILAN IX in Quito, Ecuador (October 1997). Fig. 16.6c.
SILAN X in Porto, Portugal (June 1998).
SILAN XI in La Coruña, Spain (September 1999).
SILAN XII in Punta del Este, Uruguay (December 2000).
SILAN XIII in Cartagena de Indias, Colombia (October 2001). Fig. 16.7a, b.
SILAN XIV in Pucón, Chile (November 2002).
SILAN XV in Estoril, Portugal (June 2003).
SILAN XVI in Salvador de Bahía, Brazil (November, 2004).
SILAN XVII in Lima, Perú (September 2005).
SILAN XVIII in San Juan, Puerto Rico (June 2006). Fig. 16.8c.
SILAN XIX in Seville, Spain (April 2007).
SILAN XX in Cancún, México (September 2008).

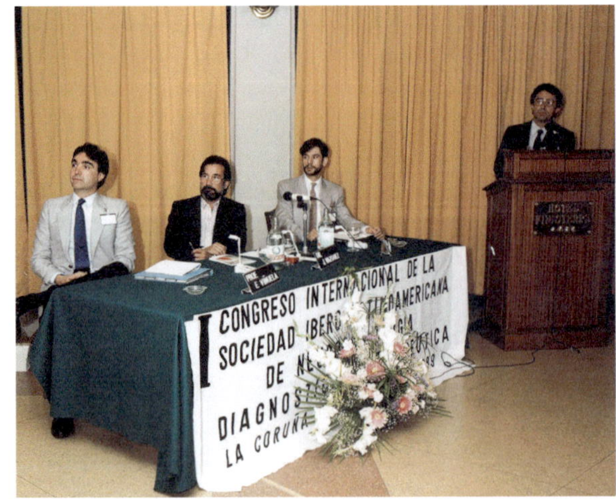

Fig. 16.3 SILAN first annual congress in La Coruña, Spain June, 1989: Presiding table on Scientific Presentations session, from left to right, Drs. Fernando Viñuela, Jorge Vazquez Rebollar, and Jorge Guedes Campos at the podium

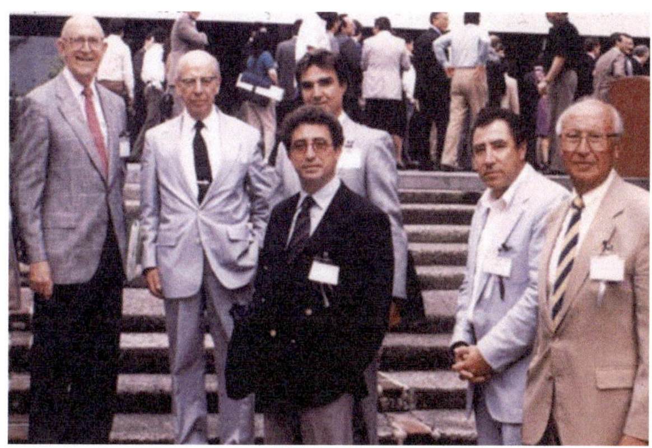

Fig. 16.4 SILAN III Annual Congress, Guadalajara, Mexico, September 1991: Meeting faculty from left to right Drs. Juan M. Taveras, Manuel Velazco Suarez (founder of the National Institute of Neurosurgery and Neurology of Mexico), Fernando Viñuela, Jorge Guedes Campos, Enrique Palacios Mayorga, and Jesús Rodriguez Carvajal, III congress president

SILAN XXI in Isla Margarita, Venezuela (October 2009).
SILAN XXII in Buenos Aires, Argentina (November 2010). Fig. 16.9a, c.
SILAN XXIII in Cascais, Portugal (October 2011).
SILAN XXIV in Quito, Ecuador (October 2012).
SILAN XXV in Ciudad de Panamá, Panamá (June 2013).
SILAN XXVI in Sao Paulo, Brazil (November 2014).
SILAN XXVII in Santiago de Compostela, Spain (June 2015). Fig. 16.10c.
SILAN XXVIII in Cartagena de Indias, Colombia (September 2016).
SILAN XXIX in San Juan, Puerto Rico (September 2017).
SILAN XXX in La Habana, Cuba (July 2018).
SILAN XXXI in Porto, Portugal (October 2019). Fig. 16.11b.
SILAN XXXII in Montevideo, Uruguay (October 2022) Fig. 16.12a.
SILAN XXXIII in Punta Cana, Dominican Republic (October 2023) Fig. 16.13b.
SILAN XXXIV in Puerto Varas, Chile (scheduled for next October 23–26, 2024).
SILAN XXXV in Barcelona, Spain (scheduled for October 2025).

SILAN as a society emphasizes the development of new neuroradiology professionals by providing opportunities to access advanced training for physicians who have completed their primary specialty training (Radiology, Neurology, or Neurosurgery) and who want to acquire advanced skills in Diagnostic or Interventional Neuroradiology. SILAN authorized the funding support for the first two initial scholarships in November 1995.

The *SILAN-MCG* visiting fellowship in Diagnostic Neuroradiology was established at the Medical College of Georgia (Dr. Ramón E. Figueroa as program director), receiving six radiology, neurology, or neurosurgery senior residents per year, each one for 2 months of intense neuroradiology training. This scholarship served as a talent screening site for further selection of potential candidates for full-length

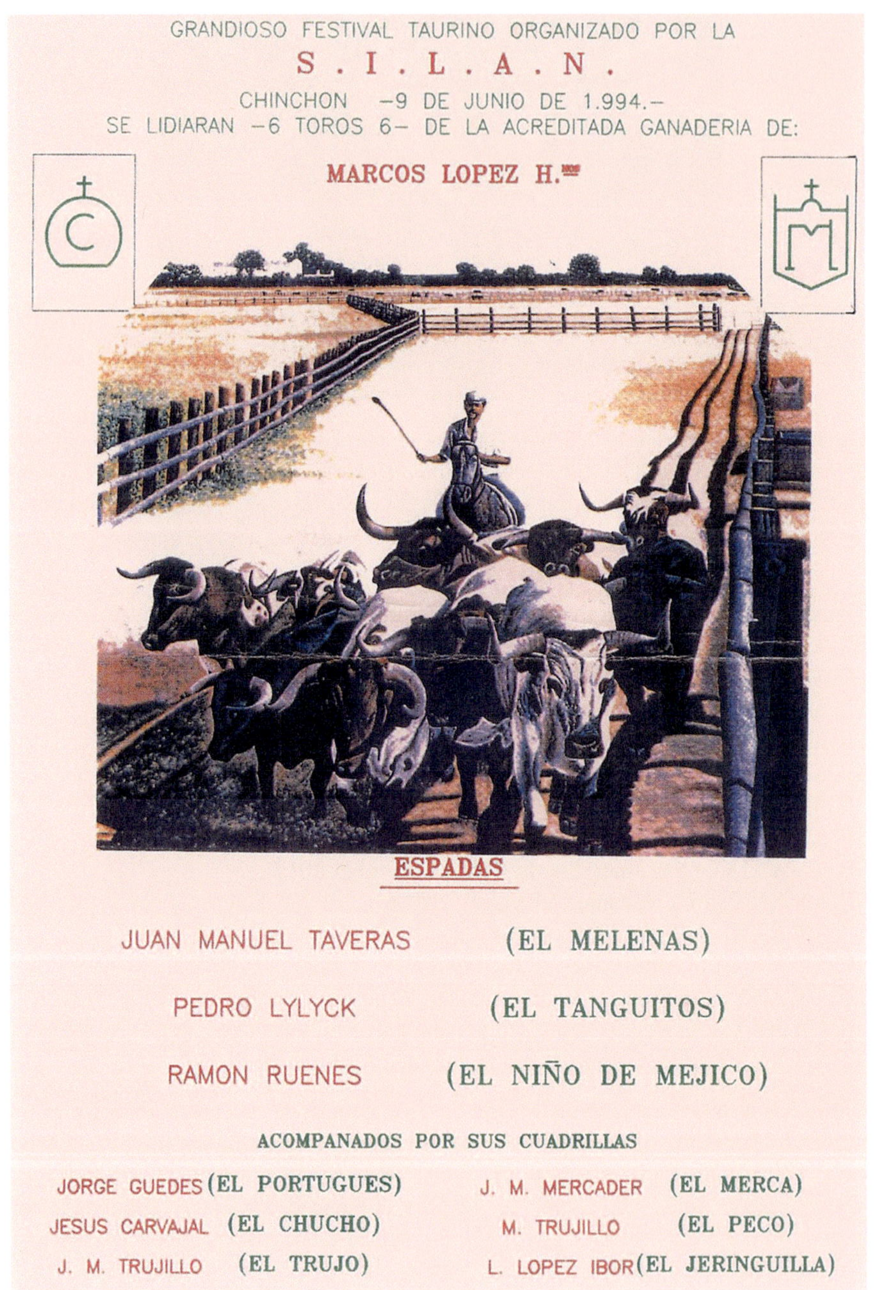

Fig. 16.5 SILAN VI Annual Congress, Madrid, Spain, June 1994: Poster for the friendship afternoon with many distinguished speakers posing as bullfighters (names in red)

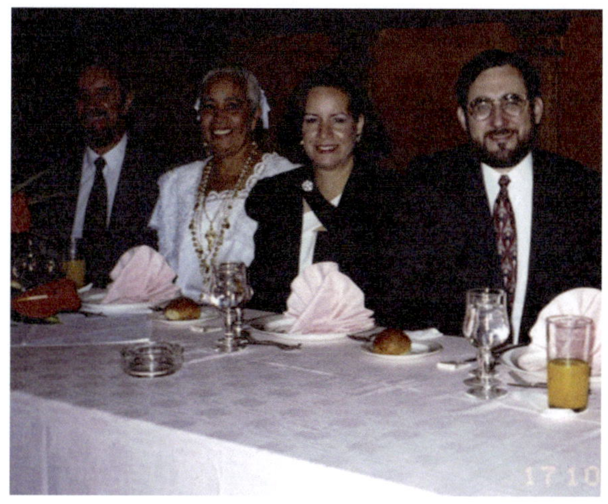

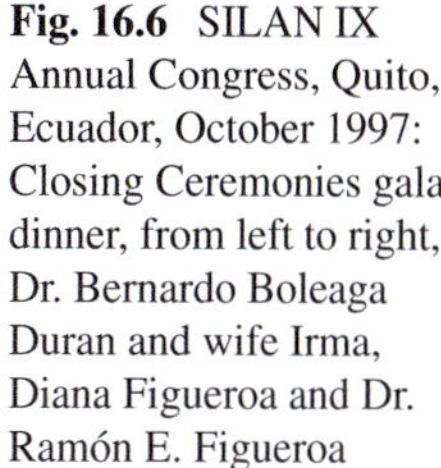

Fig. 16.6 SILAN IX Annual Congress, Quito, Ecuador, October 1997: Closing Ceremonies gala dinner, from left to right, Dr. Bernardo Boleaga Duran and wife Irma, Diana Figueroa and Dr. Ramón E. Figueroa

1-year training programs sponsored by SILAN. After 26 years of continuous training and receiving 154 SILAN fellows (of which 96 are now practicing neuroradiologists), this program closed when Dr. Figueroa retired in 2023, with the program transitioning to the University of Texas in Houston in July 2024, under the leadership of Dr. Roy Riascos as program director (Dr. Riascos himself is a former 2003 SILAN-MCG fellow and now is the chief of Neuroradiology at UT Houston).

The first 1-year interventional neuroradiology training program was the *SILAN-ENERI* fellowship at the ENERI Institute in Buenos Aires, Argentina, with Dr. Pedro Lylyk as program director, starting in 1996, with one fellow chosen per year. Due to the success of this program, it was increased to two scholarships per year shortly before the year 2000 and later expanded to a 2-year format. This program continues to the present time, with nearly 50 graduates representing a significant portion of the active neurointerventional specialists in current practice across Latin America.

Additional diagnostic and interventional neuroradiology training programs financially supported by SILAN were progressively incorporated, as new training centers and program directors were identified in various countries. The new sites were selected based on their recognition as international centers of excellence, and where SILAN members were in leadership and teaching positions, thus opening further training opportunities over the years. These programs include the following sites:

SILAN-HUGC Neurointerventional, a 1-year program established in 2003, hosted at the Hospital Universitario General de Cataluña in Barcelona, Spain, receiving one fellow per year (see Fig. 16.14). Program directors at the start of the program were Drs. Teresa Sola and Leopoldo Guimaraens. Dr. Guimaraens continues until today as program director. Approximately 20 fellows have been trained, with this program now offering an optional second year of training.

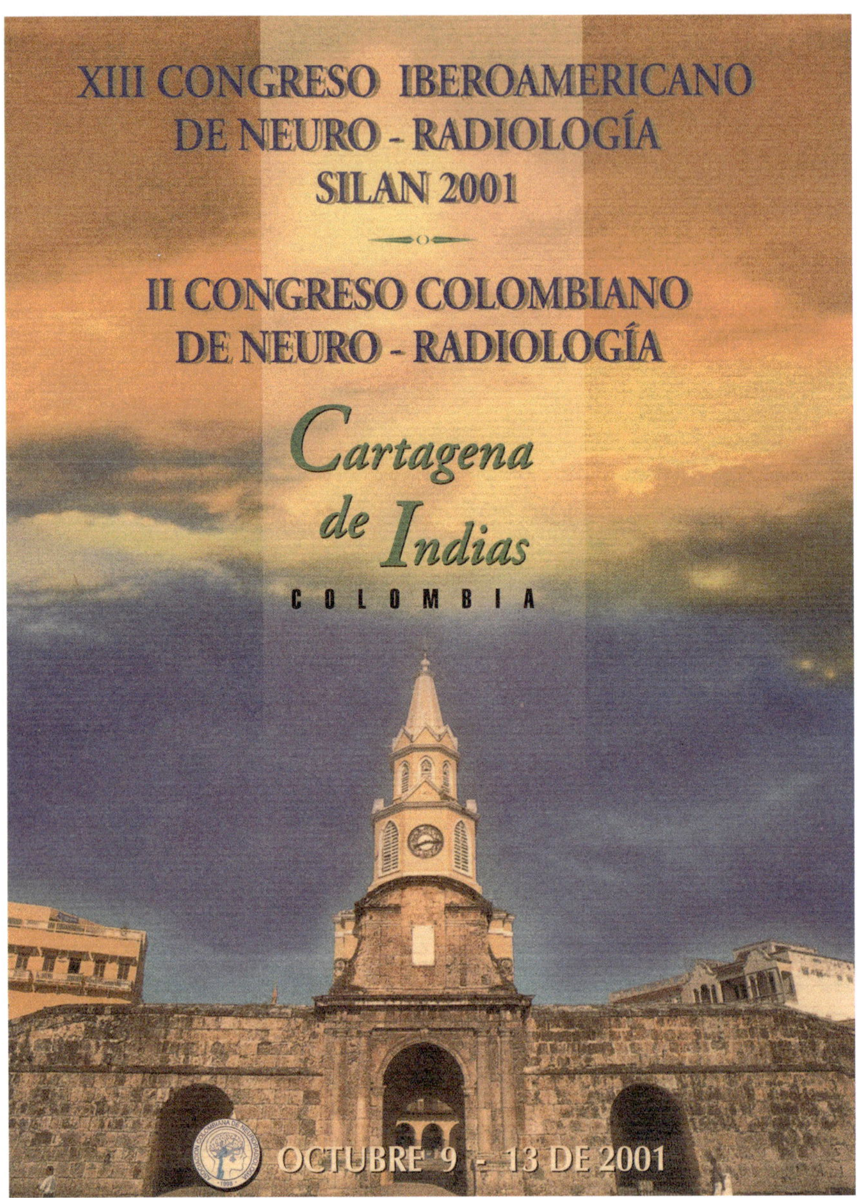

Fig. 16.7 SILAN XIII Annual Congress, Cartagena de Indias, Colombia, October 2001: Poster for SILAN XIII Annual Congress. Present and past presidents of SILAN, from left to right Dr. Fernando Gomez Villafane, president of the XII annual congress, Dr. Ramón E. Figueroa (present SILAN President 2001–2003), past presidents Dr. Pedro Lylyk (1999–2001), Dr. Jordi Ruscalleda (1997–1999), Dr. Jorge Guedes Campos (1993–1995), Dr. Jesus Rodriguez Carvajal (1991–1993) and Dr. Juan M. Taveras (1989–1991)

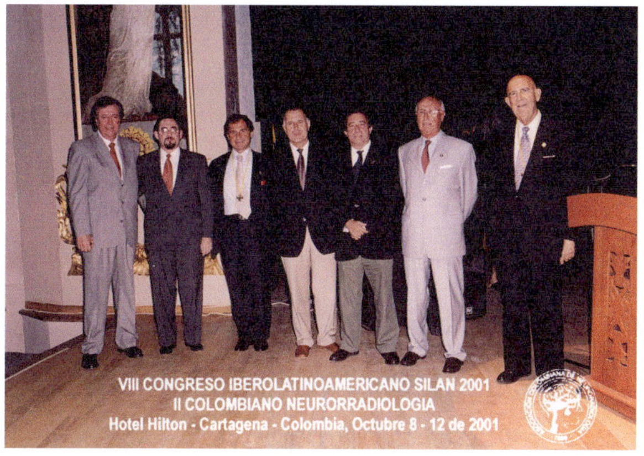

Fig. 16.7 (continued)

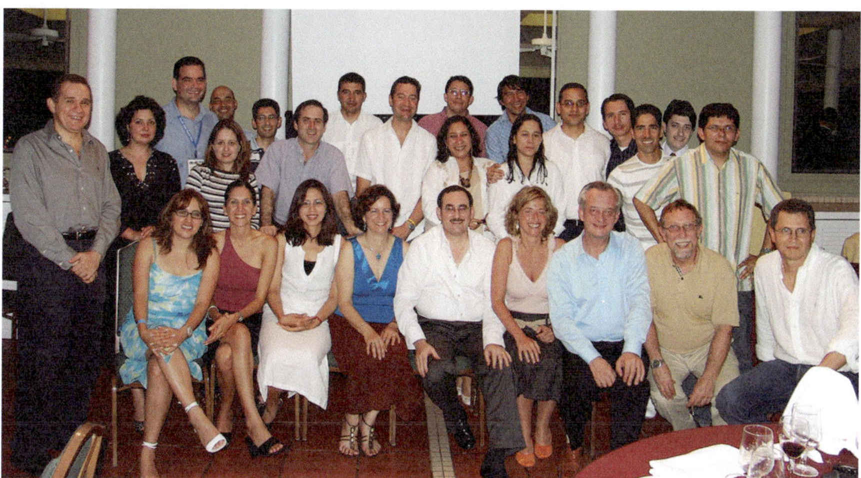

Fig. 16.8 SILAN XVIII Annual Congress, San Juan, Puerto Rico (June 2006): First annual meeting of SILAN fellows from SILAN-MCG, SILAN-ENERI, SILAN-HUGC, and SILAN-Zaragoza scholarship programs. Since the 2006 SILAN meeting, fellows present at each annual congress join for a fellowship dinner on the second night of congress

SILAN-Zaragoza Diagnostic neuroradiology, a 1-year training program sponsored by Dr. Nicolas Fayed Miguel at the Hospital Universitario Grupo Quirón, in Zaragoza, Spain. This program ran from 2004 to 2012, training eight diagnostic neuroradiologists, closing after the program director retired.

SILAN-Vall d'Hebrón Diagnostic Neuroradiology Program A 1-year diagnostic neuroradiology program with Dr. Alex Rovira as program director, chief of neuroradiology at the Vall d'Hebrón Hospital in Barcelona, Spain. This program, with

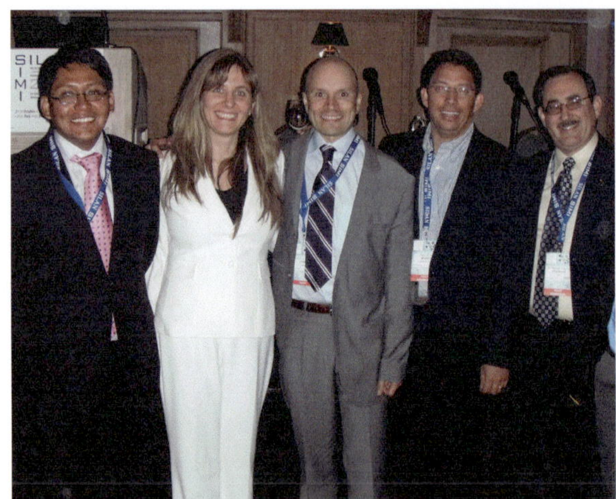

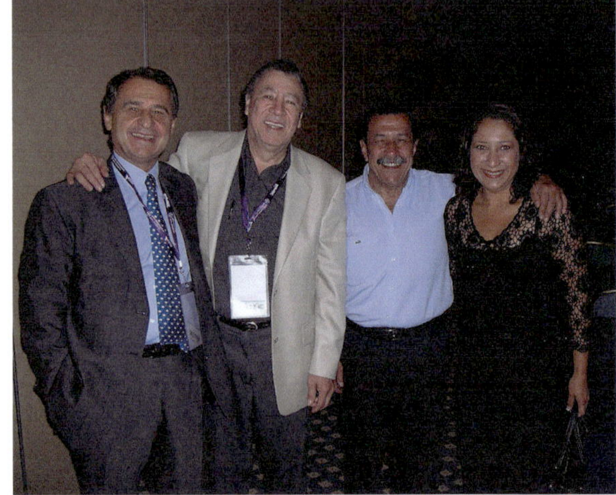

Fig. 16.9 SILAN XXII Annual Congress, Buenos Aires, Argentina (October 2010): Young Scholars Pediatric Neuroradiology faculty (from left to right) Dr. Jorge Davila (SILAN fellow in MCG and Zaragoza, now pediatric neuroradiologist in Ottawa, Canada); Dr. Elka Miller, Dr. Carlos Torres; Dr. Roy Riascos (previous SILAN-MCG fellow, currently chief of Neuroradiology at University of Texas-Houston); Dr. Ramón Figueroa (SILAN Continuous Medical Education coordinator). From left to right, Dr. Pedro Lylyk (SILAN 2010 congress president and ENERI Director), Dr. Enrique Palacios Mayorga, Dr. Alejandro Musacchio (SILAN ENERI faculty), and Dr. Guadalupe Ramirez (SILAN-MCG and SILAN-ENERI fellow)

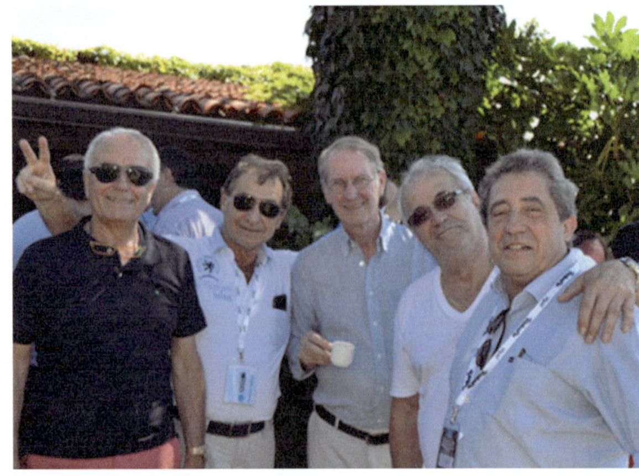

Fig. 16.10 SILAN XXVII Annual Congress, Santiago de Compostela, Spain (June 2015) Friendship afternoon relaxation among friends, from left to right: Drs. José Manuel Pumar (2015 Congress president, Spain), Pedro Lylyk (Argentina), Jacques Theron (France), Jose Maria Modenesi Freitas (Brazil), Jorge Guedes Campos (Portugal)

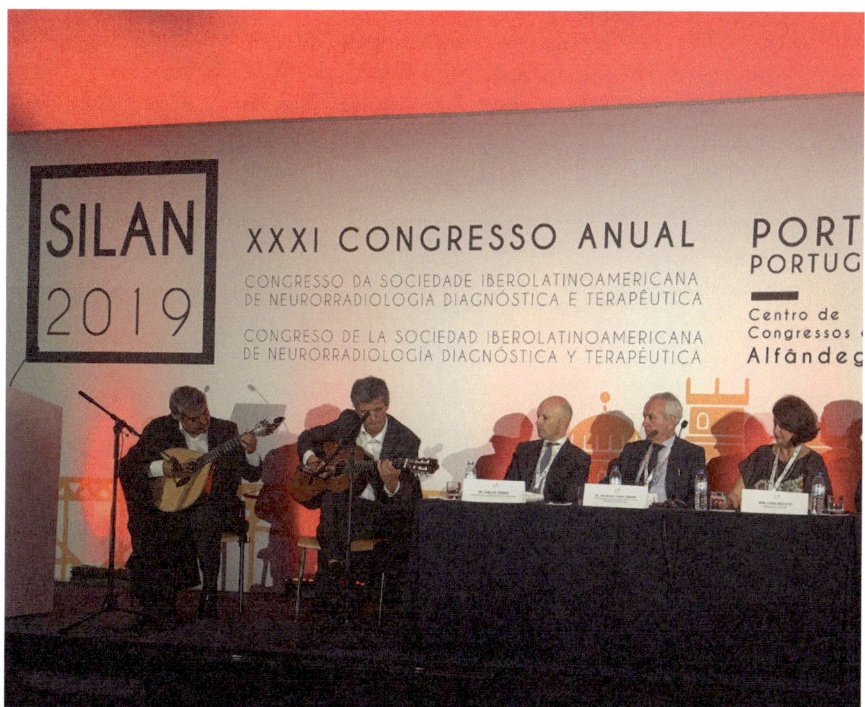

Fig. 16.11 SILAN XXXI Annual Congress, Porto, Portugal (September 2019): Opening ceremonies with Portuguese music introduction. On the presiding table, from left to right, Dr. Carlos Torres (SILAN Vice-President, Canada), Dr. Manuel Pumar (SILAN President, Spain), and Dr. Luisa Biscoito (SILAN Past President, Lisbon, Portugal)

emphasis on neuroradiology research, has trained eight diagnostic neuroradiologists since its inception in 2013, receiving one fellow per year.

SILAN-Vall d'Hebrón Neurointerventional program A 2-year interventional neuroradiology program with Dr. Alejandro Tomasello Weitz as program director, chief of interventional neuroradiology at the Vall d'Hebrón Hospital in Barcelona, Spain. This program, with strong emphasis on neuroradiology research, has trained eight interventional neuroradiologists since its start in 2013.

SILAN-Oulton Neuroradiology program: a 1-year program established in 2018, transitioning to a 2-year program in 2024, with Dr. Gustavo Foa Torres as program director, hosted by Instituto Oulton in Cordoba, Argentina. This program has trained five fellows since its inception, functioning as a mixed program where both diagnostic and interventional neuroradiology training skills are provided.

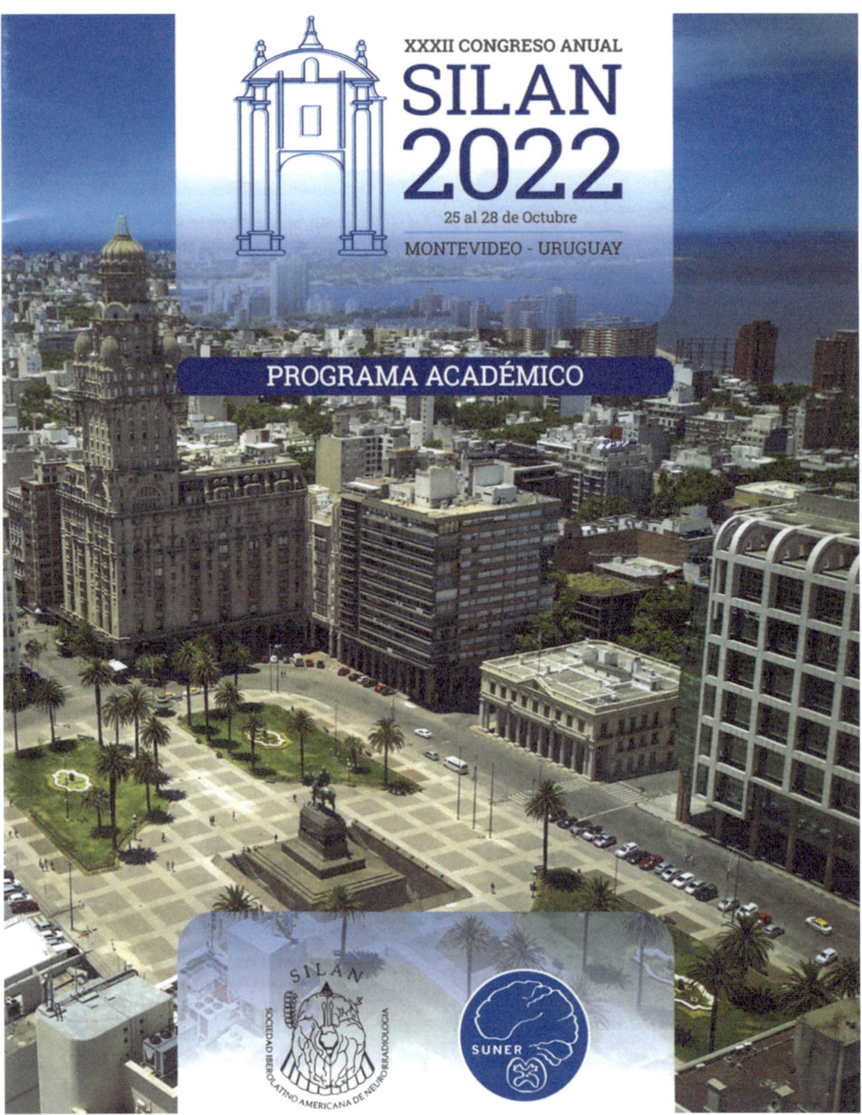

Fig. 16.12 SILAN XXXII Annual Congress, Montevideo, Uruguay (October 2022): SILAN 2022 Program Poster

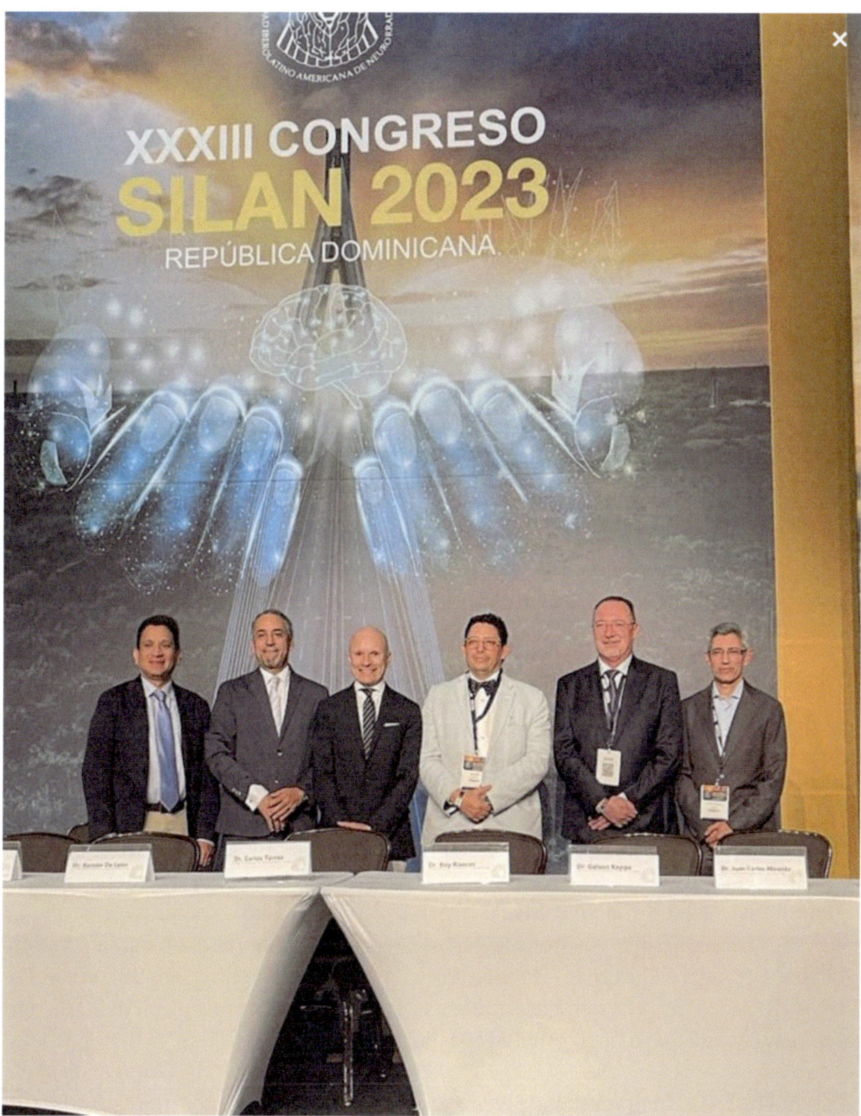

Fig. 16.13 SILAN XXXIII Annual Congress, Punta Cana, Dominican Republic (October 2023): Leadership of SILAN 2023 Congress, from left to right: Dr. Javier Romero, chief of Neuroradiology at Harvard University Massachusetts General Hospital and coordinator of SILAN 2023 scientific program; Dr. Ramón de León Berras, President of SILAN 2023 Congress: Dr. Carlos Torres Arbelaez, SILAN President; Dr. Roy Riascos, Vice-president of SILAN; Dr. Gelson Koppe, Secretary of SILAN; and Dr. Juan Carlos Miranda, Treasurer of SILAN

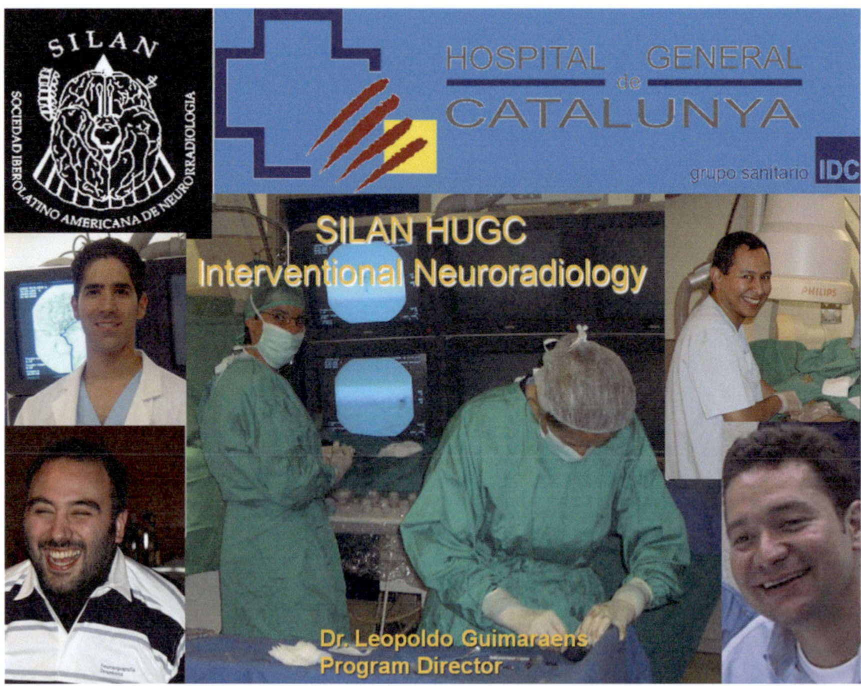

Fig. 16.14 SILAN-HUGC Interventional Neuroradiology Scholarship program is sponsored by Dr. Leopoldo Guimaraens at the Hospital Universitario General de Cataluña, Barcelona, Spain. Several of the fellows from the SILAN-HUGC program

SILAN-Garrahan Pediatric Neuroradiology Scholarship: a 2-month scholarship program to provide advanced training in pediatric neuroradiology to practicing neuroradiologists who are active SILAN members desiring to expand their scope of practice. There are three positions awarded each year (2 months each), sponsored by Hospital Pediátrico Garrahan, Buenos Aires, Argentina. The program director is Dr. Carlos Rugilo. This program has trained six fellows since its inception in 2022, and three new awards have been granted for the year 2024.

SILAN-HUFJD Interventional Neuroradiology program: the newest program established in 2022 as a 2-year interventional neuroradiology training program at the Hospital Universitario Fundación Jimenez Diaz, in Madrid, Spain. The program director is Dr. Claudio Rodríguez, with the first fellow completing his training in June 2025.

The SILAN scholarships are funded through the economic support generated from annual scientific meetings, membership dues, and unrestricted educational grants from commercial partners, channeled through the SILAN Foundation, a not-for-profit entity created to support the training programs. The sponsoring institutions in Spain also provide complementary financial support to compensate for the higher cost of living locally. Over 250 trainees from 24 countries have benefited from the SILAN programs over the span of 28 years, with a direct total investment by the SILAN society of approximately 1.2 million US dollars.

Since its humble beginnings with 24 founding members in Acapulco, Mexico, in 1988, SILAN has gone a long way and remains today the leading forum for continuous medical education and training in its member countries, with around 560 registered members from 24 countries. It currently sponsors the preeminent annual international educational and scientific meeting in the Spanish and Portuguese languages, emphasizing the presentation and discussion of cutting-edge diagnostic and interventional neuroradiology concepts and techniques. It has also served as the engine for the development and strengthening of most national neuroradiological societies in Spanish and Portuguese-speaking countries. SILAN's strong support for neuroradiologic education through the sponsorship of both diagnostic and interventional neuroradiology training programs has impacted all member countries by supplying many competent, well-trained neuroradiology practitioners, especially across Latin American countries. The graduates from our programs have continued this tradition of educational service, with many now involved in fostering local training programs in their own countries. The longitudinal growth of the SILAN society and its generous knowledge sharing continues to open opportunities for training to many deserving students within the neurosciences, building upon the vision of our founding members and leading us into a future where the practice of our discipline becomes more widely available and easily accessible to most people in our member countries.

Information Resources

SILAN society official website (www.silan.org).

SILAN: History of its Foundation, Development and Future: 1989 a 2001. Author: Jesus Rodríguez Carvajal, published as a society service for its members with support from Schering, Mexico, 2002.

Dr. Ramón Figueroa personal archives, 1993–2023.

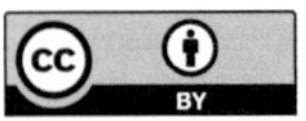

Chapter 17
History of South African Neuroradiology

Clive Wyndham Sperryn, Sally Candy, Ebrahim Kader, Andre MacDonald, Duncan David Royston, Victor Mngomezulu, Coert de Vries, Shalendra Kumar Misser, Leon Janse van Rensburg, and Linda Tebogo Hlabangana

Abbreviations

ASHNR	American Society of Head & Neck Radiology
ASNR	American Society of Neuroradiology
BSNR	British Society of Neuroradiologists

C. W. Sperryn (✉)
Neuroradiology, Morton and Partners, Cape Town, South Africa
e-mail: clive.sperryn@morton.co.za

S. Candy
Diagnostic Radiology, Groote Schuur Hospital/University of Cape Town, Cape Town, South Africa

E. Kader
General and Neuro Interventional Radiology, Morton and Partners Inc, Cape Town, South Africa

A. MacDonald
SCP Radiology, Panorama, Cape Town, South Africa

D. D. Royston
Lake Smit and Partners Radiology, Entabeni Hospital, Cape Town, South Africa

V. Mngomezulu
Diagnostic Radiology, Chris Hani Baragwanath Academic Hospital/University of Witwatersrand, Johannesburg, South Africa

C. de Vries
Scholtz and Partners, Midstream Mediclinic, Centurion, South Africa

S. K. Misser
Radiology, Lake Smit and Partners, Durban, South Africa

L. Janse van Rensburg
Division of Radiodiagnosis, Tygerberg Academic Radiology, Cape Town, South Africa

L. T. Hlabangana
Diagnostic Radiology, University of Witwatersrand, Johannesburg, South Africa

D. Birchall (ed.), *A World History of Neuroradiology*,
https://doi.org/10.1007/978-3-032-16653-1_17

CHBAH	Chris Hani Baragwanath Academic Hospital
CME	Continuing Medical Education
CUBIC	Cape Universities Body Imaging Centre
EDiHNNR	European Diploma in Head and Neck Neuroradiology
EDiINR	European Diploma in Interventional Neuroradiology
EDiNR	European Diploma in Neuroradiology
EDiPNR	European Diploma in Paediatric Neuroradiology
ESNR	European Society of Neuroradiology
GDC	Gugliemi Detachable Coil
HPCSA	Health Professions Council of South Africa
IALCH	Inkosi Albert Luthuli Central Hospital
ISMRM	International Society of Magnetic Resonance in Medicine
KU Leuven	Katholieke Universiteit Leuven
PLANET	Pierre Lasjaunias Neurovascular Education Team
PACS	Picture Archiving and Communication System
RIS	Radiology information system
RXH	Red Cross War Memorial Children's Hospital
RSNA	Radiological Society of North America
RSSA	Radiological Society of South Africa
SAMRC	South African Medical Research Council
SANIS	South African Neurointerventional Society
SASNI	South African Society of Neurological Imaging
SASPI	South African Society of Paediatric Imaging
UCT	University of Cape Town
WFNRS	World Federation of Neuroradiological Societies
WFPI	World Federation of Paediatric Imaging

The Context

South Africa has a population of 62 million with an age distribution typical for a developing country with rapid urbanisation [1]. The 2019 Global Health Index [2] ranks its healthcare 49th out of 89 countries. While occupying top position in Africa, it lags countries such as India and the Philippines. These statistics mask an unusual dichotomy of a 2-tier system, in which a beleaguered and underfunded public sector is used by 86% of the population, and a small, but high functioning private sector services the remainder [3].

A total of 750 radiologists are presently registered with the national licencing body, the Health Professions Council of South Africa (HPCSA), including 439 specialists in full time private practice, 133 in the Public Health system, and 253 registrars (residents) across ten training institutions [4]. This equates to 1.3 radiologists per 100,000 population, compared with 8.6/100,000 in the United Kingdom, 12.8 in the European Union, and ten in the USA.

Broken down further, there are 0.5 radiologists per 100,000 in the state sector compared with 4.65/100,000 in private.

The Radiological Society of South Africa (RSSA) is a stewardship umbrella body with 1086 members, including members in Namibia, Zimbabwe, and Botswana, foreign and retired members, and nuclear medicine physicians. The country comprises nine provinces with historic inequalities in health care provision, medical training, and specialisation patterns. Skills scarcity in SA requires most radiologists to function as generalists. Neuroradiology has been and remains a large component of modern imaging practice and, while many have availed themselves of subspeciality training, few practitioners have the luxury of concentrating solely on neuroimaging.

The South African Society of Neurological Imaging (SASNI), constituted in 2011, has 153 members, Paediatric Imaging (SASPI) has 106, and the SA society of Neuro-intervention (SANIS) has 21 members (0.03/100,000).

The Early Years

The Western Cape tertiary health care facilities, Groote Schuur Hospital affiliated to the University of Cape Town and Tygerberg Hospital, affiliated with Stellenbosch University, are considered to have been historically advantaged in terms of equipment and staffing.

The history of neuroradiology in the Cape is peppered with colourful characters who shaped the growth of the sub-speciality with their unique personalities and styles of teaching. Three eminent personalities stand out in the pioneering days: Prof Lenny Handler, Prof Kaye de Villiers, and Prof Richard Hewlett.

Lenny Handler was the first official South African neuroradiologist. After his Radiology training at the University of Cape Town (UCT) in 1965, he completed a Neuroradiology fellowship at Wessex Neurological Centre, Southampton under Ted Burrows, a neurosurgeon, ex Queen's Square/Great Ormond Street. He returned to South Africa to a neuroradiology post at Groote Schuur Hospital specifically created for him by the head of Neurosurgery at the time, Prof. Kaye de Villiers. Despite diametrically opposed personalities and often at loggerheads, the dynamic duo fostered the growth and recognition of the subspeciality, attending conferences and presenting lectures on new topics, such as, "How to perform an angiogram"! Prof. Handler pioneered procedures at Groote Schuur, such as direct stick carotid angiograms, air encephalography and myelography. Those who trained with him remember the days of manual subtraction cerebral angiography and myelography with a mix of amusement and high anxiety. Catheter angiography came later, under the impetus of Alan Goldin and Phil Harries Jones. Lenny remained active in registrar training well past his official retirement in 2001.

Modern neuroradiology is indebted to the physicists who made it possible. Allan Cormack, who matriculated at Rondebosch Boys High and completed an MSc in physics at the University of Cape Town in 1945 shared the 1979 Nobel Prize with Sir Godfrey Hounsfield for work he had published in 1963 and 1964 on the mathematics required to facilitate cross-sectional imaging [5]. Sir Godfrey Hounsfield developed the first EMI scanner, sharing the first results in 1972.

The genre-altering transition to cross-sectional imaging of the brain came with the installation of the first CT scanner at Tygerberg Hospital in 1976. A revolution in its time, the single slice 64 × 64 matrix EMI unit was as far removed from modern super-scanners as a model-T Ford was from a self-driving Tesla Electric Vehicle. The Groote Schuur Complex followed shortly after with its first CT installation in 1977.

The first MRI in the southern hemisphere, a 0.5 T Elscint unit, was installed at the Medical Research Council (SAMRC) Cape Town and commissioned in 1986. Selected patients were transferred by ambulance to and from their base hospitals across the Western Cape. Run by a young physicist, Bruce Spottiswood, it was used exclusively for neuroimaging and the first radiologists to be involved were Bates Alheit and Jan Lotz, both of whom later moved into private practice.

Diagnostic Neuroradiology

The SAMRC became the home for two young radiologists who would play significant roles in the advancement of the subspeciality—Roger Smith, a neurosurgeon who had spent 4 years of MRI Fellowship training under Walter Kucharczyk in Toronto, and Leon Janse van Rensburg, who completed a 2-year Fellowship in the unit, under the mentorship of Roger Smith and Richard Hewlett.

Roger and Leon were responsible for organising the first MR imaging course in Cape Town in November 1991 (Fig. 17.1). The international faculty included

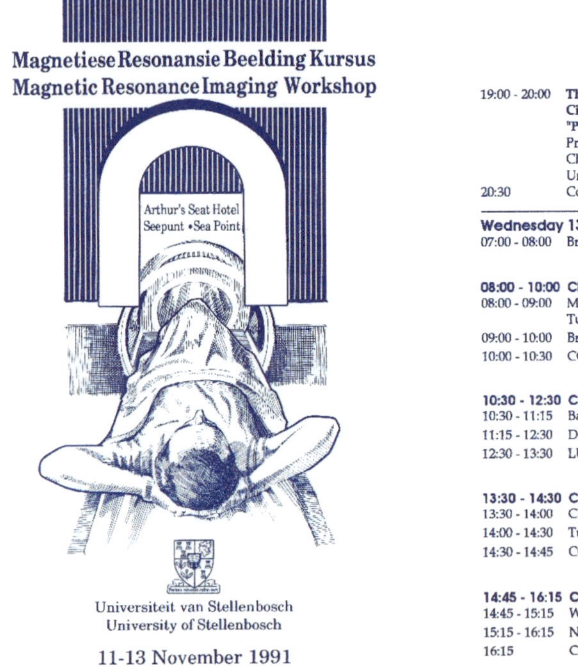

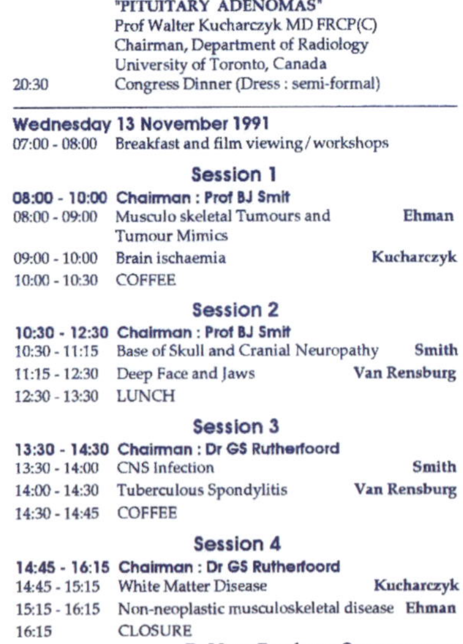

19:00 - 20:00	**The 1st JA Beyers Magnetic Resonance Lecture** **Citation : Prof AT Scher** **"PITUITARY ADENOMAS"** Prof Walter Kucharczyk MD FRCP(C) Chairman, Department of Radiology University of Toronto, Canada	
20:30	Congress Dinner (Dress : semi-formal)	
Wednesday 13 November 1991		
07:00 - 08:00	Breakfast and film viewing/workshops	
	Session 1	
08:00 - 10:00	**Chairman : Prof BJ Smit**	
08:00 - 09:00	Musculo skeletal Tumours and Tumour Mimics	**Ehman**
09:00 - 10:00	Brain ischaemia	**Kucharczyk**
10:00 - 10:30	COFFEE	
	Session 2	
10:30 - 12:30	**Chairman : Prof BJ Smit**	
10:30 - 11:15	Base of Skull and Cranial Neuropathy	**Smith**
11:15 - 12:30	Deep Face and Jaws	**Van Rensburg**
12:30 - 13:30	LUNCH	
	Session 3	
13:30 - 14:30	**Chairman : Dr GS Rutherfoord**	
13:30 - 14:00	CNS Infection	**Smith**
14:00 - 14:30	Tuberculous Spondylitis	**Van Rensburg**
14:30 - 14:45	COFFEE	
	Session 4	
14:45 - 16:15	**Chairman : Dr GS Rutherfoord**	
14:45 - 15:15	White Matter Disease	**Kucharczyk**
15:15 - 16:15	Non-neoplastic musculoskeletal disease	**Ehman**
16:15	CLOSURE	

Dr LJ van Rensburg : Course convenor

Fig. 17.1 Magnetic resonance imaging workshop. (Courtesy of Prof. Leon Janse van Rensburg)

Richard Ehman and Walter Kucharczyk and marked the official start of a subspeciality collaboration which continues to this day.

Leon Janse van Rensburg has been pivotal in the RSSA CME program in general and neuroimaging and specifically head and neck imaging. He was awarded a Doctor of Science degree by the University of the Western Cape for his groundbreaking research on correlative CT, MRI, and histopathology of Maxillofacial Tumours. As CME Chair, he brought a substantial number of neuroradiologists to South Africa and is well known internationally having been on the WFNRS committee, involved in the ISMRM, and is an Honorary member of the ESNR, in recognition of his contribution to advancing Neuroradiology training outside of Europe.

Jan Lotz worked with Richard Hewlett at the City Park Hospital and, in 1992, organised the "First African Neuroradiology" meeting with Prof. Anne Osborn as the keynote speaker.

Prof. Richard Hewlett (Fig. 17.2), locally and internationally renowned neuropathologist and correlative CT/MRI expert, was a key influence on the development and trajectory of radiologists and clinicians with an interest in CNS and head and neck imaging throughout SA. Richard grew up in East Africa, attended the Prince of Wales School in Nairobi, and studied medicine at the University of Cape Town (UCT) where, as a junior lecturer in the anatomy department, he completed a PhD on the anatomy of the rock hyrax(dassie). This was the start of a lifelong fascination with pathology of the nervous system.

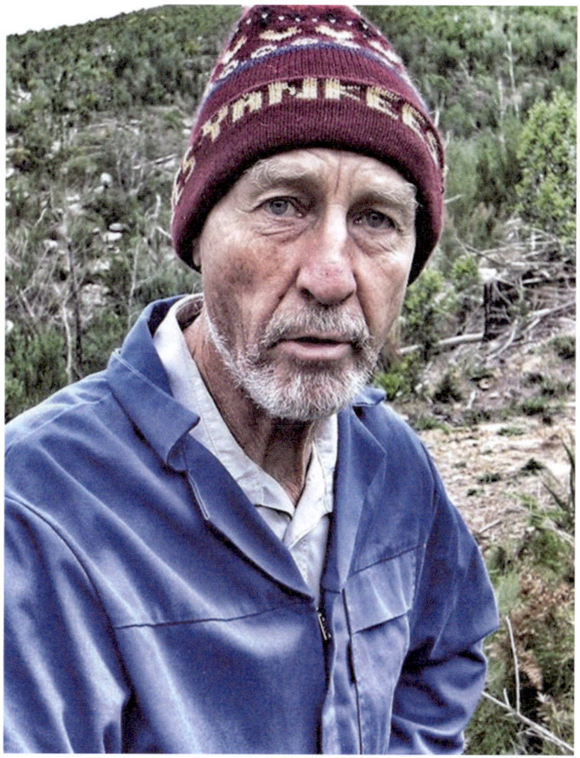

Fig. 17.2 Prof. Richard Hewlett. (Courtesy of Dr. Andre MacDonald)

After specialising in neuropathology in Bristol, he returned to South Africa, joining the Pathology department at Stellenbosch University as an Associate Professor, Depts. of Anatomical & Forensic Pathology. Early on, Richard recognised the powerful correlation between the cut brain and in vivo MR Imaging. He had the proverbial 'head start' on CT and MRI interpretation.

Recognising the unique value Richard brought to the discipline, Prof. Andre Beyers, head of Radiology at Tygerberg hospital, created a special appointment for him in the department as a neuropathologist, in 1987. Richard was an enthusiastic teacher and engaging speaker. His unique insights and skills came to the attention of Professor Anne Osborn, who herself had an interest in pathology and its radiological correlates. They co-authored several papers. "*Their shared excitement when searching through Richard's slide collection to find the perfect match for one of Anne's texts was a delight. They developed a remarkably close friendship. Richard visited the US to lecture in correlative neuropathology to the neuroradiology community, and Anne became a regular visitor to South Africa, lecturing and engaging enthusiastically with colleagues and registrars at all levels.*"

Together they were to have a huge influence on the rapidly evolving subspeciality of neuroradiology in South Africa.

Prof. Richard Hewlett and Dr. Stuart Rutherford co-authored the Atlas of Correlative Surgical Neuropathology and Imaging (Fig. 17.3). Published in 2012, it contains over 600 CT and MRI images and 400 full colour pathological images.

Prof. Sally Candy trained in radiology at the University of Cape Town/Groote Schuur Complex in 1995. Early in her training, she met Pierre Lasjaunias who visited Cape Town to perform pro-bono neuro-intervention on state patients. Impressed by Pierre's unique understanding of the role of embryology in the manifestation of pathology, as well as his extraordinary understanding of neurovascular anatomy, she became fascinated by neuroradiology and trained under Lenny Handler and Richard Hewlett. After qualifying, she completed a Diagnostic Neuroradiology Fellowship at New York Presbyterian and Memorial Sloan Kettering Hospitals. Her return to SA in 2001 coincided with the dawn of the modern era in Neuroradiology in the state sector. In this year, MRI was installed for the first time at Groote Schuur Hospital, the old manual subtraction angiography unit was replaced with a biplanar DSA suite, 4F catheters and plastic syringes replaced their previous iterations, and the first PACS/RIS was introduced. Soon, myelography was to become a scarce skill and diagnostic catheter angiography was all but supplanted by new, less invasive CT and MR techniques. Sally was elected Chair of the newly constituted SASNI in 2011 and remains actively involved in academic neuroradiology training and examining.

Meanwhile at Tygerberg Hospital, Dr. Andre Macdonald was training under the tutelage of Richard Hewlett. It was through Richard that Andre met Anne Osborn on a lecture tour to South Africa. He was selected for a 2-year Neuroradiology and Head & Neck fellowship at the University of Utah from 2001–2003 under the directorship of Professors Osborn and Ric Harnsberger. After completion of his

CURRENT HISTOPATHOLOGY
SERIES CONSULTANT EDITOR: G. AUSTIN GRESHAM
VOLUME TWENTY-FOUR

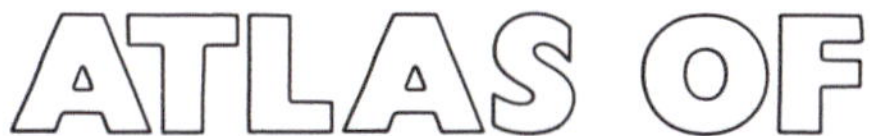

CORRELATIVE SURGICAL NEUROPATHOLOGY AND IMAGING

BY G. S. RUTHERFOORD AND R. H. HEWLETT

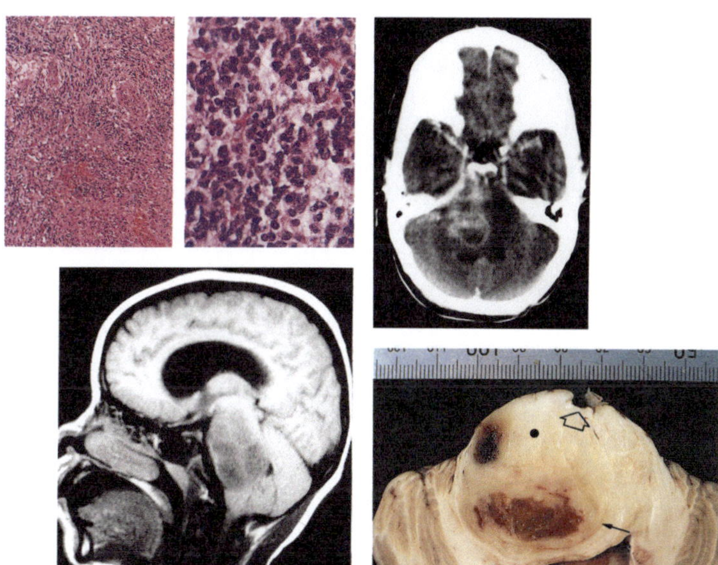

Fig. 17.3 Atlas of correlative surgical neuropathology and imaging. (G. Stuart Rutherfoord, R. H. Hewlett, Atlas of Correlative Surgical Neuropathology and Imaging, 1994, Springer Nature. Reprinted with permission. Image courtesy of Prof. Leon Janse van Rensburg)

fellowship, he remained in the University of Utah academic orbit working at the Veterans Affairs Hospital. During this period, he contributed extensively to several Amirsys neuroradiology texts and to the online portal, STATdx. He returned to South Africa in 2015, bringing specialist expertise in all aspects of neuro/head and neck imaging.

In 2020, Prof. Christelle Ackermann, Head of the Department of Clinical Oncology and Imaging, Stellenbosch University and Tygerberg Hospital, completed a PhD: "Neuroimaging in HIV, an MRI/DTI study."

Dr. Elias Pretorius completed a 2-year Neuroradiology Fellowship in Calgary, Canada and having returned to Cape Town is active in Head, Neck, and Skull base imaging.

In Kwazulu Natal, specialists Peter Corr (UCT trained) and Jay Maharajah were influential in shaping and fostering registrars to become familiar with new imaging modalities and less invasive catheter angiography techniques. In 1995, Peter recruited Duncan Royston to Wentworth Hospital. Duncan, too, had trained under Steve Beningfield and Lenny Handler and would be tasked with heading the Radiology Department and establishing and maintaining the MRI service, focusing on neuroradiology. Wentworth Hospital had the distinction of being the first state-run hospital to acquire an MR scanner, and Duncan would be responsible for training radiology registrars from the Nelson Mandela School of Medicine. The opening of the Inkosi Albert Luthuli Central Hospital in 2002 on the outskirts of Durban with state-of-the-art equipment marked the beginning of a new era in neuro- imaging in the province.

In 2010, Dr. Shalen Misser commenced the European Society of Neuroradiology Pierre Lasjaunias Courses and was awarded the European Diploma in Neuroradiology. He was followed initially by Dr. Thami Mngoma and subsequently many others. These two went on to complete the EDiPNR and the EDiHNNR. Shalen since completed a PhD under Prof. James Barkovich on "Neonatal Hypoxic Ischaemic Brain Injury." Wonder-boy Mbatha returned to Durban in 2018 after completing a Neuroradiology Fellowship at University College London, Queens Square under Prof. Tarek Yousry and Prof. Rolf Jager.

Dr. Clive Sperryn, a past President of the RSSA, has been the SASNI Chair since 2018. His brief time in Neurosurgery with Prof. James van Dellen at Wentworth Hospital, Durban before commencing radiology training stimulated an interest in neuroradiology further strengthened by visiting Fellowships at UCSF. He completed the EDiNR and EDiPNR and has been involved in collaborations with the ESNR, specifically the RSSA SASNI ESNR Spine Course, co-convened with Prof. Pia Maly Sundgren, and the 2024 Brain Imaging course. During this tenure, SASNI has grown from 56 to 153 members.

Many South African radiologists now have European Diplomas: (EDiNR 46, EDiPNR 10, EDiHNNR 5, EDiINR 2.) Prof. Linda Tebogo Hlabangana and Dr. Marc Jordaan will be part of the Young Leaders Forum at the World Federation, an initiative of Dr. Daniel Birchall (BSNR).

Paediatric Neuroradiology

In South Africa, Paediatric Neuroradiology forms part of the work of general radiologists. Until recently, few were fellowship trained.

Cape Town's Red Cross War Memorial Children's Hospital (RXH) opened as the only dedicated paediatric hospital in the Southern Hemisphere in 1956. Paediatric neuroradiology developed organically with the requirements of the clinical discipline until the introduction of a formal 12-month subspeciality training programme introduced in 2009 leading to a postgraduate diploma in paediatric radiology by the University of Cape Town. Similar fellowship training is now available at the Nelson Mandela Children's Hospital/Witwatersrand Academic Complex in Johannesburg.

Since 2018, the World Federation for Paediatric Imaging (WFPI), under the auspices of the William Shiels memorial foundation, has offered a 3-month funded paediatric radiology observership in South Africa, at either Red Cross War Memorial or the Nelson Mandela Children's Hospital. These programs have a strong neuro emphasis and course content.

Several South African Radiologists Have Made an International Name in Paediatric Neuroradiology

Prof. Derek Harwood Nash was a graduate of the University of Cape Town who specialised at the Hospital for Sick Children in Toronto and established the discipline of Paediatric neuroradiology. His three-volume publication with Charles Fitz *Neuroradiology in Infants and Children in 1976* was an authoritative reference. He was the founding President of the WFNRS 1994–1998 [6]. His legacy lives on in the RSNA Derek Harwood-Nash International Fellowship.

Prof. Bryan Cremin headed radiology at RXH and published widely on the use of ultrasound in the diagnosis of neonatal CNS haemorrhage, tuberculous meningitis and comparison of transcranial ultrasound and computed tomography of the infant brain. He and Dr. Douglas Jamieson co-authored *Childhood Tuberculosis: Modern Imaging and Clinical Concepts* published by Springer-Verlag in 1995.

Prof. Caroline Robson, ex RXH, has had a stellar career in paediatric neuroradiology with a special interest in Head and Neck at Boston Children's Hospital. She is Past President of the ASHNR and the ASPNR.

Prof. Savvas Andronikou began his paediatric radiologist career at RXH in 1998. An inspiring teacher and prolific researcher, he was responsible for the manual, *Baby Steps into Paediatric Neuroradiology* published in SA in 2004 (editors Savvas Andronikou, Nicky Wieselthaler, Ebrahim Kader). He chaired the SA society of Paediatric Imaging and having completed 2 PhD's on neuroradiological topics and published widely on neuro-imaging topics of importance in the developing world, he now occupies the vice chair of radiological research at the Children's Hospital of Philadelphia (CHOP) in the USA.

Dr. Tracy Kilborn, who headed the department of radiology at RXH until 2022, has been a regular speaker at international meetings, including the ESNR annual meeting.

Dr. Marc Jordaan is a US trained radiologist who completed a Paediatric Radiology Fellowship at Harvard Medical School, Boston's Children's Hospital where his focus was paediatric neuroradiology. After serving as an Assistant Professor in Clinical Radiology at Columbia University Medical Center, he has joined a private practice in Cape Town. He recently completed the EDiNR.

Dr. Gopolang Mndebele has the distinction of having completed a paediatric neuroradiology fellowship at the Hospital for Sick Children and University of Toronto and now heads the Nelson Mandela Children's Hospital. The department is small, with three radiologists, one of whom is currently completing a fellowship in paediatric intervention in Toronto and, one junior medical officer. There is approved accreditation for two registrar posts who will rotate through the Witwatersrand academic circuit. All consultants have honorary affiliation with Witwatersrand, participating in teaching and research supervision.

Neuro-intervention

Despite its size and geographic location, South Africa has the distinction of early adoption and progress in the field of Neurointerventional Radiology (Neuro-IR), in parallel with large centres in Europe and North America. This is due to the close personal ties and working relationships between local practitioners and the international pioneers in the field.

Derek Sables kick-started general Interventional Radiology at Groote Schuur Hospital with minimally invasive urological procedures. His tenure from 1968–1971 overlapped partially with that of Alan Goldin (1970–1978). Goldin introduced interventional techniques for vascular occlusion using catheter-delivered cyanoacrylate glue to control haemorrhage, years ahead of its widely accepted use. Toronto-trained Phil Harries-Jones (1981–1988) succeeded Goldin and formalised the interventional radiology (IR) service at Groote Schuur Hospital.

Phil introduced additional angiographic techniques such as angioplasty. Used routinely today, this was a pioneering procedure at the time. Up until this point, practitioners were limited by conventional fluoroscopic equipment for most procedures, and manual subtraction angiography for cerebral work.

In the 1980s, neuro-intervention was developing rapidly. The French anatomist and radiologist, Pierre Lasjaunias conceptualised a new way of thinking about neurovascular disease and, together with Alex Berenstein in December 1986, published one of the seminal works in the field, the imposing three volume, *Surgical Neuroangiography* (Springer Heidelberg).

In the same year, the installation of a digital subtraction angiography suite in the new Groote Schuur Hospital provided a technological leap for radiology in Cape

Town. Despite its geographic isolation at the southern tip of Africa, there was recognition of the immense potential of Neuro-IR and registrars were encouraged to embark on training in the burgeoning field.

On a visit to the United States, Phil Harries-Jones met Grant Hieshima in San Francisco and Alejandro Berenstein in New York, further fuelling his enthusiasm to grow the IR service in Cape Town. On his return, he performed and taught a wide range of procedures, including diagnostic cerebral and spinal angiograms, intra- and extracranial artery embolisation, aneurysm occlusion, and traumatic AV fistula closure. The recently launched Guglielmi detachable coil which was to bring about a seismic shift in neuro-interventional practice was not yet available in South Africa.

Steve Beningfield was one of the first radiologists in the country to close CCFs using detachable latex balloons, a technique he had observed in San Francisco in the early 1990s. A quiet visionary, superb radiologist, and the newly appointed head of Radiology at Groote Schuur and Red Cross Children's Hospital, he recognised the potential for intervention and oversaw its implementation. Under his watch, Pierre Lasjaunias visited Groote Schuur Hospital, where he lectured on and demonstrated Vein of Galen and spinal AV malformation intervention, highlighting the use of microcatheters, cyanoacrylate, and lipiodol.

With Steve's support, the formal neurointerventional unit was set up at Groote Schuur in 2001. Prof. Allan Taylor, a neurosurgeon who had completed the International master's degree in Neurovascular Diseases convened by Pierre Lasjaunias at the Universities of Paris Sud and Chiang Mai and spent practical observerships with several doyens of the speciality, notably Pierre Lasjaunias, Karel ter Brugge, George Rodesch, and In Sup Choi, was ideally positioned to head the unit. At the same time, Lenny Handler returned to play a final part, encouraging a newly graduating Radiologist, Ebrahim Kader, to complete the same master's degree. Ebrahim, who had been running the Interventional Radiology unit at Groote Schuur Hospital, briefly joined Professor Taylor, but departed shortly thereafter to establish an interventional service in the private sector in Cape Town. He was replaced by neurosurgical colleague, Prof. David le Feuvre, who had followed a similar trajectory into the neurointerventional sphere as Allan and Ebrahim. The Cape Town Neurointerventional unit is one of the busiest in SA, and the Stroke unit is the busiest in the country. Internationally renowned, it provides neuro-interventional training and support at home and abroad.

Pieter Fourie kicked off the Neuro-IR practice at the Unitas Hospital in Pretoria. Pieter had GDC training with Jacques Moret in Switzerland in 1995 and was the first in South Africa to treat an intracranial aneurysm with the GDC coil system. A founder member of the Interventional Peer Review Group, Pieter, together with a neurosurgical colleague, Joachim Mennem, provided a service to the private sector in his region over several decades. Dr. Sandra Basson, after a 6-month fellowship at UCLA in 1990, collaborated with Prof. Fourie in the early years but has relocated to the Eastern Cape and is no longer active. The service continues in the capable hands of his trainees: Stefan Steyn and Francois Potgieter. Arthur Winter has since relocated to the Western Cape.

Coert de Vries and Duncan Royston set up units in the central plains, Bloemfontein, and in the East Coast, Durban, respectively.

Coert de Vries headed the respected academic radiology training program at the University of the Free State between 1996 and 2017 having completed the GDC course in Oxford in Dec 1995. He launched a general and neuro-interventional service in 1996 with Dr. Eugene Loggenberg. Cases were initially done on a general screening table until a dedicated angiography suite was commissioned in 1998. Coert established the first neurointerventional fellowship program in the country. Although designed Initially as a 1-year advanced diploma, it was later expanded to a 2-year MPhil degree in Interventional Radiology, in line with other subspeciality training in South Africa. The European Board of Interventional Radiology examination was used as the exit exam for this degree.

Radiologists, Peter Nataniël, Matthys van Wyk, Jacques Janse van Rensburg, Francois Potgieter and Werner van Straaten graduated from this program. Werner gained further experience in acute stroke treatment in Bern, Switzerland, and now works with Duncan Royston in private practice in Durban.

Duncan Royston, also inspired by Pierre Lasjaunias while in training at GSH, completed his Neuro IR fellowship in Oxford with James Byrne and Andy Molyneux. In 1998, he returned to Durban, South Africa and established a neurointerventional service at Wentworth Hospital and in private practice at Entabeni Hospital. Dr. Karel Ter Brugge of the Toronto Hospital for Sick Children—a close friend and colleague of Pierre Lasjaunias, provided valuable mentorship and support during this early phase. In 2002, the flagship academic Inkosi Albert Luthuli Central Hospital (IALCH) in Durban was opened and Duncan was appointed to train registrars in Interventional Neuroradiology. In 2011, Dr. Rohen Harrichandparsad, a recently qualified neurosurgeon, began interventional neuroradiology training under Duncan Royston's tutelage.

Dr. Indheresan Moodley completed a 1-year INR fellowship at the University of Zürich under the late Prof. Anton Valavanis and set up an interventional practice at Ethekwini Hospital also in Durban in 2011.

An interventional neuroradiology fellowship was established at IALCH in 2020, by Dr. Rohen Harrichandparsad and has graduated four fellows to date, all of whom are running neurointerventional services in state hospitals.

The first, Dr. Phila Mpanza from Department of Neurosurgery, Sefako Makgatho Health Sciences University qualified in 2020 and now runs a busy academic neurointerventional service at Dr. George Mukhari Academic Hospital in Ga-Rankuwa.

The second, Dr. Rambelani Khohomela, is currently Head of Unit and Consultant Neurovascular Surgeon at Chris Hani Baragwanath and Charlotte Maxeke Hospitals as well as servicing the public/private Donald Gordon Medical Centre in Johannesburg.

The third (2022), Dr. Bradley Moshokoa, also a neurosurgeon, is currently co-director of the Neurovascular Unit at Dr. George Mukhari Hospital.

The fourth and most recent fellow, Dr. Thembani Hina, provides neurointerventional services in the public sector in Gqeberha (Port Elizabeth).

The most densely populated province in SA, Gauteng, initially trailed behind the rest of the country. A key driving personality in the region was Prof. Victor

Mngomezulu. After a brief stint in private practice, Victor returned to the public sector as the Head of Department of George Mukhari Hospital which formed part of the University of Limpopo. After completing the PLANET course and international observerships, Victor established two neurointerventional units in the Wits University Academic complex, at Chris Hani Baragwanath (CHBAH) and Charlotte Maxeke Hospitals. He had a close collaboration with Profs. Taylor and Le Feuvre. He has been a driving force in growing the subspeciality in SA, advocating for a multidisciplinary team approach, encompassing neurologists, neurosurgeons, and radiologists. He has played a significant role in training active and key members in the discipline, including Thandi Buthelezi and Werner van Straaten.

During the period of rapid growth in the 1990s, the practice of Neuro-IR was based on anecdote. Meetings tended to be collegial discussions of techniques based on limited local experience. It was only after publication of the ISAT trial in 2002, demonstrating the superiority of endovascular coiling over surgical clipping in the treatment of ruptured intracranial aneurysms, that Neuro-IR took its first tentative steps into the practice of evidence-based medicine. SA saw the launch of an annual peer review meeting in 1998, arranged by Pieter Fourie, Coert de Vries, Eugene Loggenberg, Joachim Mennen, Ian Duncan, and Duncan Royston. This meeting has provided the much-needed support for the expansion of a national neurointerventional service.

Currently the local Neuro-IR efforts are stewarded by the South African Neurointerventional Society (SANIS) with 21 members with backgrounds in radiology and neurosurgery. *Pieter Fourie, Allan Taylor, David le Feuvre, Coert de Vries, Rohen Harrichandpersad, Arthur Winter, Ebrahim Kader, Victor Mngomezulu, Francois Potgieter, Stefan Steyn, Duncan Royston, Indheresan Moodley, Mogwale (Sam) Motebejane, Eugene Loggenberg, Armin Gretschel, Werner van Straaten, Rambelani Khohomela, Bradley Moshokoa, Phila Martin Mpanza, Theo Nel, Moaaz Omar, Thandi Buthelezi.*

Academic Support and Continuing Medical Education

Having developed close relationships with American and European luminaries in the field of Neuroradiology over years and, cognisant of the need for ongoing specialist training and exposure to the latest advances in the field, Prof. Leon Janse van Rensburg formulated the CME branch of the RSSA in 2006. Under the banners of the various subspeciality groups (SASNI /SASPI and SANIS), annual international conferences, courses, and topic updates are held on home soil.

In addition, regular webinars on a wide variety of neuro-related topics are held for RSSA members.

Fellowships in Canada have become sought after since no additional entrance examination is required.

Because of the close European ties, subspecialisation has become accessible and affordable to South African radiologists, many of whom have completed accredited European Society courses.

In addition, the ASNR affiliated Anne G. Osborn ASNR International Outreach Program has, since 2017, recruited US-trained senior neuroradiologists chosen for their teaching skills to spend several weeks each year teaching in South African academic centres. This program is mutually beneficial, exposing American neuroradiologists to the idiosyncrasies of the South African context while providing trainees with insights into neuroimaging trends in countries with less stringent fiscal and logistical constraints.

Through the invitation of Dr. Daniel Birchall, our academic departments have had the opportunity to participate in and present cases at the BSNR Grand Rounds.

At present, Radiology training in SA adequately covers most aspects of brain and spine imaging for generalist needs. Advanced neuroimaging is, however, either not available or underutilised. This is due to a combination of factors, including non-reimbursement by medical insurance and the perception that it does not add significantly to clinical management.

The Cape Universities Body Imaging Centre (CUBIC) is a medical imaging research facility focusing on problems specific to South Africa and Africa [7]. Located within the recently completed Neuroscience Institute next to Groote Schuur Hospital in Cape Town, this 3 T magnet has been operational since 2015. Headed by US-trained MRI physicist, Professor Ernesta Meintjies, CUBIC has established itself as the centre for advanced imaging of psychiatric, neurocognitive, developmental, and psychosocial pathologies in Africa. The unit is active in the development and refinement of novel MR sequences, particularly in MR motion reduction.

Prof. Mngomezulu is exploring the establishment of a centre of excellence at CHBAH which will encourage teaching and training of registrars and consultants from both neurosurgical and radiological departments. The centre will collaborate with neurointerventional departments both locally and internationally.

The Future

The future presents a challenge for research and training in an environment rich in research material and opportunities. Mounting resource constraints and dormant/unfilled posts in the state sector pose a threat to training. Original research, which tends to be done in academic centres, has suffered under the pressures of service delivery. Research, as it is, has tended to be clinical in its concerns, with expected emphasis on HIV and Tuberculosis—both disappointingly prevalent in SA. For neuroradiology to grow beyond diagnostics in SA, there are various socioeconomic, political, bureaucratic, and academic challenges to overcome.

Broadly, these issues relate to the geographic distribution of the population, the widening wealth gap, poor healthcare leadership and hospital management in a struggling public sector. Some academic departments which previously had international recognition are now shadows of their former selves. Unfortunately, the exceptional formally accredited interventional training established by Prof. Coert de Vries at the University of the Free State was terminated.

Restoring these crumbling institutions is no easy task but not beyond the scope of imagination. It requires an increased commitment to state hospital service and academic endeavour to grow the pool of subspeciality trained neuroradiologists in SA.

Given the lack of adequate government support for public services, as with other spheres in South Africa, alternative and creative strategies need to be developed. Teleradiology and the use of artificial intelligence-generated diagnostic algorithms could be key to providing a more uniform access to neuroradiology reporting in underserviced areas of the country. Public-private partnerships with funded registrarships, fellowships, and/or stewarded training could be a way forward. There is a precedent for this model with certain private hospital groups partnering with universities to complete undergraduate medical student training. Additionally paediatric fellowship training posts have in the past been sponsored by private radiology firms. The rich, character-driven history of our subspeciality has left a legacy of partnerships with academic institutions in other parts of the world. International exchange programs at registrar and post qualification level should be fostered and expanded. Research collaborations with respected international colleagues would serve to strengthen academic endeavour, expand the scope of the discipline, and incentivise this important and exciting career choice.

Acknowledgements We would like to acknowledge the international societies and individuals who have contributed to the development of Neuroradiology in South Africa.

ISMRM, KU Leuven, ESNR, ASNR, WFPI, RSNA, BSNR, ASHNR, PLANET
Prof. Pierre Lasjaunias
Dr. Karel ter Brugge
Prof. Anne Osborn
Prof. Walter Kucharczyk
Prof. Jan Casselman
Dr. Roger Smith
Prof. Savvas Andronikou
Dr. Vincent Chong
Prof. Howard Rowley
Dr. David Saloner
Prof. James Barkovich
Prof. Pia Maly Sundgren
Prof. Majda Thurner
Prof. Rob Hermans
Dr. Berit Verbist
Dr. Yannick De Brucker
Prof. Frank Parmeijer
Dr. Ilona Schmalfuss
Dr. Herve Tanghe
Prof. Turgut Tali
Prof. Johan Van Goethem
Prof. Davide Farina
Prof. Ann King
Prof. Roberto Maroldi
Prof. Alex Rovira
Prof. Paul Parizel

Prof. Bruno Policeni
Prof. Cem Calli
Prof. Luigi Manfre
Prof. Chiara Zini
Richard H Wiggens III
Prof. Caroline Robson
Dr. Daniel Birchall

Links

Chris Hani Baragwanath Academic Hospital https://www.chrishanibaragwanathhospital.co.za/
Cape Universities Body Imaging Centre https://cubic.uct.ac.za/
Health Professions Council of South Africa https://www.hpcsa.co.za/
Inkosi Albert Luthuli Central Hospital https://www.ialch.co.za/
Red Cross War Memorial Children's Hospital https://www.childrenshospitaltrust.org.za/the-hospital/
Radiological Society of South Africa https://rssa.co.za/
South African Medical Research Council https://www.samrc.ac.za/
South African Neurointervention Society http://www.sanis.co.za/
University of Cape Town https://uct.ac.za/

References

1. https://www.statssa.gov.za/?p=16716#:~:text=The%20Census%202022%20results%20show,is%20the%20largest%20since%201996.
2. https://www.numbeo.com/health-care/rankings_by_country.jsp.
3. https://businesstech.co.za/news/finance/639147/red-flags-for-south-africas-overburdened-tax-base/.
4. Radiological Society of South Africa data https://rssa.co.za/.
5. Banerjee D, Johnston A, Bell D, Allan Macleod Cormack. Reference article, Radiopaedia.org. Accessed on 12 May 2024. https://doi.org/10.53347/rID-60244.
6. Huckman MS. Derek F. C. Harwood Nash, MB, ChB, DSc, FRCPC, FACR, FC RAD (SA). AJNR Am J Neuroradiol. 1997;18(10):1803–12. https://www.ajnr.org/content/18/10/1803.
7. CUBIC | University of Cape Town. https://cubic.uct.ac.za/.

Chapter 18
The History of Swiss Neuroradiology

Karl-Olof Lövblad, Isabel Wanke, Luca Remonda, and Daniel Rüfenacht

The Swiss Society for Neuroradiology (SGNR/SSNR)

The Swiss Society for Neuroradiology (called in German: Schweizerische Gesellschaft für Neuroradiologie [SGNR] and in French: Société Suisse de Neuroradiologie [SSNR]) was founded in 1988 by a group of Swiss Neuroradiologists composed of Anton Valavanis and Othmar Schubiger from Zurich, Peter Huber from Bern, and Ernst Radu from Basel [1]. This was finalized on July 25, 1989 in Zurich at the Hotel Schweizerhof. These early pioneers would constitute the nucleus that would create neuroradiology as we know it today in Switzerland. Initially, two main centers would form the nucleus for training and Science, Bern and Zurich. The first president of the society was therefore Peter Huber (1989–1993), followed by Anton Valavanis (1993–1999) and Othmar Schubiger (1999–2001), followed by Anton Valavanis again (2001–2010), then by Luca Remonda (2010–2018), Jan Gralla (2018–2020), Karl-Olof Lövblad (2020–2022), then today Isabel Wanke. Currently, the SGNR has a committee with ten members that meet at regular

K.-O. Lövblad (✉)
Division of Neuroradiology, Département diagnostique, Hôpitaux Universitaires de Genève, Genève, Switzerland
e-mail: karl-olof.lovblad@hcuge.ch

I. Wanke
Swiss Society of Neuroradiology, Swiss Neuro Institute, Zurich, Zurich, Switzerland
e-mail: Isabel.wanke@hirslanden.ch

L. Remonda
Division of Neuroradiology, Kantonsspital Aarau, Aarau, Switzerland
e-mail: luca.remonda@ksa.ch

D. Rüfenacht
Swiss Neuro Institute, Zurich, Zurich, Switzerland
e-mail: daniel.rufenacht@hirslanden.ch

D. Birchall (ed.), *A World History of Neuroradiology*,
https://doi.org/10.1007/978-3-032-16653-1_18

intervals and are appointed every 2 years. The society has two awards: The yearly Peter Huber award, which is given for the best original research by a young neuroradiologist, and the Anton Valavanis Medal, which honors a leading neuroradiologist who will have furthered the specialty along the lines defined by Anton Valavanis. The Valavanis Medal has been given twice to Professors Luc Picard and Georges Rodesch from France. The society also provides support in the form of help to organize fellowships in both diagnostic and interventional neuroradiology. The society is currently presided over by Professor Isabel Wanke from Zurich, and the committee has Profs Jan Gralla, Luca Remonda, and Karl Olof Lövblad as past presidents. Initial honorary members of the society were Professors Josef Wellauer, Gazi Yasargil, and Ugo Fisch, all from Zurich due to their immense contributions and support to the Society and the Specialty. The Society additionally has working groups that deal with various thematics of neuroradiology: there are working groups for Advanced neuroimaging (chaired by Prof Roland Wiest from Bern), Head and Neck Radiology (Prof Franca Wagner, Bern), interventional neuroradiology (Prof Pasquale Mordasini, St. Gallen), Spinal imaging (Dr Alessandro Cianfoni, Lugano), Pediatric Neuroradiology (Aikaterina Fitsiori, Geneva). The Society is affiliated with the ESNR and the WFNRS.

Before the Swiss Society of Neuroradiology

Before becoming a clearly defined and regulated subspecialityin Switzerland, Neuroradiology had been performed in various forms, in an especially innovative way, even before the systemic structure that we know today [2]. Especially, angiographic techniques had been developed in great part by the neurosurgeon MG Yasargil at the University Hospital in Zurich under the guidance of Professor Hugo Krayenbühl [3–5]. Additionally, techniques such as myelography were widely used for diagnostic procedures of the CNS [6]. It was with the advent of axial imaging techniques that radiology, especially neuroradiology, would see great advances: the first CT would be installed in Basel at the Bürgerspital [7] in 1973, and the first MR units would appear in 1982 in Geneva and Zurich [2].

The first Swiss professor for Neuroradiology was Peter Huber from Bern [8, 9], who was a neurosurgeon by training and who had written the final version of the classic Krayenbuhl monograph on angiography: Peter Huber had won the Robert Bing Prize in 1968 and would retire in 1992; Peter Huber would be succeeded by Professor Gerhard Schroth [10]. The division, which would become the institute it is today under the leadership of Gerhard Schroth, a specialist in Neurology and Neuroradiology who had trained in Tübingen in Germany; Gerhard Schroth had also spent 2 years in Zürich with Anton Valavanis, and he would therefore develop intensively interventional techniques in Bern, especially for the treatment of stroke, as well as the use of MR techniques for improved diagnosis and management of patients with neurological diseases. The current chair of Neuroradiology in Bern is Prof Jan Gralla, who trained with Gerhard

Schroth. Functional imaging would be implemented with the installation of the Siemens Vision echo-planar scanner in the 1990s and would allow the clinical implementation of techniques such as DWI and fMRI.

Neuroradiology in the Various Institutions and Cantons

Neuroradiology would develop in a structured way in the German-speaking part of Switzerland, initially around interventional centers and specialists. The first independent Institute for Neuroradiology was established in Switzerland under Prof Anton Valavanis [11, 12]; soon Bern would follow and the Neuroradiology Unit would become also an Institute of Neuroradiology under Prof G Schroth, who succeeded P Huber, the first Swiss Professor of Neuroradiology. Full professorships with independent divisions would be established in Geneva, Bern, and Zurich. The first privately owned independent neuroradiology institute would be founded in Zurich by Professors Daniel Rüfenacht and Isabel Wanke, first at the Hirslanden Klinik and then co-jointly at the Swiss Neuro Institute (SNRI).

The Zurich history of a close interaction between the basic and clinical Neurosciences and Neuroradiology is long: while Yasargil and Krayenbuhl perfected cerebral angiography, Prof Wellauer would do the same for myelography: and as early as 1973, Dr. Othmar Schubiger would devote himself to neuroradiology and, as of 1977, exclusively; Othmar Schubiger would become the head of neuroradiology in Aarau between 1980 and 1986. Othmar Schubiger would then move to the Klinik, im Park in Zurich [13], being later succeeded in Aarau by A Mironov and L Remonda successively. The institute of Neuroradiology in Zurich would focus heavily on interventions of brain vascular malformations, the use of advanced MR techniques and Head and Neck imaging [14, 15], under the leadership of Prof Valavanis, Werner Wichmann; Spyros Kollias would introduce modern MR techniques such as fMRI and DTI at the Zurich institute [16]. Thierry Huisman would move to the USA as a pediatric neuroradiologist, first at Johns Hopkins then at the Texas Children's Hospital. Due to the high visibility achieved in interventional neuroradiology by the Zurich institute [17–20], a yearly course on interventional neuroradiology was established by Anton Valavanis that helped establish Zurich as a center for neuro-vascular interventions. Building on the Zurich tradition in neurosciences, Anton Valavanis would help create the Zurich Clinical Neurocenter that he would direct for many years. The current head of Neuroradiology in Zurich is Dr. Zsolt Kulcsar who had trained in Hungary and in Switzerland with Daniel Rüfenacht in Geneva. The Institute in Bern would be a pioneer in the use of intra-arterial treatments of ischemic diseases such as stroke, using either at first intra-arterial thrombolysis or later thrombectomy. The Division in Geneva would concentrate efforts on the minimal invasive treatment of among others aneurysms and also of diseases of the spine. In Basel, EW Radü was the director of the unit of neuroradiology at the Kantonsspital Basel as of 1984, and became Privat docent in 1986 and finally professor; EW Radü would concentrate his academic efforts on the study of inflammatory diseases of the CNS such as Multiple Sclerosis, being succeeded by Christoph Stippich from Heidelberg who would leave for Zurich. The current professor in neuroradiology in Basel is Professor Marios Psychogios.

In the French part of Switzerland, Neuroradiology was structured initially slightly differently; in Geneva, neuroradiology was established at first in the neurology department as early as 1963 and, after a succession of three neuroradiologists, in 1972, Dr. Marcelle Megret was nominated chief of this division [21]. At the Cantonal Hospital of Geneva initially, the CT was installed on the second floor of the Geneva Cantonal Hospital in Neurology and the division was held by Drs. Marcelle Megret and Jacqueline Delavelle; upon the nomination of François Terrier in radiology, the CT was integrated in radiology; this, together with the acquisition of the MR unit, would allow full diagnostic work-up of neurological patients and neuroradiology would become a clearly defined unit of the division of radiology in 1989. With the growth of newer techniques, it became necessary also to establish knowledge in interventional neuroradiology: hence Daniel Rüfenacht, a scholar of Peter Huber in Bern and Jean-Jacues Merland in Paris [22–24], and who was working in Minnesota would be recruited to Geneva in 1992 and would be the first academic division head and professor in neuroradiology in the French part of Switzerland. In Lausanne, neuroradiology was integrated in Radiology under the direction of Drs. Antoine Uske and Reto Meuli. Reto Meuli, a neuroradiologist with an extensive background in MR physics, would eventually also become the head of the radiology division of the CHUV in Lausanne. A notable trainee from Lausanne is Max Wintermark who is currently at the MD Anderson Institute and editor-in-chief of the AJNR. Prof Daniel Rüfenacht and Antoine Uske, who had both worked in Parie with Jean-Jacques Merland, would thus establish interventional neuroradiology in the French-speaking part of Switzerland and would collaborate closely during the establishment of their respective divisions. This was also central to the establishment of the "centre romand de neurochirurgie" (neurosurgical center of the French-speaking area (Romandie). The excellence in MRI in Geneva and Lausanne would help establish the Centre d'imagerie Bio-médicale (CIBM.ch) that exists to this day as a platform for basic and clinical research and for translational imaging in the Romandie. Professor Daniel Rüfenacht would introduce a prototype flat panel angiography room in 2008, the salle 37, which remained in function until 2023. Daniel Rüfenacht also would introduce and popularize minimally invasive techniques such as vertebroplasty in Switzerland and also establish the international intracranial Stent meeting that runs until this day as well as founded the ESMINT society [25]. Among his notable trainees is Philippe Gailloud, currently at the Johns Hospkins University. He would briefly found the Service Neuro-interventionnel at the HUG, before moving to Zurich. Upon his departure, the Neuro-interventional division would be re-fusioned with diagnostic neuroradiology and the division would be led by Prof Karl-Olof Lövblad as of 2008; Karl-Olof Lövblad, having trained in Bern under the supervision of Gerhard Schroth, would do a fellowship in Boston with Professors Robert Edelman and Steven Warach, during which he would participate in the early pioneering studies on the clinical use of diffusion-weighted MR imaging. Additionally, after moving to Geneva and working for Daniel Rüfenacht, under his leadership, distinct units for diagnostic and interventional neuroradiology would be created. The interventional unit would be led by Prof Vitor Mendes Pereira (now in Toronto), Dr. Zsolt Kulcsar (nor in Zurich) and is currently led by Paolo Machi; the diagnostic Unit was led successively by Drs. Jacqueline Delavelle, Karl Olof Lövblad, and Maria Vargas and is now led by Professor Felix Kurz. In the italian part of Switzerland, the Tessin, in Lugano, Neuroradiology was led by Claude Merenda (1941–2022), who introduced interventional neuroradiology techniques; upon the creation of the Neurocenter in Lugano under the auspices of Professor Claudio Bassetti, Neuroradiology as a division was formalized by Alessandro Cianfoni, who built up an impressive team encompassing all modalities of diagnostic and interventional neuroradiology; Professor Cianfoni has a strong focus on spinal interventions.

The Swiss Title in Neuroradiology

In 1991, the subtitle of Neuroradiology was created and validated by the FMH (Foederatio Medicorum Helveticorum, the Swiss Medical Society), thereby offering physicians trained in radiology the possibility to subspecialize according to a clear curriculum. Neuroradiology was thus quickly recognized as a subspecialty and board examinations were established, the first being held in Zurich in 1997. Initially this subspecialty comprised all of neuroradiology, both diagnostic and interventional. Due to a reform of the Swiss medical specialty system, in 1997, neuroradiology was elevated to a full specialty and remained so for 4 years until 2001. When the final revision of the Swiss medical specialties was finalized in 2001, Neuroradiology became composed of two subspecialities (Schwerpunkt in German; formation approfondie in French) of radiology, one for diagnostic and one for interventional (called invasive). Both subspecialities require initially to have obtained a certification as a specialist in radiology with additionally 2 years of sub-specialization both in diagnostic and interventional neuroradiology at a postgraduate level with an oral exam for each sub-specialty; the prerequisite for obtaining the title in invasive neuroradiology being having first obtained the sub-specialty in diagnostic neuroradiology. Training time in the subspecialty is at the moment 4 years with, as stated above, 2 years each in diagnostic and interventional neuroradiology, 1 year in diagnostic neuroradiology can be accounted for during the training in diagnostic radiology if the curriculum is organized accordingly. The exact number of examinations and procedures performed are guided by a log-book. The Swiss Society of Neuroradiology manages the invasive (interventional) neuroradiology and co-manages the one in diagnostic Neuroradiology with the Swiss Society for Radiology. The training centers in Switzerland are recognized by the SIWF (the Swiss Institute for medical training) which is a branch of the Swiss medical association (the FMH; fmh.ch). Currently the curricula are being reevaluated.

Building on a high technical expertise and clinical experience, Swiss neuroradiologists have helped advance the field to become a fully established specialty that uses highly specialized techniques to improve patient outcomes. This has been done by the early clinical implementation of MR techniques and endovascular treatment modalities. Swiss neuroradiology thus works within the well-established confines of the Highly specialized Medicine concept in Switzerland and is present as a leader in all stroke centers. Currently, there are 8 stroke centers in Switzerland that can provide all diagnostic and therapeutic modalities for patients with diseases of the vessels of the CNS; additionally, there are currently 5 ultra-high-field (7 T) scanners in operation in Switzerland, which are in part devoted to research and clinical activities for the benefit of local patients.

Neuroradiology and Research

The Swiss Society of Neuroradiology has always had a high academic profile, with a large and varied output in scientific publications by all its members [26, 27]. The Swiss Society of Neuroradiology has held Congresses initially alone and more and more in cooperation with the various societies that now compose the SFNCS (Swiss Federation of clinical Neurosciences) [28]. Neuroradiology also had an important role in the birth of the SFCNS: indeed, in 2009, under the leadership of Anton Valavanis, Claudio Bassetti Christian Hess, and Hildebrandt, the SFCNS was founded as a society covering all Swiss specialties involved in clinical neuroscience; the SFCNS hold its conference every 3 years with all societies being present. In October 1989, the first congress of the Swiss Society of Neuroradiology would take place at the University Hospital in Zurich. These congresses would take place on a yearly basis in different cities in Switzerland, with the local institution hosting them. Since the early 2000s, the meetings are organized jointly with other clinical neuro-societies. Switzerland has hosted the year's ESNR congress four times: in 1983, in Bern with Professor Huber as president; in 1991, in Zurich with Anton Valavanis as President; in 2006, in Geneva with Daniel Rüfenacht; and in 2021, in Geneva again with Karl-Olof Lövblad [29]. Daniel Rüfenacht was one of the founding members of the ESMINT in 2007. Additionally, a training course in neuroradiology organized by the SSNR is held annually in Bern since 2005, which was initiated by Karl-Olof Lövblad in 2005.

The Swiss Society of Neuroradiology would edit its own yearly journal for a decade, *Neuroradiologia Helvetica*, before adopting *Neuroradiology* and *Clinical Neuroradiology* as its official journals [30]. Current news of the Society are published on the website www.swissneuroradiology.ch. The society is also closely associated with the Journal *Clinical and Translational Neurosciences* that Anton Valavanis would help establish.

While the local academic specialties that existed initially (stroke in Bern, aneurysms and spine in Geneva, head and neck and AVM's in Zurich, and inflammatory diseases in Basel) that allowed for world class excellence in these centers due to their high visibility, these differences have almost entirely resolved with all centers offering today a full array of diagnostic and interventional techniques [31], the high level of expertise offered by the centers is an all-time high. This has allowed neuroradiology in Switzerland to position itself strongly within the areas of Highly Specialized Medicine (HSM) specialties [32].

References

1. Valavanis A. Die Schweizerische Gesellschaft für Neuroradiologie: ihre Gründung und Entwicklung. Neuroradiol Helvet. 2005;10:4–9.
2. Wieser C, Etter H, Wellauer J. Radiologie in der Schweiz. Verlag Hans Huber; 1989.
3. Yasargil MG. Die vertebralisangiographie. Springer; 1962.
4. Krayenbühl H, Yaşargil MG. Percutaneous vertebral angiography. Acta Radiol Diagn (Stockh). 1966;5:263–6.
5. Huber P. Zerebrale Angiographie für Klinik und Praxis. Georg Thieme Verlag; 1979.
6. Wellauer J. Die myelographie mit positiven Kontrastmiteln. Georg Thieme Verlag; 1960.
7. Radü EW, Kendall BE, Moseley IF. Computertomographie des Kopfes. Thieme; 1994.
8. Obituary Peter Huber 2.3.1926–2.6.1999. Neuroradiology. 1999;41(10):709–710. https://doi.org/10.1007/s002340050829.
9. Huber P. der Subspezialist. Schweiz Arzteztg. 1992;73:1645.
10. Ozdoba C. Retirement of prof Dr Gerhard Schroth. Clin Neuroradiol. 2014;24(1):3. https://doi.org/10.1007/s00062-014-0296-4.
11. Wanke I, Lövblad KO, Grossmann H, Bassetti CLA, Remonda L. In memory of professor Valavanis. Neuroradiology. 2023;65(10):1561–3.
12. Wanke I, Lövblad KO, Remonda L. Professor Antonios Valavanis. AJNR Am J Neuroradiol. 2023;44(8):E33–4.
13. Valavanis A. Othmar Schubiger. Neuroradiology. 2017;59(6):537–8.
14. Valavanis A, Schubiger O, Wellauer J. Computed tomography of acoustic neuromas with emphasis on small tumor detectability. Neuroradiology. 1978;16:598–600. https://doi.org/10.1007/BF00395374.
15. Wichmann W, Valavanis A, Haller D. Use of high performance nuclear magnetic resonance tomography in neuroradiology. Experience with 2,000 studies. Schweiz Med Wochenschr. 1987;117(47):1841–52.
16. Wanke I, Lövblad KO, Remonda L, Schroth G, on behalf of Swiss Society of Neuroradiology SSNR. In Memory of Prof. Werner Wichmann. Clin Neuroradiol. 2023; https://doi.org/10.1007/s00062-023-01330-x.
17. Valavanis A. The role of angiography in the evaluation of cerebral vascular malformations. Neuroimaging Clin N Am. 1996;6(3):679–704.
18. Valavanis A, Yaşargil MG. The endovascular treatment of brain arteriovenous malformations. Adv Tech Stand Neurosurg. 1998;24:131–214.
19. Valavanis A, Pangalu A, Tanaka M. Endovascular treatment of cerebral arteriovenous malformations with emphasis on the curative role of embolisation. Interv Neuroradiol. 2005;11(Suppl 1):37–43. https://doi.org/10.1177/15910199050110S107.
20. Valavanis A, editor. Interventional neuroradiology. Springer Verlag; 1993.
21. Megret M. A landmark for the choroidal arteries of the fourth ventricle–branches of the posterior inferior cerebellar artery. Neuroradiology. 1973;5(2):85–90.

22. Rüfenacht DA, Merland JJ, Guimaraens L, Reizine D. A simple propulsion-chamber-system for the 16 gauge approach. Neuroradiology. 1986;28(4):355–8.
23. Rufenacht D, Merland JJ. A new and original microcatheter system for hyperselective catheterization and endovascular treatment without risk of arterial rupture. J Neuroradiol. 1986;13(1):44–54. PMID: 3746438
24. Rüfenacht D, Merland JJ. Superselective catheterization using very flexible, formed catheters. Acta Radiol Suppl. 1986;369:600–2.
25. Wanke I, Rüfenacht DA. European Society of Minimally Invasive Neurological Therapy (ESMINT). Clin Neuroradiol. 2015;25(Suppl 2):135–6.
26. Valavanis A, Bassetti C. Im Dienste der Neurowissenschaften. 910. Schweizerische Aerztezeitung. 2015;96:910–2.
27. Lövblad KO. Neuroradiology and neuroimaging. J Neuroradiol. 2014;41(4):217–9.
28. Bassetti C. Swiss federation of clinical neurosciences, SFCNS. Schweiz Arzteztg. 2010;91(8):296.
29. Sundgren P, Lövblad KO. The ESNR Congress recovers from COVID! Neuroradiology. 2022;64(1):3–4.
30. Bassetti C, Valavanis A. Clinical and translational neuroscience (2017–): a 100-year-old newborn former Swiss archives of neurology and psychiatry (1917–2016). Clin Transl Neurosci. 2017;1(1):15. https://doi.org/10.1177/2514183x17725631.
31. Pereira VM, Vargas MI, Marcos A, Bijlenga P, Narata AP, Haller S, Lövblad KO. Diagnostic neuroradiology for the interventional neuroradiologist. World J Radiol. 2013;5(11):386–97.
32. Lövblad KO. Highly specialized neuroradiology. J Neuroradiol. 2015;42(4):191–2.

Chapter 19
The Neuroradiological Society of Taiwan

Chao-Bao Luo, Wan-Yuo Guo, and Michael Mu-Huo Teng

The Neuroradiological Society of Taiwan (hereinafter referred to as NRST) is considered one of the youngest subspecialty medical societies within the Taiwan Neurological Society. Originally, the NRST stemmed from the Neuroradiology Group of the Taiwan Neurological Society. In those years, members from the group were appointed as representatives or elected as directors and supervisors to attend relevant meetings of the Neurological Society.

In 1994, Professor Tsuen Chang, Professor Takahashi from Japan, Professor Sage from Australia, and Professor Chang from South Korea, jointly deliberated on the formation of the Asian-Oceanian Congress of Neuroradiology and Head & Neck Radiology (AOCNHNR). At that time, national membership was a prerequisite for joining the World Federation of Neuroradiological Societies. Therefore, under the leadership of Professor Tsuen Chang and in collaboration with the leading neuroradiology experts in Taiwan at the time, a preparatory committee for the NRST was formed to establish a formal society and actively participate in international academic and organizational activities.

After several meetings and with the assistance of the Department of Social Affairs of the Ministry of the Interior, the NRST was officially established in March 1995. At the time of establishment, the society had 64 founding members, with Professor Tsuen Chang elected as the first chairperson. Professor Tsuen Chang also represented Taiwan in attending the first AOCNHNR held in Kumamoto, Japan in the same year. Additionally, the society was honored to obtain the hosting rights for the second conference, which was scheduled to be held in Taipei in 1997.

In 1997, the second AOCNHNR conference held in Taipei witnessed the participation of approximately 260 attendees from both domestic and international regions.

C.-B. Luo (✉) · W.-Y. Guo
Department of Radiology, Taipei Veterans General Hospital, Taipei, Taiwan
e-mail: cbluo@vghtpe.gov.tw; wyguo@vghtpe.gov.tw

M. M.-H. Teng
Department of Radiology, Cheng-Hsin General Hospital, Taipei, Taiwan

D. Birchall (ed.), *A World History of Neuroradiology*,
https://doi.org/10.1007/978-3-032-16653-1_19

The event was unprecedentedly successful, featuring over ten experts from Europe, America, and Asia delivering keynote speeches. It was the most attended conference by international scholars at the time.

In 1998, Professor Michael Mu Huo Teng was elected as the second chairperson. During his tenure, multiple lectures, seminars, and live demonstrations on interventional neuroradiology were organized. Invitations extended to international experts spurred a surge of interest in this field in Taiwan. The third AOCNHNR conference, held in Adelaide, Australia in 1999, saw over ten Taiwanese participants who presented more than ten research papers, showcasing significant advancements in Taiwan's neuroradiology.

In 2001, Dr. Hon-Man Liu was elected as the third chairperson, continuing to actively promote academic development and adapting to changes in the medical society by establishing a specialist physician system. In 2004, Dr. Sandy Cheng-Yu Chen was elected as the fourth chairperson. During his tenure, he established a society newsletter and enriched our official website. Additionally, a specialist physician examination was introduced to enhance the connectivity between members and the society.

Subsequent chairpersons included Professor Michael Mu Huo Teng (2007), Professor Wan-Yuo Guo (2010), Professor Ho-Fai Wong (2013), Professor Sandy Cheng-Yu Chen (2016), and Professor Chao-Bao Luo (2019 to 2025). Each chairperson has been committed to enhancing the teaching and research of neuroradiology and increasing its international visibility, aspiring to keep pace with advanced countries around the world.

In addition to these achievements, the society has also promoted neuroradiology interventional treatments in response to the rapid development of minimally invasive neurovascular interventions. Currently, the society boasts 320 active members. Its organizational structure is composed of one chairperson, 15 directors, and five supervisors. It holds three 1-day academic conferences and a 2-day annual conference each year, providing a platform for academic exchange among its members. Additionally, an annual examination for specialist physicians is conducted. The society also accredits the specialties of acute ischemic stroke thrombectomy and neuroradiology intervention in the country.

Significant Milestones of the NRST

1. Organized the 1997 Asian-Oceanian Congress of Neuroradiology and Head & Neck Radiology, chaired by Professor Tsuen Chang.
2. Established the training requirements of intravascular interventional neuroradiology, and capability requirements to obtain a certificate of subspecialty of intravascular interventional neuroradiology, and obtain a certificate of proctor of intravascular interventional neuroradiology in 2004. The NRST began to issue certificates of subspecialty of intravascular interventional neuroradiology, and certificates of proctor of intravascular interventional neuroradiology in January 1, 2005 to those who meet the requirements. After this step, diagnosis and intravascular intervention are equally important for neuroradiology training.

3. Organized the 2008 eighth Meeting of the Asian-Australasian Federation of Interventional and Therapeutic Neuroradiology (AAFITN 2008), chaired by Professor Michael Mu Huo Teng.
4. Organized the 2009 Asian-Oceanian Neuroradiology Interventional Treatment Forum, chaired by Professor Michael Mu Huo Teng.
5. Organized the 2018 Asian Oceanian Society of Neuroradiology and Head & Neck Radiology Annual Conference, chaired by Professor Sandy Cheng-Yu Chen.
6. Organized the 2018 Symposium Neuroradiologicum, chaired by Professor Wan-Yuo Guo.
7. Since 2019, the society has held a 2-day academic conference as its annual meeting.
8. In 2022, Professor Wan-Yuo Guo was elected the President of the World Federation of Neuroradiological Societies.

The Asian-Australasian Federation of Interventional and Therapeutic Neuroradiology (AAFITN 2008)

The eighth Meeting of the Asian-Australasian Federation of Interventional and Therapeutic Neuroradiology was held from April 5 to April 8, 2008 in the Grand Hotel, Taipei. The Cross-Strait Interventional and Therapeutic Neuroradiology symposium was held in the evening of April 5, 2008, too.

There were 391 registered attendees, including Taiwan 173, China 43, Japan 40, Thailand 32, USA 14, Australia 13, and other countries or regions with less than ten attendees. Totally, 58 invited lectures, 104 free papers (oral 23, poster 81). Six more invited lectures from Chinese Mainland and two from Taiwan for the Cross-Strait Interventional and Therapeutic Neuroradiology symposium.

XXI SNR in Taiwan

The XXIst SNR (The World Congress of Neuroradiology 2018) was hosted by the Neuroradiological Society of Taiwan (NRST). Professor Wan-Yuo GUO was elected as the President of the XXIst SNR in 2010 during the XIXth SNR in Bologna, Italy. After 8 years of preparation, the XXIst SNR under the Presidency of Prof Wan-Yuo GUO started on March 19 and lasted until March 23 at Taipei International Congress and Exhibition Center (TICC), Taipei, Taiwan. Totally, more than 1000 attendees from 50 countries of five continents and 39 industry sponsors participated in the XXIst SNR. The 5-day Congress consisted of 74 sessions with 6 themes, including Brain, Head & Neck, Pediatric, Spine, Intervention, Highlights, and special sessions such as "Master to Master" and "Junior Meets Junior."

In addition to the comprehensive scientific program, the XXIst SNR Organizing Committee unprecedentedly invited famous Taiwanese artists to join the Congress and exhibit their artworks, as well as hosted tea art performances throughout the Congress at the Congress Venue of TICC. It is the true form of realization and unification of "The Art of Healing, the Healing of Art." And as for the attendees, the Organizing Committee hosted a "Photography Exhibition Competition" that allowed the attendees to submit their photographs and which were displayed during the congress.

Below are some of the photos taken at the XXIst SNR and links to multiple video clips summarizing XXI SNR (Fig. 19.1).

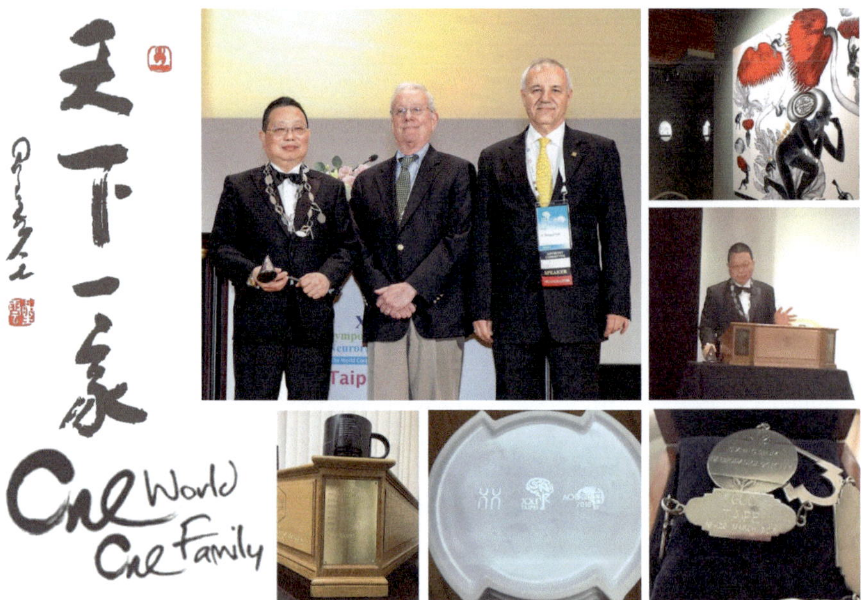

Fig. 19.1 The 21st Symposium Neuroradiologicum (XXI SNR) was inaugurated under the noble theme "One World, One Family," a spirit that united scholars and practitioners of neuroradiology from across the globe. The calligraphy of these four words, bestowed by Venerable Master Hsing Yun, founder of Fo Guang Shan, stood as a symbol of universal fellowship and as a tribute to the worldwide contributions of the World Federation of Neuroradiological Societies (WFNRS). The opening ceremony was solemnly presided over by three consecutive WFNRS Presidents Wan-Yuo Guo, Nick Bryan, and Turgut Tali. In keeping with the time-honored tradition of the congress, President Wan-Yuo Guo, adorned with the ceremonial chain of past congress presidents, struck the historic gavel to herald the commencement of the proceedings. The gathering was further enriched by the presence of celebrated Taiwanese contemporary artists, whose works lent cultural and artistic brilliance to the scientific assembly. To honor its legacy, the congress presented delegates with commemorative black and white mugs, specially crafted in the form of the podium that has been passed down since 1955 (IV SNR, London), leaving a lasting impression of dignity, culture, and fraternity upon all who attended

1. https://youtu.be/3E-I83STCH8?si=2dsWs6uvWqLLgsdV
2. https://youtu.be/E6krP_w2mqU?si=yw5-Ydlr3b97Nkca
3. https://youtu.be/8zLfP0ZMcXs?si=MWONe2u7TaZwrk7L
4. https://youtu.be/zMr1PG1lK38?si=sloJmW4EvWAk_mJV

Written by Professors Chao-Bao LUO, Wan-You GUO, and Michael Mu Huo TENG, Dec. 12, 2023, Taipei, Taiwan.

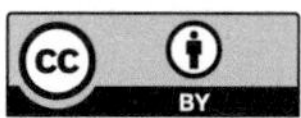

Chapter 20
Neuroradiology in Türkiye

E. Turgut Tali

There exists no comprehensive record detailing the evolution of neuroradiology in Türkiye. However, based on personal communications, it is believed that vascular neuroradiology began at Istanbul University's Capa Medical School in 1955. A small cohort of neurosurgeons conducted pneumoencephalography and carotid angiography, initially through open dissection of the carotids and later via percutaneous puncture. These initial cerebral angiographic views were obtained by manual changers at Towne and lateral head projections and most of the catheters were custom-made. Among the trailblazers of modern neurosurgery clinics in Türkiye, Prof. Dr. Bülent Tarcan from Istanbul University Faculty of Medicine, Prof. Dr. Nurhan Avman from Hacettepe University Faculty of Medicine in Ankara, and neurologist Prof. Dr. Sabahattin Kerimoglu from Istanbul University Cerrahpasa Medical Faculty Department of Neurology can be acknowledged as the pioneers of neuroradiology in our country [1–4] (Fig. 20.1).

These early pioneers were subsequently joined by radiologist Prof Dr. Hadi Ozer from Hacettepe University Faculty of Medicine Department of Radiology, neurologist Prof. Dr. Okay Saribas from the Department of Neurology, radiologist Prof. Dr. Uluhan Berk from the Department of Radiology at Ankara University Faculty of Medicine, neurologist Prof. Dr. Gencay Gürsoy from the Department of Neurology at Istanbul University Faculty of Medicine, and neurologist Prof. Dr. Hayrünnisa Denktas from the Department of Neurology at Istanbul University Cerrahpasa Medical Faculty, along with their respective teams (Fig. 20.2).

As modern neuroradiology began to take shape in the 1960s, particularly in the United States of America and Europe, notably Scandinavia, Prof. Dr. Gencay Gürsoy undertook neuroradiology training in Norway between 1967 and 1969. Upon his return to Istanbul University Faculty of Medicine, he initiated the practice of contemporary diagnostic and interventional procedures along with his team [4].

E. T. Tali (✉)
Department of Radiology, Lokman Hekim University Faculty of Medicine, Ankara, Turkey

D. Birchall (ed.), *A World History of Neuroradiology*,
https://doi.org/10.1007/978-3-032-16653-1_20

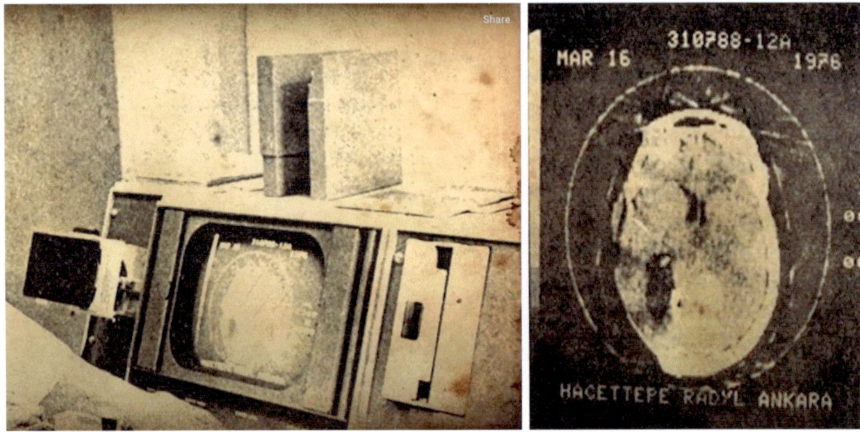

Fig. 20.1 The CT unit of Hacettepe University and one of its images. Permission and courtesy of Prof. Oguz Dicle.Yuzyillik Yolculuk: Baslangicindan Gunumuze Turk Radyolojisi. 1995, 5G Matbaacılık Ltd. Sti. Istanbul

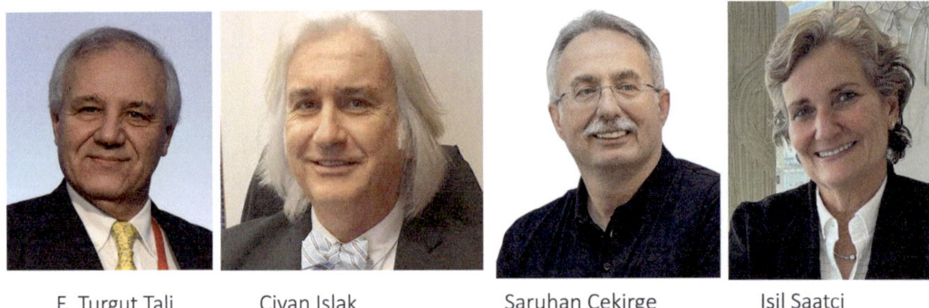

Fig. 20.2 Early pioneers

The growing popularity of neuroradiology spurred interest from both neurologists and radiologists, leading to turf battles within the field. Concurrently, the number of individuals seeking neuroradiology training abroad from various institutions surged.

In Türkiye, neuroradiology was established as a clinic or division for the first time in 1975. With the decision of the Faculty Board of Istanbul University Istanbul Medical Faculty, the Neuroradiology Division became a part of the Department of Neurology. Subsequently, plans were set in motion for an "Institute of Neurological Sciences" within the Capa campus of Istanbul University, which would encompass the Departments of Neurology and Neurosurgery, as well as the Neuroradiology Division. Construction of this facility, outfitted with state-of-the-art equipment for the period, was finalized in 1982 and inaugurated by the Prime Minister at the time. Around the same period, propelled by the foresight of Prof.

Dr. Abdullah Kenanoglu, the Chair of the Department of Radiology at Hacettepe University Faculty of Medicine in Ankara, and under the auspices of Rector Prof. Dr. Ihsan Dogramaci, the 6th (some sources suggest the 11th) EMI Computed Brain Tomography worldwide was installed in the Department of Radiology at Hacettepe University Faculty of Medicine in April 1976 (Fig. 20.1) (6-13). This device could complete each image in a 64x90 matrix in 4.5 minutes. It took approximately two hours for an examination to appear. Following cerebral angiography and pneumoencephalography, this equipment heralded a new era in neuroradiology not only within our country but globally as well. In 1980, Istanbul University published the first cranial angiography book in Türkiye authored by Prof. Dr. Hayrünnisa Denktas and Prof. Dr. Sabahattin Kerimoglu. The year 1982 marked a significant milestone as Prof. Dr. Reha Tolun returned from neuroradiology training in France and conducted the inaugural "balloon embolization" in a patient afflicted with carotico-cavernous fistula. During the early 1980s, Prof. Dr. Münci Oran, following his training in Glasgow, UK commenced the application of contemporary diagnostic neuroradiology techniques at the Department of Radiology, Hacettepe University Faculty of Medicine. Concurrently, Prof. Dr. Baki Göksan, from the Department of Neurology at Istanbul Cerrahpasa Medical Faculty, pioneered the utilization of Doppler ultrasonography in neuroradiology.

The inception of the first digital subtraction angiography (DSA) device in Türkiye was installed in 1986 within the Department of Radiology at Gazi University, Faculty of Medicine. The diversification of interventional neuroradiological procedures ensued through the endeavors of Prof. Dr. Olcay Cizmeli and Prof. Dr. Erhan Ilgit, who worked to facilitate and to assist the importation of those materials from foreign companies to our country [5–13].

In 1986, during the restructuring in the university, efforts were made to transition the Neuroradiology Division of the Department of Neurology at Istanbul University Faculty of Medicine into a section. However, disagreements arose, primarily from radiologists seeking involvement in neuroradiology, leading to protracted discussions. Ultimately, in 1988, the decision was made to found Neuroradiology as an independent department instead of a section of a department, with Prof. Dr. Cahit Babuna from the Department of Radiology appointed as its chair. Prof. Dr. Reha Tolun from the Department of Neurology and Prof. Dr. Ozenc Minareci from the Department of Radiology were also designated faculty members. Nonetheless, in 1989, the Council of Higher Education dismantled the Department of Neuroradiology, relegating Neuroradiology back to a section within the Department of Radiology.

With the visionary leadership of Prof. Dr. Abdullah Kenanoglu, this time as the founding Dean of Dokuz Eylül University Faculty of Medicine in Izmir and Chair of the Department of Radiology, the first Magnetic Resonance Imaging (MRI) device was installed in the Department of Radiology. This marked a significant breakthrough for our country in the field of neuroradiology. Subsequently, in the same year, three more MRI devices were introduced, with two in Istanbul and one in Ankara, elevating neuroradiological diagnostic capabilities to a new level.

As technological advancements in neuroradiology and radiology accelerated globally, in 1990, proactive steps were being taken in Türkiye to acquaint itself with

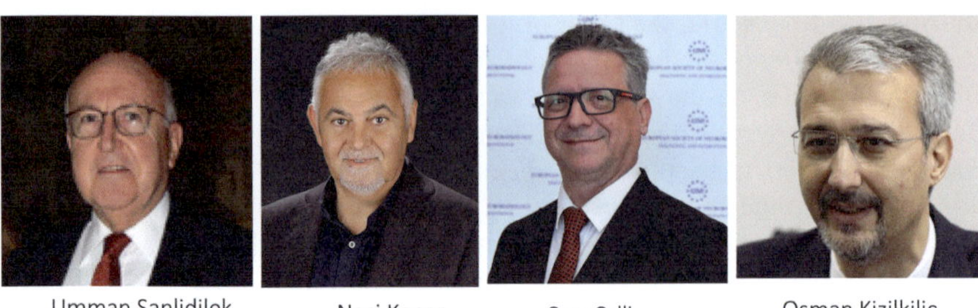

Fig. 20.3 The inaugural cranial arteriovenous malformation (AVM) embolization was performed in 1990

these new technological innovations in both diagnostic and interventional neuroradiology. In 1990, Prof. Dr. E. Turgut Tali embarked on diagnostic neuroradiology training at the University of Iowa in the USA, while Pro. f Dr. Civan Islak pursued training in both diagnostic and interventional neuroradiology in Nancy, France. Subsequently, in 1991, Prof. Dr. Isil Saatci underwent similar training at Georgetown University in the USA, followed by Prof. Dr. Saruhan Cekirge, who pursued interventional neuroradiology training at Pittsburg University in the USA in 1992 (Fig. 20.2).

The history of Turkish neuroradiology is marked by a series of events peculiar to Türkiye. Türkiye was among the first European countries in which interventional neuroradiology developed as a strong discipline, overcoming the obstacles presented by the notorious political situation. In spite of many obstacles, modern diagnostic and interventional neuroradiology suites established in many Radiology Departments, where nowadays, all kinds of neuroradiology techniques for treatment of cerebrovascular disease are routinely performed.

Meanwhile, the inaugural cranial arteriovenous malformation (AVM) embolization was performed in 1990 by Prof. Dr. Umman Sanlidilek from the Department of Radiology, Ankara University Faculty of Medicine (Fig. 20.3) [12]. Upon the return of Dr. Civan Islak, followed by Dr. Isil Saatci and Dr. Saruhan Cekirge from their overseas training, advanced techniques in interventional neuroradiology were seamlessly integrated into routine practice and research, fostering international collaborations in the field.

In 1991, the Turkish Society of Neuroradiology (TSNR) was founded in Istanbul, under the leadership of Prof. Dr. Oktay Cokyüksel, the Chair of the Department of Radiology at Istanbul Cerrahpasa Medical Faculty, uniting individuals dedicated to advancing this field. Dr. Oktay Cokyüksel assumed the role of the first President of the Society. Currently, TSNR has 221 full, 140 junior members actively practicing neuroradiology in Türkiye. TSNR is a member of the World Federation of Neuroradiological Societies, the Asian and Oceanian Society of Neuroradiology and Head and Neck Radiology, and an institutional member of the European Society of Neuroradiology. TSNR also collaborates with numerous international societies such as the American Society of Neuroradiology, the American Society of Spine

Radiology, WFITN, and ESMINT. Initially, "Rivista di Neuroradiologia," indexed in major indexes such as SCI and Index Medicus, was the official journal of the society alongside the Italian Society of Neuroradiology. Since 2012, "Neuroradiology" has become the official journal of the society.

In 1994, Dr. Oktay Cokyüksel founded the Section of Neuroradiology within the Department of Radiology at Istanbul University Cerrahpasa Faculty of Medicine. This section transitioned to its independent facility in 2004 with brand new equipment. Subsequently, Neuroradiology Sections were established within the Departments of Radiology in numerous universities.

In the same year, the treatments of cerebral aneurysms with Guglielmi detachable coils were performed by Dr. Civan Islak from Istanbul University Cerrahpasa Faculty of Medicine, Department of Radiology and with MDS and IDC detachable coils by Dr. Isil Saatci and Dr. Saruhan Cekirge from Hacettepe University Faculty of Medicine, Department of Radiology for the first time.

The inaugural event of the Turkish Society of Neuroradiology took place in 1997 as the "Symposium on White Matter Diseases Imaging" featuring the participation of esteemed experts such as Dr. James Barkovich and Dr. Jan Brismar.

In 1998, Dr. Isil Saatci introduced the intranidal long Onyx injection technique, pioneering the concept of curative treatment in arteriovenous malformations (AVMs); it gained global acceptance. In 1999, the treatment of aneurysms with liquid ONYX began to gain prominence, with Dr. Cekirge and Dr. Saatci in Hacettepe University being the first Turkish team to collaborate with European and US centers involved in FDA trials on this subject. Their publications on the use of Onyx in AVM and aneurysm treatment received over 1000 citations reflecting their impact in the field. During the same years, Dr. Cekirge pioneered the concept of advanced reconstruction of the aneurysm neck with intracranial stenting associated with coiling and/or Onyx, marking a global breakthrough. This group also initiated aneurysm treatments with coronary stents for the first time worldwide, in collaboration with several international centers.

The international engagement of the Turkish Society of Neuroradiology and neuroradiologists expanded significantly. In 2001, the first certification course of the European Society of Neuroradiology, sixth Cycle third course, was convened in Antalya (Fig. 20.4). Subsequently, in 2003, the 12th Advanced Course and 28th Annual Congress of the European Society of Neuroradiology, organized by Dr. E. Turgut Tali in Istanbul, achieved resounding success (Fig. 20.5).

In 2006, under the leadership of the Chairman Prof. Dr. Aytekin Besim, Dr. Isil Saatci, and Dr. Saruhan Cekirge from Hacettepe Medical Faculty, Department of Radiology, Dr. Civan Islak and Prof Dr. Naci Kocer from Cerrahpaşa Medical Faculty Section of Neuroradiology, and Dr. E. Turgut Tali from Gazi University Medical Faculty Section of Neuroradiology, organized the first international interventional neuroradiology live course with the name of "Anatolian Course in Interventional Neuroradiology" (Fig. 20.6).

In the same year, Dr. E. Turgut Tali took a role in the Executive Committee of the European Society of Neuroradiology and subsequently served as its president from 2012 to 2014.

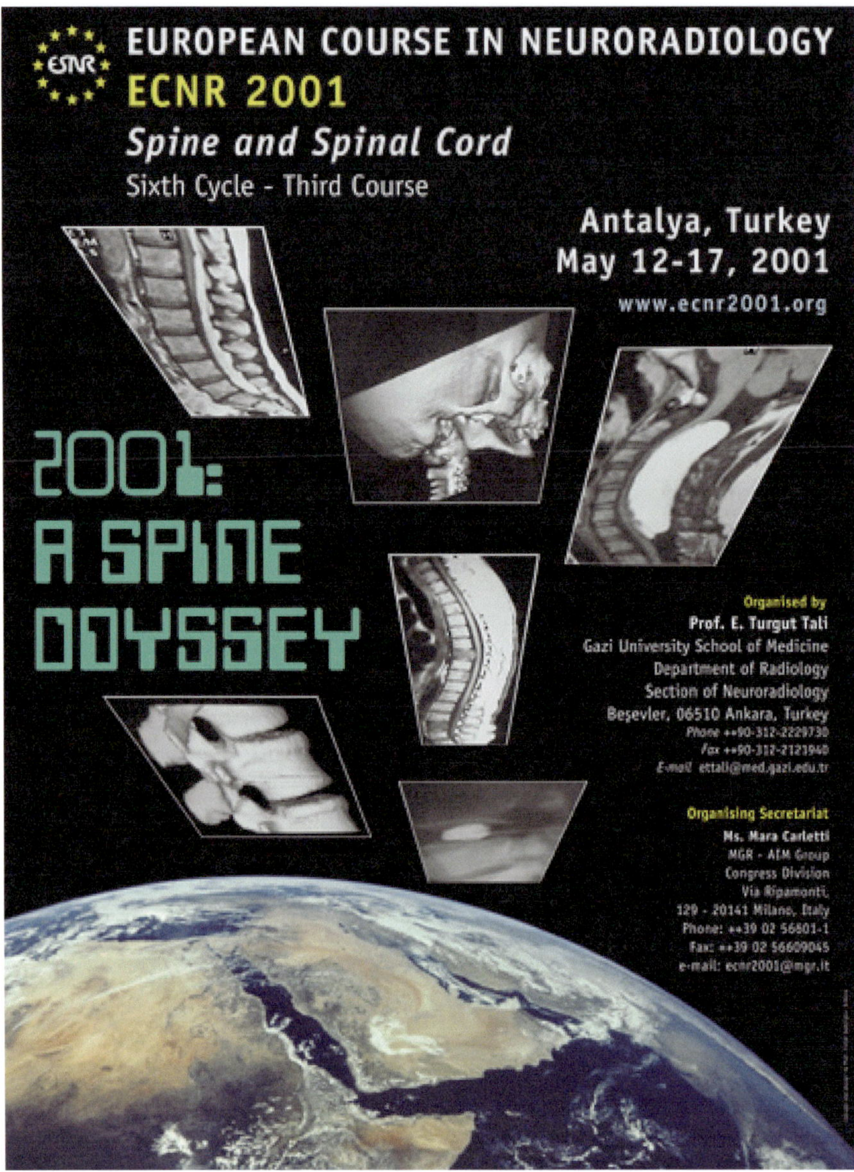

Fig. 20.4 The international engagement of the Turkish Society of neuroradiology and neuroradiologists

By the end of 2008, following the introduction of the Pipeline device, Drs. Cekirge, Saatci, and their team in Hacettepe University participated in the FDA Trial for Pipeline (PUFS) alongside eight major USA centers, earning recognition as the center with the highest number of cases in the trial. Following FDA approval of the Pipeline device, Hacettepe University Faculty of Medicine Department of

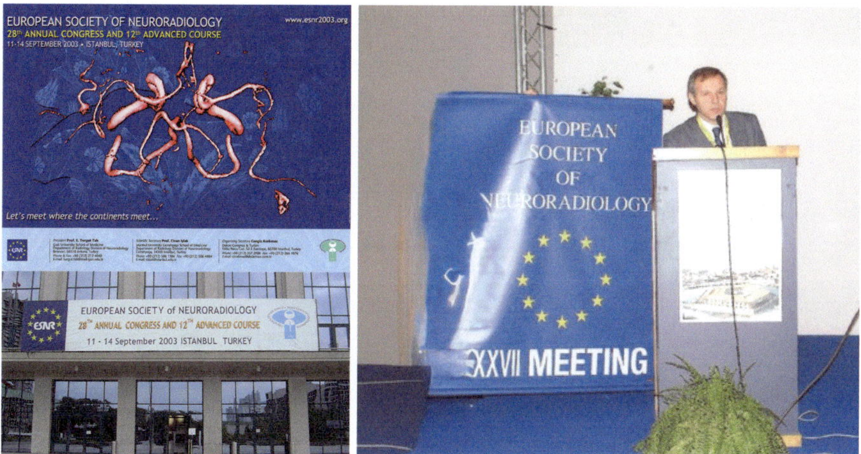

Fig. 20.5 The 12th Advanced Course and 28th Annual Congress of the European Society of Neuroradiology, 2003

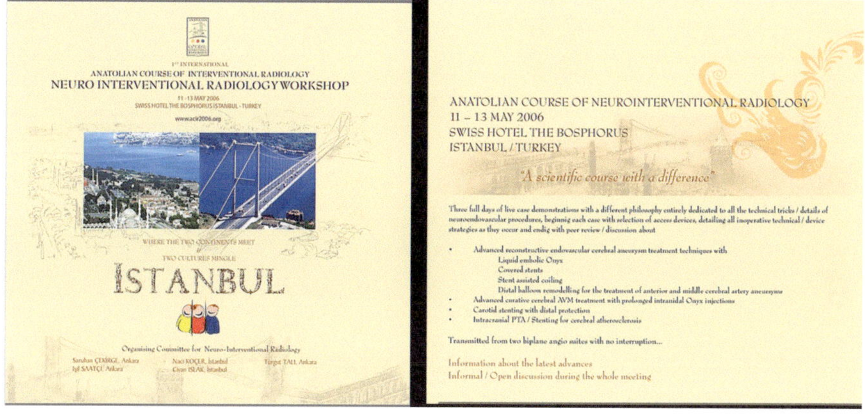

Fig. 20.6 Anatolian course of interventional radiology

Radiology became a hub for training in this technique. Physicians from numerous interventional neuroradiology centers across the USA, including prestigious universities, attended courses organized at Hacettepe University, contributing to the widespread adoption of this technique. Between 2001 to 2012, more than 400 physicians from USA to Japan visited Ankara to learn advanced cerebral aneurysm and AVM treatment techniques. Under the leadership of Dr. Islak, Dr. Kocer, and Prof Dr. Osman Kizilkilic, Istanbul University Cerrahpasa Faculty of Medicine Section of Interventional Neuroradiology has also become a training side for many physicians visiting from all over the world. Over the years, the team of the "Anatolian Course in Interventional Neuroradiology" gained prominence and the Anatolian Course in Interventional Neuroradiology collaborated with the LINNC

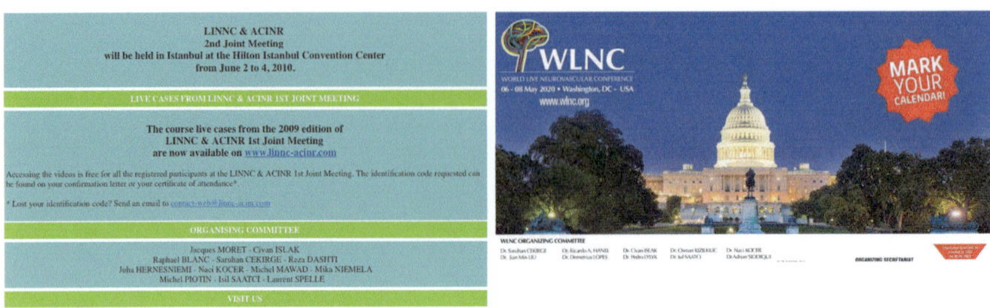

Fig. 20.7 Conference event held in different continents globally

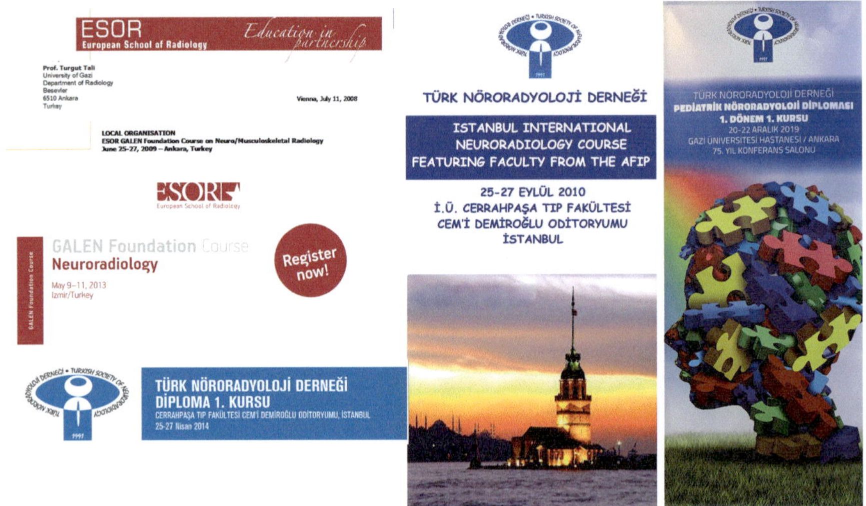

Fig. 20.8 Galen neuroradiology course

course organized by the renowned Dr. Jacques Moret and his team from France between 2009 and 2012. In 2013, Dr. Saatci, Dr. Cekirge, Dr. Islak, Dr. Kocer, and Dr. Kizilkilic, along with the eminent interventional neuroradiologists Pedro Lylyk and Demetrius Lopez from Argentina and the USA established the "World Live Neurovascular Conference" (WLNC) and it has become empowered with the participation of several other world-renowned neurointerventionists, such as Drs. Hanel, Liu, Mounier, and Siddiqui in 2020. This conference is now being held in different continents every year and has become the foremost event in the field globally (Figs. 20.3 and 20.7).

On the other hand, with respect to diagnostic neuroradiology events, the Galen Neuroradiology course, one of the basic courses of the European Society of Radiology, was organized by Dr. E. Turgut Tali in Ankara in 2009 and Dr. Cem Calli in Izmir in 2013 (Fig. 20.8).

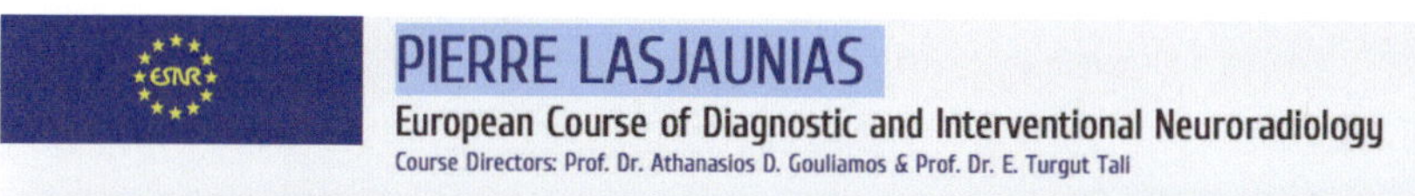

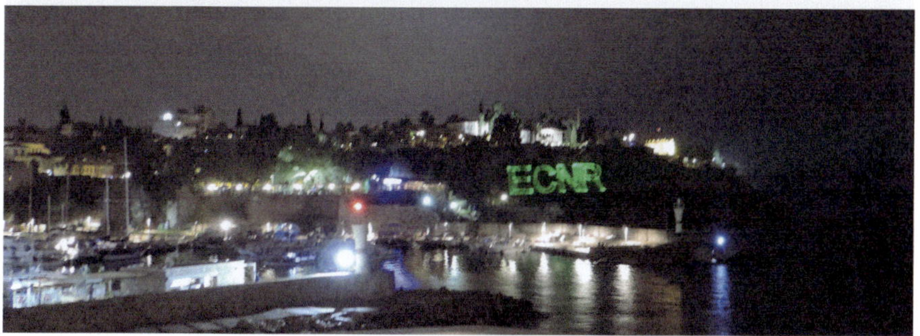

Fig. 20.9 12th and 13th cycles of the European course in neuroradiology-ECNR, Antalya-Athens, 2012–2016

Dr. Tali was elected as a member of the Board of Directors of the World Federation of Neuroradiological Societies in 2010 after fulfilling various committee roles.

In 2010, Dr. Tali organized the Istanbul Neuroadiology Course in collaboration with the Armed Forces Institute of Pathology (AFIP), USA (Fig. 20.8). This was followed by the Erasmus Pediatric Neuroradiology Course in 2011, also held in Istanbul. Additionally, the Turkish Neuroradiology Society commemorated its 20th anniversary with the organization of the tenth Anniversary Neuroradiology Meeting in Antalya in the same year.

Between 2011 and 2014, Dr. Tali organized together with Prof Dr. Athanassios Gouliamos the European Courses in Neuroradiology, the diploma courses of the European Society of Neuroradiology, in Antalya and Izmir in Türkiyeu and Athens and Rhodes in Greece (Fig. 20.9).

Since 2014, the Turkish Diploma in Neuroradiology courses have been organized in collaboration with the European Society of Neuroradiology twice a year (Fig. 20.8). These courses, mirroring the rules and program of the European Course in Neuroradiology (ECNR), have garnered substantial interest. In the same year, the Turkish Board of Neuroradiology was founded, with Dr. Naci Kocer elected as its first chair. Additionally, Turkish Pediatric Neuroradiology Diploma courses, following similar criteria and program, have been introduced in 2019 (Fig. 20.8), the Turkish Diploma in Pediatric Neuroradiology courses have been held annually. Both diplomas received endorsement from the European Society of Neuroradiology and the European Society of Radiology in 2015. Currently, 281 members hold the Turkish Diploma in Neuroradiology, and 68 neuroradiologists have obtained the Turkish Diploma in Pediatric Neuroradiology. TSNR has organized numerous certification courses and educational activities related to neuroradiology. In 2016, the annual "Stroke and Treatments" courses were initiated in collaboration with the Society of Interventional Radiology.

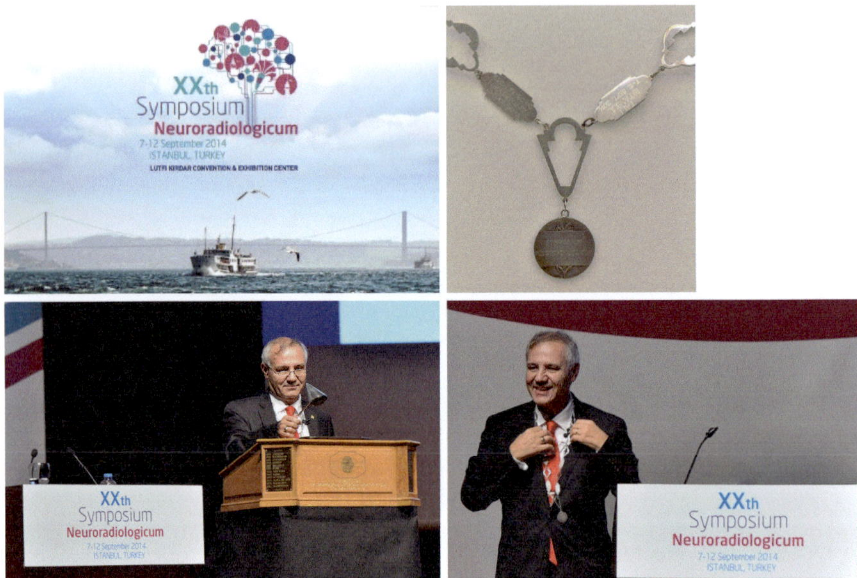

Fig. 20.10 The XXth symposium neuroradiologicum

The XXth Symposium Neuroradiologicum, esteemed as one of the traditional and paramount gatherings in neuroradiology, was meticulously organized by Dr. Tali in Istanbul in 2014, drawing the participation of internationally renowned neuroradiologists (Fig. 20.10). At this congress, Dr. Tali was elected as the president-elect to the Board of Directors of the World Federation of Neuroradiological Societies and subsequently served as president from 2018 to 2022.

In 2014, Prof Dr. Cem Calli from Ege University Faculty of Medicine, Department of Radiology, was elected to the board of directors of the European Society of Neuroradiology and currently holds the position of treasurer (Fig. 20.3).

Meanwhile, Dr. Cekirge and Dr. Saatci participated in another FDA Trial (WEB-IT STUDY) for the intrasaccular flow modifier Web device in 2016, with their center being one of the two non-US sites in the world. Subsequently, they provided training on this device's application in numerous centers, including significant ones in the USA, serving as proctors.

Prof Dr. Serdar Geyik has established the nation's largest stroke center in Istanbul in the recent years. With his team, they have been participating in several international stroke researches; they are organizing the international ICure Stroke meeting with their very well-known global partners every year in Istanbul since 2021.

Since 2016, the Turkish Society of Neuroradiology has annually organized congresses with international participation in Istanbul every February (Fig. 20.11).

Dr. Tali is one of the founders of the European Board of Neuroradiology in 2016 and served as its CEO until 2018.

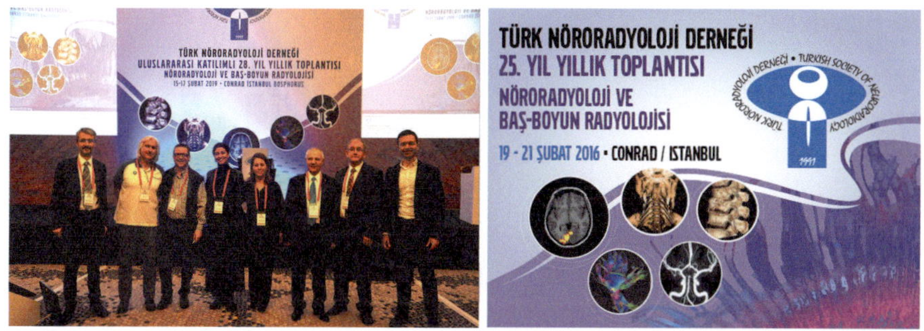

Fig. 20.11 Turkish Society of Neuroradiology organize congresses with international participation in Istanbul every February

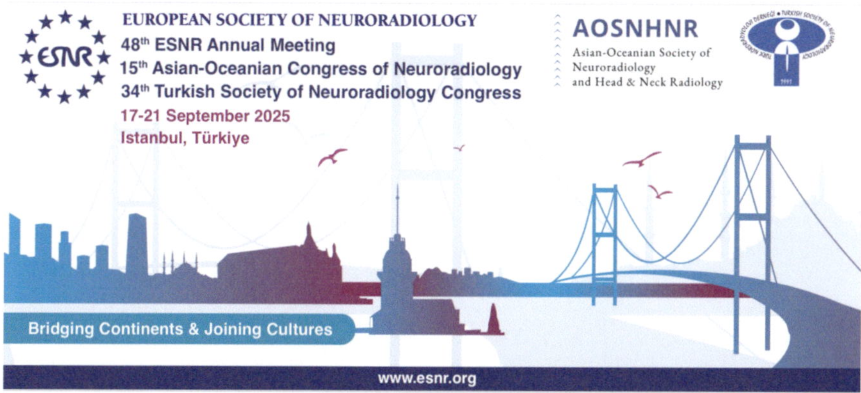

Fig. 20.12 Bridging continents and joining cultures

In 2017, Dr. Naci Kocer from Istanbul University Cerrahpasa Faculty of Medicine, Section of Neuroradiology, was elected to the Executive Committee of the European Society of Neuroradiology to chair the Interventional Neuroradiology. In 2019, he started the organization of European Course in Interventional Neuroradiology on behalf of ESNR with the ultimate target of offering European Diploma in Interventional Neuroradiology, endorsed by the UEMS, to the qualified individuals.

In 2023, Dr. Isil Saatci was elected to the Executive Committee of the European Society of Neuroradiology and took over the leadership of the organization of the European Course in Interventional Neuroradiology.

Dr. Cem Calli was elected President of the Annual Congress of the European Society of Neuroradiology in 2025, while Dr. E. Turgut Tali was elected President of the Congress of the Asian and Oceanian Society of Head Neck Radiology and Neuroradiology in the same year. They will jointly organize the "Bridging Continents and Joining Cultures" congress in Istanbul (Fig. 20.12).

References

1. T. Pirnar, O. Dicle, Yüz yillik yolculuk. Baslangicinden günümüze Türk Radyolojisi. 5 G Matbaacilik. Istanbul, 1995.
2. Ince F, Keskinbora HK. Overview of the history of Turkish Radiology in the light of archives documents (1896–1933). Mersin Universitesi Tip Fakültesi Lokman Hekim Tıp Tarihi ve Folklorik Tıp Dergisi. 2023;13(2):303–13. https://doi.org/10.31020/mutftd.1238285.
3. Istanbul Universitesi Nöroloji web page.
4. Tolun MR. A shorth history of neuroradiology and interventional neurology in the world and in Turkey. Turk J Neurol. 2019;25:260–2.
5. Olcay C. Girisimsel Nöroradyolojiye Nasil Basladik. TRD Sem. 2022;10(1):154–9.
6. Personal communications with Prof. Dr. Hadi Ozer.
7. Personal communications with Prof. Dr. Erdem Gökmen.
8. Personal communications with Prof. Dr. Oktay Cokyüksel.
9. Personal communications with Prof. Dr. Aytekin Besim.
10. Personal communications with Prof. Dr. Ersin Lüleci.
11. Personal communications with Prof. Dr. Dinç Ozaksoy.
12. Personal communications with Prof. Dr. Umman Sanlidilek.
13. Personal communications with Prof. Dr. Baris Diren.

Chapter 21
History of the Swedish Society of Neuroradiology and Swedish Neuroradiology 1990–2024

Isabella M. Björkman-Burtscher, Ida Blystad, Tobias Granberg, and Pia Maly Sundgren

Neuroradiology in Sweden during 1990–2024, and thus the national society's agenda, is marked by the main methods developed and used in modern diagnostics and intervention: CT, MRI, and angiography. However, the history of the speciality and the society is based on technical developments of a far more historic character. Thus, a brief retrospection is needed to set the stage for the events that followed.

The formation of the Swedish Society of Neuroradiology (SSNR) in 1971 was preceded by many decades where Swedish neuroradiology was characterized by a pioneering spirit that already struck a chord far beyond the country's borders. Only 1 year after the discovery of X-rays in 1895, Thor Stenbeck used the technique to localize a bullet in the brain of a patient, who later was successfully operated on [1]. In the 1930–1940s, the Serafimer Hospital in Stockholm became a research and teaching centre for neuroradiology well known far outside Sweden. Also referred to as the "Stockholm School of Neuroradiology," Stockholm was visited by many international guest researchers and colleagues. The same applied to other academic institutions in Sweden, where former colleagues from Stockholm established their centres: Ingmar Wickbom moved to Gothenburg, and Sten Cronquist to Lund [2, 3].

I. M. Björkman-Burtscher (✉)
University of Gothenburg, Gothenburg, Sweden
e-mail: isabella.bjorkman-burtscher@gu.se

I. Blystad
Linköping University, Linköping and President of SSNR, Linköping, Sweden
e-mail: ida.blystad@regionostergotland.se

T. Granberg
Karolinska Institutet, Stockholm, Sweden
e-mail: tobias.granberg@ki.se

P. M. Sundgren
Lund University, Lund, Sweden
e-mail: pia.sundgren@med.lu.se

D. Birchall (ed.), *A World History of Neuroradiology*,
https://doi.org/10.1007/978-3-032-16653-1_21

Refinements in the use of X-rays in neuroradiology were not least achieved by Erik L.R. Lysholm, who showed technical aptitude and was a driving force in the technological development of radiology and neuroradiology—e.g. "the Lysholm grid" and "the Lysholm skull table" [4, 5]. Angiography also quickly found its place in Swedish neuroradiology. The Sven-Ivar Seldinger technique [6] and Torsten Almén's work with non-ionic contrast agents [7] are two Swedish pioneering achievements that were especially important for the breakthrough of angiography and interventional neuroradiology.

Computed Tomography was introduced in Sweden in 1973, the first CT scanner in mainland Europe and the third in the world outside of the United Kingdom [2] was placed at the Karolinska Hospital in Stockholm, only 2 years after the first patient was examined with the technique. Notably, this gave rise to the first publications on CT cisternography, CT angiography, dynamic CT, and stereotactic CT. This pioneering installation sparked national collaborations on CT techniques and was soon followed by installations at other major academic hospitals in Sweden. Magnetic resonance imaging began its victory streak in Swedish neuroradiology during the early 1980s, with in-house manufactured installations, early clinical systems, and a paper in Swedish on "Medical applications of nuclear spin resonance—NMR" published in 1982 [8].

The Swedish Society of Neuroradiology, SSNR (Svensk Förening för Neuroradiologi, SFNR)

The idea to form a Swedish Society of Neuroradiology (SSNR) was born in 1969 when the European Society was formed. SSNR was established in 1971, one year prior to the formation of the Nordic Society of Neuroradiology, with Erik Lindgren as president, Torgny Greitz as vice-president, and Bengt Liliequist as secretary.

SSNR has always focused on the scientific development of neuroradiology as a speciality, and on education for members and health professionals working within or close to neuroradiology. To support educational and scientific goals of the society, SSNR has promoted appointments of professorships within the field. Currently, six of the seven Universities with medical faculties have, or have had, appointed professorships in neuroradiology. Current active full professors in neuroradiology and/or interventional neuroradiology are Johan Wikström, Uppsala, Staffan Holmin, Stockholm, Pia Maly Sundgren, Lund, and Isabella Björkman-Burtscher, Gothenburg. Presidents of SSNR during the last 20 years were Elna-Marie Larsson, Lars Gustafsson, Anders Lilja, Birgitta Ramgren, Tommy Andersson, Birgitta Leiram, Johan Wikström, Roger Siemund, and the current president Ida Blystad.

Early members of the board strongly promoted the establishment of neuroradiology as a medical speciality in Sweden. The history of neuroradiology in Sweden and the SSNR from 1990 and onwards is greatly influenced by the fact that neuroradiology was established as a medical subspeciality by the Swedish National Board of Health and Welfare in 1991.

On the request of the National Board of Health and Welfare, the society has outlined and revised the training curricula for the speciality in collaboration with the Swedish Society of Radiology and adhering to the European training curriculum for radiology and for subspecialisation. From the beginning of the millennium, SSNR has, for more than a decade, awarded grants for participation in the European Course of Neuroradiology (ECNR) to support young neuroradiologists in their ambition to certify internationally. Today employers endorse the participation in the ECNR series for neuroradiologists in training and the courses as well as the European Diploma in Neuroradiology (EDiNR) are part of the recommended education of young neuroradiologists. The society has further awarded travel grants to meetings such as ESNR, Symposium Neuroradiologicum, ASNR, and ISMRM.

Funding for research and visits abroad is also facilitated by The Erik Lysholm Foundation (Stiftelsen för Medicinsk Bildering till Erik Lysholms Minne), founded in 1995 and since managed by SSNR.

The society has, during the last decades, increased its international partnerships and SSNR is today affiliated with the Swedish Society of Radiology (SFMR) and the Swedish Society of Medicine (SLS), a member organization of the World Federation of Neuroradiological Societies (WFNRS), a member society of the World Federation of Interventional and Therapeutic Neuroradiology (WFITN), and an institutional member of the European Society of Neuroradiology (ESNR). Further, SSNR has representation in the European Union of Medical Specialists (UEMS) Section of Radiology, Division of Neuroradiology with two delegates.

According to the statutes, SSNR is open to all who work in and/or have an interest in neuroradiology. Its purpose is to represent the speciality's scientific interests, to promote the development of neuroradiology by organizing meetings with scientific lectures and discussions, to conduct and support education in the field, and to constitute a referral body for the Swedish Medical Society and other national health care and governmental bodies.

For more than four decades, educational courses have been arranged or endorsed by the society covering basic and advanced diagnostic neuroradiology, spine imaging, head and neck imaging, paediatric neuroradiology, interventional radiology, and MR physics. A much-appreciated concept was courses held, for example, on Cyprus and Mallorca, gathering neuroradiologists and clinicians such as neurologists and neurosurgeons as members of the teaching faculty, that discussed and taught course participants not only imaging findings but also the relevance of radiological examinations, how they are performed, how they are read, and how they are reacted upon. These courses were also exceptional as they invited different professions to participate—radiologists, neuroradiologists, clinicians, radiographers, and physicists. The exchange of knowledge at these meetings has also been driving the development of clinical neuroradiology in Sweden. Due to economic and sustainability requirements, these courses are today held in Sweden with the driving aim of gathering a multidisciplinary faculty for a few days.

In addition to these educational efforts, the SSNR arranges annual meetings with scientific and educational programmes that reflect both contemporary aspects of neuroradiology and honour national and international achievements in the field.

SFNR honorary lecturers and former Torgny Greitz lecturers between 1991 and 2024 are:

1991: Professor Makthar Gado, Bethesda, USA; 1992: cancelled; 1993: Professor Pierre Lasjaunias, Paris, France; 1994: Professor Ian Isherwood, Manchester, UK; 1995: Professor Danielle Balériaux, Bruxelles, Belgium; 1996: Professor Derek C. Harwood-Nash, Toronto, Canada; 1997: Assoc. Professor Sten Cronqvist, Lund, Sweden; 1998: Professor Ivan Moseley, London, UK; 1999: Professor Guiseppe Scotti, Milan, Italy; 2000: Professor Ingar Skalpe, Oslo, Norway; 2001: Professor A. James Barkovich, USA; 2002: Professor Carsten Gyldensted, Århus, Denmark; 2003: Professor Isabelle Berry, Toulouse, France; 2004: Professor Michael Sage, Australia; 2005: Professor Anne Osborn, Utah, USA; 2006: Professor Luc Picard, Nancy, France; 2007: Tomas Hindmarsh, Stockholm, Sweden; 2008: Pål Svendsen, Gothenburg, Sweden; 2009: Dan Greitz, Stockholm, Sweden; 2010: Professor Rüdiger von Kummer, Dresden, Germany; 2011: Professor Raili Raininko, Uppsala, Sweden; 2012: Professor Daniela Prayer, Vienna, Austria; 2013: Professor Karel Terbrugge, Toronto, Canada; 2014: Professor Sven Ekholm, Rochester, USA and Gothenburg Sweden; 2015: Professor Sven Haller, Geneva, Switzerland; 2016: Professor Tommy Andersson, Stockholm, Sweden; 2017: Professor Ric Harnsberger, Utah, USA; 2018: Professor Elna-Marie Larsson, Uppsala, Sweden; 2019: Professor Pia Maly Sundgren, Lund, Sweden; 2020 and 2021: cancelled; 2022: Assoc. Professor Michael Söderman, Stockholm Sweden; 2023: Professor Meike Vernooji, Rotterdam, The Netherlands; 2024: Assoc. Professor Birgitta Ramgren, Lund, Sweden.

The international perspective of the Society and its members is further reflected by the huge number of contributions to the field that individual members from Sweden have achieved during these decades. It is impossible to list all. Neuroradiologists and radiographers in Sweden and members of SSNR have served amongst other achievements as presidents of ESNR, ESMRMB, ISMRM, ISMRT, UEMS division of neuroradiology, and WFITN. Not least the relation to ISMRM and ESMRMB shows the close relationship between neuroradiology and physics and technology in Sweden, which is also evident by the fact that neuroradiological departments in Sweden always closely collaborate with medical radiation physicists both regarding CT and MR. Frequently, MR physicists are either employed by or directly affiliated with the radiology/neuroradiology department. Further, at several university departments, neuroradiologists nowadays also build bridges to nuclear medicine and cover reading also of SPECT and PET-CT/MR. A further fruitful symbiosis in clinical practice is the many multidisciplinary conferences neuroradiologists in Sweden participate in, building bridges between different specialities and ensuring a focus on the patient's actual needs.

There is a strong national collaboration in Swedish neuroradiology. Employers of SSNR board members represent all Swedish University Hospitals and thus the whole country. Further, the board includes clinical and academic neuroradiologists with an interest in diagnostic and interventional neuroradiology, head and neck radiology, and nuclear medicine, the latter mainly among head and neck radiologists.

The broad national representation of the board and its diversity in areas of interest allows SSNR to address national questions of interest and anchor decisions broadly within national health care. For example, a current focus of the society is to publish national recommendations on neuroradiological MRI protocols and reporting templates for main diseases and patient groups. Members of the society publish white papers and guidelines and are involved in the development of national care programmes and national clinical guidelines that include diagnostic and/or interventional neuroradiology.

SSNR has 231 members (45 retired) per October 2024, including 15 honorary members. According to statistics from the Swedish National Board of Health and Welfare (Table 21.1), the number of certified neuroradiologists employed within healthcare has increased from 46 in 1995 to 145 in 2022. However, the number of colleagues working at private departments or smaller public hospitals (no data available) who are not specialized specifically in neuroradiology has also increased. The latter potentially means that specialist competence is not necessarily used adequately.

Sweden has a population of 10.5 million inhabitants on a land area of 450,000 km^2 and a length from north to south of 1550 km. In 2018, Sweden had approximately 225 MRI scanners installed at approximately 90 sites (numbers are based on communication with vendors; according to OECD Data Explorer [data-explorer.oecd.org] 14.9 scanners per million) and according to OECD, 19 CT scanners per million inhabitants. For radiology at large, these produced approximately 1,501,000 CT scans and 548,000 MR examinations in 2018, compared to 651,000 CT scans and 268,000 MR examinations in 2005. This is an increase of approximately 130% for CT and 100% for MR over 13 years and these numbers have continued to increase since [9]. For neuroradiology, there is a continuous shift from CT to MRI. This is heavily noticeable in the clinical workflow and implies a huge challenge due to the limited number of neuroradiologists. Further, the number of neuro-interventionists among neuroradiologists has increased and today 26 interventionists perform approximately 4000 interventions per year at seven neuro-interventional centres.

Table 21.1 Statistics on neuroradiologists working in health care in Sweden 1995–2022

	Neuroradiologists[a] (n, %) employed:		
Year	In public healthcare	In private healthcare	Total
2022	123 (85%)	22 (15%)	145
2012	97 (84%)	18 (16%)	115
2002	61 (88%)	8 (12%)	69
1995	46	No data available	46

[a]Including neurointerventionists; data collected from the statistical database of the Swedish National Board of Health and Welfare

The national health care development has also contributed to an increased availability of advanced radiological imaging modalities available for diagnostic and interventional radiology and thus neuroradiology, including amongst others two 7 Tesla MR installations (Lund and Stockholm) allowing both clinical imaging and research; four PET-MR installations (Umeå, Uppsala, Stockholm, and Gothenburg); intra-operative MR systems; several installations with high performance gradient MR systems; multinuclear MR systems; and 14 photon-counting CT scanners (including one system in pre-authorization trials) in addition to a modern CT-scanner infrastructure with multiple dual energy scanners.

Current Swedish neuroradiological research spans a wide range of topics (Fig. 21.1). On the neuro-interventional side, this includes the participation in multiple randomized controlled trials, the introduction of AI software tools in stroke diagnosis, and the development of an inverted Seldinger technique, referred to as an "extroducer," for intraparenchymal access and localized treatments and biopsies. On the diagnostic side, Sweden continues its pioneering work in CT diagnostics, leveraging its considerable fleet of photon-counting CT scanners. This includes optimized cerebral CT angiographies with spatial resolution non-invasively matching that of conventional angiography. Notably, usage of dual-source high-pitch photon-counting CT has also expanded the boundaries of neuroradiology when the heart can be imaged without ECG gating at the primary CT examination for stroke

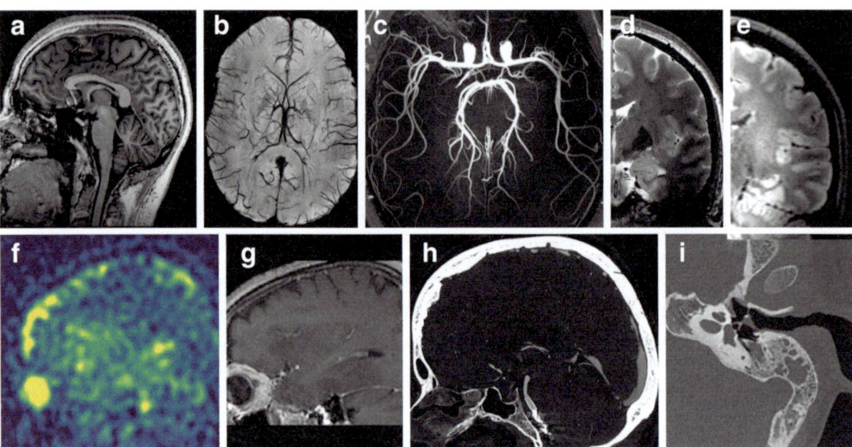

Fig. 21.1 Swedish neuroradiological research spans a wide range of topics and implementation of new technologies is one of the fundamental driving forces. Sweden has, for example, two 7 Tesla MR installations despite its population of only ten million inhabitants—T1-weighted (**a**) and SWI (**b**) 7 Tesla MR scans from Stockholm and TOF angiogram (**c**) and T2-weighted (**d**) and FLAIR scans (**e**) from Lund. Sodium MR imaging is implemented for clinical trials in Gothenburg (**f**—illustrating ^{23}Na MRI in a low-grade glioma, **g**—corresponding contrast-enhanced T1-weighted imaging), and the currently 14 PCCT installations are used for both routine outpatient and emergency care (**h**—PCCT cerebral angiography in a patient with coiling due to a giant vertebral aneurysm and a flow diverter with patent lumen; **i**—pre-surgical planning temporal bone scan of a cholesteatoma)

calls. Another example of strong national collaborations, in conjunction with the unique opportunities of Swedish quality registers, is where photon-counting CT of the brain will be acquired at multiple sites as part of the national nationwide, population-based Swedish Cardiopulmonary bioimage study (SCAPIS). Notable research within MRI includes the clinical optimization of PET-MR for neuroradiology, clinical implementation of 7 Tesla MRI, and advanced motion-correction allowing for high-quality imaging even in small children without sedation. Future aspirations include diversifying clinical use of CT and MRI also to the bedside of paediatric and adult patients. This work will likely change our way of providing neuro-intensive care, with more informed and targeted decisions. Several centres focus on the development of advanced diffusion imaging techniques in the central nervous system and in peripheral nerves. Other development areas include metabolic MRI, where efforts into levering GlucoCEST for non-ionizing quantification of the brain glucose metabolism are ongoing in both Lund and Stockholm. Also, APTw imaging is evaluated in several studies, including multicentre studies. Clinical sodium MR research in brain diseases is further ongoing in brain tumour and epilepsy cohorts in Gothenburg.

Sweden is widely known for its many and comprehensive quality registers. For example, the Swedish Neuro registry has excellent coverage and is the foundation of a vast amount of research studies. The tight integration with standardized neuroradiological reporting, for example, in neuroinflammatory and neurodegenerative disorders, has been the basis for several post-authorization studies. This has, for example, been used in proving the efficacy of anti-CD20 therapy for multiple sclerosis, which is now considered an essential drug by the WHO. Nationwide registries for neurointerventional procedures are a further example of close collaboration within the nation. Sweden is also a nation of early adopters of new IT tools. This has been reflected in the early implementation of digital PACS systems in the 1990s and hospitals can today share images nationwide. Swedish neuroradiologists also pioneer the efforts in introducing brain volumetrics, AI decision support tools, and quantitative MRI in clinical practice.

In conclusion, the Swedish Society of Neuroradiology (SSNR) has played a pivotal role in shaping the landscape of modern neuroradiology, not just in Sweden but also globally. From pioneering advancements in diagnostic techniques like CT and MRI to fostering a spirit of international collaboration and education, SSNR's contributions have been profound. The society has consistently pushed the boundaries of neuroradiological practice, ensuring that Sweden remains at the forefront of innovation in both diagnostics and intervention. As we look to the future, SSNR's commitment to research, training, and multidisciplinary collaboration will continue to shape the field, making it not only a leader in technology but also a beacon of clinical excellence. The legacy of the SSNR is a testament to the power of vision, dedication, and collaboration in advancing medical science. On behalf of the board of SSNR, the authors would like to express their gratitude to everybody contributing to this legacy (Fig. 21.2).

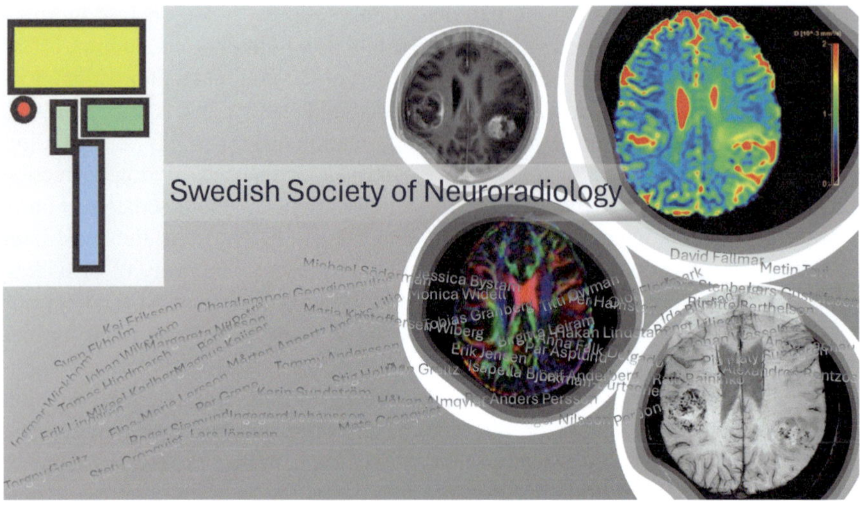

Fig. 21.2 SSNRs tribute to its members and colleagues contributing to the society's legacy of the last decades

References

1. Wikipedia. Thor Stenbeck. (in Swedish). https://sv.wikipedia.org/wiki/Thor_Stenbeck. Accessed 10 Oct 2024.
2. Lindgren E, Greitz T. The Stockholm school of neuroradiology. Am J Neuroradiol. 1995;16(2):351–60.
3. Hindmarsh T, Kaijser M. One hundred years of neuroradiology in Acta Radiologica: a Swedish perspective. Acta Radiol. 2021 Nov;62(11):1451–9.
4. Lindgren E, Erik L, Lysholm R. Dictionary of Swedish National Biography. urn:sbl:9979. Accessed 10 Oct 2024.
5. Gordon D. A note on the use of the Lysholm skull table. Br J Radiol. 1947;20(234):238–9.
6. Greitz T, Seldinger S-I. Dictionary of Swedish National Biography. urn:sbl:5858. Accessed 10 Oct 2024.
7. Nyman U, Ekberg O, Aspelin P. Torsten Almén (1931–2016): the father of non-ionic iodine contrast media. Acta Radiol. 2016 Sep;57(9):1072–8.
8. Persson BR. Medicinska tillämpningar av kärnspinnresonans – NMR. Lund: Studentlitteratur Lund; 1982. (Libris 7277025)
9. Swedish Radiation Safety Authority Report 2020:14 – Radiologiska undersökningar i Sverige under 2018. Swedish Radiation Safety Authority 2020. ISSN: 2000-0456.

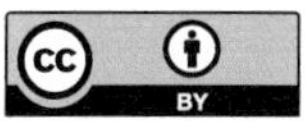

Part II
Women in Neuroradiology

Introduction

This part of the book represents a milestone in the history of medicine, particularly neuroradiology, by bringing to light the often invisible contributions of women to the advancement of this medical specialty on all continents.

The chapters are divided by continent to provide a comprehensive overview of the trajectories of pioneers and leaders who, with their expertise and dedication, shaped the field of neuroradiology worldwide.

Neuroradiology, an area dedicated to the diagnosis and treatment of diseases of the central nervous system through imaging, is a complex and constantly evolving field. In this context, women have played a fundamental role, overcoming gender barriers and contributing significantly to the development of new techniques, technologies, and care protocols.

The women doctors who chose neuroradiology as a specialty studied and worked hard, overcoming many barriers and often overcoming prejudices. In their profession, they know that medicine, like life, is a constant learning process and they never stop learning and teaching. In their constant search for accurate imaging diagnoses that guide precise treatments, female neuroradiologists are able to fulfill the main function of the profession, which is to try to save lives or at least try to alleviate the suffering of patients and their families.

By exploring the life stories and scientific contributions of female neuroradiologists from different cultural backgrounds and socioeconomic contexts, we seek not only to celebrate their achievements, but also to promote gender equality in the health field and inspire future generations of female doctors to follow in their footsteps.

This book is the result of meticulous research and a collaborative effort by neuroradiologist researchers from different parts of the world, who came together with the goal of rescuing and valuing the history of women in neuroradiology. We believe that this work will contribute to enriching knowledge about the history of medicine and to fostering discussion about the importance of diversity and inclusion in the health field.

I would like to take this special moment to thank God first for everything and our families for their unconditional support. I would also like to thank all the colleagues and friends who joined and accepted the idea of writing and including the History of Women Neuroradiologists on each Continent as part of the book on the History of World Neuroradiology that was already being written, although our initial idea was to write a separate book. Our special thanks to the Executive Board of the WFNR, especially the WFNRS President Prof. Dr. Wan-Yuo Guo and the WFNRS President-Elect and editor of this book Prof. Dr. Daniel Birchall, as well as the Executive Secretary of the WFNRS Prof. Dr. Pia Sundgren, the Member at Large Prof. Dr. Paul M. Parizel and Ms. Karen Lyp (WFNRS Director of Administration) for their support in ensuring that this part of the book on Women Neuroradiologists was accepted and implemented. I would like to thank from the bottom of my heart all the main authors from the continents (Prof. Dr. Kumiko Ando, Prof. Dr. Pamela Schaefer, Prof. Dr. Clive Sperryn, Prof. Dr. Pia Sundgren and Prof. Dr. Maria Isabel Vargas) and all our co-authors and collaborators for agreeing to collect information and write in an extremely short time frame of 1 month extended to 3 months. Thus, with enthusiasm, great good will, and determination, we were able to join forces and collect information about the History of the most influential Women Neuroradiologists in the world that will be presented here.

With fraternal greetings

WFNRS
Recife, Pernambuco, Brazil

Maria de Fátima Viana Vasco Aragão

Chapter 22
Women in Neuroradiology in Africa

Clive Wyndham Sperryn, Napo Kasirye-Mbugua, Sally E. Candy, Sahar Saleem, Amal Saleh Nour, Hafisatu Gbadamosi, Sheila Waa, Phyllis Mezue, Hamdi Mohamed Isse, Thandi Eunice Buthelezi, Gopolang Mndebele, Ugumba Mussa Kwikima, Valeria Nabossa, Rita Nassanga, and Sarah B. Nshimbi

Abbreviations

AKUHN	Aga Khan University Hospital Nairobi
ASHNR	American Society of Head & Neck Radiology
ASNR	American Society of Neuroradiology
BMGF	Bill and Melinda Gates Foundation
BSNR	British Society of Neuroradiologists

C. W. Sperryn (✉)
Morton and Partners Inc., Vincent Pallotti Hospital, Cape Town, Western Cape, South Africa
e-mail: clive.sperryn@morton.co.za

N. Kasirye-Mbugua
Department of Radiology, Foothills Medical Centre, Calgary, Alberta, Canada

S. E. Candy
Department of Diagnostic Radiology, Groote Schuur Hospital/University of Cape Town, Cape Town, Western Cape, South Africa

S. Saleem
Department of Radiology, Kasr Al Ainy Faculty of Medicine-Cairo University, Cairo, Egypt
e-mail: saharsaleem@kasralainy.edu.eg

A. S. Nour
Department of Radiology, School of Medicine, College of Health Sciences, Addis Ababa University, Tikur Anbessa Specialized Hospital, Addis Ababa, Ethiopia
e-mail: amal.saleh@aau.edu.et

H. Gbadamosi
Department of Radiology, Korle Bu Teaching Hospital, Accra, Ghana

Department of Radiology, University of Ghana Medical School, Accra, Ghana
e-mail: hgbadamosi@ug.edu.gh

S. Waa
Department of Radiology, Aga Khan University Hospital, Nairobi, Kenya
e-mail: Sheila.ponda@aku.edu

D. Birchall (ed.), *A World History of Neuroradiology*,
https://doi.org/10.1007/978-3-032-16653-1_22

CAMERA	Chan Zuckerberg funded Consortium for Advancement of MRI Education and Research in Africa
CHBAH	Chris Hani Baragwanath Academic Hospital
CME	Continuing Medical Education
CUBIC	Cape Universities Body Imaging Centre
EDiHNNR	European Diploma in Head and Neck Neuroradiology
EDiINR	European Diploma in Interventional Neuroradiology
EDiNR	European Diploma in Neuroradiology
EDiPNR	European Diploma in Paediatric Neuroradiology
ESNR	European Society of Neuroradiology
GCPS	Ghana College of Physicians & Surgeons
GDC	Guglielmi Detachable Coil
HPCSA	Health Professions Council of South Africa
IALCH	Inkosi Albert Luthuli Central Hospital
ISMRM	International Society of Magnetic Resonance in Medicine
KBTH	Korle Bu Teaching Hospital
PACS	Picture Archiving and Communication System
RIS	Radiology information system
RSNA	Radiological Society of North America
RSSA	Radiological Society of South Africa
RXH	Red Cross War Memorial Children's Hospital

P. Mezue
Everlight Radiology, London, UK

H. M. Isse
Department of Radiology, Sahan Diagnostic Center, Mogadishu, Banadir, Somalia

T. E. Buthelezi
Department of Diagnostic Radiology, Chris Hani Baragwanath Academic Hospital, Johannesburg, South Africa

University of the Witwatersrand, Johannesburg, South Africa
e-mail: Thandi.Buthelezi@wits.ac.za

G. Mndebele
Department of Radiology, Nelson Mandela Children's Hospital, Johannesburg, South Africa
e-mail: gopolang.mndebele@nmch.org.za

U. M. Kwikima
Department of Radiology, Lugalo Military Hospital & Muhimbili University of Health and Allied Sciences, Dar es Salaam, Tanzania

V. Nabossa · R. Nassanga
Department of Radiology, Uganda Cancer Institute and Makerere University College of Health Sciences, Kampala, Uganda
e-mail: valeria.nabbosa@uci.or.ug

S. B. Nshimbi
Department of Radiology, University Teaching Hospitals – Adult Hospital, Lusaka, Zambia

SANIS	South African Neurointerventional Society
SASNI	South African Society of Neurological Imaging
SASPI	South African Society of Paediatric Imaging
SNOSSA	Society for Neuro-Oncology subSaharan Africa
UCT	University of Cape Town
VGH	Vancouver General Hospital
WACS	West African College of Surgeons
WFNRS	World Federation of Neuroradiological Societies
WFPI	World Federation of Paediatric Imaging

Africa is the continent with the smallest number of radiologists per capita. This chapter is an incomplete window on remarkable women in neuroradiology in Africa which highlights success and challenges. These women function as crucial role models. There is tremendous opportunity for wealthier countries where neuroradiology is well established to support institutions and individuals in the developing world through subsidisation of online teaching and evaluation platforms, attendance at international conferences and collaborative research and training endeavours. The real benefits of collaborations are illustrated in the stories from Ethiopia and Tanzania where collaborative Neuroradiology Fellowships have been established. Uganda is on the threshold of establishing a collaborative Neuroradiology Fellowship. Ghana is taking early steps. Kenya has one Fellowship trained neuroradiologist and one in head and neck. There is just one in Nigeria. Bold radiologists in Somalia and Zambia provide a remarkable service despite the absence of formal neuroradiology fellowships. In South Africa, despite a greater number of neuroradiologists, much of the neuroradiology work is still done by general radiologists. This chapter highlights that there is enormous potential for future collaborations, emulating those already established to make a real difference in numerous countries in Africa.

Egypt

The science and art of medicine have long been integral to Egypt's rich history, with ancient practices highlighting some of the most advanced medical knowledge of their time. Women like Peseshet, a physician from the 5th Dynasty (2494–2345 BC), exemplified this legacy, serving as overseers of female physicians and significantly contributing to medical practice. This historical backdrop paved the way for modern medical education in Egypt, notably with the establishment of institutions like Kasr Al-Ainy Medical School in 1827. Today, this legacy continues through exemplary figures like Dr Sahar Saleem (Fig. 22.1), a prominent Egyptian neuroradiologist, whose work has significantly advanced the field both locally and globally. Dr Saleem began her journey at Kasr Al-Ainy, where she earned her master's and Medical Doctorate in Radiology, culminating in a PhD focused on Neuroradiology.

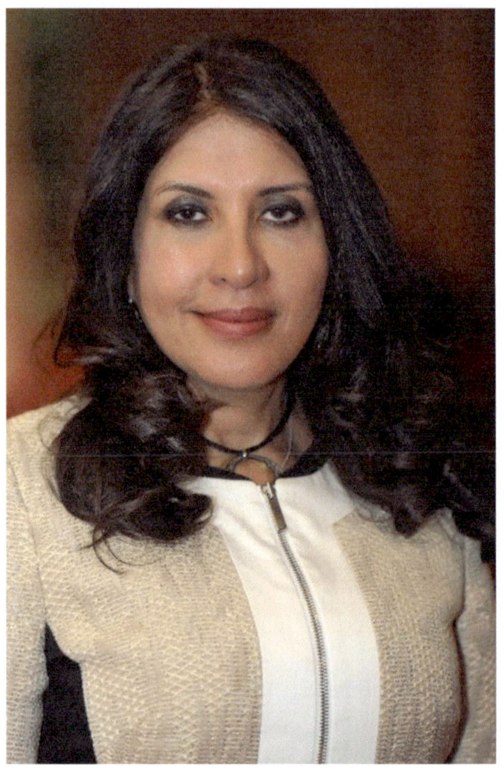

Fig. 22.1 Prof Sahar Saleem. (Copyright holder: All Fig. 22.3 Rights Reserved)

Further honing her skills, she completed fellowships in Neuroradiology and Medical Education at the University of Western Ontario in Canada. As a professor at Cairo University, she has held leadership roles, including heading the Neuroradiology unit and later the Radiology department.

Professor Saleem's clinical practice at Cairo University Hospitals—where over two million patients are treated annually—reflects the commitment to advancing patient care in Egypt. Her innovative research has led to the identification of several novel syndromes within the genetic landscape of neuroradiology and foetal MRI, enhancing diagnostic capabilities and treatment options. In 2012, she founded and directed the Egyptian School of Radiology, a non-profit organisation affiliated with the Egyptian Society of Radiology (EgSR), dedicated to promoting education and professional development in the field. A pioneer in paleoradiology, Dr Saleem employs advanced imaging techniques to study mummies (Fig. 22.2) and antiquities, making significant discoveries, including insights into the cause of death of King Tutankhamun. With over 100 scientific publications and 12 authored or co-authored books, her influence extends beyond academia. She also serves as Faculty Member of several Scientific Societies such as RSNA. Saleem is a key member of the Membership Committee at the World Federation of Neuroradiological Societies (WFNRS), advising on the development of

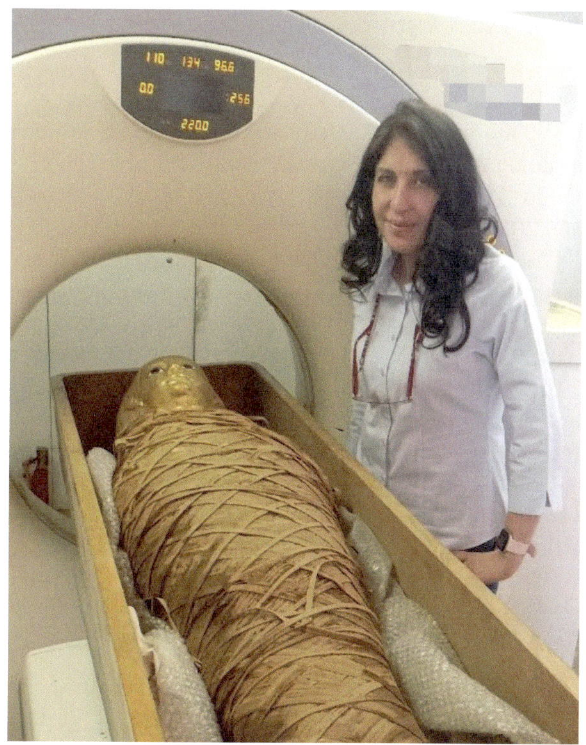

Fig. 22.2 Prof Sahar Saleem with Mummy in CT scanner. (Copyright holder: Prof. Sahar Saleem, All Rights Reserved)

neuroradiology worldwide, with a focus on Africa. Professor Saleem's numerous accolades, including the Cum Laude award from the Radiological Society of North America (RSNA), and both Summa Cum Laude honours from the American Society of Neuroradiology (ASNR) and the British Society of Neuroradiology (BSNR). The Egyptian Presidential Award for Iconic Successful Woman underscores her exceptional contributions and leadership in the medical community. Sahar Saleem stands out as a model of success for neuroradiologists in Egypt and Africa, embodying innovation and leadership in her field and inspiring future generations of women in medicine.

In Egypt, there are around 50 women neuroradiologists, with experience spanning from 5 to 30 years. All have successfully completed their PhD theses in Egypt, specialising in neuroradiology, and have undergone local training. Additionally, at least seven of these professionals possess international diplomas in neuroradiology and/or specialised fellowships from institutions in Europe or North America. Their credentials include fellowships from Canada, the USA, the UK, and Switzerland, as well as European Diplomas in Neuroradiology (EDiNR). Some notable female neuroradiologists in Egypt, listed alphabetically, include: Aya Abdel Galil, Eman Darwish, Eman Geniedi, Radwa Kamel, and Habeba Mostafa.

Ethiopia

Dr Tequam Debebe Weldehawariat (Fig. 22.3) completed her neuroradiology training in the Czech Republic in 2002. She returned as the first Ethiopian female neuroradiologist. She has served in the School of Medicine, Addis Ababa University for the last 20 years where she became dean of the School of Medicine between 2018 and 2022.

As the departmental chair of radiology, she advocated for the procurement and installation of the first 1.5T MRI in the institution's teaching hospital. This has provided invaluable support in the diagnosis of neurological conditions and improved patient care, particularly to the financially disadvantaged.

Her efforts have led to the establishment of MDT and research collaborations and the advancement of education and training in neurosurgery and neurology and the expansion of neuroradiology services in Ethiopia.

Notably, Dr Weldehawariat established a local 2-year neuroradiology fellowship programme in collaboration with Prof. Patricia Hudgins of Emory University, Atlanta.

Dr Amal Saleh (Fig. 22.4) was the first graduate of this programme. She has served as neuroradiology unit head, departmental chair of radiology and as dean of the School of Medicine since her specialisation in 2022. She has participated in

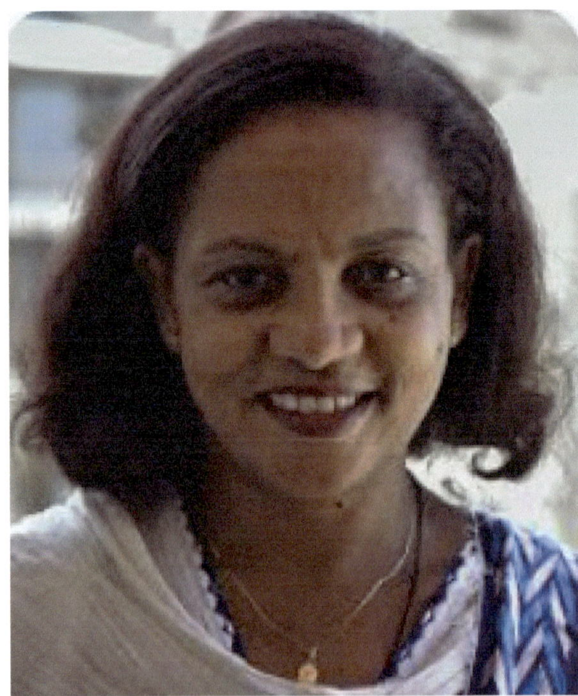

Fig. 22.3 Dr Tequam Debebe Weldehawariat

Fig. 22.4 Dr Amal Saleh

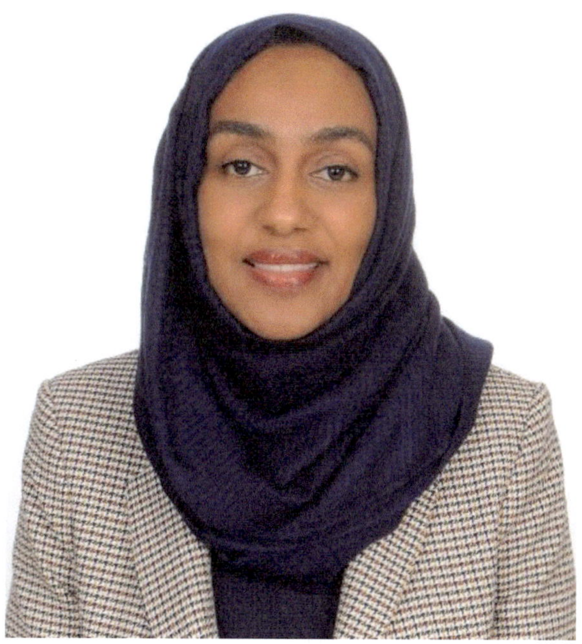

multiple local, regional, and international societies and has helped establish further overseas collaboration for neuroradiology fellowship training.

Three more female graduates have recently completed the neuroradiology fellowship programme, Dr Etsehiwot Demeke, Dr Ilili Amin, and Dr Metti Kuma, bringing the number of female neuroradiologists in Ethiopia to five.

Although their number is small, these women have shown remarkable resilience and determination in the face of challenges such as equipment procurement and maintenance, a rising population and demand for focused healthcare.

They feel the future is bright for women in neuroradiology and are optimistic that with new collaborative opportunities in education and research they will be well positioned to improve service delivery and healthcare within Ethiopia and more broadly on the African continent.

Ghana

Radiology in Ghana, though still relatively young, has evolved over the past 70 years of its introduction in mainstream medicine, revolutionising how diseases are diagnosed and treated. Amidst this transformative journey, there have been notable highs and lows, highlighting the challenges and triumphs experienced by those at the forefront of radiology in Ghana.

The West African College of Surgeons (WACS) and the Ghana College of Physicians & Surgeons (GCPS) are mandated to train radiologists in Ghana. WACS was established in1960 and has authority over the West African Sub-region. Radiologists began training in Ghana in 1999, examinations initially being held in Nigeria. The GCPS was established locally in 2003, with training starting a year later. The two colleges have churned out a total of 100 radiologists. For a population of over 30 million, this is still quite inadequate; this lack of radiologists is further compounded by the shortage of specific subspecialisations.

The progress chalked in the field of radiology in Ghana is a testament to the collective efforts of dedicated women and men who are committed to advancing the field.

Some of the most influential women in our time include Professor Millicent Obajimi, a renowned Nigerian radiologist who spent a yearlong sabbatical in the year 2000 at the Korle Bu Teaching Hospital (KBTH) in the capital, Accra. Her mandate, to consolidate the progress of our infant residency programme. She remains one of the major contributors to radiology research in the country and left an indelible mark in that space. Undoubtedly, her tenure contributed to the graduation of some of the most influential female alumni, including the first female Ghanaian-trained radiologist, Professor Klenam Dzefi-Tettey (Fig. 22.5), and Vice-President, Association of Radiologists in West Africa (ARAWA). Others, like Drs

Fig. 22.5 Professor (Mrs) Klenam Dzefi-Tettey

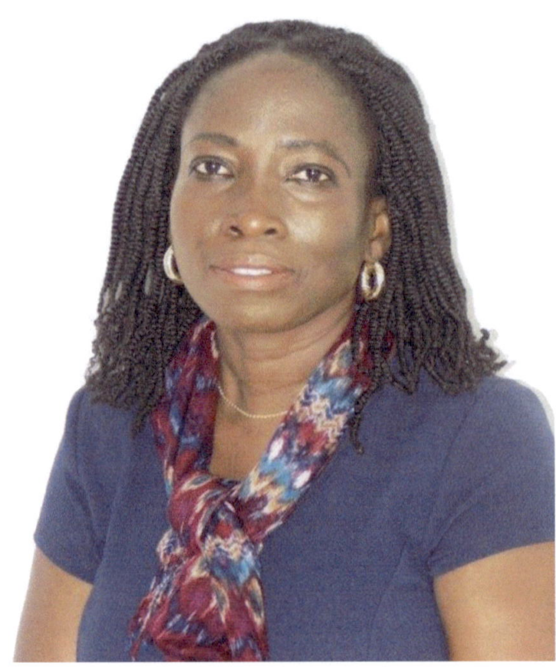

Augustina Badu Peprah (Fig. 22.6) and Ewurama Andam Idun (Fig. 22.7), both former Presidents, Ghana Association of Radiologists, have held institutional leadership positions. They continue to serve as excellent role models and magnets to a profession that was previously male dominated.

In the early part of 2012, the radiology department of the Korle Bu Teaching Hospital (KBTH) in Ghana welcomed a retired neuroradiologist, Dr Joselyn Lapointe, formerly of the Vancouver General Hospital (VGH) in Canada, who

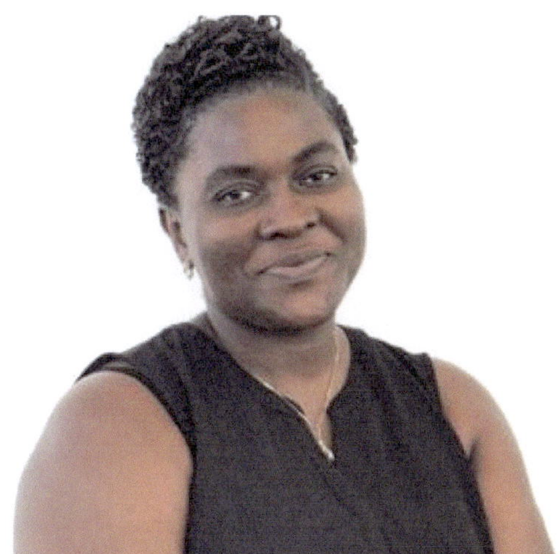

Fig. 22.6 Dr Augustina Badu-Peprah

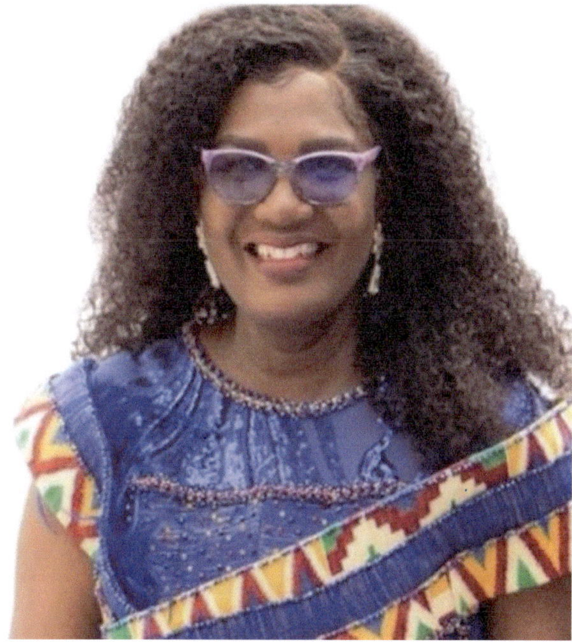

Fig. 22.7 Dr Ewurama Andam Idun

opened the gates to the world of neuroradiology. In the words of Dr Hafisatu Gbadamosi, *"She is what I will call the mother of neuroradiology in Ghana. I was fortunate to learn at her feet during this very exhilarating year of her tutelage."* Her tenure culminated in a legacy of a yearly observership for residents in Neuroradiology at VGH via a Canadian neuroscience foundation. Dr Gbadamosi (Fig. 22.8) was a first among several other beneficiaries of this initiative which led to a bigger desire and interest in the field of neuroradiology. Another female beneficiary, Dr Rosemond Aboagye (Fig. 22.9) went on to complete a paediatric radiology fellowship from the BC Children's Hospital, Canada, and has subsequently contributed significantly to our management of paediatric conditions in Ghana.

The teaching faculty in all our teaching hospitals are quite diverse, with every consultant having a stake in moulding the next generation of radiologists.

While most of our members are still general radiologists, recent growth has made it possible for some level of subspeciality training to be achieved.

First, for the country, neurointerventional procedures and pain management are provided for by Professor Benjamin Dabo Sarkodie and Dr Emmanuel Jackson who are fellowship-trained in interventional radiology and neuroradiology, respectively. Some minor interventional procedures are, however, provided by

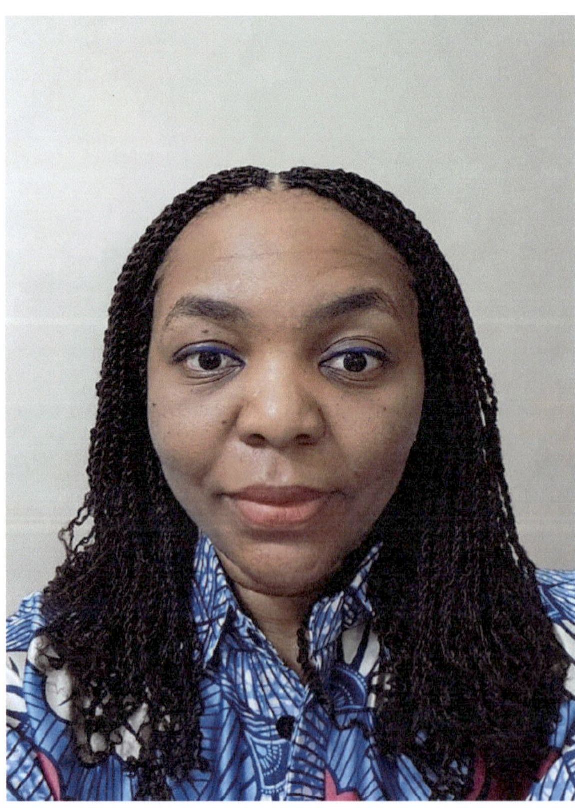

Fig. 22.8 Dr Hafisatu Gbadamosi

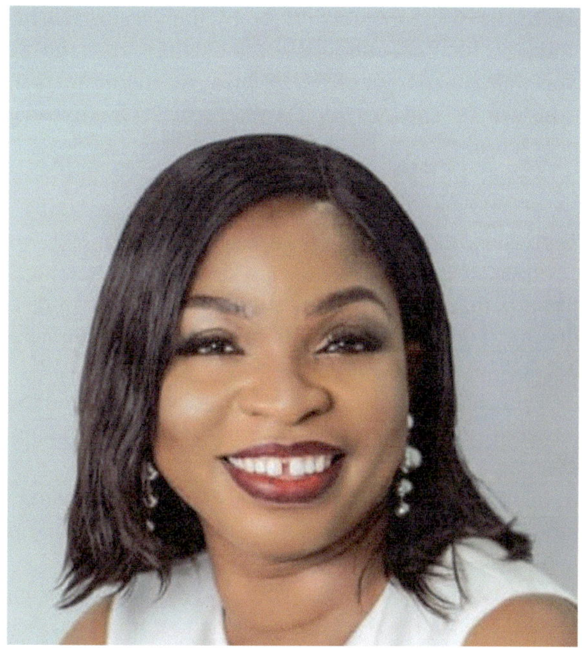

Fig. 22.9 Dr Rosemond N. D. Aboagye

non-interventionists. This capacity growth was harnessed to create a new faculty of interventional radiology with one product so far, and a soon-to-be-graduated first female interventional radiologist. The Faculty of Radiology, Oncology & Radiotherapy of the Ghana College of Physicians and Surgeons—with collaboration from some international partners—is in the final stages of approving our local neuroradiology curriculum, which will be another profound milestone for us. Our struggle with the lack of foreign fellowship opportunities over the years as well as the burning need for growth in the area has fuelled this drive of faculty towards internal development.

Dr Gbadamosi is currently training as a neuro/head and neck radiologist at the Singapore General Hospital. Though delayed by many years, it will be a fulfilled dream which will contribute to the development of Neuroradiology in Ghana. This will bring the number of neuroradiologists in Ghana to only two.

While advanced imaging tools may not be equitably distributed all over Ghana, there is access to high resolution ultrasound and Computerised Tomography (CT) scan machines. Magnetic Resonance Imaging (MRI) is done using 1.5T magnets with one 3T magnet available in the country. Equipment for interventional studies is also available in a few facilities. We have a Dual-Energy X-ray Absorptiometry (DEXA) scan facility available, and plans are underway to set up the first Positron Emission Tomography (PET) scanner in the country. The government of Ghana, however, remains the major provider of equipment nationwide with consistent growth of private sector investment.

Research in Ghana is driven by the various teaching hospitals and affiliations with the medical schools. Organisations like the Society for Neuro-Oncology Sub-Saharan Africa (SNOSSA) have encouraged multi-stakeholder collaborations for us and provided a platform for increased research collaboration and peer learning.

As one of the lead radiologists on the paediatric radiology and paediatric neuroradiology multidisciplinary teams, Dr Gbadamosi benefited from a St Jude's neuro-oncology training seminar workshop in 2022 which provided a platform for sustained growth for the team as well as increased our appetite for research. Despite these positives, we are unable to play in the space of advanced research due to the lack of the requisite technology such as advanced sequences and the needed support.

Unfortunately, many of our successes are limited to the major teaching hospitals, emphasising the need for scalability to the other major and regional hospitals in the country.

Things we can improve on locally include sustained development as far as collaborations in the neurological, adult neurosurgical, ophthalmology and Ear, Nose, and Throat (ENT) services are concerned.

There is a need to expand our scope of neuroradiological studies, institute strong imaging workflows, improve access to advanced neuroimaging technology, and provide more comprehensive on-the-job training for our technologists. These would require a concerted effort from governments, healthcare institutions, and international partners to strengthen radiological services and improve patient care across our country and continent.

> On the whole, despite our inexperience with these new territories we seek to chart, there remains an equal level playing field for all irrespective of gender. I hope that I can inspire more women, to develop an interest in this intimidating but exceptional specialty of neuroradiology. Hopefully, together we can create a great neuroradiology community to deepen our knowledge and create a new generation of impactful Global leaders—Dr Hafisatu Gbadamosi.

Kenya

Neuroradiology practice in Kenya dates back to 1967 when direct carotid angiography was first introduced by a neurosurgeon and thereafter taken up by radiologists.

Women pioneers in the field of neuroradiology were Dr Agola Onyango-Akena and Dr Milcah Wambugu who from 1977 to 1978 conducted direct carotid angiograms during their radiology training and thereafter as faculty at Kenya's largest public hospital, Kenyatta National. The two as part of a team would later transition to femoral puncture carotid angiography in the early 1980s.

With the arrival in Kenya of CT in 1982 and MRI in the late 1990s scanners, neuroradiological studies have mostly been reported by general radiologists.

In the past decade, the subspeciality practice of Neuroradiology has grown with women making an impact.

Dr Sheila Waa (Fig. 22.10), following Residency at Aga Khan University Hospital Nairobi (AKUHN), Neuroradiology Research Fellowship at University Health Network, Toronto, and the only registered Neuroradiologist in Kenya, has provided imaging training and support for acute stroke care programme (JCIA certified; 2021, 2024), neuro-oncology imaging and dementia imaging (MRI, FDG-PET). Also, at AKUHN since 2019, Dr Jacqueline Mavuti, a fellowship-trained Head and Neck imaging specialist, has developed a service that spans oncology, skull base evaluation, emergency imaging, and other broad non-oncologic multimodality imaging.

Dr Jane Thinwa, formerly of Kenyatta National Hospital (KNH), was one of the first radiologists to provide head and neck oncological imaging. Although a general radiologist, Dr Rose Nyabanda, also of KNH, has been heavily involved in neuroradiology teaching of radiologists and radiologists-in-training in CMEs. Dr. Wangari Maina, a KNH based Interventional Radiologist, conducts a few neurointerventional procedures, in particular aneurysm coiling.

A major challenge for neuroradiology practice has been the lack of neuroradiology fellowship programmes. The dilemma of whether to bolster neuroradiology in

Fig. 22.10 Dr Sheila Waa

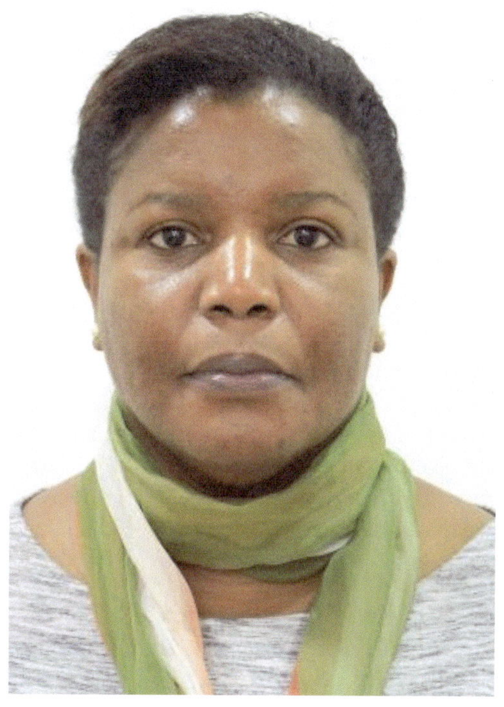

residency programmes as opposed to starting fellowship programmes, given the small size of neuroradiology practice in the country, is one major factor. Another is the paucity of Neuroradiologists, given the difficulty of attracting internationally fellowship-trained Kenyan Neuroradiologists, including Interventionists, back to Kenya.

Nigeria

Nigeria is the largest and most populous country in Africa. As with many developing countries, the healthcare of the population is underserved with approximately one doctor per 9000 population.

An even more acute shortage of radiologists means that most serve as generalists. Interventional radiology is provided by expat or visiting specialists.

Dr Aisha Umar completed her Neuroradiology fellowship in Zurich and became the first female neuroradiologist in Nigeria after her return in the early 2000s. During her tenure at the biggest government hospital in the capital, National Hospital (Abuja), she has provided both a comprehensive radiological service as well as contributing extensively to teaching and training of residents.

Her inspiration to pursue neuroradiology stemmed from the desire to improve the clinical outcome of her patients. Some of the drawbacks she identifies are the lack of resources, e.g. insufficient MRI scanners, underfunding for training, and insufficient role models to inspire and guide future radiologists into the subspeciality.

Having made a significant positive impact over many years at both local and national levels, she has transitioned to an administrative role in the hope that she will be able to address at least some of the structural difficulties affecting radiology in Nigeria.

There are many challenges for female radiologists wishing to pursue subspecialisation in Nigeria and neighbouring countries. Dr Umar's vision is directed at finding workable and sustainable solutions by collaborating with other radiological communities in West Africa and further afield.

Dr Phyllis Mezue (Fig. 22.11) is a consultant Radiologist with an interest in Head and neck, currently working with a globally established teleradiology provider. Prior to this, she worked in the UK National Health service.

She completed her radiology training in the United Kingdom. During her training, she had the opportunity to travel to Nigeria for an out-of-programme experience, which is where her passion for Neuroradiology and Head and Neck imaging became established. She has been accepted into a 2-year Neuroradiology fellowship programme in Canada and is looking forward to it.

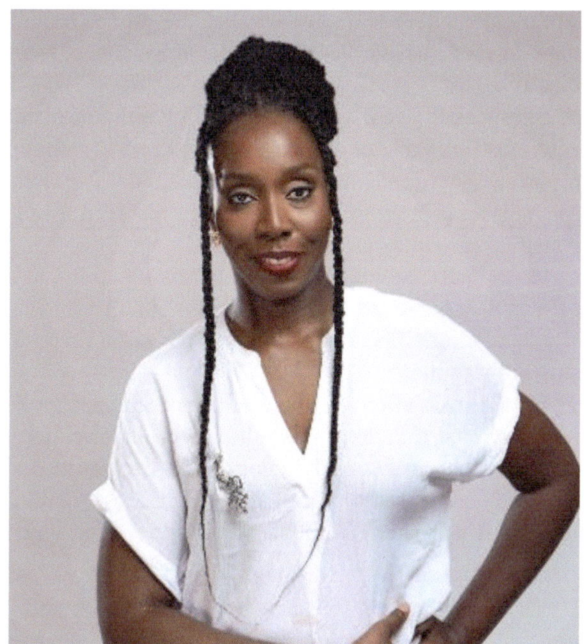
Fig. 22.11 Dr Phyllis Mezue

Somalia

In Somalia, in the field of neuroradiology, women are underrepresented, with only three female radiologists practising nationwide: Hamdi Mohamed Isse and Haliema Abdullahi (Sahan Diagnostic Centre, Mogadishu), Degmo Ali Mohamed, (Hayat Diagnostic Centre, Hargesia). There are no registered female neuroradiologists. Despite this, female radiologists in Somalia frequently encounter and report on a variety of neuroimaging cases using different modalities.

Common cases include neurodegenerative disorders, dementia, brain abscesses, TB meningitis, and neoplasms such as meningiomas and glioblastomas. Additionally, congenital anomalies are regularly encountered in practice.

Although there are no registered female neuroradiologists in the country at present, there is a growing interest in this speciality among female radiologists. We are hopeful that in the coming years, Somalia will see the emergence of female neuroradiologists who will further advance the field.

South Africa

In South Africa, women represent 31% of the radiology workforce. The South African Society of Neuroradiology (SASNI) boasts 49 women members out of a total of 129 members (38%). Women account for 50% of the SASNI leadership committee. These statistics parallel the global feminisation of medicine, though they conceal the hurdles to subspeciality and advancement within the academic hierarchy.

Subspeciality in diagnostic radiology remains uncommon in South Africa (as it is in most subSaharan African countries). Most radiologists function as generalists, reporting neuroimaging as part of their daily practice. Formal accredited post-specialisation programmes are costly and are not seen as a priority in a resource constrained health care environment.

Historically, South African radiologists wishing to subspecialise in neuroradiology have done so in academic institutions in Canada and Australia, countries for which additional local examinations are not a prerequisite for entry into a fellowship programme.

Notable exceptions in South Africa are the postgraduate diploma programmes in interventional radiology (including neurointervention) set up at the University of the Free State in 2002, the Diploma in Paediatric Radiology (which has a strong emphasis on neuroradiology) at the Red Cross Children's Hospital attached to the University of Cape Town and the Fellowship in Neurointervention at Chris Hani Baragwanath Hospital (CHBAH), attached to the University of the Witwatersrand (WITS).

Paediatric Neuroradiology

The Paediatric radiology diploma programme was initiated by Prof. Tracy Kilborn who completed her radiological training in the UK and returned in 2005, heading the Radiology division at The Red Cross Children's hospital from 2011–2022. Her research interests include the imaging of paediatric CNS infection and neuro-oncology. Together with a small team of dedicated paediatric radiologists, including Dr Nicky Wieselthaler, she has provided high level neuropaediatric training. To date, five female radiologists have graduated from this programme. Their expertise is now spread throughout South Africa.

Dr Gopolang Mndebele (Fig. 22.12) is the current head of the radiology unit at the prestigious Nelson Mandela Children's Hospital (NMCH). In her words, "*This role is not just a title but a platform for me to significantly influence the field of paediatric radiology and paediatric neuroradiology in particular.*" The Children's Hospital provides quaternary medical services to both state and private patients, dealing with complex and challenging cases that require the expertise it houses in various departments.

She completed her radiology training at The University of Witwatersrand University (WITS) and worked as a general radiologist at Chris Hani Baragwanath Hospital (CHBAH)before joining the team at Nelson Mandela Children's Hospital in 2020. Her passion for paediatric imaging and neuroradiology led her to pursue a fellowship in Paediatric Neuroradiology at The Hospital for Sick Children in Toronto, which she completed in 2022.

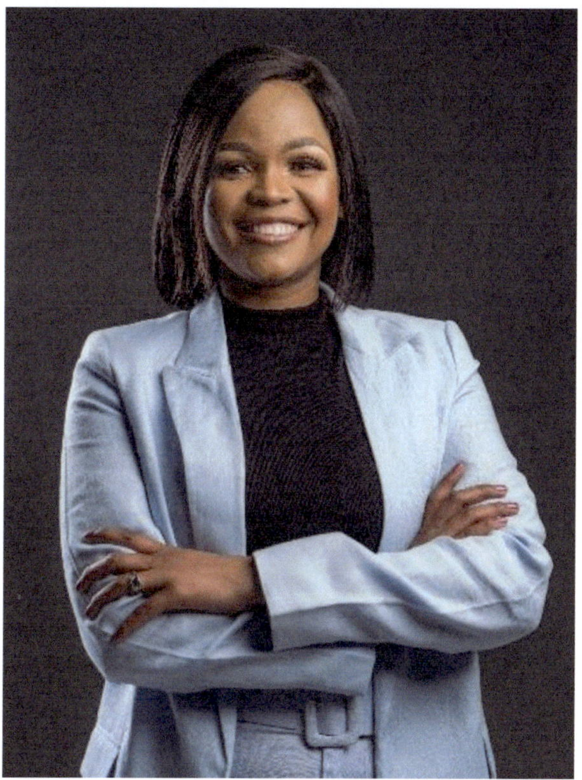

Fig. 22.12 Dr Gopolang Mndebele

She is a joint staff member at the Wits Diagnostic Radiology Department, supervising three radiology MMed registrars, participating in registrar lectures, and mentors two young radiology students.

One of the low points of her career has been recognising the lack of dedicated, paediatric imaging services in South Africa. *"It is disheartening that we cannot meet this need due to the shortage of paediatric radiology trained personal. However, this realization drives my passion for teaching even more and speaks to my dream to one day pass the knowledge through a fellowship training program at NMCH"*—Dr Gopolang Mndebele.

University of Cape Town graduate, Prof Caroline Robson/Levitt obtained her paediatric neuroradiology specialisation with a particular interest in head and neck imaging in the US and has had an illustrious career at Boston Children's Hospital where she is now vice-chair of radiology.

Interventional Neuroradiology

Dr Sandra Basson is recognised as a pioneer in the discipline of neuroradiology, particularly neurointervention in South Africa. Having qualified as a radiologist in 1989, she pursued a 6-month observership in neurointervention at UCLA. The unit was at the forefront of detachable ballon development, evaluating the Guglielmi detachable coil and the use of Onyx in the treatment of cerebral AVM. In her own words: *"these were exciting times."* Returning to South Africa, she accepted a consultant position at the Universities of the Free State and Pretoria where she continued her diagnostic and interventional work.

Dr Thandi Eunice Buthelezi (Fig. 22.13), affectionately known as "Mumsy," stands as a trailblazer in the field of neuroradiology and interventional neuroradiology (INR) in South Africa. She joined the INR team at Chris Hani Baragwanath Hospital in June 2021 where she completed a Fellowship in Neuro-intervention. In 2024, she joined the South African Neuro-intervention Society (SANIS) becoming the only registered active female member.

She credits her mentor Prof. Victor Mngomezulu for sparking her interest in interventional neuroradiology. His patience, dedication, and meticulous approach to INR cases were an inspiration in her passionate pursuit of the speciality. Prof. Samia

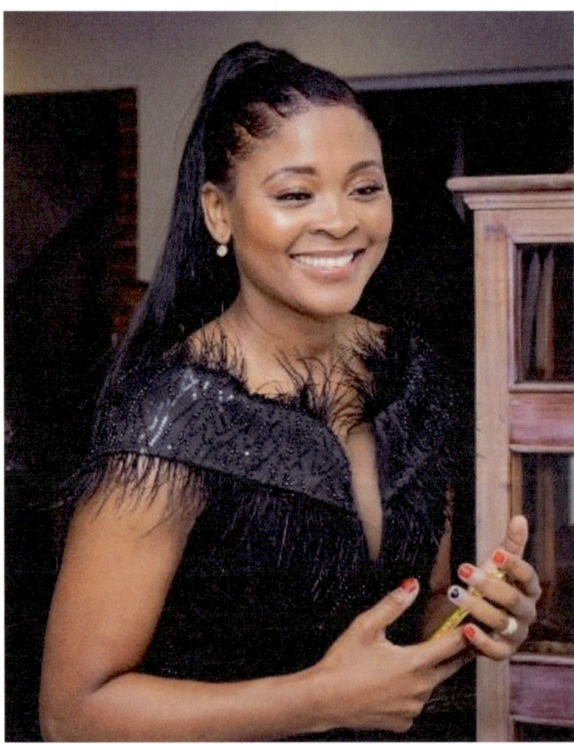

Fig. 22.13 Dr Thandi Buthelezi

Amed from the University of Pretoria was one of few women in the field of neurointervention at the time. The presence of another female at the table provided her with a sense of comfort and inspiration, reinforcing her determination to succeed in a male-dominated field.

Dr Buthelezi has made significant contributions to neuroradiology and INR in South Africa. She has applied advanced knowledge to improve patient outcomes, enhancing the quality of care in her practice. She is affiliated with the University of the Witwatersrand (WITS). Her teaching efforts, through multidisciplinary team meetings and on-floor training sessions, demonstrate her commitment to skill transfer and education.

Her continued presence at the institution has sparked significant interest in Neurointervention, leading to a waiting list for the Neurointervention fellowship programme. One of their current fellows is female, Dr Boitumelo Khoza (Fig. 22.14), which is a source of immense pride and a testament to the possibilities for others like her.

One of Dr Buthelezi's most significant achievements is her role as a pioneer for Black women in neuroradiology. Her success serves as a powerful example that background does not limit potential. This realisation fuels her commitment to working in the public sector, ensuring that skilled healthcare is accessible to all, regardless of class.

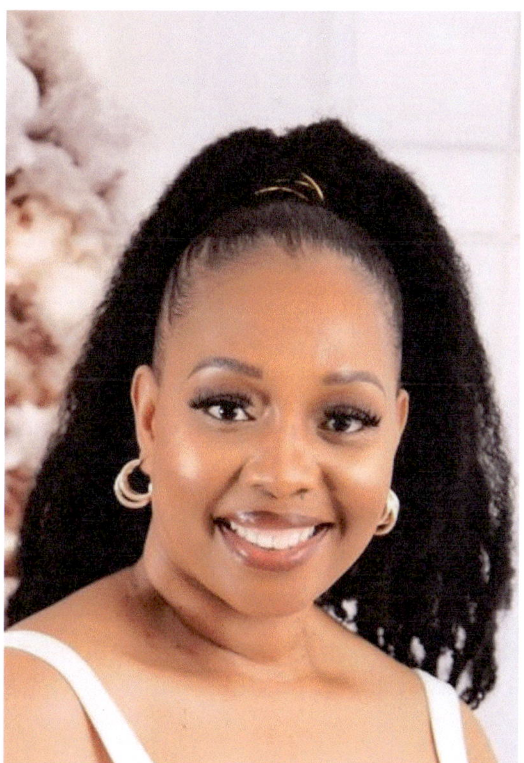

Fig. 22.14 Dr Boitumelo Khoza

Diagnostic Neuroradiology

In South Africa, in the field of Neuroradiology**,** Professor Sally Candy (Fig. 22.15) as the first chair of the South African Society of Neuroimaging is well known and respected for her contributions to the discipline. She attributes her love of neuroradiology to her local mentor at Groote Schuur Hospital, Prof. Lenny Handler, but her role model was the visionary Professor Anne Osborne whose frequent visits to Cape Town inspired her to uproot her family to New York City in 2000/2001. Here she completed fellowship training at the New York Presbyterian and Memorial Sloan Kettering Hospitals.

As the clinical head of neuroradiology at Groote Schuur Hospital, Cape Town, and an examiner at the Colleges of Medicine South Africa (CMSA), she has been involved in the education and development of radiologists for over 20 years. She believes strongly in the importance of interdisciplinary cross pollination, ensuring regular interdisciplinary meetings between the departments of radiology, oncology, neurology, ophthalmology, neurosurgery, neuropathology, and neurointervention. Her research has centred on neuroimaging of Tuberculosis and in HIV/AIDS. Her wish is to have passed on an appreciation of the particularity of neuroimaging in the

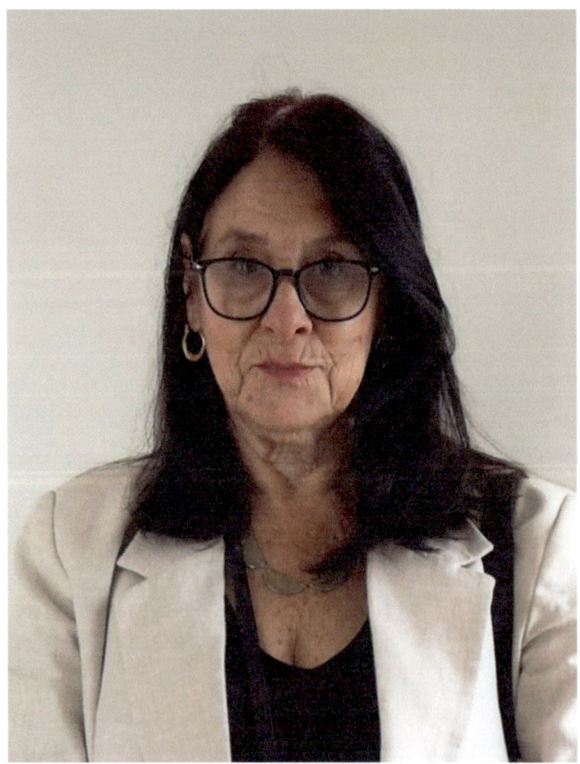

Fig. 22.15 Prof Sally Candy

South African context and hopes that she provides a positive academic role model for her female trainees.

Dr Kathleen Jacobs (Fig. 22.16) completed her radiology training at the University of Witwatersrand, Johannesburg in 2017 under the supervision of Victor Mngomezulu and worked as a consultant at Chris Hani Baragwanath Hospital (CHBAH), Soweto, before pursuing a 2-year Neuroradiology Fellowship at Foothills Medical Centre/University of Calgary, in Canada, in 2019. Her motivation to complete subspeciality training was the desire to understand more about the complexities and intricacies of the central nervous system. Currently, she is a Clinical Assistant Professor at the University of Calgary specialising in Head and Neck imaging.

Dr Napo Kasirye-Mbugua (Fig. 22.17) completed her radiology training at the University of Cape Town in 2019 under the supervision of Prof. Sally Candy, whom she credits for kindling her interest in neuroradiology. She worked as a general radiologist in the private sector where she was exposed to increasing subspecialisation in clinical referral, prompting her decision to pursue a Neuroradiology Fellowship. A 24-month stint at Foothills Medical Centre/University of Calgary has increased her depth and understanding of CNS pathology, has expanded her research

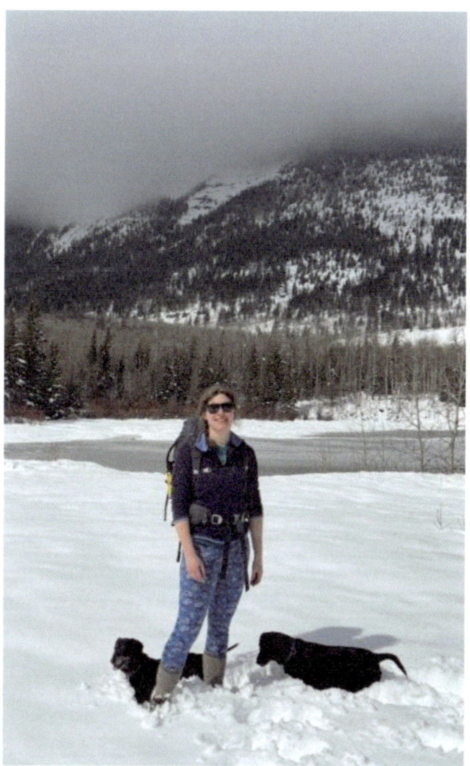

Fig. 22.16 Dr Kathleen Jacobs

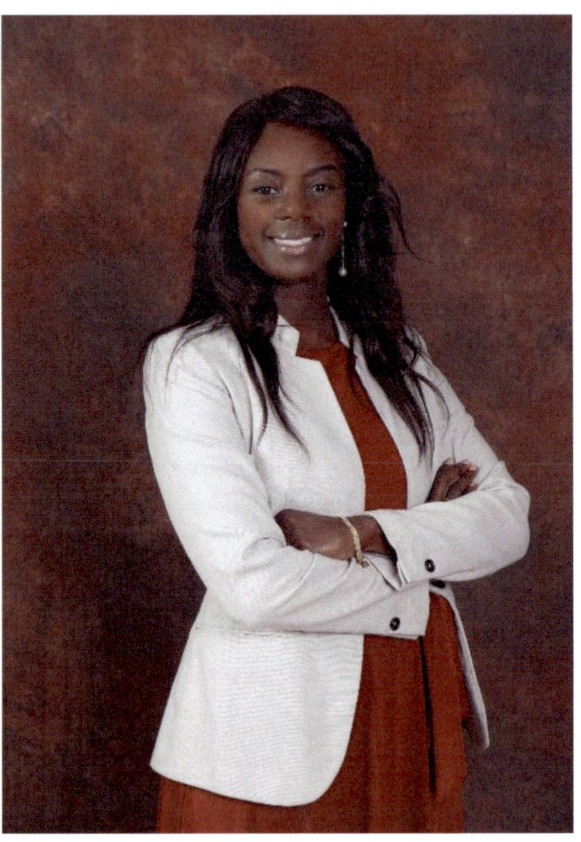

Fig. 22.17 Dr Napo Kasirye-Mbugua

interests into Myelin Oligodendrocyte Glycoprotein Antibody associated Disease (MOGAD) and given her the opportunity to present at international conferences.

While these (usually 24 month) International Fellowship programmes have the advantage of complete immersion in the sub-discipline, they are associated with significant financial and social cost and are often not practical for many women with families.

Dr Christelle Ackerman presently heads the Department of Radiology at Tygerberg Hospital (Stellenbosch University). She is one of very few radiologists in South Africa, and one of only two women, who have completed their PhD in neuroradiology. She is an inspirational teacher of the subspeciality and a long-standing examiner of the Colleges of Medicine of South Africa (CMSA).

Internationally accredited conferences and, more recently, part-time diplomas in neuroradiology (EDiNR) and paediatric neuroradiology (EDiPNR) offered by the European Society of Neuroradiology (ESNR) have facilitated subspecialisation without the disruption that full-time overseas study demands.

At present, 12 women members of the South African Society for Neuroimaging (SASNI) hold diplomas in adult neuroradiology, including Kerryn Devy, Mariane

Kuehnast, and Jeanine Owen who hold key membership roles in the organisation. Dr Christelle Ackerman is the only female member of SASNI with a diploma in Head and Neck imaging.

Despite the increasing number of radiologists and subspeciality trained radiologists in South Africa, the challenge of a low ratio of radiologists per capita remains. South Africa has a total of seven postgraduate medical training programmes. Upon completion of registrar training, radiologists will hold a fellowship of the Colleges of Medicine of South Africa (CMSA) and a Masters of Radiology (MMed). At present, 54% of all radiology trainees (residents) are women. The number or female radiologists registered with the Health Professions Council of South Africa has increased two-fold between 2002 and 2019 and the number is growing at an annual rate of 14%.

The healthcare system in South Africa is divided into private and public sectors with notable discrepancies in funding and the number of people accessing care. The underfunded public sector serves a larger proportion (84%) of the population of South Africa. This unfortunate discrepancy can result in delayed or absent access to advanced imaging techniques and procedures, resulting in delayed diagnoses and poor patient outcomes.

High patient loads and understaffed departments can result in frustration and burnout, creating a problem of retention. “Brain drain” is a common issue faced by many African countries as radiologists seek educational and or career opportunities out of the African continent.

The radiological society of South Africa (RSSA) includes South African trained radiologists but also radiologists from multiple countries in subSaharan Africa. Together with SASNI and SANIS, they create forum for education, training, and networking which opens doors for collaboration amongst radiologists based in South African and internationally.

By identifying and acknowledging the role of women in radiology, we hope to unveil the potential to which women can be elevated in a historically male dominated profession. We hope to provide mentors and positive role models for women in training so that they can meet the realisation that *“you belong in every room that you are in”* —Shond Rhimes.

Tanzania

Dr Ugumba Mussa Kwikima, (MD, MMed-Radiology, Msc-Neuroradiology) (Fig. 22.18) is a Neuroradiologist at Lugalo General Military Hospital and Honorary Lecturer at Muhimbili University of Health and Allied Sciences, Dar es Salaam.

She completed her radiology residency at MUHA and her interest in neuroradiology was sparked by a visiting neuroradiologist, Dr Frank Minja. Originally of Tanzanian origin, Dr Minja received under- and postgraduate training in the USA and is attached to Emory University, Atlanta.

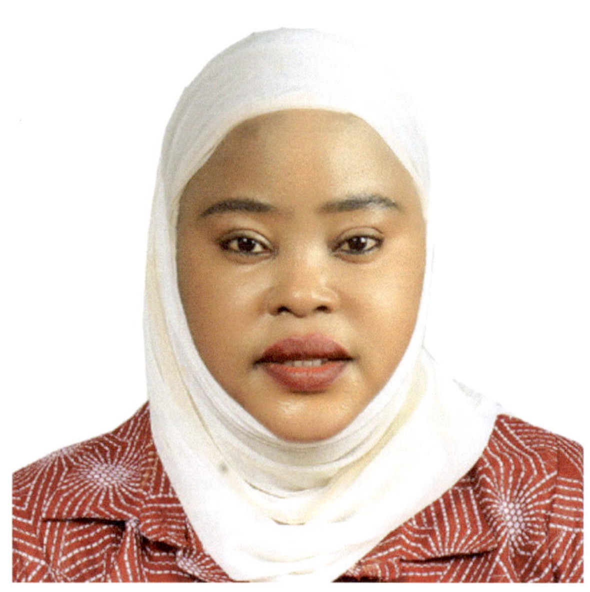

Fig. 22.18 Dr Ugumba Mussa Kwikima

Together with a colleague, Dr Mwajabu Saleh (Fig. 22.19), she secured admission to the first neuroradiology training programme at MUHAS in 2020. This fellowship was set up and supported by RSNA as a Global Learning Centre programme.

This 2-year programme emphasises competency-based clinical training. It has didactic components, a clinical apprenticeship, longitudinal clinical research project/publication, and three formal evaluations per semester (Figs. 22.20 and 22.21).

Post fellowship, Dr Kwikima was selected for the 2022 Derek Harwood Nash Scholarship observership programme at Emory University Hospital in Atlanta.

In her words: “Being an RSNA GLC fellow significantly expanded my networking opportunities in the field and has facilitated my involvement in various multidisciplinary collaborations.”

One such important collaboration has been engagement with SNOSSA, the Society of neuro-oncology of subSaharan Africa. A broad umbrella body comprising radiologists, radiotherapists, neurosurgeons, and neuro-oncologists, SNOSSA was formed with the vision of enhancing diagnosis and management of CNS tumours and to reduce this burden in Sub Saharan Africa. Through engagement with SNOSSA, SIOP (International Society of Paediatric Imaging), and the recently formed ISMRM African Chapter, Dr Kwikima and colleagues have enhanced their clinical, diagnostic and research skills. An international conference will be held in Dar es Salaam in September 2024 with an emphasis on AI and Machine learning in the African context.

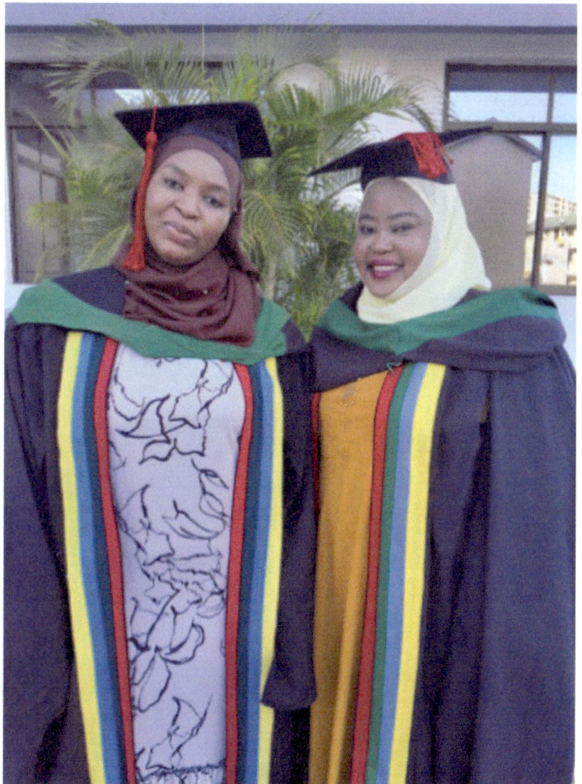

Fig. 22.19 First cohort graduates 2022 (Ugumba Mussa Kwikima and Mwajabu Saleh)

As pioneers of first Neuroradiology training programme in the country, she and colleagues have, with the guidance of RSNA neuroradiology faculty, begun to teach more neuroradiology fellows within Tanzania. Currently, there are four attending neuroradiologists in Tanzania, three of whom are women.

By 2027, Tanzania will have trained 11 neuroradiologists locally, eight of whom will be women. This is an extraordinary achievement and emblematic of what is possible on our continent.

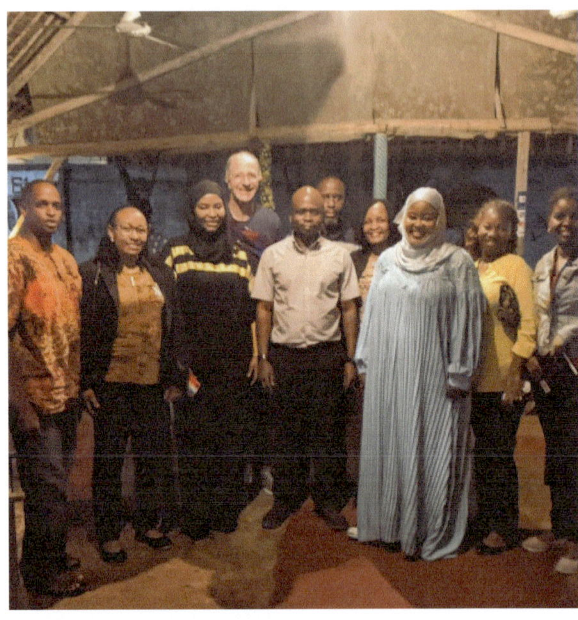

Fig. 22.20 2022 Graduation Dinner (RSNA GLC and MUHAS Faculty, Fellows, and Graduates)

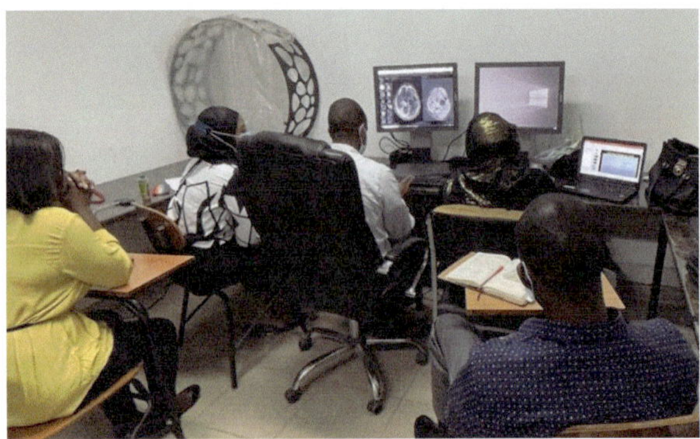

Fig. 22.21 Case review session with Professor Minja (RSNA Faculty)

Uganda

Prof. Elsie Kigule Malwadde (Fig. 22.22), former Chair of Radiology at Makerere University and currently the Director of Health Workforce and Development at the African Centre for Global Health and Social Transformation, established a supportive environment for training women radiologists, mentoring young women in radiology, and encouraging their professional growth.

Dr Rosemary Byanyima, former clinical head of Radiology at Mulago National Referral Hospital and current Executive Director of the Mulago National Referral Hospital, advocated for government funding to train radiologists and secure

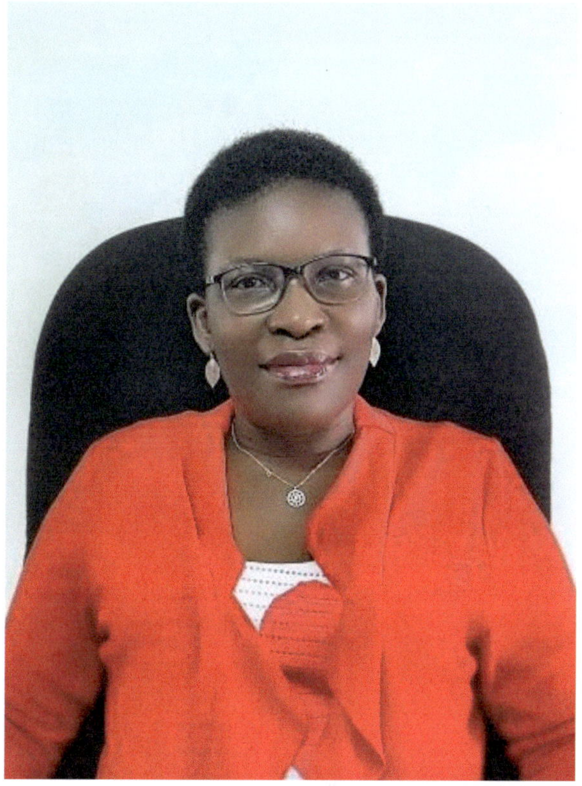

Fig. 22.22 Prof Elsie Kiguli Malwadde

advanced equipment like the 1.5 Tesla MRI magnet. As Executive Director, she ensures the Radiology department receives necessary supplies and funds. She also obtained funding for training radiologists, radiology technologists in subspecialties and MRI techniques.

Dr Rita Nassanga (Fig. 22.23), the current Chair of Radiology and Radiotherapy at Makerere University since 2020, focuses on neuroradiology and is pursuing a PhD in brain MRI for dementia. Under her leadership, collaborations with the University of Utah, University of Vermont, and Vanderbilt University Medical Centre have been established, bringing experts to train residents and radiologists. She successfully applied for the RSNA International Visiting Professors programme, leading to a two-week training session in head and neck radiology in 2018. Dr Nassanga is negotiating with these universities to establish a local neuroradiology fellowship in Uganda. Additionally, she is working with Dr Joyce Nayiga and the MRI Online team to provide affordable neuroradiology courses for local radiologists. She says:

> As a medical student at Mbarara University of Science and Technology, I developed right upper quadrant pain, I was sent for an abdominal sonar which revealed a gallstone. I was fascinated by the technology and decided to complete a masters in radiology after my degree in human medicine. In 2015 a radiology elective at McMasters University gave me

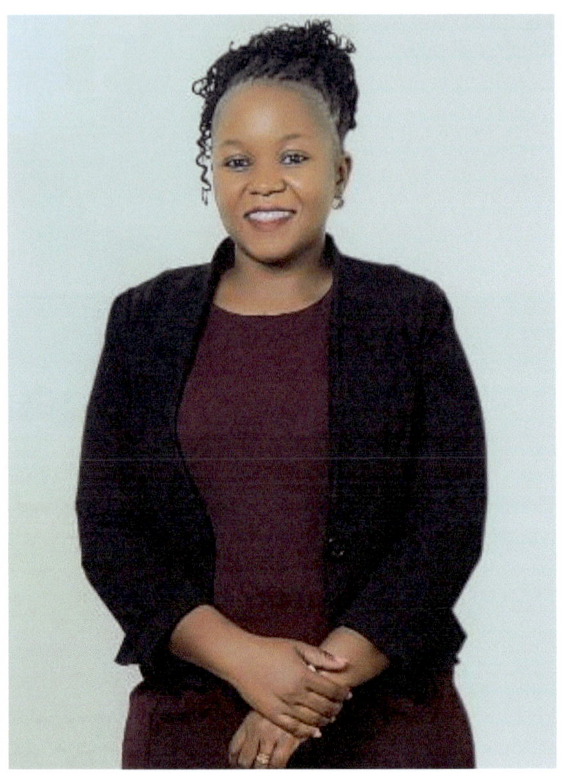

Fig. 22.23 Dr Rita Nassanga

exposure to neuroradiology. I subsequently met Prof Andrea Rossi and Prof James Barkovich at a conference in South Africa (SASPI) in February 2020 and I am currently enrolled in a PhD in MR imaging in dementia.

Paediatric Neuroradiology

Dr Valeria Nabbosa (Fig. 22.24), radiologist at the Uganda Cancer Institute, specialising in paediatric oncology of the brain, head, and neck CT studies, chairs the paediatric neuro-oncology tumour boards and trains radiology residents in neuro-oncology.

Her radiology journey began in her third year of undergraduate medical school at St. Petersburg University in Russia when she saw cardiac catheterisation. On returning to Uganda, she enrolled for a master's degree in radiology at Makerere University and developed an interest in paediatric oncology. In 2021, at a South African Society of Paediatric Imaging conference in Johannesburg, South Africa, she was inspired by a lecture given by Prof. Andrea Rossi on paediatric neuro-oncology. She now

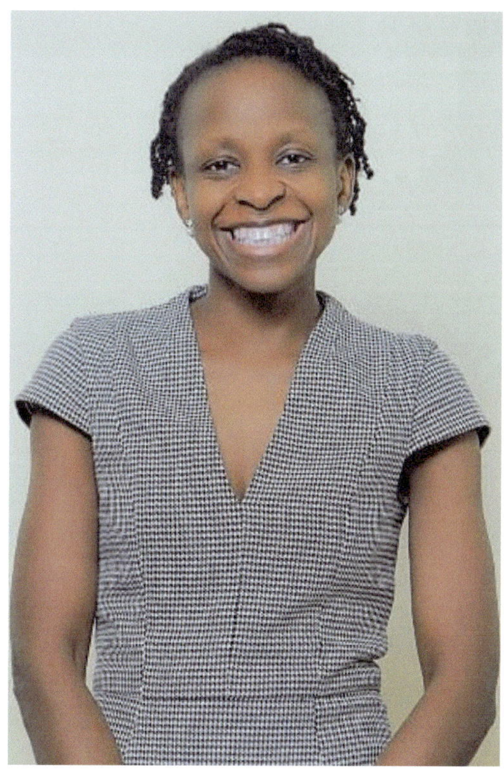

Fig. 22.24 Dr Valeria Nabbosa

trains radiology residents in neuro-oncology at Makerere University. Her immediate plans include the establishment of a formal fellowship in Paediatric Neuro-oncology, to set up a paediatric brain tumour registry in Uganda and to pursue a PhD.

Interventional Neuroradiology

Dr Eva Nabawanuka (Fig. 22.25) led the first Interventional Radiology (IR) fellowship in Uganda, started in August 2023. This programme is accredited by the Medical Council of Uganda, hosted by Makerere University and Mulago National Referral Hospital, and is supported by 'Road to IR' international faculty. She says:

> Growing up I had a grandmother who was hypertensive and called me her doctor because I always reminded her to take her oral medication, hospital appointments, etc. She was the first person who inspired me to become a doctor. Before I took my high school examination, a radiologist came to our school for a career guidance session. Later I found out that he was the first radiologist in the country. I remember listening to him so intently, fascinated by his description of x-rays that go through metal, form images but cannot be seen or felt. It was sheer fascination that made me list radiography as one of the options I could take at college.

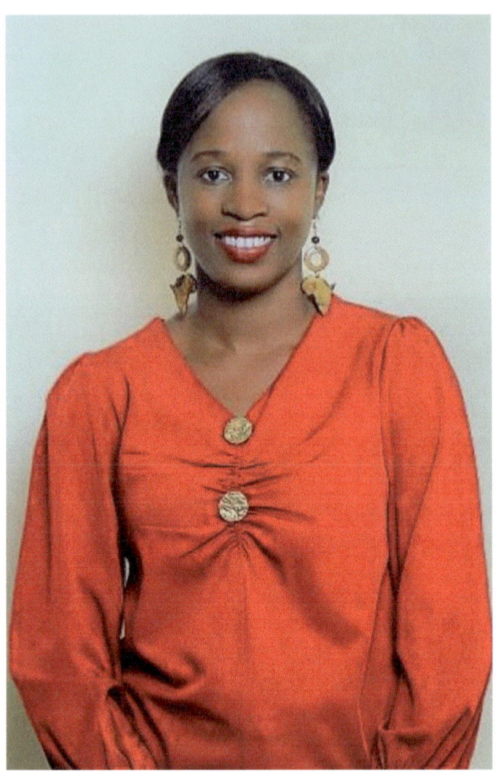
Fig. 22.25 Dr. Eva Nabawanuka

Months later I found out that I had a government scholarship to study radiography in Makerere University. In the radiology department at Mulago hospital, the training facility for Makerere university, I met many amazing women at various stages of their careers in radiology from residents to the chair of the department, Prof. Elsie Kiguli. I graduated top of my class and was beyond excited when I got the offer to practice in the same department. I would later know these women radiologists more personally and the grace with which they did their work not only inspired me but also re-awakened my dream of pursuing a career in medicine. Around the same time, my beloved grandmother had a stroke, and it was the helplessness that made me determined to go back to medical school. The wonderful women radiologists continued to support my journey throughout my undergraduate and post graduate training. My interest in neuroradiology was triggered by the difficulty I had in interpreting CNS imaging. As I became more familiar with diagnostic neuroimaging, I discovered the possibility of offering interventions to improve clinical outcomes in patients like my grandmother. This pursuit motivated me to build Uganda's first radiology subspecialty fellowship training in Interventional radiology (IR). The pioneer class of three trainees (me included) will graduate in August 2025. I look forward to a time I can do mechanical thrombectomies in patients with stroke at my institution! We are still a long way from achieving this dream as an institution, but I have learnt that scarcity breeds innovation. And as we journey along, others are inspired.

Zambia

Zambia has a total of 18 registered radiologists, ten of whom are women, including four recent graduates who are in the process of registration. To date, none holds a subspeciality qualification in neuroradiology.

Two female radiologists, both generalists and foreign nationals, Drs Rheka and Dilya, practised in Zambian University Teaching Hospitals between 1980 and the early 2000s. Both have since retired.

Dr Veronica Sunkutu-Sichizya (Fig. 22.26) is the first Zambian radiologist. She obtained her diagnostic radiology fellowship at The University of Cape Town and moved back to Zambia where she became consultant radiologist at the University Teaching Hospitals in Zambia. At the same time, she served as the national coordinator of medical imaging at the Ministry of Health Zambia for 18 years. Dr Sichizya has made significant contributions to the development of radiology in Zambia. Her most far-reaching achievement has been the development of the first fellowship in diagnostic radiology in Zambia in 2018. To date, this fellowship has graduated a total of ten diagnostic radiologists, six of whom are women.

Dr Jane Shawa (Fig. 22.27) is another influential female radiologist. She is Zambian-born and trained as a diagnostic radiologist at the University of

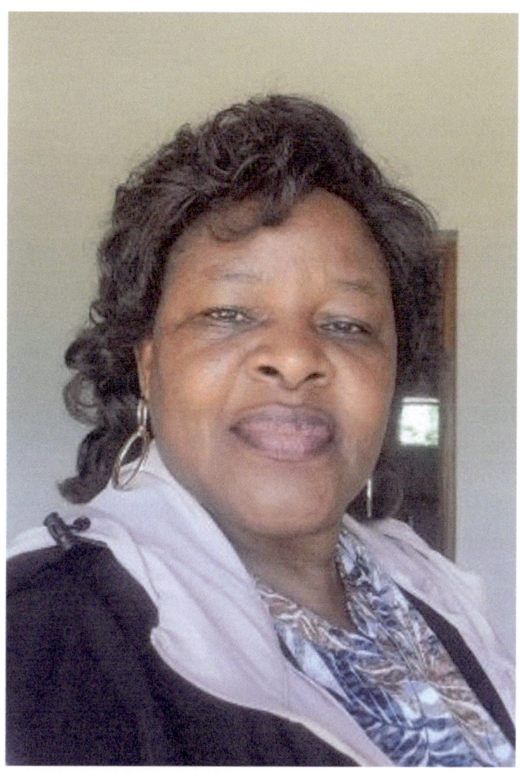

Fig. 22.26 Dr Veronica Sunkutu-Sichizya

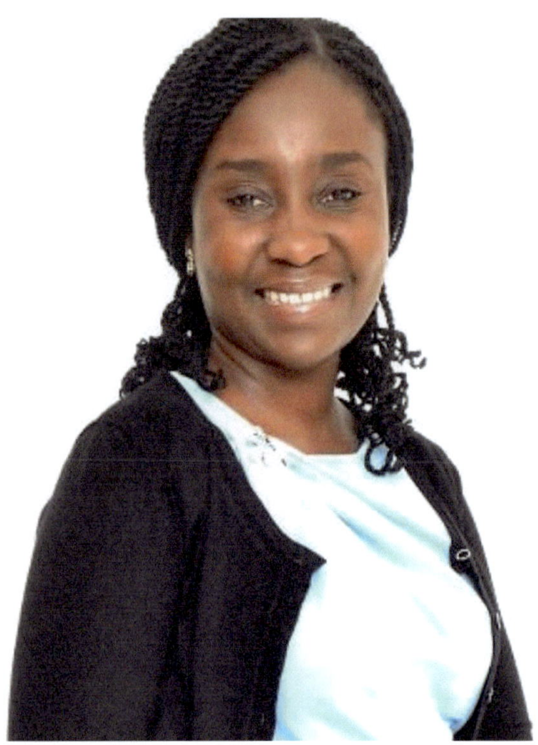

Fig. 22.27 Dr Jane Shawa

Stellenbosch in South Africa, where she was trained and inspired by Prof. Christelle Ackerman. Since her return, she has been instrumental in supporting diagnostic radiology in the Levy Mwanawasa University Hospital in Lusaka.

The first graduating class of the Fellowship in Diagnostic Radiology under the Zambia College of Medicine and Surgery comprised four graduates—all women!

These 'home-grown' female radiologists are Drs Lena Lambart (Fig. 22.28), Ruth Phiri (Fig. 22.29), Juliet Mulopwe (Fig. 22.30), and Sarah Nshimbi (Fig. 22.31), who currently head radiology departments of three major public hospitals in Zambia. Despite not having had dedicated subspeciality training, they feel competent to report on most aspects of neuroradiology. They credit consultant neuroradiologists, Drs Michael Pochen (University of Rochester University, NY) and Doris Lin (Johns Hopkins, Baltimore), and Drs Jill Wruble and Professor Gretchen Birbeck, who were founders of the local Zambian radiology training programme. They refer particularly to Professor Pochen's dedication and consistency (he remains very actively involved, conducting in-person neuroradiological mentorship on his annual visits to Zambia and twice weekly online case conferences with local radiologists and residents).

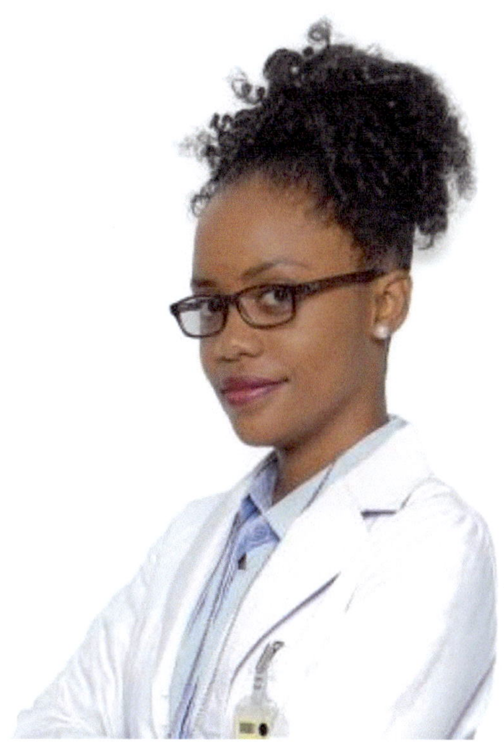

Fig. 22.28 Dr Lena Lambart

Dr Lambart: "*Despite not being specialized in Neuroradiology, I believe that I have been able to be of assistance to the Zambian population, together with my colleagues in the other tertiary hospitals. However, there is still a need to encourage specialization in neuroradiology and other disciplines.*"

Dr Sarah Nshimbi describes her excitement at being awarded the 2024 American Society of Paediatric Neuroradiology educational scholarship (ASPNR): "*This is an online resource that gives me access to the latest advancement in paediatric neuroradiology. Interacting with the international community through webinars and visiting the radiology department on a 2-month observership at University of Rochester in Rochester New York and interacting with residents and radiologists in their normal work environment.*"

Referring to the problems encountered in their home country (which may be common to all countries which lack the IT infrastructure necessary to optimise what imaging is available), she adds: "*The systemic inefficiencies that make timely diagnosis and communication of results so protracted that it impedes appropriate clinical management.*"

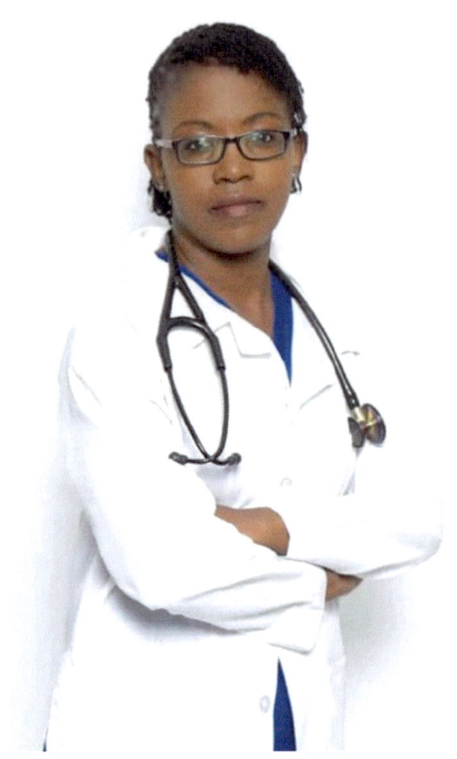

Fig. 22.29 Dr Ruth Phiri

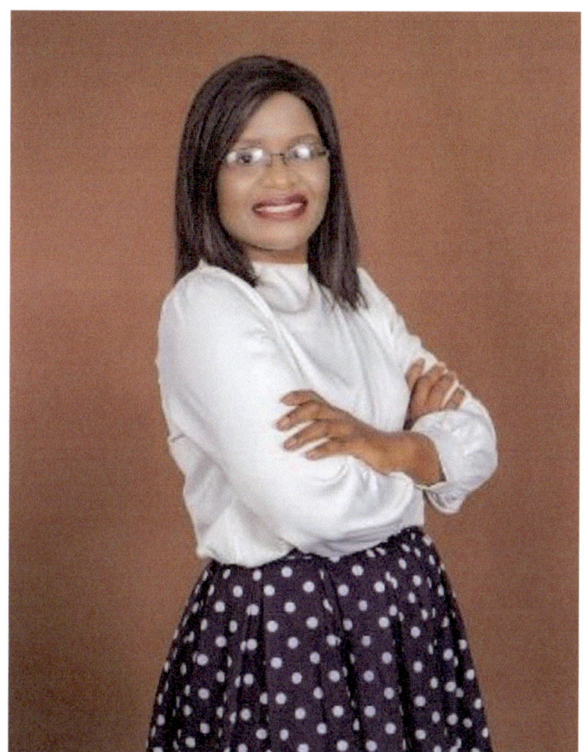

Fig. 22.30 Dr Juliet Mulopwe

Summary

Women are achieving more in terms of academic accomplishment and are increasingly seen in positions of leadership and influence. This provides mentorship and inspiration for younger women as they rise in their careers.

As in other demanding professions, women can achieve only if they have strong support systems. Childcare and domestic responsibilities still lie with women. Despite the relative increase in women in medicine, hospitals and employers are not required by law to provide adequate childcare facilities. In Africa, affordable childcare exists but sets up a continued system of exploitation, undermining the advancement of women in society. Job-sharing and working from home are suited to the practice of neuroradiology but are uncommon.

The demand for imaging far outstrips the capacity for specialist reporting. Most neuroimaging, both in private and government practice in Africa, is and will continue to be reported by generalists.

Plain film is not routinely reported in state hospitals in South Africa. Many state institutions have no radiologist. Increasingly, CT scanners are being installed in government-run/public hospitals which are unable to attract adequate radiology staffing. Widespread subspecialisation is unlikely in this environment.

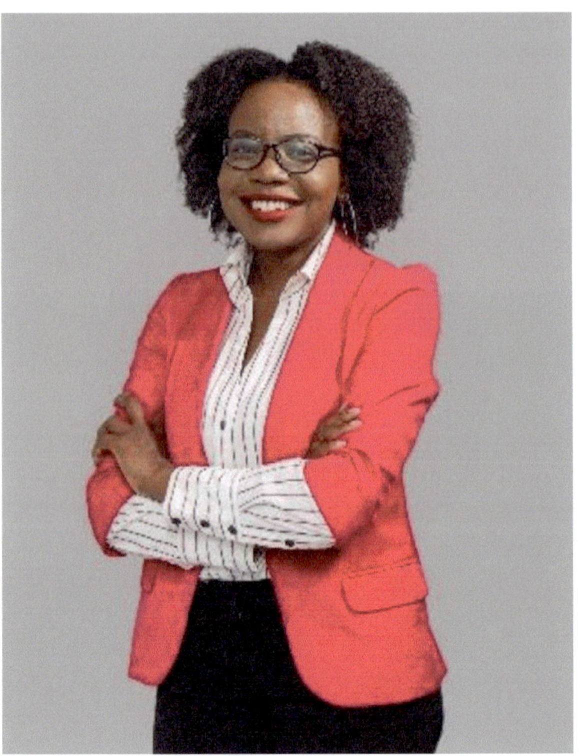

Fig. 22.31 Dr Sarah Nshimbi-Makaliki

However, as seen by the examples given, there has been a slow but definite shift towards female subspecialisation in several African countries. Despite the difficulties described, women are finding opportunities for networking that allow the development of professional and educational relationships which open pathways for further education and skill development. It behoves wealthier countries where neuroradiology is well established to support institutions and individuals in the developing world. This may be in the form of subsidisation of online teaching and evaluation platforms, attendance at international conferences, and collaborative research endeavours.

Programmes such as the Anne G. Osborn International Outreach Professor Program supported by ASNR have the advantage of exposing the visitor first-hand to the societal and healthcare problems and radiological priorities.

A major step forward has been the formation of the 2022 ISMRM African Chapter. This was the culmination of several years of work on the part of a subcommittee of Africa-based academics in the Mbarara University of Science and Technology Mbarara, Uganda and made possible by the Chan Zuckerberg funded Consortium for Advancement of MRI Education and Research in Africa (CAMERA). Strategic partnerships have been forged between the Bill and Melinda Gates Foundation (BMGF) and the ISMRM aimed at enhancing global access to MR education with a focus on bridging the gap between developed and developing countries.

Acknowledging the financial constraints facing African academics, Phase 1 brought together 100 fully funded delegates to attend the 2023 ISMRM in Toronto. Fifty of these were from the Gates 'Unity Project' and 50 from the Africa Chapter (chosen by the founders of the chapter) and representing equal numbers of male and female, MDs and PhDs, radiographers, and technicians, senior and juniors and representing the entire African continent.

Phase 2 will be the establishment of 'Knowledge Exchange Fellowships' where members from high income countries will partner with sites in the LMIC to improve MRI technology education and patient care in the Global South.

In the words of one of the founders, Dr Udunna Anazondo, a female Nigerian neuroscientist presently working in Montreal *"The ISMRM African Chapter represents tenacity in the face of complex challenges. It stands as a testament of the capacity to mobilize a global scientific community to effect transformative change."*

And a colleague based in Zambia adds: "*As an African I am proud of this bold step in ISMRM leadership to change the narrative about Africa and contribute to the MRI knowledge base of scientists in the region. The journey of a thousand miles starts with a step and you have taken a leap.*"

The first meeting of the ISMRM African chapter was held in Ghana in Sept 2023; the next will be in Tanzania in Sept 2024 and the annual ISMRM meeting is scheduled to take place at the Cape Town International Conference Centre in South Africa in 2026. This is expected to draw a wide audience of scientists, academics, and clinicians from all over the world. With careful planning, this may provide the ideal platform to highlight women's contributions to neuroradiology both on the African continent and abroad.

The future (of women in neuroradiology) is 'bright', a phase reiterated by all the women interviewed for this piece. We must ensure that the light never dims—aluta continua!

Acknowledgements Anne G. Osborn International Outreach Professor Program

Bill and Melinda Gates Foundation

Chan Zuckerberg funded Consortium for Advancement of MRI Education and Research in Africa

Derek Harwood Nash Scholarship

Emory University, Atlanta.

ISMRM African Chapter

American Society of Paediatric Neuroradiology educational scholarship (ASPNR).

McMasters University

'Road to IR' international faculty

RSNA International Visiting Professors programme

RSNA Global Learning Centre

University of Rochester, New York

University of Utah

University of Vermont

Vanderbilt University Medical Centre

Dr Frank Minja (Emory University)

Prof. Patricia Hudgins (Emory University)
Drs Michael Pochen (University of Rochester University, NY),
Prof Doris Lin (Johns Hopkins, Baltimore)
Dr Jill Wruble (Johns Hopkins, Baltimore)
Prof. Gretchen Birbeck (University of Rochester)
Prof. Andrea Rossi
Prof. James Barkovich

References

Links

Aga Khan University Hospital Nairobi: http://hospitals.aku.edu/nairobi/Pages/default.aspx
Cairo University: https://cu.edu.eg/Home
Cape Universities Body Imaging Centre: https://cubic.uct.ac.za/
Chris Hani Baragwanath Academic Hospital: https://www.chrishanibaragwanathhospital.co.za/
Health Professions Council of South Africa: https://www.hpcsa.co.za/
Inkosi Albert Luthuli Central Hospital: https://www.ialch.co.za/
Kenyatta National Hospital: https://knh.or.ke/
Levy Mwanawasa University Hospital, Lusaka: https://lmmu.ac.zm/
Makerere University: https://www.mak.ac.ug/
Mbarara University of Science and Technology: https://www.must.ac.ug/
Muhimbili University Dar es Salaam: https://www.mnh.or.tz/
National Hospital Abuja: https://nationalhospital.gov.ng/
Radiological Society of South Africa: https://rssa.co.za/
Red Cross War Memorial Children's Hospital: https://www.childrenshospitaltrust.org.za/the-hospital/
Sahan Diagnostic Centre, Mogadishu: https://sahandiagnostic.com/
School of Medicine, Addis Ababa University: https://www.aau.edu.et/chs/
Soc. of Neuro-oncology of subSaharan Africa: https://snossa.org/
South African Medical Research Council: https://www.samrc.ac.za/
South African Neurointervention Society: http://www.sanis.co.za/
Uganda Cancer Institute: https://uci.or.ug/
University of Cape Town: https://uct.ac.za/

Chapter 23
History of Women in Neuroradiology in Asia Oceania

Kumiko Ando, Patrcia Desmond, Lou Xin, Christina Andica, Sri Andreani Utomo, Mohit Agarwal, Won-Jin Moon, Norlisah Mohd Ramli, Ling Ling Chan, Chao-Bao Luo, Nitaya Suwanwela, Laetitia de Villiers, Lee-Anne Slater, Lesley Cala, and Patricia Desmond

Introduction

Kumiko Ando

Hello, my name is Kumiko Ando. First of all, I would like to express my deep gratitude to everyone who contributed to the creation of this chapter. I am not an active researcher but rather a clinical neuroradiologist. However, I had the chance to meet Professor Maria de Fátima Aragão, who is leading the *History of Women Neuroradiologists* project, when I was at Mt. Sinai Hospital in New York in 2007, and now I have the opportunity to work on the Asia and Oceania chapter. At that time, Mt. Sinai welcomed students from various regions around the world, regardless of gender. Now, as I compile the Asia and Oceania chapter, it has been a great pleasure to learn about the remarkable achievements of some of these individuals.

K. Ando (✉)
Department of Diagnostic Radiology, Kobe City Medical Center General Hospital, Kobe, Japan

P. Desmond · P. Desmond
Royal Melbourne Hospital, University of Melbourne, Melbourne, VIC, Australia
e-mail: Patricia.Desmond@mh.org.au

L. Xin
Department of Radiology, Chinese People's Liberation Army General Hospital, Beijing, China

C. Andica
Faculty of Health Data Science, Juntendo University, Bunkyo, Tokyo, Japan

Department of Radiology, Juntendo University Graduate School of Medicine, Bunkyo, Tokyo, Japan

S. A. Utomo
Department of Radiology, Dr. Soetomo General Hospital, Surabaya, Indonesia
Faculty of Medicine, Universitas Airlangga, Surabaya, Indonesia

D. Birchall (ed.), *A World History of Neuroradiology*,
https://doi.org/10.1007/978-3-032-16653-1_23

In this chapter, we introduce the history of women in neuroradiology in Asia and Oceania. Asia and Oceania are vast regions, with numerous countries and regions, each facing significantly different circumstances. In some areas, the subspecialty of neuroradiology is not yet fully recognized. However, it is clear that women in radiology and neuroradiology across the region have overcome various challenges to reach their current positions. While we may not be able to cover every region comprehensively, we hope this chapter will help more people learn about the history of women in neuroradiology in Asia and Oceania, contribute to addressing ongoing challenges, and support the future development of the field.

We will introduce each region in alphabetical order.

M. Agarwal
Department of Radiology, Medical College of Wisconsin, Milwaukee, WI, USA

W.-J. Moon
Department of Radiology, Konkuk University Medical Center, Konkuk University School of Medicine, Seoul, Republic of Korea

N. M. Ramli
University Malaya, Kuala Lumpur, Wilayah Persekutuan Kuala Lumpur, Malaysia

College of Radiology, Academy of Medicine of Malaysia and Malaysian Society of Radiologists, Kuala Lumpur, Wilayah Persekutuan Kuala Lumpur, Malaysia

Asian Oceanian Society of Radiology Akriti Baral, MD,
Kuala Lumpur, Wilayah Persekutuan Kuala Lumpur, Malaysia

L. L. Chan
Department of Neuroradiology, Division of Radiological Sciences, Singapore General Hospital, Singapore, Singapore

Duke-NUS Medical School, Singapore, Singapore

C.-B. Luo
Department of Radiology, Taipei Veterans General Hospital, Taipei, Taiwan

N. Suwanwela
Department of Radiology, King Chulalongkorn Memorial Hospital and Chulalongkorn University Medical School, Bangkok, Thailand

L. de Villiers
Department of Radiology, Monash Health and School of Clinical Sciences Monash University, Clayton, VIC, Australia

Department Neurointerventional Radiology, Gold Coast University Hospital, Southport, QLD, Australia

Qscan Radiology Clinics, Neutex Image Guided Surgical and Robotics Training Centre, Southport, QLD, Australia
e-mail: laetitia.devilliers@health.qld.gov.au

L.-A. Slater · L. Cala
Department of Radiology, Monash Health and School of Clinical Sciences Monash University, Clayton, VIC, Australia

Women in Neuroradiology and Neurointervention in Australia

Laetitia de Villiers, Lee-Anne Slater, Lesley Cala and Patricia Desmond

Neurointerventional radiology has a rich history in Australia with Australian neurointerventionists generally regarded as innovative, highly skilled, and early adopters of new technology and evidence-based research while maintaining high ethical standards and patient care. Although the specialty is predominantly male dominated in Australia and New Zealand, there are several women who early on recognized the wide scope, exciting technology, incredible challenges, and rewards interventional neuroradiology brings along with the amazing results that can be achieved for patients. These women, early on in the specialty's existence, actively pursued advanced training, grasped available opportunities, and created opportunities where there were none, and as a result became an integral part of neurointervention in Australia and worldwide. The first woman in Australia to pursue a fellowship and career in neurointervention was Dr Rebecca Scroop who gained an advanced fellowship in neurointervention at the University of Washington and Harbor view in Seattle, USA and then returned to the Royal Adelaide Hospital in 2003 and was integral in establishing and is the director of the neurointerventional service at the Royal Adelaide Hospital.

Dr Laetitia de Villiers

Dr Laetitia de Villiers, inspired by her colleagues, and excited by the emerging specialty, initially completed a fellowship in Interventional Radiology at the Princess Alessandra Hospital in 2006. She then went on to gain an advanced fellowship in neuroradiology and neurointervention in 2007 at Mount Sinai Medical Center, New York, and on her return to Australia initially worked as a consultant at Princess Alexandra Hospital in Brisbane but shortly afterward joined her colleague Dr Hal Rice at the Gold Coast University Hospital, Gold Coast, Queensland where she pursued her interest in new technologies. Dr de Villiers and Dr Rice contested and won a bid to cohost the World Federation of Interventional and Therapeutic Neuroradiology (WFITN) 13th World Congress on the Gold Coast in 2015, a hugely successful conference that had never before been held in Australia. 2015 was the year that the trials confirming that endovascular thrombectomy with intravenous lysis was superior to intravenous lysis alone in treating acute ischemic stroke, resulting in one of the greatest advancements in medicine in recent history changing the lives of patients suffering from an acute stroke. One of these pivotal trials was performed in Australia (Extend IA, Campbell et al)) run from the Royal Melbourne Hospital with multiple centers across Australia contributing. This changed the specialty of neurointervention dramatically across the world with a sudden increase in demand for time sensitive acute thrombectomy in AIS, resulting in exponential service demand being placed on the INR workforce.

The specialty of neurointervention at this stage was growing and rapidly advancing across the world and in Australia and New Zealand, and together with her colleague, Dr Hal Rice, they established the Gold Coast University Hospital as an international site for introducing cutting edge technologies in neurointervention, collaborating in research and with industry, in device development, first in human and post market trials. It was therefore a natural choice for the neurointervention department at the Gold Coast Hospital to become the second site in the world to receive the first endovascular robotic system used in neurointervention and Dr de Villiers was the first women in the world to perform a robotic endovascular intracranial aneurysm treatment.

Being relentlessly curious and dissatisfied with the status quo, Dr de Villiers remains passionate about neurointervention as a specialty and what it brings to patients and physicians alike. As a result, she cohosts regular training workshops in Advanced Neuroendovascular Techniques for national and international neuroendovascular specialists, and cofounded the Gold Coast Fellows Training Course for Australian and New Zealand Neurointerventional advanced trainees. In 2009, the annual Australian and New Zealand Neurointerventional M&M meeting, NeuroExchange, was established by her colleague Dr Hal Rice (Gold Coast) and Dr Jason Wenderoth (Sydney) and she has co-hosted this meeting for the past 5 years. This conference brings INRs from across Australia and New Zealand together, where their most challenging and difficult cases are discussed and learned from in a collegiate environment. Dr de Villiers is currently a member of the RANZCR Interventional Radiology Committee and involved in other RANZCR committees developing the new training pathways and curriculum, and accreditation, for interventional and neurointerventional radiology in Australia and New Zealand and sits on the ANZSNR council. She is a regular invited keynote speaker at national and international meetings.

Dr de Villiers recently co-founded NeuTex (Image Guided Therapy, Surgical and Robotics Training center) at the Gold Coast Health and Knowledge Precinct. A facility dedicated to innovation, research, and training that utilizes state-of-the-art medical imaging equipment and 3D printing to precisely replicate surgical treatments for training and biomedical innovation. The NeuTex center regularly hosts specialists from across Australia and throughout the Asia Pacific region for hands on training and workshops enabling international collaboration bringing together colleagues from the Asia Pacific region and introducing new technology.

Dr Lee-Anne Slater (Fig. 23.1)

Dr Lee-Anne Slater completed fellowships at Monash Health in Victoria, Australia from 2012 to 2014 under the guidance of Dr Winston Chong, Dr Michael Holt and Dr Ronil Chandra. She then went to Toronto, Canada to gain further experience in adult neurointervention, but to also gain invaluable exposure to pediatric neurointervention to bring back to Monash Health and the Monash Children's hospital. She completed her fellowship through the University of Toronto with placements at Toronto Western Hospital and The Hospital for Sick Children. In addition to the endovascular component of her fellowship, Dr Slater received a broad experience in vertebroplasty and was able to bring that skillset back to Australia. She returned to Australia to take on a full-time position at Monash Health in July 2015 and has been

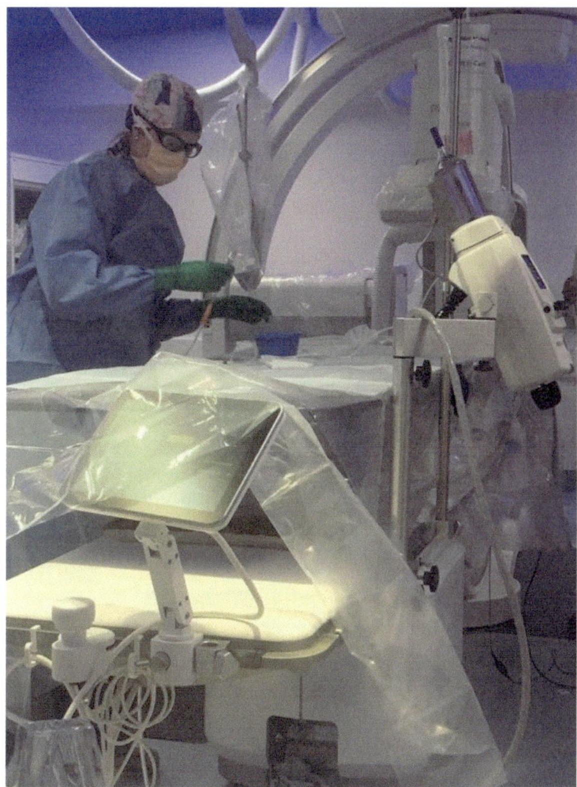

Fig. 23.1 Dr Lee-Anne Slater

growing an adult and pediatric service since then in addition to a busy vertebroplasty service. Inspired by Dr de Villiers academic and research activity and portfolio, she too began to develop her own academic career with a particular interest in new technologies. She completed her first trial as coordinating phase one (PI) with Dr de Villiers one of the site PI's of this study, speaking of the collaboration that exists and is being fostered amongst the women in neurointervention in Australia. She currently sits on the ANZSNR council and has a role in committees helping establish the accreditation of training programs for neurointervenion and is a director of training for the diagnostic radiology program at Monash Health.

Dr Kate Mahady

These three leading women in neurointervention in Australia, established a trend which helped inspire and encourage other women to consider joining the specialty and to be empowered to contribute to the interventional neuroradiology community across the country. Dr Kate Mahady came from the UK to Australia, for a fellowship in neurointervention at the Royal Brisbane and Women's Hospital and is now the director of neurointervention at that hospital. She has a strong interest in pediatric neurointervention. Dr Grace Aw (Royal Brisbane Hospital), Dr Alice Ma (Royal North Shore Hospital), and Dr Ruchi Kabra (Royal Perth Hospital) subsequently joined the growing number of women who are now also part of this group of pioneering women, each making huge contributions to their neurointerventional teams, communities, and patients. Dr Anh Do achieved an advanced fellowship in neurointervention at Monash Health, Royal Adelaide Hospital, and then in Vienna with Dr Monica Keller. She was a neurointerventionalist at Royal Adelaide hospital until 2023 when she sadly passed away. She is remembered as a loving mother and member of the small community of Australian women in neurointervention.

As of now women represent less than 10% of interventional neuroradiologists in Australia; however, these women are contributing well over and above this percentage to research, first in human studies, training, education, and patient care.

Dr Lesley Cala

Dr Lesley Cala's life in neuroradiology started 60 years ago (Fig. 23.2)

Dr Lesley Cala was one of the original neuroradiologists in Australia, going back 60 years. A major milestone was the invention of the CT head scanner, and this was installed at SCGH (the first in the Southern Hemisphere) where Dr Cala examined patients and gave a diagnosis. Neurosurgical treatment was thus enhanced. Also, she noted that one could show multiple sclerosis plaques and so separated the condition from others with similar symptoms.

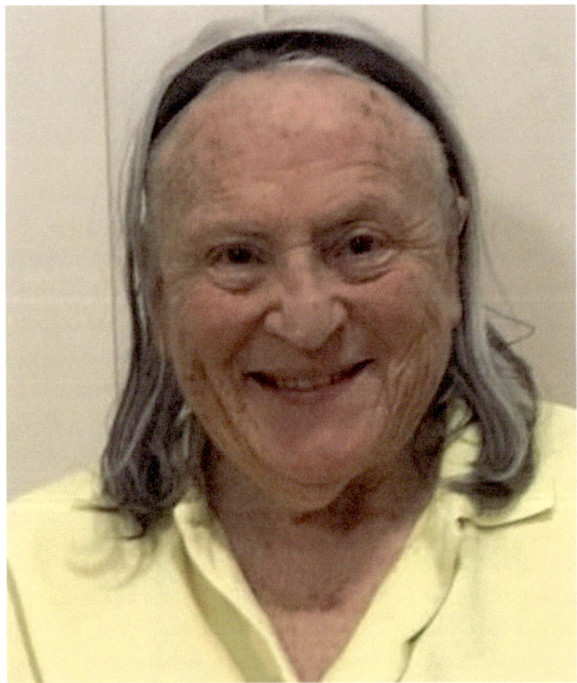

Fig. 23.2 Dr Lesley Cala

Next Dr Cala supervised the new magnetic resonance imaging (MRI) that was installed, improving diagnosis and treatment even more, including the evolution of multiple sclerosis (MS) plaques.

Doctors came from overseas to see the MRI with a view to getting a machine in their country.

One non-clinical task Dr Cala performed was imaging deceased patients for the coroner for 30 years using plain films and CT outside of normal working hours.

Dr Tricia Desmond

Tricia Desmond is a neuroradiologist with clinical and research expertise in neuroimaging, magnetic resonance imaging, and MR-based analysis. She and her research team have a strong emphasis on translation of imaging findings into clinical practice.

She grew up in Melbourne, with her three brothers and sister, attending private schools in the area. Her favorite subjects were Maths and Physics. She continued with her chosen subjects in a Science degree at the University of Melbourne, obtaining first class honors and first place in her year. After completing an Honors year, she started a Master's degree in Biophysics at the Howard Florey Institute but found dealing with live sheep with electrodes somewhat confronting and returned to main Physics to complete an MSc in Particle Physics. Unsure of her next step, she started to see the possibilities that a research career in Medicine might offer. She applied to and started in Medicine at University of Melbourne in 1981. From her second year of Medicine, she had felt that radiology was her particular area of interest. Her MBBS was followed by subspecialization in radiology (FRANZCR). She completed a Research Fellowship at UCSF and upon return in 1991 was appointed to staff position in Department of Radiology at RMH. In 1992, she was appointed as Director of MRI. In 2002, she was instrumental in the development of the Department of Radiology as research site for GE and assisted in development of Brain Imaging Laboratory. In 2003, she was appointed Associate Professor University of Melbourne Department of Radiology and in 2007, Edgar Rouse Chair of Radiology, The University of Melbourne and Director of Imaging, The Royal Melbourne Hospital. She is currently Head, Radiology University of Melbourne and a consultant radiologist at Royal Melbourne Hospital

She has a strong history of clinical translation of research imaging findings with applications in stroke, dementia, epilepsy, and brain tumors. She has been the lead imager on multi-site clinical trials in stroke and led the development of imaging post processing at the Royal Melbourne Hospital. Professor Desmond is a Fellow of the Royal Australian and New Zealand College of Radiologists, immediate past Chair of the Radiology Research Committee and supports the discipline as an Examiner of the College, by extensive committee memberships including as past Secretary of the Australian and New Zealand Society of Neuroradiology, past Associate Editor of Journal of Medical Imaging and Radiotherapy (JMIRO) and as a reviewer of clinical neuroscience publications and research grants. Her peer review involvement includes; Review of Radiology Services at Alfred Hospital (2013); Review of Neurointerventional Services in South Australia (2012); Associate Editor,

Australasian Radiology (2006–2013), Associate Editor, Journal of Clinical Neuroscience (2008–2015).

She has publications totaling more than 272 peer-reviewed original papers in high quality radiological, neurological, neuroscience, neuropsychology, psychiatric, and geriatric journals. Professor Desmond has attracted sustained funding from the National Health and Medical Research Council in clinical neuroscience, acute stroke, dementia, and schizophrenia and has significant funding from other sources.

She has been an invited speaker at many national and international scientific meetings and conferences. She enjoys teaching and mentoring students and has received outstanding teacher awards from the University of Melbourne.

She is married and has four grown children. Out of work, she enjoys spending time with family and friends, walking along the beach and/or sharing simple meals with friends; either in Melbourne or at their beach house. She is thankful to the mentoring she received in her career especially from the previous Head of Department Professor Brian Tress. She feels very lucky to have had such a full and exciting career in Radiology.

Women in Neuroradiology and Neurointervention in China

Lou Xin

Lou Xin, MD, PhD, is a Professor and Director of Department of Radiology in the Chinese People's Liberation Army General Hospital (Fig. 23.3). She graduated from Chinese PLA Medical School with a doctoral degree in 2005 and has worked at Chinese PLA General Hospital up till now. From 2014 to 2017, she served as a visiting scholar at Reagan Medical Center at the University of California, Los Angeles, and the Stanford University School of Medicine. She had been awarded as ESMRMB/ISMRM Certified Teacher in clinical MRI in 2016.

She has long been dedicated to the innovation and clinical application of neuroimaging techniques, being the first to propose the imaging paradigm of "atherosclerotic plaque-cerebral blood flow-collateral circulation" triad for ischemic stroke. She had led the formulation of the first publication of Chinese guideline for standard utilization of imaging for cerebrovascular diseases. In China, she was among the first to launch clinical trials using MRI-guided focused ultrasound (MRgFUS) technology for the treatment of neurological disorders such as essential tremor and Parkinson's disease. As a pioneer in the clinical application of ultra-high field 7T MRI, she has provided critical evidences for its clinical implementation in various nervous system diseases. She actively engages in the clinical translation of state-of-art technology in artificial intelligence and big data in medicine, and has proposed a novel contrast-free CT angiography approach and a general intelligent diagnostic model for brain diseases powered by deep learning. In the past 5 years, she has published 96 articles in SCI-indexed journals, with representative works appearing in renowned journals such as JAMA neurology, radiology, Lancet digital health, and

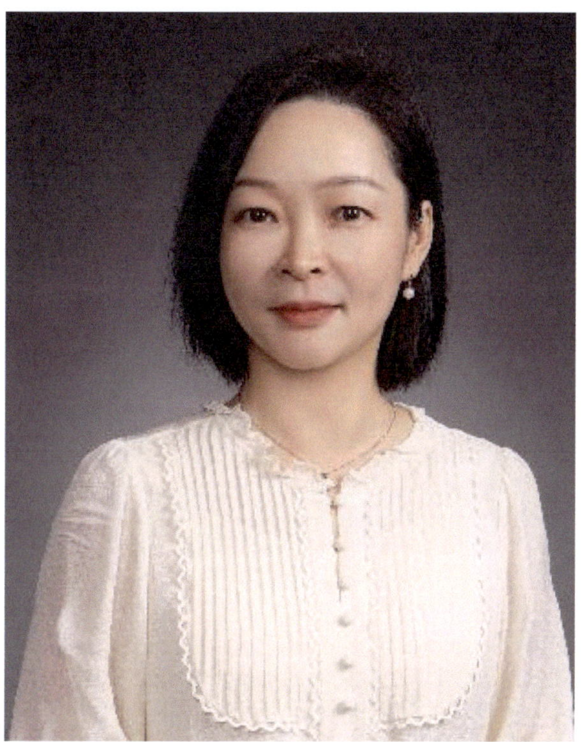

Fig. 23.3 Lou Xin MD. PhD.

stroke. She has published six monographs related to neuroimaging and participated in the formulation of international guideline for the clinical application of arterial spin labeling perfusion. She has led more than ten projects, including the National Science Fund for Distinguished Young Scholars of China. She serves as a member of the editorial board for the English edition of the Investigative Radiology and Stroke & Vascular Neurology. She has given keynote lectures multiple times at international conferences such as annual meeting of The International Society for Magnetic Resonance in Medicine (ISMRM) and Asian Oceanian Congress of Neuroradiology (AOCNR).

Prof. Geng Daoying

Prof. Geng Daoying is a radiologist and has been engaged in medical diagnostic imaging for nearly 40 years. She received her PhD from Fudan University in 1996. She later pursued postdoctoral studies (1996–1998) and was a senior visiting scholar in neuroimaging at the University of Southern California Keck School of Medicine (2004). In 2011, she attended a management training course at the Harvard School of Public Health. In addition, she has served as the Deputy Secretary of the Party Committee (2011–2019) and Vice President (2020–2023) of Huashan Hospital affiliated with Fudan University. She has always focused on solving difficult clinical problems and has created key CT/MRI imaging techniques for major brain diseases, and won the second prize of National Science and Technology Progress Award in 2015. By combining medicine and engineering to develop new intelligent imaging products, she is committed to improving the reading efficiency and accuracy of radiologists. She led the team to develop artificial intelligence diagnostic software for major diseases such as brain tumors and cerebrovascular diseases. One of the intelligent diagnostic software programs for cerebral aneurysms has obtained the National Medical Products Administration Class III Medical Device Registration Certificate, leading neuroimaging into a new field of intelligence.

Dr Minming Zhang

Dr Minming Zhang is a professor and chief physician in the Zhejiang University School of Medicine. Dr Zhang graduated with a bachelor's degree in Medicine from Zhejiang University School of Medicine in 1982. She completed her Medical Residency in Radiology, and meanwhile obtained her master's degree in Radiology and Nuclear Medicine in 1989 from the same institution. She further pursued her PhD in Clinical Medicine at Kobe University in Japan, completing it in 1998, and conducted her postdoctoral research in Neurology at Emory University in USA from 2001 to 2003. Since then, she came back to China working in the field of neuroradiology at Affiliated Hospital of Zhejiang University School of Medicine. Beginning in 2009, Dr Zhang served as the director of the Department of Radiology at the Second Affiliated Hospital of Zhejiang University School of Medicine. In March 2021, she was appointed as the head of the Clinical Medical Imaging Research Center at the same hospital.

Dr Zhang's contributions to the field of medical imaging are extensive. She has authored over 300 research papers and has been a principal investigator for several national and provincial key research projects. Her research interests include the imaging biomarkers for Parkinson's disease and Alzheimer's disease, disease mechanism study of cognitive impairment, and cerebral small vessel disease. She has won the First Prize in the Huaxia Medical Science and Technology Award and several Zhejiang Provincial Science and Technology Progress Awards. Dr Zhang is highly respected for her contributions to medical education and research, having supervised over 100 PhD and master's students. As an active member of the academic community, Dr Zhang holds several prestigious positions. She is a committee member of the Radiology Branch of the Chinese Society of Radiology, a member of the Chinese Society of Biomedical Engineering, and Former Chairman of the Radiology Branch of the Zhejiang Medical Association.

Feng Feng, MD

Feng Feng, MD is a Chinese neuroradiologist. She is a Professor of Radiology and Chair of Department of Radiology, Peking Union Medical College Hospital (PUMCH) in Beijing, China. Dr Feng graduated from Peking University Medical School with a MD degree in 1990. Subsequently, she completed residency in radiology and served as Chief Resident at PUMCH. Immediately after her residency, she became an attending radiologist at the same hospital and quickly advanced through the ranks of Lecturer, Associate Professor and Professor. In the early

1990s, Dr Feng was among the first to adopt MRI for radiologic diagnosis in China and was instrumental in introducing MR spectroscopy to clinical practice. For more than three decades, Dr Feng has dedicated her career to the advancement of diagnosis and treatment of neurological diseases. She and her team have applied cutting-edge medical imaging technologies to enhance the accuracy and efficacy of several diagnostic imaging methods. Their contributions are exemplified by improving the diagnosis of Cushing's disease, neurodegenerative diseases, epilepsy, cerebrovascular diseases, and brain tumors. Dr Feng is well published in medical journals and has trained a large number of medical students and radiology residents. She presently serves as Associate Editor-in-Chief of Chinese Journal of Medical Imaging Technology, a Deputy Editor of Journal of Magnetic Resonance Imaging, and a board member of Chinese Journal of Radiology and Chinese Journal of Neurology. Dr Feng is the president of Chinese Women's Physician Association in Radiology and the vice-chair of Chinese Society of Imaging Technology. She also serves as a standing member or board member of several organizations, including Beijing Society of Radiology, the MRI Division of the Chinese Society of Radiology, Chinese Stroke Association, and Hypothalamus-Pituitary, Chinese Alliance of Rare Diseases.

Zhang Hui MD, Professor and Doctoral tutor, is a well-known neuroradiologist in China. She was admitted to Shanxi Medical University in 1979 and received a Bachelor's degree of Clinical Medicine in 1984. She has completed her residency at the First Hospital of Shanxi Medical University. In 1995, she obtained a Master's degree of Medicine from Shanxi Medical University (SXMU), and her MD of Medical Imaging and Nuclear Medicine from the Medical College of Fudan University in 2002. Over the years, she is mainly engaged in clinical, teaching, and research work in medical imaging. She served as the Vice President of SXMU, Dean of the School of Medical Imaging at SXMU, and Director of the Department of Radiology at the First Hospital of Shanxi Medical University. She is awarded the special government allowance, and the title of National Excellent Science and Technology Worker. Currently, she serves as the Standing Committee Member of the Radiology Branch of the Chinese Medical Association, the Deputy Director of the Neuroimaging Professional Committee, the Standing Committee Member of the Radiology Branch of Chinese Medical Doctor Association, and the Director of the Neuroimaging Professional Committee. She is the person in charge of the "Intelligent Imaging and Nanomedicine" Key Laboratory and the "Intelligent Imaging Big Data and Functional Nanoimaging" Engineering Research Center of Shanxi Province. Her primary research focuses on neuroradiology, functional magnetic resonance imaging (fMRI), and intelligent imaging. She has dedicated herself to the imaging diagnosis and intelligent image analysis of central nervous system diseases, such as brain tumors, cerebrovascular diseases, and dementia. She has remarkable achievements in the fMRI studies on ultra-early diagnosis of cerebral infarction, dementia, and cerebral degenerative changes; and in the multimodal radiogenomics on the genotypes of brain tumors. She has given more than 100 lectures in the fields of radiology, neuroimaging, and oncology internationally and domestically. Dr Zhang currently hosts one key project and three general projects funded by the National Natural Science Foundation of China, and over 20 provincial and ministerial-level research projects. She is the editor in chief of "Approach to Clinical Application of Magnetic Resonance Imaging" and "Variations of Human Anatomy on MR Imaging". She has published over 180 professional papers, of which 68 have been indexed by SCI. Guided over 40 doctoral and postdoctoral students, over 80 master's students, and trained a large number of outstanding talents in the field of radiology nationwide.

Jie Lu, MD, PhD
Jie Lu, MD, PhD, the Director of Department of Radiology and Nuclear Medicine, Xuanwu Hospital, Capital Medical University, mainly engaged in brain function and molecular imaging research.

Jie Lu graduated from Capital Medical University (Beijing, China) with a doctoral degree in 2004. In 2005, she embarked on postdoctoral research at Beijing Normal University in China, focusing on the application of functional MRI in neurological diseases. From 2006 to 2008, she served as a visiting scholar at Massachusetts General Hospital, Harvard University, mainly engaged in individualized brain function studies. Upon her return to China, her team took the lead in the use of positron emission tomography (PET)/MR in neurological diseases, developing new technologies and innovative scanning sequences for brain function analysis. To facilitate the clinical use of multi-modal neuroimaging methods, she further developed series of AI-based technologies and several full-process automatic platforms for the fast and accurate diagnosis of brain diseases. In the past 5 years, she has published more than 80 SCI articles as the first or corresponding author, with the representative works published in international authoritative journals such as Radiology, Brain, Nat Commun, and EJNMMI. Among them, the most cited article being cited 629 times, listed in the top 1% ESI highly cited papers. Prof. Jie Lu was also the main editor of 6 PET/MR monographs, authorized 7 related patents, chaired or participated in 12 expert consensuses, presided over 20 research projects in China. Till now, she has delivered several keynote speeches at international academic meetings, such as the International Society of Magnetic Resonance in Medicine (ISMRM) annual meeting in 2018. Currently, she holds a membership in ISMRM Perfusion Study Group and the editorial board of several academic journals, such as EJNMMI and JMRI.

Prof. Bing Zhang
Prof. Bing Zhang graduated from Nanjing Railway Medical College in 1997 with a medical degree in Medical Imaging. She subsequently joined the Department of Radiology, The Affiliated Drum Tower Hospital, Medical School of Nanjing University, where she engaged in radiological diagnosis. During this period, she obtained both a Master's degree and a PhD in Medicine from Southeast University Medical School. From 2012 to 2013, Prof. Zhang conducted postdoctoral research in neuroimaging at the Aging and Dementia Imaging Research Laboratory (ADIR), Department of Radiology, Mayo Clinic, under the mentorship of Clifford R. Jack, Jr., MD, a renowned scientist in Alzheimer's disease (AD) brain imaging. In 2015, she was appointed as a Chief Physician and established renowned expert clinics in

medical imaging and cognitive impairment MDT clinics. She conducts over 1,040 consultations for difficult cases annually, with more than 50% of these being external cases. Prof. Zhang has long been dedicated to applying new imaging technologies in the clinical diagnosis and treatment of major neurological diseases, particularly AD. She has developed highly specific fMRI techniques targeting the entorhinal cortex and identified its significant value in the early diagnosis of AD. Additionally, she advanced the clinical application of neuroimaging artificial intelligence (AI) technology, established screening and follow-up protocols for the entorhinal cortex fMRI, and facilitated the application of AI technology in real-world scenarios. These efforts advanced the diagnostic window for AD and pioneered a new research field in intelligent neuroimaging diagnosis and intervention specifically targeting the entorhinal cortex. She has published over 100 scientific papers in international journals in radiology and neuroimaging, edited and translated monographs such as "High Field Magnetic Resonance Imaging" and "Essentials of Osborn's Brain: A Fundamental Guide for Residents And Fellows," contributed to the writing of eight textbooks including "Cranial Imaging Diagnosis" for People's Medical Publishing House, as well as reviewed and edited the translation of book titled "Introduction to Resting State fMRI Functional Connectivity." Prof. Zhang has led the development of two industry standards for image quality control and published an expert consensus in an international journal. Her work has been incorporated into four domestic and international expert consensuses on dementia diagnosis and treatment, and she holds nine patents (including one US invention patent) and 14 software copyrights.

Chen Feng, MD. PhD

Chen Feng, MD. PhD, graduated from Wuhan University in 2006 and has worked at Hainan General Hospital ever since. In March 2017, she began postdoctoral research at the Institute of Automation, Chinese Academy of Sciences. From January 2018 to January 2019, she participated in a visiting study at the Magnetic Resonance Center of Johns Hopkins University in the United States. She currently serves as the professor, chief physician, doctoral supervisor, deputy director of Hainan General Hospital, director of the Medical Imaging Center and the Radiology Department, as well as director of the Department of Medical Imaging at Hainan Medical University. She is a committee member of the Radiology Branch of the Chinese Medical Association and vice leader of the Neurology Group, a committee member of the Radiology Physician Branch of the Chinese Physician Association, and chair of the Radiology Specialty Committee of the Hainan Medical Association, where She is also the leader of the Neurology Group, as well as the director of the Hainan Radiology Diagnosis Quality Control Center. In recent years, she has focused on functional magnetic resonance research, conducting in-depth studies on neuroimaging, particularly for neurological cognitive diseases. She has presided over four National Natural Science Foundation projects (two general and two regional), subprojects of Hainan Province's major science and technology program, key research and development plans in Hainan, Hainan Natural Science Foundation projects, and Hainan Social Development Fund projects, among others. She has published more than 100 research papers, with 56 of them as the first or corresponding author in SCI journals. She has edited or translated four monographs as the chief editor and four more in a deputy role. She has won four first prizes for provincial science and technology progress (ranking first, second, second, and seventh, respectively) and three second prizes (ranking first, second, and second). In 2012, she was recognized as one of the "Outstanding Young and Middle-aged Medical Talents in Hainan," became a "First-tier Candidate" in Hainan's 515 Talent Program in 2015, received the Hainan Province May Fourth Youth Medal in 2016, was named a "Leading Talent" in Hainan in 2018, selected as a reserve candidate for "Key Experts Serviced by the Hainan Provincial Committee" the same year, recognized as an "Outstanding Expert with Notable Contributions" by Hainan Province in 2018, awarded the "Nanhai Celebrity" Educational Talent Plan in 2019, granted special government subsidies in 2020, and honored as an advanced individual in the national fight against COVID-19 by the Ministry of Science and Technology in 2021. She received the May Day Labor Medal from the Hainan Provincial Federation of Trade Unions in 2022, the National May Day Labor Medal from the All-China Federation of Trade Unions in 2023, and the title of "Most Beautiful Doctor" from the Publicity Department of the CPC Central Committee and the National Health Commission in 2023.

Fei-Yun Wu

Fei-Yun Wu is a neuroradiologist from Nanjing City, Jiangsu Province of China. She graduated from Southeast University School of Medicine, and obtained the bachelor's degree in 1995. Then, she was admitted as a staff of Radiology Department, The First Affiliated Hospital of Nanjing Medical University. Whereafter, she obtained her master's and doctor's degrees from Nanjing Medical University in 2001 and 2012, respectively. In 2013, she visited Columbia University in New York City of USA, and got the research training for 1 year. From 2018, she started working as a professor of radiology in Nanjing Medical University. Now, she is the Director of Radiology Department, The First Affiliated Hospital of Nanjing Medical University, and dean of Medical Imaging School of Nanjing Medical University.

As to the specialty societies, Dr Wu currently serves as the member of Chinese Society of Radiology, the vice chairman of Chinese Society of Head and Neck Radiology, and the vice chairman of Jiangsu Province Association of Radiologist. Until 2024, Dr Wu has authored more than 70 scientific papers in peer-reviewed journals, contributed to more than five books, and given more than 100 lectures in the fields of radiology.

Xia Shuang MD

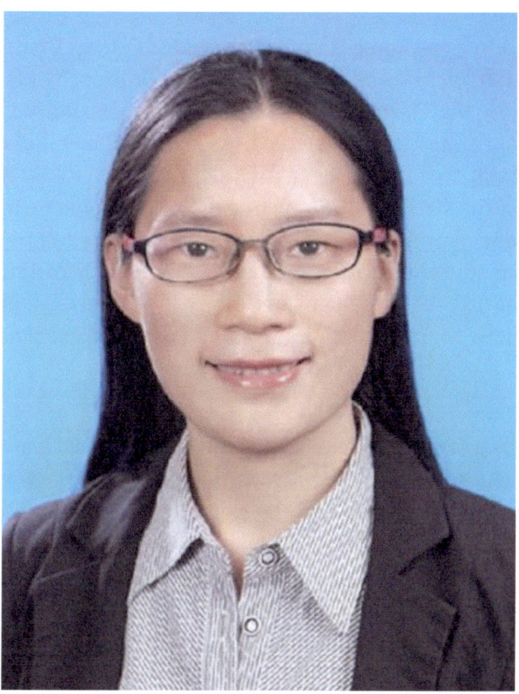

Xia Shuang MD. Chief Physician of the Radiology Department at Tianjin First Central Hospital, engaged in clinical and research work in neurology and head and neck imaging medicine. Graduated with a PhD from Tianjin Medical University in 2005. Currently serving as a doctoral supervisor at Tianjin Medical University and Nankai University. She went to Wayne University in the United States for a 3-month training program in 2012. She went to the American College of Radiology for 1 month residency teaching training from March to April 2019. She was selected as the first level candidate for the Tianjin "131" Innovative Talent Training Project and passed with excellence in 2014. She was awarded the first batch of "Jinmen Medical Talents" by the Tianjin Health and Family Planning Commission and the Teaching Excellence Award by Tianjin Medical University in 2018. She has received the title of "Excellent Teaching Teacher" from the Chinese Medical Association in 2019. She has received the "Tianjin Science and Technology Progress Second Prize" twice in 2020 and 2023. She has hosted one key research and development project of the Ministry of Science and Technology of China, three projects funded by the National Natural Science Foundation of China, one major science and technology plan and special project of Tianjin, one project supported by the China Postdoctoral Fund, one major science and technology special project and engineering project of Tianjin, one project supported by the China Postdoctoral Science Foundation, and three projects supported by the National Social Science Fund of China. She has published 58 papers in internationally authoritative journals, with a cumulative impact factor of over 100 points.

She currently serves as youth member of the Radiology Branch of the Chinese Medical Association, member of the Medical Imaging Branch of the Chinese Stroke Society, member of the Head and Neck Imaging Professional Committee of the Radiology Branch of the Chinese Medical Association, member of the Radiology Branch of the Tianjin Medical Association, member of the Radiology Branch of the China Association for the Promotion of International Exchange in Healthcare, and member of the Council of the China Medical Imaging Integration Alliance. She currently serves as an editorial board member for "Radiology of Infectious Disease," "International Journal of Medical Radiology," "Chinese Journal of Clinical Medicine," "Chinese Journal of Radiology," "Magnetic Resonance Imaging," and "Medicine.

Yongmei Li, MD

Yongmei Li, MD, is a female professor at Chongqing Medical University and serves as the deputy director of the Radiology Department in the university's First Affiliated Hospital in China. She is a member of the Neurology Group of the Chinese Society of Radiology, the Radiology Branch of the Chinese Medical Association, and vice chairman of the Radiology Branch of the Chongqing Medical Association. She earned her doctoral degree from Chongqing Medical University in 2008. In 2010, she was a visiting fellow in the Neuroradiology Department at New York University Medical College for 6 months. Dr Li has specialized in neuroradiology for approximately 20 years, focusing on demyelinating and cerebral small vessel diseases of the central nervous system. She has published numerous articles in reputable journals, including European Radiology, J Magnetic Imaging, J Neuroradiology, J Neurol, Neuroradiology, Academic Radiology, Cerebral Cortex, and Multiple Sclerosis and Related Disorders. Additionally, she has served as a peer reviewer for several journals such as Multiple Sclerosis and Related Disorders, Academic Radiology, Insights into Imaging, and the Chinese Journal of Radiology. She is also the communicating editor for the Chinese Journal of Radiology, a leading journal in the field. As a member of expert consensus working groups, including the Diagnostic Criteria for Multiple Sclerosis Imaging and Standardized Application of Multiple Sclerosis MRI, she has contributed to the development of multiple sclerosis guidelines. She has co-authored several books, including Brain Imaging Diagnosis (Third edition), Imaging of Central Nervous System Demyelinating Diseases, and Imaging of Central Nervous System Infections and Neuroimmunology, published by People's Health Publishing House. As a mentor for master's and doctoral candidates, she has trained numerous successful radiologists. She has been awarded Academic Leader and Chongqing innovative talents leader.

Yunjing Xue MD.

Yunjing Xue MD is a Chinese neuroradiologist, a Professor and Doctoral supervisor at the Fujian Medical University. She currently serves as the chairperson of the department of radiology at Fujian Medical University Union Hospital, imaging technology of Fujian Medical University and the Fujian Society of Radiology in China. She graduated with a degree in medicine from Fujian Medical University in 1995. She did her residency in radiology at the Fujian Medical University Union Hospital. She received her doctorate from the Capital Medical University of Beijing in 2007. She spent 1 year at the University of Washington Medical Center—in the vascular radiology laboratory as a visiting fellow from 2010 to 2011. That was a great experience for her, becoming part of the cardiovascular radiology and neuroradiology staff from then on. With a career from 2007 to the present, she brings extensive experience and expertise to her role. Her work focuses on medical radiology, particularly in cardiovascular radiology and neuroradiology. The paper "Preliminary Study on Computational Fluid Dynamics of Carotid Bifurcation Hemodynamic State" was honored as the fifth Outstanding Academic Paper by the Journal of China Association for Science and Technology. Her project "The Establishment and Promotion of MRI Precision Diagnosis System for Major Brain Diseases" won the second prize of the Fujian Medical Science and Technology Award. This system serves the clinical practice of a variety of high-incidence and high-risk of major brain diseases such as stroke, brain tumors, and neurodegenerative disorder, which has significantly improved the cure rate and reduced the mortality and disability rate.

Yan Zhou MD.

Yan Zhou MD is a Chinese neuroradiologist. Yan Zhou received her MD from Shanghai Jiao Tong University, Shanghai, China, in 2007. She is the director of the Department of Radiology at Renji Hospital, School of Medicine, Shanghai Jiao Tong University. Her research interests lie in Neuroimaging. She was a visiting scholar at the University Hospital of KU Leuven in Belgium and the University of Washington in the US in 2005 and 2011, respectively. Since 2021, she has been the administrative director of the Department of Radiology at Renji Hospital. She is also a professor and doctoral supervisor at the School of Medicine, Shanghai Jiao Tong University. She serves as a member of the Neuroimaging Group of the Chinese Society of Radiology and the Neuroimaging Group of the Chinese Medical Doctor Association, among other roles. She and her research group have published 70 papers focusing on functional imaging of cardiovascular and cerebrovascular diseases. Her work has received coverage from mainstream media outlets domestically and internationally, including CNN, China Daily, and People's Daily Online.

Zhiyun Yang

Zhiyun Yang, graduated from Sun Yat-sen University of Medical Sciences and got her bachelor degree in 1988, after which, she specialized in the diagnostic imaging of head and neck, ophthalmic and otorhinolaryngologic and neurological diseases with celebrated Professors Chen Junlu and Professor Meng Quanfei and was granted the master degree and doctoral degree, respectively.

As the chief physician in the radiology department of the first affiliated hospital of Sun Yat-Sen university, supervisor of PhD and the vice-director of diagnostic radiology, she devoted her life to diagnostic radiology of the head and neck and the central nervous system. In addition, she has been awarded various kinds of titles in many academic organizations, such as the member of neurological and head and neck specialized group of Chinese Society of Radiology, and the chairman of head and neck specialized group of Radiological Society of Guangdong province.

She actively engages in numerous professional activities, regularly participating in academic conferences and continuing education events. Throughout her career, Prof. Yang has been a proponent of innovative imaging techniques, diagnostic approaches, and new ideas, generously sharing her clinical experiences and insights with her peers and young doctors. Her work has significantly advanced the field of imaging diagnostics and techniques in China, particularly within Guangdong province.

Over the years, Prof. Yang has authored and co-authored over 100 scientific research papers published in both domestic and international journals.

Women in Neuroradiology in Indonesia

Christina Andica and Sri Andreani Utomo

Christina Andica

Christina Andica, MD, PhD, is an Indonesian Junior Associate Professor at the Faculty of Health Data Science, Juntendo University, and the Department of Radiology at Juntendo University Graduate School of Medicine, Tokyo, Japan (Fig. 23.4). She completed the Indonesian Board Examination in Radiology and graduated as a Diagnostic Radiologist from Padjadjaran University in Bandung, Indonesia, in 2014. In 2020, she earned her PhD from Juntendo University and then served as a postdoctoral fellow under the Japan Society for the Promotion of Science for 2 years. Her research focuses on leveraging advanced diffusion MRI and myelin imaging to explore brain microstructural changes in neuropsychiatric diseases. She has published over 90 peer-reviewed papers and has received multiple prestigious awards from both Japanese and international radiological societies, including the Kato Prize from the Japanese Society of Neuroradiology, the Magna Cum Laude from the International Society for Magnetic Resonance in Medicine, and a Certificate of Merit from the Radiological Society of North America.

Here is a message from Christina Andica:

In Indonesia, women have made notable progress in the field of neuroradiology, with many female radiologists holding key positions in academic and clinical environments. However, one area that still requires improvement is the involvement of female neuroradiologists in research. I view research as a critical component in advancing patient care, especially in early diagnosis and personalized treatment strategies. This belief motivated me to pursue my research career in Japan, where I

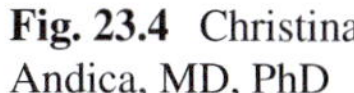

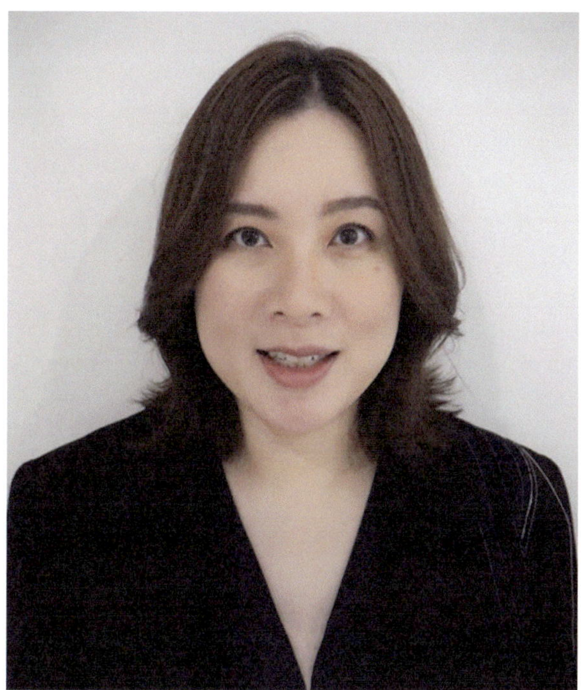

Fig. 23.4 Christina Andica, MD, PhD

have had the privilege of learning from leading experts in the field. In Japan, while neuroradiology remains predominantly male-dominated, there is a growing awareness of the need for greater gender diversity. My experience here has been incredibly enriching, providing me with invaluable skills and knowledge. Now, I feel it is time to give back to my home country, Indonesia, by fostering research collaboration between Japan and Indonesia, particularly by empowering female researchers. I firmly believe that by strengthening research ties, we can not only enhance the field of neuroradiology but also inspire more women to take on leadership roles in this important area.

Sri Andreani Utomo, Dr, Sp.Rad (K)N-KL.

Dr Sri Andreani Utomo, Sp.Rad (K)N-KL. is a Staff and senior lecturer in Dept. of Radiology, Dr. Soetomo General Hospital, Faculty of Medicine, Universitas Airlangga, Surabaya, Indonesia (Fig. 23.5)

She is a Member of The Indonesian Radiology Society, Secretary of The Indonesian Neuroradiology Society, Member of Neuroradiology Team, Dr. Soetomo Academic General Hospital, Surabaya, Indonesia, Member of AOSNHNR (Asian Oceanian Society of Neuroradiology and Head & Neck Radiology), Member of AMS (Asian Musculoskeletal Society), Member of The Oncology Musculoskeletal Team (Pertumsi), Dr. Soetomo Hospital, Surabaya, Indonesia.

She has published 18 papers and 4 reviews mainly on advanced MRI.

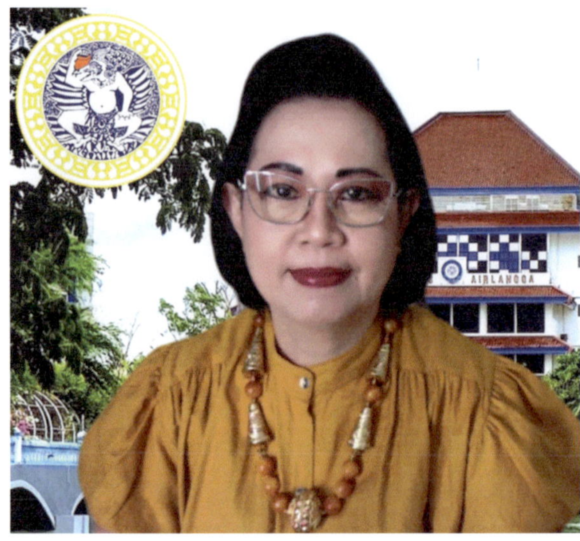

Fig. 23.5 Sri Andreani Utomo, Dr, Sp.Rad (K)N-KL

Here are some of her recent papers:

1. Apparent Diffusion Coefficient Values and Dynamic Contrast-Enhanced Magnetic Resonance Perfusion are Potential Predictors for Grading Meningiomas: Sri Andreani Utomo, Abdul Hafid Bajamal, Yuyun Yueniwati, Irfan Deny Sanjaya, Dyah Fauziah, International Journal of Medical Sciences, 2022; 19(9): 1364–1376. doi:10.7150/ijms.75092
2. The role of apparent diffusion coefficient in differentiating typical from atypical meningioma: Sri Andreani Utomo, Abdul Hafid Bajamal, Yuyun Yueniwati Prabowowati Wadjib, Irwan Barlian Immadoel Haq, Vivid Umu Varidha, Dyah Fauziah, Bali Medical Journal 2022; 11(1): 455–459. doi:10.15562/bmj.v11i1.3244
3. Advanced MRI prediction of meningioma histopathological classification: A literature review and case presentations: Sri Andreani Utomo, Abdul Hafid Bajamal, Yuyun Yueniwati PW, Irwan Barlian Immadoel Haq, Dyah Fauziah, Eunike Serfina Fajarini, Bali Medical Journal 2022; 11(1): 23–27. doi:10.15562/bmj.v11i1.3100

Here is a message from Dr Sri Andreani Utomo:

It is interesting for the female neuroradiologists in Indonesia.

I have been a neuroradiologist since 2002, at that time the number of neuroradiologists in Indonesia was just only six persons, three females and three males.

Since then, the number of female neuroradiologists increased; now, in Indonesia we have 26 neuroradiologists, mostly females with only 8 male neuroradiologists.

Not just neuroradiologists, the radiologists in Indonesia right now are mostly females rather than males.

History of Women Neuroradiologists in India

Mohit Agarwal

Dr Sneh Bhargava

Dr Sneh Bhargava was the first woman radiologist in India. She was born in 1930 and received her medical degree from Lady Hardinge Medical College, New Delhi, India. Dr Bhargava completed a fellowship in diagnostic radiology from the Imperial College, London, UK, and was awarded a DMRD from the Royal College of Physicians and Surgeons. She joined the All India Institute of Medical Sciences (AIIMS), the apex medical institute in India, as assistant professor, and in due course ascended to the rank of Professor and was appointed Chair of the department of radiology. She was the first and the only woman to be named the Director of this premier institute. She has served many national and international radiology committees including the Indian Radiology and Imaging Association, of which she was the president. During her career, she has worked relentlessly for the advancement of education and patient care at her institute and in the country at large, which includes the establishment of the first ever CT scanner in India in the year 1978. She was instrumental in advancing neuroradiology during her leadership at AIIMS. She has been awarded the Padma Shri, the fourth highest civilian award in India, and was awarded honorary membership of the RSNA in the year 2018.

Other prominent radiologists who have worked or are working in the field of Neuroradiology in India are Prof. Neera Kohli (Chair at Chhatrapati Shahuji Maharaj University, Lucknow India), Prof. Manorama Berry (former Chair at AIIMS), Prof. Sima Mukhopadhyay (former Chair at AIIMS), Prof. Sushma Vashisht (former Chair at AIIMS), Prof. Ratni Gujral (former Chair at SGPGIMS, Lucknow), Prof. Sudha Suri (former Chair at PGIMS, Chandigarh), Prof Veena Chaudhary (former Chair Mualana Azad Medical College, Delhi), and Prof. Meher Ursekar (Mumbai).

Dr Varsha Joshi is another prominent Neuroradiologist in India who is currently a senior consultant at Vijaya Diagnostic Center, Hyderabad. She is the past President of the Indian Society of Head and Neck Radiology and is now the international liaison officer for the society. Other prominent current women neuroradiologists in India are Prof. Rose Dawn Bharath (NIMHANS), Prof. Hima Pendharkar (NIMHANS), Dr Rashmi Saraf (Mumbai), Dr Sunithi Mani, Dr Arpita Sahu, and Dr Manisha Joshi.

History of Woman in Neuroradiology in Japan

Kumiko Ando

I am Kumiko Ando, MD, PhD I graduated from Saga Medical School in 1990, worked at Hyogo College of Medicine Hospital, and now serve as the Director of the Department of Diagnostic Radiology at Kobe City Medical Center General Hospital (Fig. 23.6). Like many radiologists in Japan, I practice as a general radiologist with a specialty in neuroradiology, particularly pediatric neuroradiology.

I am not an active researcher, and my scientific contributions are limited.

Ando K, Ishikura R, Ogawa M, et al. MRI tight posterior fossa sign for prenatal diagnosis of Chiari type II malformation. Neuroradiology. 49: 1033–9, 2007.

However, perhaps because I have been fortunate to have several good friends in Japan and across Asia and other parts of the world, I am honored to compile the Japan Chapter for the Chapter of Women in Neuroradiology in Asia Oceania of the WFNRS.

The history of female membership in the Japanese Society of Neuroradiology (JSNR) shows that the first presentation by a female lead presenter was given by Yuko Ono (Saito) in 1978 at the seventh Annual Meeting on CT and angiography in cerebellopontine angle tumors. By 2024, about 20% of JSNR members are women.

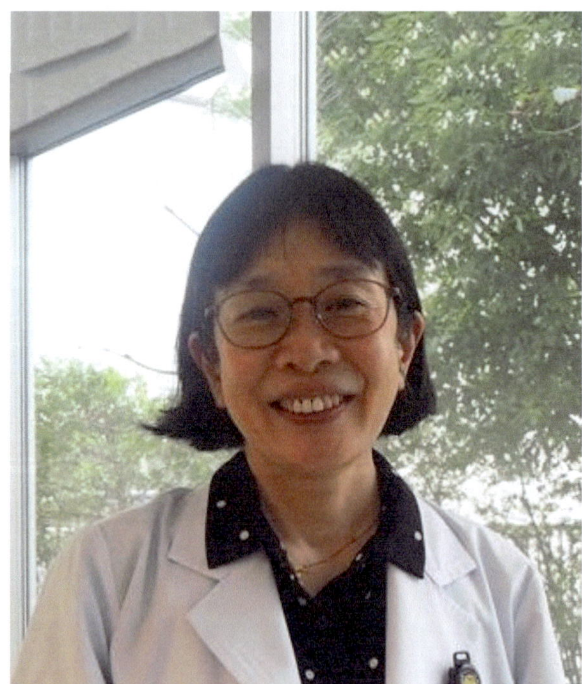

Fig. 23.6 Kumiko Ando

Women have recently represented 23–30% of presentations and lectures. Among the 75 council members, 11 are women, and of the 17 board members, 2 are women.

In 2015, Dr Yoko Kato from Fujita Health University Neurosurgery became the first female president of the JSNR Annual Meeting. In 2017, the Diversity Promotion Committee was established, with me as chair, aiming to create an inclusive environment for women and people from diverse backgrounds.

I have not felt that I have faced any discrimination as a woman when participating in academic activities at the Japanese Society of Neuroradiology or any other neuroradiology society worldwide, yet men still dominate leadership roles especially in Japan.

This is partly because household, childcare, and caregiving duties often fall on women, and support systems like babysitters are lacking in Japan. And as a result, female doctors in their 30s and 40s are often forced to interrupt their careers due to childcare responsibilities. Encouragingly, younger generations increasingly embrace shared caregiving responsibilities.

As a result, many young female neuroradiologists continue their careers even after marriage and childbirth. And more women are becoming leaders in hospitals and research institutions, contributing to clinical practice, research, and mentoring. The number of female university professors in neuroradiology is increasing.

I believe that supporting radiologists facing various challenges, regardless of gender, will contribute to the development of neuroradiology. Let each of us offer small acts of support to them!

Below, I introduce some female neuroradiologists in Japan who have been active over the past 60 years, limited to those I have interacted with. Many more are contributing significantly, including those who succeeded after studying in Japan, such as Dr Tha Khin Khin from Myanmar (Hokkaido University) and Dr Andica from Indonesia (Juntendo University).

Pioneers

Yuko Ono, MD, PhD.

Prof. Yuko Ono graduated from Tokyo Women's Medical University and later studied at the University of Mainz in Germany (Fig. 23.7). She became a professor in the Department of Radiology at Tokyo Women's Medical University and was the first female lead presenter at a JSNR meeting. She has published 142 original papers, 92 review articles, and 20 textbooks. Her research using various imaging techniques, such as angiography, CT, MRI, and MRS, has significantly contributed to understanding conditions like cerebrovascular disease, gliomas, normal pressure hydrocephalus, and multiple sclerosis.

Her notable studies include the assessment of cerebrospinal fluid flow patterns using the time-spatial labeling inversion pulse technique with 3T MRI, the usefulness of 4D-CTA in detecting cerebral dural sinus occlusion or stenosis with

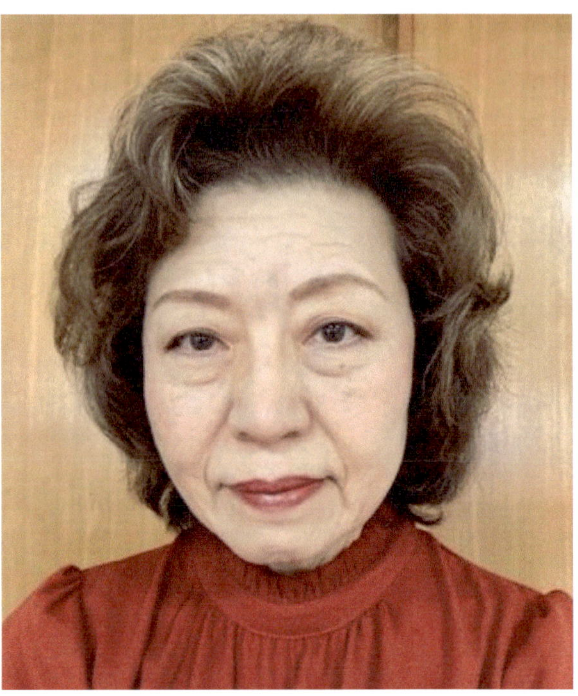

Fig. 23.7 Yuko Ono, MD, PhD

collateral pathways, and the optimal visualization of multiple brain metastases for gamma knife radiosurgery.

Here is a message from Yuko Ono:

After 2 years of training in radiation therapy, diagnostic radiology, and nuclear medicine, I began training in the Department of Neuroradiology in 1975 at the Neurological Institute in Tokyo Women's Medical University Hospitals, where there are Departments of Neurosurgery, Neurology, and Neuroradiology. At that time, brain imaging relied on skull X-rays, cerebral angiography, and pneumoencephalography. In August 1975, the Japanese first clinical CT scanner was installed at our facility. The first case involved a patient with malignant melanoma, and the CT images revealed multiple small metastases that they could not detect by previous cerebral angiography. This marked the beginning of a new era in neuroradiological diagnosis.

From then on, CT became a routine method alongside other imaging techniques. Managing each type of examination, patient care, reporting, and research presentations were simultaneously challenging but enriching. It was a great experience for me to learn many diverse and important cases in the only one Institute of Neurology in Tokyo.

During my practical studies in the Mainz University Hospital in Germany in 1982, I attended the first European MR Conference. At that time, the utility of MRI was still debated, but it soon became a crucial diagnostic tool alongside CT.

Experiencing various diagnostic techniques and studying classical methods provided a strong foundation for my career as a neuroradiologist. Although some traditional techniques, like pneumoencephalography, are no longer used, they helped me understand the modern diagnostic tools easily, considering the dynamic state of the cerebrospinal fluid or detail anatomical knowledge of the arteries and veins. I believe that this knowledge remains invaluable.

There are few independent neuroradiology departments in Japan, which was a source of pride for my mentor, Dr Kobayashi. However, due to hospital restructuring, the Department of Neuroradiology was merged into diagnostic imaging. Although the nature of the work remains the same, this change felt like a loss of identity for those of us in neuroradiology.

After retiring in 2014, I have been working at Ebina General Hospital, specializing in diagnostic neuroradiology. Remote image reading has also become possible, which I have started using as needed.

At the JRS Annual Meeting, I see the incredible advancements in imaging technology and AI, which motivate me to continue working as a neuroradiologist.

Imaging diagnosis is an excellent profession for women, as much of the work can be done remotely. However, obtaining a specialist qualification alone is not enough; continuous training is essential to take responsibility for diagnoses. In neuroradiology, trust between radiologists, neurosurgeons, and neurologists is crucial, requiring knowledge and communication skills to aid in treatment decisions.

Women often face the challenges of balancing childcare and professional duties, but being a physician also offers a stable economic foundation; therefore, it could be possible to have a maid or a sitter. I hope my experiences serve as a reference for women who wish to continue their careers in medicine and leadership.

Prof. Noriko Aida, MD, PhD.

Prof. Noriko Aida graduated from Yokohama City University in 1984, and since the 1990s, has been actively working at the Kanagawa Children's Medical Center (Fig. 23.8). As a leader in pediatric neuroradiology in Japan, she has made numerous research contributions to the field and mentored many pediatric neuroradiologists. She also served as the President of the Japanese Society of Pediatric Radiology.

Among her many published papers, the following received the Kato Award from the Japanese Society of Neuroradiology (JSNR):

Aida N, Tamagawa K, Takada K, et al. Brain MR in Fukuyama congenital muscular dystrophy. AJNR Am J Neuroradiol. 17:605–13, 1996.

She was the first female recipient of the Kato Award.

Other notable works include her research on MR imaging of perinatal brain damage, and 1H-MR Spectroscopy of the pediatric brain.

- Aida N, Nishimura G, Hachiya Y, et al. MR imaging of perinatal brain damage: Comparison of clinical outcome with initial and follow-up MR findings. AJNR Am J Neuroradiol. 19:1909–21, 1998

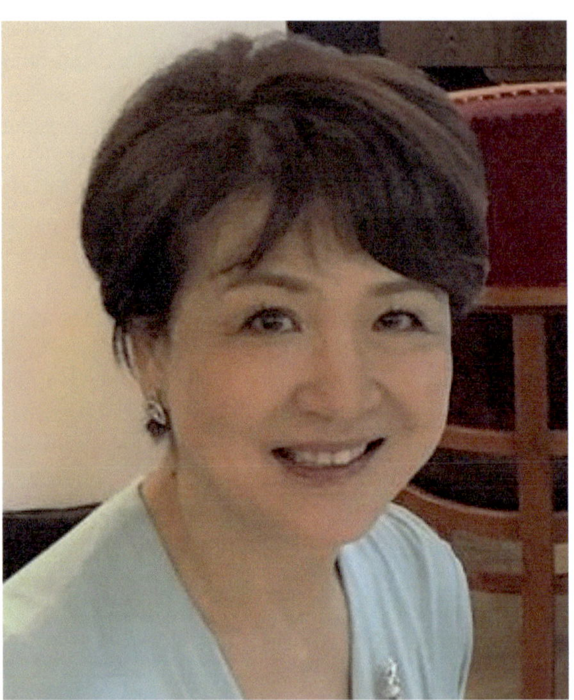

Fig. 23.8 Noriko Aida, MD, PhD

- Tomiyasu M, Aida N, Watanabe Y, et al. Monitoring the brain metabolites of children with acute encephalopathy caused by the H1N1 virus responsible for the 2009 influenza pandemic: A quantitative *in vivo* 1H MR spectroscopy study. Magn Reson Imaging. 30:1527–33, 2012.
- Aida N. ^{1}H-MR Spectroscopy of the Early Developmental Brain, Neonatal Encephalopathies, and Neurometabolic Disorders. Magn Reson Med Sci. 21:9–28, 2022.

Here is a message from Noriko Aida:

When I started working at a large children's hospital in the 1990s, I struggled because there were almost no textbooks or teachers for pediatric neuroradiology in Japan. Furthermore, pediatric neuroradiology papers were seldom presented even at neuroradiology conferences, making it almost impossible to have discussions with experts in Japan. So, I tried to present pediatric neuroradiology papers almost every year, initially at RSNA and then at ASNR. The discussions and many presentations there encouraged me to continue practicing neuroradiology at the Children's Hospital. Over time, many younger radiologists have thankfully become interested in pediatric neuroradiology, and recently there have been many pediatric neuroradiology presentations at radiology conferences in Japan.

In my 40s and 50s, I became concerned about the social weakness and small presence of the pediatric radiology field, including pediatric neuroradiology, in Japanese radiology. Therefore, I continued to work for the Japanese Pediatric

Radiology Society and the Japanese Neuroradiology Society as a board member, director, and president. Later, I became a board member of the Japanese Radiological Society and worked consistently to improve its status. Finally, I became the first woman to serve on the JRS Board of Directors and worked hard to promote diversity, including introducing a quota system for representative and director elections.

Many female neuroradiologists are now active both clinically and academically in Japan, so I am not worried about that. However, socially speaking, in terms of promotions and roles within facilities, I do not think that women radiologists and neuroradiologists have yet achieved a status commensurate with their efforts. Therefore, it is necessary for everyone to continue to cooperate and make steady efforts.

Personally, as I have reached retirement age, I have received the honor of becoming an honorary member of the Japanese Society of Neuroradiology. I would like to continue to support and encourage my dear junior colleagues by sharing my experience, even if only in a small way.

Akiyo Sadato, MD, PhD.

Professor Akiyo Sadato graduated from Kyoto University in 1986 and initially joined the Department of Neurosurgery. She furthered her training in neuroradiology at the University of Rochester and in neurosurgery at the State University of New York at Buffalo. Currently, she serves as a Professor of Neurosurgery at Fujita Health University. Her area of specialization is neuroendovascular surgery. Some of her representative papers are as follows:

- Sadato A, Hayakawa M, Adachi K, Nakahara I, Hirose Y. Large Residual Volume, Not Low Packing Density, Is the Most Influential Risk Factor for Recanalization after Coil Embolization of Cerebral Aneurysms. PLoS One. 11: e0155062, 2016.
- Sadato A, Adachi K, Hayakawa M, Kato Y, Hirose Y. Effects of anatomic characteristics of aneurysms on packing density in endovascular coil embolization: Analysis of a single center's experience. Neurosurg Rev. 39: 109–114, 2016.
- Sadato A, Wakhloo AK, Hopkins LN. Effect of low concentrated n-butyl cyanoacrylate (NBCA)-Ethiodol mixture on tissue reaction and permanency of arterial occlusion after embolization. Neurosurgery. 47: 1197–1205, 2000.
- Sadato A, Taki W, Ikada Y, Nakahara I, Matsumoto K, Tanaka M, Kikuchi H. Immediately detachable coil for aneurysm treatment. AJNR Am J Neuroradiol. 16: 1459–1462, 1995.
- Sadato A, Taki W, Ikada Y, Nakahara I, Yamashita K, Matsumoto K, Tanaka M, Kikuchi H, Doi Y, Noguchi T, Inada I. Experimental study and clinical use of poly(vinyl acetate) emulsion as liquid embolization material. Neuroradiology. 36: 634–641, 1994.

Here is a message from Professor Akio Sadato

Over the past 30 years, I have specialized in research and clinical practice in endovascular surgery. During this period, I have witnessed the remarkable advancements in the treatment of cerebrovascular disorders thanks to the development of new devices. I expect further advancements in the future. Specializing in cerebrovascular disorders often involves emergency work, which may be seen as a deterrent to some, regardless of gender. However, I hope that the participation of many young individuals will lead to further progress in this field.

Noriko Sato, MD, PhD.
Noriko Sato graduated from Gunma University in 1987. After studying at Yale University and making significant contributions at Gunma University, she became the Director of the Department of Radiology at the National Center of Neurology and Psychiatry (NCNP) in Japan (Fig. 23.9). She has greatly contributed to mentoring her juniors, providing guidance not only to radiologists but also to many young doctors in psychiatry, pediatrics, neurology, and neurosurgery.

She has published 234 papers and authored 10 books. Her awards are too numerous to mention, but in 2021, she received the Top Cited Article 2020–2021 award from the Journal of Neuroimaging.

Her notable studies include:

- Iijima K, Fujii H, Suzuki F, et al., and Sato N. Genotype-relevant neuroimaging features in low-grade epilepsy-associated tumors. Front Neurol. 15:1419104, 2024.
- Nakaya M, Sato N, Matsuda H, et al. Free water derived by multi-shell diffusion MRI reflects tau/neuroinflammatory pathology in Alzheimer's disease. Alzheimers Dement (N Y). 8(1), 2022.

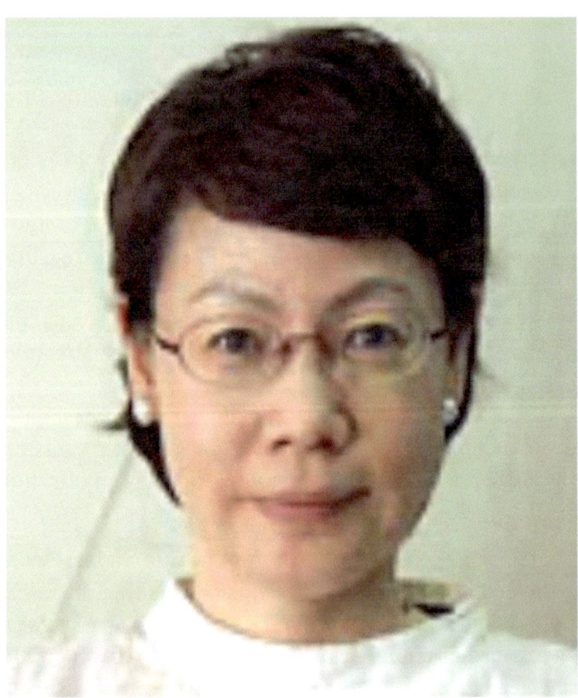

Fig. 23.9 Noriko Sato, MD, PhD.

- Hirasawa-Inoue A, Sato N, Shigemoto Y, et al. New MRI findings in Fukuyama congenital muscular dystrophy: Brain stem and venous system anomalies. AJNR Am J Neuroradiol. 41(6):1094–1098, 2020.
- Sato N, Ota M, Yagishita A, et al. Aberrant midsagittal fiber tracts in patients with hemimegalencephaly. AJNR Am J Neuroradiol. 29(4):823–7, 2008.
- Sato N, Ishizaka H, Yagi H, et al. Posterior lobe of the pituitary in diabetes insipidus: dynamic MR imaging. Radiology. 186:357–60, 1993.

Here is a message from Noriko Sato:

I have supervised the doctoral theses of 14 students so far. Additionally, regardless of their degree status, I have provided guidance on research and papers to many young doctors in radiology, psychiatry, pediatrics, neurology, and neurosurgery. Working with young doctors from various fields has been enjoyable, as I have learned a lot from them as well. I am also grateful that Japanese neuroradiologists maintain good relationships across institutions, and I am glad I chose this specialty. I hope to see further dynamism among young doctors.

I would like to continue to provide education, conduct research, and supervise papers, as I have done so far. I believe that gender does not influence one's ability to excel in the fields of diagnosis and research, and therefore, anyone can succeed in every aspect of this field regardless of gender.

Aya Tokumaru, MD, PhD.

Aya Tokumaru graduated from the Medical College of Mie University in 1985 (Fig. 23.10). After studying under Dr A. James Barkovich at the San Francisco Medical Center of the University of California, she became the Director of Diagnostic Radiology at the Metropolitan Medical Center of Gerontology in 2005. She has published 67 papers, particularly on imaging diagnostics of dementia, focusing on the correlation between brain pathology.

Here is a message from Aya Tokumaru

Personal Statement

- I strive to be a well-rounded physician, aiming for excellence in the "three-legged stool" of clinical service, education, and research. I believe that a doctor must use pioneering research and observation, built on a foundation of best-practice clinical patient interaction, to impart a vision to all stakeholders. To this end, I have endeavored to build consultative clinical credibility, leading to research, then education and administration.

I have the expertise, leadership, training, expertise, and motivation necessary to successfully carry out the proposed research project. I have a broad background in diagnostic radiology with specific training and expertise in neuroradiology. I have pursued the significance of clinic-radio-pathological correlationship especially in neurodegenerative diseases. In this unprecedented aging society, appropriate medical interventions are crucial for the diagnosis of neurodegenerative disease that may cause dementia, disturbance of active daily life, the disease course, which extends over several decades, and there is now an urgent need for countermeasures. Our team have contributed to clarify specific pathophysiologi-

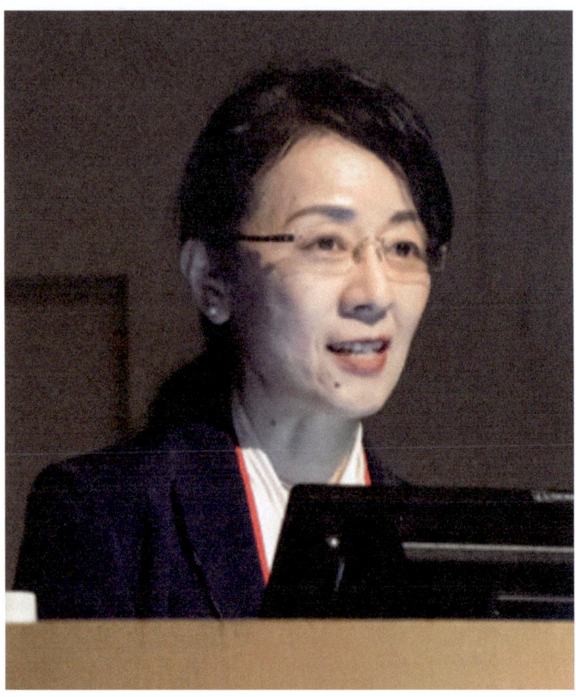

Fig. 23.10 Aya Tokumaru, MD, PhD.

cal processes of neurodegenerative diseases (argyrophillic grain disease, corticobasal degeneration syndrome, progressive supranuclear palsy, etc.) by analyzing the high-resolution volumetric MRI correlating with neuropathology.

In addition, I successfully administered the projects collaborated with other researchers, and produced several peer-reviewed publications from each project. As a result of these previous experiences, I am aware of the importance of frequent communication among project members and of constructing a realistic research plan, timeline, and budget.

Contribution to Science

- My early publications directly addressed the significance of clinico-radiogico-pathological correlations of central nervous system (CNS) diseases especially in neurodegenerative disorders. In actual medical practice, an incorrect judgment may be made if making a diagnosis is prioritized. It is very difficult to assume the background pathology in a very early stage of neurodegenerative disease in many cases. From the background pathology of serial biopsy specimens from 1212 patients with degenerative dementia, we have analyzed the correlation of clinic-radio-pathological correlationships. The prevalence of Alzheimer's disease (AD) was high when the concomitant pathologies of dementia with grains (DG), neurofibrillary tangle disease (NFTD), progressive supranuclear palsy

(PSP), and corticobasal degeneration (CBD) were included. Senile tauopathy reached 33% in the group with CDR > 0.1 and 57% in the group with CDR = 0.5. To succeed in clinical trials in the treatment strategy of neurodegenerative disease, it is necessary to obtain images consistent with the background pathology. By providing evidence and creating more accurate clinical diagnostic criteria of CB D and PSP, we would play an important role of this body of works.

Selected publications

- Sakurai K, Tokumaru AM, Aiba I, et al. Conventional magnetic resonance imaging key features for distinguishing pathologically confirmed corticobasal degeneration from its mimics: A retrospective analysis of the J-VAC study. Neuroradiology. 66: 123–30, 2024.
- Tokumaru AM, Saito Y, Murayama S. Diffusion-weighted imaging is key to diagnosing specific disease. Magn Reson Imaging Clin N Am. 29: 163–83, 2021.
- Tokumaru AM, Saito Y, Murayama S, et al. Imaging-pathologic correlation in corticobasal degeneration. AJNR Am J Neuroradiol. 30: 1884–92, 2009.
- Tokumaru AM, et al. Optic tract hyperintensity on T2-weighted images among patients with pituitary macroadenoma: Correlation with visual impairment. AJNR Am J Neuroradiol. 27: 250–54, 2006.
- Tokumaru AM, et al. Prominent meningeal enhancement adjacent to meningioma on Gd-DTPA enhanced images: Histopathologic comparison. Radiology. 175: 431–33, 1990.

Keiko Toyoda, MD, PhD.

Keiko Toyoda graduated from The Jikei University School of Medicine in 1986 and joined the Department of Radiology at the same university (Fig. 23.11). The Jikei University School of Medicine has produced many head and neck radiologists. In 1997, she studied abroad at the Service Hospitalier Frédéric Joliot (SHFJ), Commissariat à l'énergie atomique (CEA) in France. Since then, she has been active as a head and neck radiologist and is currently a Professor in the Department of Radiology at The Jikei University School of Medicine.

She is a leader among Japanese head and neck radiologists, having published more than 20 papers and contributed to 14 textbooks. Some of her representative works include:

- Toyoda K, Ida M, Fukuda, K. Fluid-attenuated inversion recovery intraarterial signal: an early sign of hyperacute cerebral ischemia. AJNR Am J Neuroradiol. 22: 1021–9, 2001.
- Toyoda K, Kitai S, Ida M, et al. "Usefulness of high-b-value diffusion-weighted imaging in acute cerebral infarction. Eur Radiol. 17:1212–20, 2007.
- Toyoda K, Oba H, Kutomi K, et al: "MR Imaging of IgG4-Related Disease in the Head and Neck and Brain. AJNR Am J Neuroradiol.33: 2136–2139, 2012.

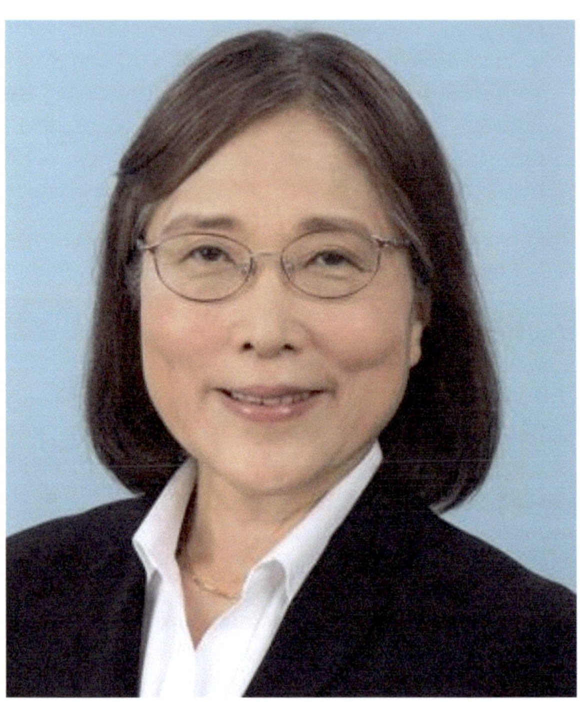

Fig. 23.11 Keiko Toyoda, MD, PhD.

Her book, "MARUWAKARI: Diagnostic Imaging of the Head and Neck Region" (Shujun Sha, Tokyo, JPN p.895), published in 2015, is considered a bible for head and neck radiologists in Japan, known as "Pink Book" (Fig. 23.12).

Here is a message from Dr Keiko Toyoda:

I have been blessed with many teachers, seniors, peers, and juniors, and I am grateful for these connections. Throughout my career, I have been deeply involved in diagnostic imaging, like a craftsman, teaching, and being taught. I have faced many challenges, but I have come this far thanks to these mentors and the support of others. During the most intensive period of my career, I often lost track of time while interpreting images, and soon, doctors from other departments began to support and encourage me.

Moreover, I was fortunate to have colleagues not only within my institution but also outside of it, which enabled me to create the "MARUWAKARI" textbook. I believe the most important thing is having such long-standing friends and colleagues who share the same passion.

Looking ahead, I hope to pass on to future generations the joy of neuroradiology and head and neck radiology and to ensure that valuable cases are properly documented.

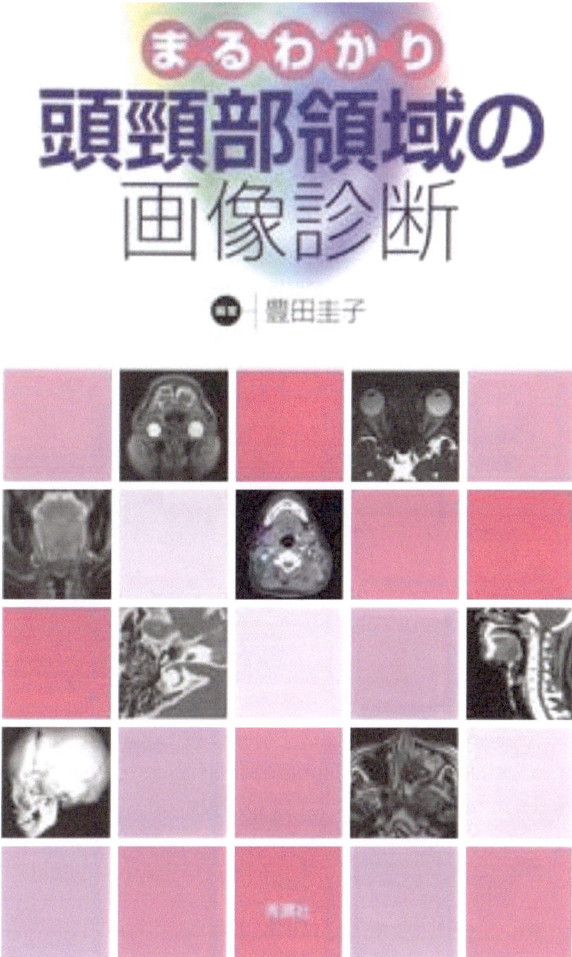

Fig. 23.12 MARUWAKARI: Diagnostic Imaging of the Head and Neck Region

Noriko Kurihara, MD, PhD.
Dr Noriko Kurihara graduated from Tohoku University in 1988 (Fig. 23.13). She has worked in National Hospital Organization Sendai Medical Center about 30 years and has educated many residents and interns on emergency cases that are rarely seen in university hospitals.

The Tohoku region of Japan has a high prevalence of cerebrovascular diseases, and she has primarily published papers on imaging diagnostics of cerebrovascular diseases. Here are some of her representative papers:

Here is the formatted version:

– Kurihara N, et al. Hemorrhage owing to cerebral cavernous malformation: imaging, clinical and histopathological considerations. JJR. 38: 613–621, 2020.

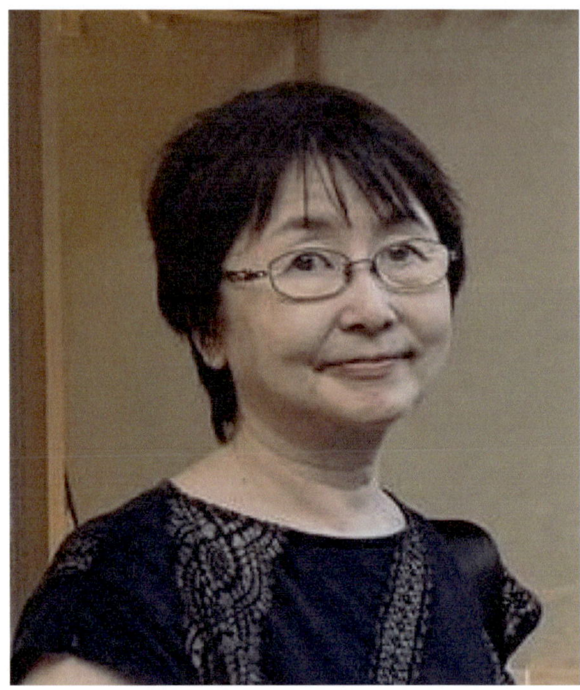

Fig. 23.13 Noriko Kurihara, MD, PhD.

- Kurihara N, et al. Edema in the retropharyngeal space associated with head and neck tumors: CT imaging characteristics. Neuroradiology. 47: 609–615, 2005.
- Tamura H, Kurihara N, et al. How does water diffusion in human white matter change following ischemic stroke? Magn Reson Med Sci. 8: 121–34, 2009.
- Kurihara N, et al. Investigation of hydrocephalus with three-dimensional constructive interference in steady state MRI. Neuroradiology. 42: 634–638, 2000.
- Kurihara N, et al. Hemorrhage in pituitary adenoma: correlation of MR imaging with operative findings. Eur Radiol. 8: 971–976, 1998.
- Kurihara N, et al. Evaluation of large intracranial aneurysm with three-dimensional MRI. J Comput Assist Tomogr. 19: 707–712, 1995.

Here is a message from Noriko Kurihara:

I have spent most of my career in community hospitals and have no particularly notable achievements. However, I feel truly fortunate to have encountered neuroradiology. I did not have a female role model nearby, and I navigated my career path by trial and error. However, because neuroradiology is a relatively narrow field, by persistently participating in regular conferences and study groups, I was able to meet many respected female doctors and envision the direction I wanted to take and my future.

Balancing work with raising children has been the most challenging part of my career. When my children were young, it was physically exhausting, and during their teenage years, it was mentally draining. Still, I believe that having my work allowed me to reset my mind and spirit, which helped me get through those tough times.

I believe that imaging diagnostics suits women who are detail-oriented and persistent. As I am nearing retirement, I want to support and nurture young doctors. Although it is not my strong suit, I have become a delegate this year to help connect with the next generation.

Salamon Noriko, MD, PhD.

Professor Noriko Salamon is currently a Professor of Radiology and the Section Chief of Neuroradiology at UCLA. She has published 290 papers in neuroradiology and has hosted many students from Japan. Many of these students have gone on to successful careers in Japan and abroad. In recognition of her contributions, the Japanese Society of Neuroradiology awarded her honorary membership in 2024.

Some of her representative papers are:

- *DTI of tuber and perituberal tissue can predict epileptogenicity in tuberous sclerosis complex*. Neurology. 85: 2011–5, 2015.
- *The clinicopathologic spectrum of focal cortical dysplasias: A consensus classification proposed by an ad hoc Task Force of the ILAE Diagnostic Methods Commission*. Epilepsia. 52: 158–74, 2011.
- *FDG-PET/MRI coregistration improves detection of cortical dysplasia in patients with epilepsy*. Neurology. 71: 1594–601, 2008.
- *Contralateral hemimegalencephaly and Clinical-Pathological Correlations in Children with hemimegalencephaly*. Brain. 129: 352–65, 2006.

Here is a message from Noriko Salamon:

My name is Noriko Salamon. I am a neuroradiologist born in Japan and now practicing in the US. During medical school, I was drawn to psychiatry and neuroscience. Around the time of my graduation, MRI technology was advancing significantly in imaging diagnosis, especially in neuroradiology. This led me to pursue training in Diagnostic Radiology, which I found to be the most appealing. It is worth noting that, as a woman in Japan, entering radiology was initially challenging due to the “allergy to Radiation” mentality influenced by Japan’s history with the atomic bomb. I was inspired by my mentor, Dr Munechika, who trained at Yale in the 1970s and supported me in becoming a diagnostic radiologist. I started as a body interventional radiologist, but my passion for the neuro field led me to neurointerventional radiology. I was fortunate to receive a French government scholarship to train in France, which was a life-changing experience and solidified my dedication to neuroradiology.

There was no equivalent exam to transfer a Japanese medical license to the French system in the 1990s, so I decided to move to the United States in 1995 with my husband, Georges Salamon. I completed another Radiology Residency at Northwestern University, Chicago, and became a faculty member at UCLA in 2003. I am now in my 21st year at UCLA, serving as a Professor of Radiology and Section Chief of Neuroradiology.

For the past 21 years, I have been dedicated to teaching and mentoring in neuroradiology. I devote 2 hours daily to teaching students, residents, and fellows, alongside reviewing cases. My primary research focus is epilepsy, and I have published over 250 peer-reviewed papers. I have also co-investigated five NIH-funded grants and published an epilepsy imaging atlas in 2023. I have received the UCLA Leo Rigler Outstanding Teaching Award seven times and was the first recipient of the Women in Neuroradiology Leadership Award in 2012. In 2024, the Japanese Society of Neuroradiology awarded me honorary membership.

I have developed a research program for radiologists, neurosurgeons, and neurologists from other countries, assisting in career development and serving as a research advisor. Since 2012, I have hosted 20 Japanese doctors (7 women) and published over 50 papers with them. I have also hosted 19 researchers (10 women) from countries including France, Portugal, Germany, Sweden, Russia, Hungary, Korea, Thailand, China, Iran, and India since 2005.

Working with researchers worldwide, I discovered that international collaboration is incredibly valuable. It helps us expand our ideas and maintain a scientifically open-minded approach. I aim to further pursue and promote this concept. This requires solid infrastructure, team effort, departmental support, clinical and research collaboration, and a reliable track record. Becoming a successful woman in any field continues to be challenging. I am committed to helping more women in neuroradiology gain international recognition and become leaders in the field.

Chihiro Takahashi, MD, PhD.
Dr Chihiro Takahashi graduated from Hokkaido University in 1989. After initially training in neurology, she became a radiologist. Following her time at the University of Rochester in the United States, she has been serving as the Chief of the Department of Radiology at Hakodate Central General Hospital since 2003. Despite being the sole neuroradiologist in a vast area, she manages a demanding workload while also presenting at national and international conferences. Every summer, she organizes the Neuroradiology Workshop in Hakodate, which gathers doctors from all over Japan. She is also known as a runner who always participates in early morning runs at conferences.

Representative Papers

- Kanayama M, Togawa D, Takahashi C, et al. Cross-sectional magnetic resonance imaging study of lumbar disc degeneration in 200 healthy individuals. J Neurosurg Spine. 11: 501–7, 2009.
- Ashton EA, Takahashi C, Berg MJ, Goodman A, Totterman S, Ekholm S. Accuracy and reproducibility of manual and semiautomated quantification of MS lesions by MRI. J Magn Reson Imaging. 17: 300–8, 2003.
- Terae S, Takahashi C, Abe S, et al. Gd-DTPA-enhanced MR imaging of injured spinal cord. Clin Imaging. 21: 82–9, 1997.
- Takahashi C and Miyasaka K. Intradural ventral nerve root enhancement in diseases of conus medullaris. Neuroradiology. 37, 1995.

Here is a message from Chihiro Takahashi:

I am the only neuroradiologist in the vast southern Hokkaido region, and I often feel anxious about daily practice. Over the past 20 years, I have not been able to take long vacations.

I hope to strengthen the imaging interpretation system in regional cities by increasing the number of full-time radiologists and enhancing the remote imaging interpretation and consultation systems.

Mika Kitajima, MD, PhD.

Dr Mika Kitajima graduated from Oita Medical University in 1990 and joined the Department of Radiology at Kumamoto University (Fig. 23.14). After studying at the University of California, San Francisco, and Massachusetts General Hospital in 2002, she became a professor in the Department of Diagnostic Imaging Technology, Faculty of Life Sciences, Kumamoto University, in 2020. Her main interest lies in advanced MR imaging of the brain, particularly in optic structures such as the lateral geniculate body and optic radiation. She has authored 99 original research papers and published over 30 review articles and book chapters. Some of her representative papers include:

- Kitajima M, Hirai T, Yoneda T, et al. Visualization of the medial and lateral geniculate nucleus on phase difference enhanced imaging. *Am J Neuroradiol.* 36:1669–74, 2015.
- Kitajima M, Korogi Y, Kakeda S, et al. Human subthalamic nucleus: Evaluation with high-resolution MR imaging at 3.0 T. *Neuroradiology*. 50:675–81, 2008.

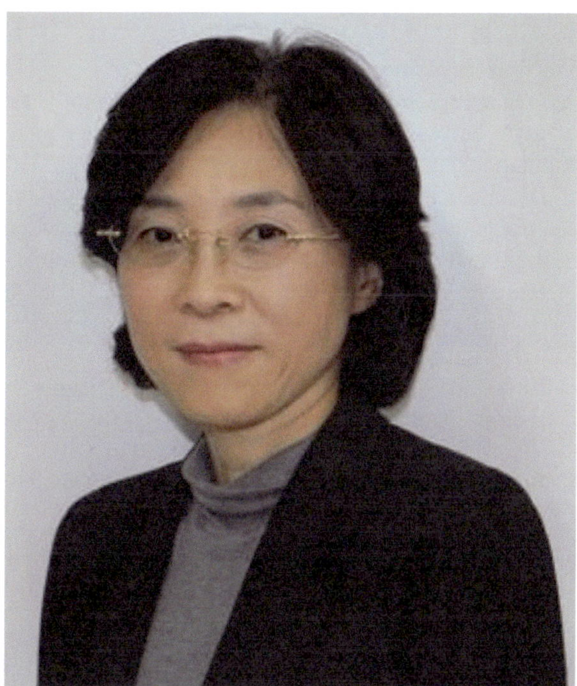

Fig. 23.14 Mika Kitajima, MD, PhD.

- Kitajima M, Korogi Y, Shigematsu Y, et al. Central nervous system lesions in adult T-cell leukemia: MRI and pathology. *Neuroradiology*. 44:559–67, 2002.
- Kitajima M, Korogi Y, Takahashi M, Eto K. MR signal intensity of the optic radiation. *Am J Neuroradiol*. 17:1379–83, 1996.
- Kitajima M, Korogi Y, Shimomura O, et al. Hypertrophic olivary degeneration: MR imaging and pathologic findings. *Radiology*. 192:539–43, 1994.

Here is a message from Dr Mika Kitajima:

What I consider fortunate is that I have met good supervisors and mentors, not just in neuroradiology. Having the chance to study abroad, even for a short time, was a valuable experience. For several years now, I have been teaching in the School of Health Sciences (training radiological technologists), which allows me more flexibility to allocate my work hours, unlike my full-time hospital work. I appreciate this flexibility, and it might benefit clinical doctors if they could work this way, though it seems challenging under current conditions.

My current situation may not serve as a reference for young doctors specializing in neuroradiology. My current important task is to train the students to become radiological technologists, so my goal is to provide quality education to students and cultivate their ability to think independently. Additionally, it would be great if they develop an academic interest in radiology and a research mindset.

I do not believe there is a specific role for women simply because they are women. Ideally, both men and women would share life and work equally. Some tasks might generally suit women better, but I believe that every individual has unique strengths. It would be beneficial to have a society (and workplace) where people can develop those strengths. As a supervisor or teacher, I think it is important to find the strengths of young doctors and students and help them grow.

Yoshiko Hayashida MD, PhD.

Associate Professor Yoshiko Hayashida is currently an Associate Professor of radiology in university of occupational and environmental health. She graduated from Kumamoto University in 1994.

Despite being a neuroradiologist in Kumamoto University, her current teaching and research needs have led her to undertake a wide range of research in areas such as the spinal cord, bone and soft tissue and abdominal areas, using her knowledge of neuroradiology.

Representative Papers

- Hayashida Y, Kakeda S, Korogi Y, et al. Diagnosis of intracranial hemorrhagic lesions: Comparison between 3D-SWAN (3D T2*-weighted imaging with multi-echo acquisition) and 2D-T2*-weighted imaging. Acta Radiol. 55: 201–7, 2014.
- Hayashida Y, Hirai T, Yamashita Y, et al. Diffusion-weighted imaging of metastatic brain tumors: Comparison with histologic type and tumor cellularity. Am J Neuroradiol. 27: 1419–25, 2006.
- Hayashida Y, Hirai T, Korogi Y, et al. Usefulness of measurement of the temporal stem on magnetic resonance imaging in the diagnosis of frontotemporal dementia. Acta Radiol. 47: 603–8, 2006.

- Hayashida Y, Hirai T, Yamashita Y, et al. Positional lumbar imaging using a positional device in a horizontally open-configuration MR unit – initial experience. J Magn Reson Imaging. 26: 525–8, 2007.

Here is a message from Yoshiko Hayashida. First of all, I would like to thank my seniors who have guided and mentored me to this point and who have left behind many great achievements. I would also like to thank my good colleagues who have made it possible for me to enjoy my work in radiology every day.

Recently, I have started to supervise young doctors in surgery, cardiology, and urology, as well as in radiology, which has given me a lot of stimulation in my daily life. Thanks to these young doctors, I am able to update myself. In the future, I would like to tell young doctors how interesting the fields of radiology and neuroradiology are. To this end, (although it is sometimes difficult), I would like to show younger colleagues that research is fun by showing them how I myself enjoy research.

Promising Talents

Miho Gomyo, MD, PhD
After graduating from Kyorin University School of Medicine in 2003, Dr Miho Gomyo is currently a senior lecturer in the Department of Radiology, Kyorin University Faculty of Medicine. She has presented research on cerebrovascular imaging using ultra-high-resolution CT and arterial spin labeling-based MRDSA, vessel wall imaging and MR bone imaging and has received cum laude awards at ECR, RSNA, and International Recognition Award at ASNR. Some of her representative papers are listed below:

- Gomyo M, Tsuchiya K, Yokoyama K. Vessel Wall Imaging of Intracranial Arteries: Fundamentals and Clinical Application. Magn Reson Med Sci. 22: 447–458, 2023.
- Takahashi S, Gomyo M, Tsuchiya K, Yoshioka T, Kobayashi K, Nakanishi A, Yokoyama K. Anatomical information of the lenticulostriate arteries on high-resolution 3D-TOF MRA at 3 T: Comparison with 3D-DSA. Surgical Radiol Anat. 45: 1287–1293, 2023.
- Gomyo M, Tsuchiya K, Goto S, Hosoi S, Tahara T, Yokoyama K. Usefulness of black-blood magnetic resonance angiography generated from vessel wall imaging after the stent-assisted treatment of intracranial arterial diseases. Neuroradiol J. 35: 36–41, 2022.

Here is a message from *Miho Gomyo*:

The most significant aspect of my career as a radiologist has been the diverse experiences I gained under excellent mentors. From my first year, I had the opportunity to engage in research and present at conferences under the supervision of Professor Kazuhiro Tsuchiya. I was also fortunate to interact with distinguished neuroradiologists from Japan and abroad, gaining invaluable experience.

When I attended a workshop where experts presented challenging neuroradiology cases, I was struck by the complexity and depth of the discussions. Even now, I am impressed by the high standards of this workshop. After my supervisor left Kyorin University, I felt an immense void but worked to fill it by validating new technology and developing scanning methods useful in clinical practice. This made me aware of my knowledge gaps, providing a valuable opportunity to study more.

With advancements in technology enabling high-speed scanning for CT and MRI, the number of examinations has increased. Balancing the improvement of diagnostic skills and research activities while managing daily tasks remains a major challenge.

With the development of high-speed imaging technology for MRI, scans can be performed in an extremely short time. This will allow for less painful examinations for patients who cannot maintain their posture for long periods after surgery or due to bone metastases. However, it is important to optimize conditions to ensure no information is lost due to high-speed scanning and to explore imaging parameters that are clinically useful.

Since photon-counting CT and radiogenomics face challenges related to post-processing time and case accumulation in single institutions, expanding collaborative research both domestically and internationally could provide significant benefits. I am eager to participate in such research if given the opportunity.

Furthermore, improving the mentoring system for junior radiologists is crucial, just as I was mentored. Securing human resources is essential to balance clinical practice, education, and research. I hope that diverse work systems, such as remote image reading and online mentoring, will be established.

Shiori Amemiya, MD, PhD.

Shiori Amemiya graduated from the University of Tokyo in 2004, where she later obtained her PhD in Radiology and Biomedical Engineering (Fig. 23.15). She is currently an Associate Professor in the Department of Radiology at the Graduate School of Medicine, University of Tokyo. Specializing in fMRI methodology and MRI (neuroradiology), she has been the principal investigator for 13 public grants, author for 70 papers, and has received numerous awards both domestically and internationally. Some of her representative papers are listed below.

- Amemiya S, Takao H, Watanabe Y, Miyawaki S, Koizumi S, Saito N, Abe O. Reliability and sensitivity to altered hemodynamics measured with resting-state fMRI metrics: Comparison with (123)I-IMP SPECT. Neuroimage. 2022;263:119654.
- Amemiya S, Takao H, Abe O. Origin of the Time Lag Phenomenon and the Global Signal in Resting-State fMRI. Front Neurosci. 14:596084, 2020.
- Amemiya S, Takao H, Abe O. Global vs Network-Specific Regulations as the Source of Intrinsic Coactivations in Resting-State Networks. Front Syst Neurosci. 13:65, 2019.

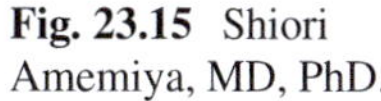

Fig. 23.15 Shiori Amemiya, MD, PhD.

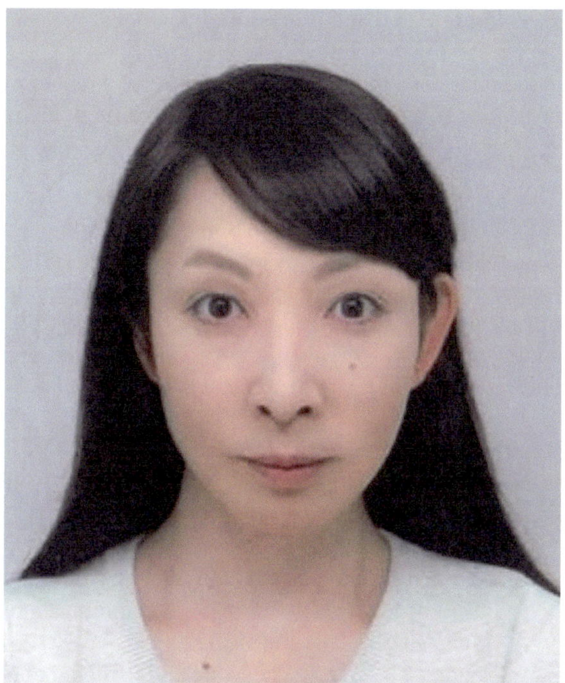

- Amemiya S, Takao H, Hanaoka S, Ohtomo K. Global and structured waves of rs-fMRI signal identified as putative propagation of spontaneous neural activity. Neuroimage. 133:331–40, 2016.
- Amemiya S, Kunimatsu A, Saito N, Ohtomo K. Cerebral hemodynamic impairment: assessment with resting-state functional MR imaging. Radiology. 270:548–55, 2014.

Here is a message from Shiori Amemiya

Despite its prominence in cognitive neuroscience, fMRI's clinical utility still needs to be improved. My initial studies on patients with hemodynamic impairment highlighted discrepancies between neural activity and expected fMRI signals. This led to a focus on understanding the relationship between hemodynamic status and the blood oxygen level-dependent (BOLD) fMRI signal. I found that the time lag of the BOLD signal accurately reflects hemodynamic status throughout the brain in health and disease. Additionally, I have shown the time lag of the physiological noise, which causes systemic fluctuations in the BOLD signal is closely and fundamentally associated with the organization of the functional resting-state networks. I have been studying the causes of these phenomena, which are necessary for enabling spatiotemporal analysis of spontaneous neural activity.

I am dedicated to furthering the development and clinical application of functional brain imaging techniques. Fortunately, I have never felt hindered in my career due to my gender. However, I am well aware of the underrepresentation of women in STEM research and professorial positions. I am deeply grateful for the efforts of the pioneering women who paved the way for us, as well as for the supportive colleagues and mentors I have encountered. I am determined to contribute to expanding opportunities for future generations through my research and teaching.

Mikako Enokizono, MD, PhD.
Mikako Enokizono graduated from Nagasaki University School of Medicine in 2004 (Fig. 23.16). She then trained at various institutions in Japan, including Nagasaki University, the Kanagawa Children's Medical Center, and the National Center of Neurology and Psychiatry, to study pediatric neuroradiology under various mentors. She is considered one of the most trusted pediatric neuroradiologists among the younger generation of radiologists in Japan. She is actively engaged in clinical practice, research, and education.

Representative Papers

- Enokizono M, Kurokawa R, Yagishita A, et al. Clinical and neuroimaging review of monogenic cerebral small vessel disease from the prenatal to adolescent developmental stage. Jpn J Radiol. 42: 109–125, 2024.
- Enokizono M, Aida N, Yagishita A, et al. Neuroimaging findings of inborn errors of metabolism: Urea cycle disorders, aminoacidopathies, and organic acidopathies. Jpn J Radiol. 41: 683–702, 2023.
- Enokizono M, Sato N, Ota M, et al. Disrupted cortico-ponto-cerebellar pathway in patients with hemimegalencephaly. Brain Dev. 41: 507–515, 2019.

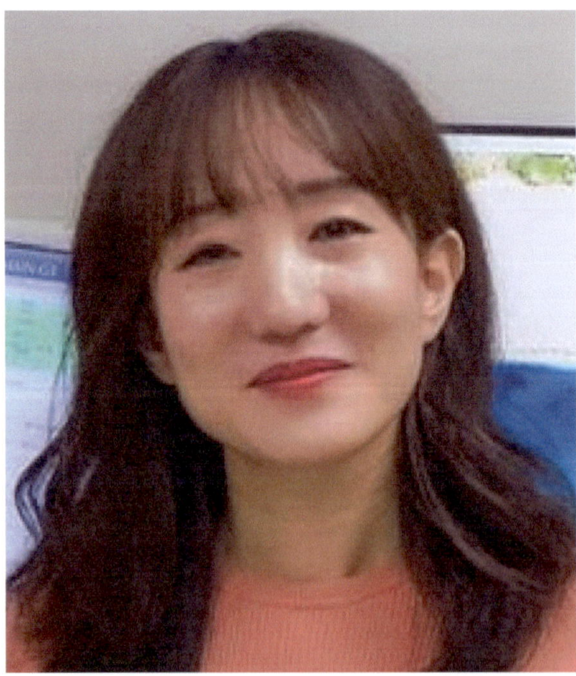

Fig. 23.16 Mikako Enokizono, MD, PhD.

Here is a message from Mikako Enokizono:

I have built an 18-year career as a radiologist. Important turning points include choosing neuroradiology as my specialty during my time as a graduate student at Nagasaki University's Department of Radiology, studying under Dr Noriko Aida, a leading expert in pediatric neuroradiology at the Kanagawa Children's Medical Center, and currently working at the Tokyo Metropolitan Children's Medical Center, specializing in pediatric imaging diagnostics.

At the university hospital, I engaged in imaging diagnostics and research, especially in neuroradiology, learning extensively from my mentors and earning my diagnostic radiology certification. Although I felt somewhat confident in interpreting adult imaging, my transition to a children's hospital brought new challenges as I encountered pediatric diseases and imaging characteristics I had never seen before. Witnessing the expertise of pediatric radiologists like Dr Noriko Aida was enlightening. This experience deepened my interest in pediatric imaging, and I have continued to pursue this field by reading research papers and understanding developmental and pathological contexts.

Currently, I work at a children's hospital where I am fortunate to have a collaborative environment. Pediatricians, surgeons, and neurosurgeons are approachable and trust my imaging reports. I have also broadened my network by participating in joint conferences with neuroradiologists and pediatric neurologists.

One of the challenges in pediatric radiology is its niche nature, requiring specialized knowledge and experience, which can deter many from entering the field. Increasing interest and attracting more specialists to pediatric radiology and pediatric neuroradiology is an urgent need.

My future goals are to further enhance my expertise in pediatric neuroradiology and to mentor the next generation. There have been remarkable advances in diagnostic techniques for genetic disorders, leading to a better understanding of previously unexplained conditions and developing new treatments. I aim to compile and share insights about imaging findings of newly diagnosed genetic disorders and their correlation with treatment effects. I also plan to actively share knowledge through national and international conferences and publications to advance this field.

As for the role of women, I have worked similarly with my male colleagues, so I have no specific stance on this topic. However, I believe some women may feel disadvantaged because they have focused on household duties or childcare. Radiology offers flexible working conditions and remote diagnostic systems, creating a favorable environment for career continuity. Such an environment benefits both men and women, enabling them to maximize their potential and contribute to the future of medicine.

Emiko Morimoto, MD, PhD

After graduating as MD from Osaka University and getting PhD from Kyoto University Graduate School of Medicine, Dr Emiko Morimoto worked at the David Geffen School of Medicine at UCLA, National Center of Neurology and Psychiatry, Chiba University, and Osaka Metropolitan University. She is currently at Osaka City General Hospital, specializing in diagnostic imaging of epilepsy (Fig. 23.17).

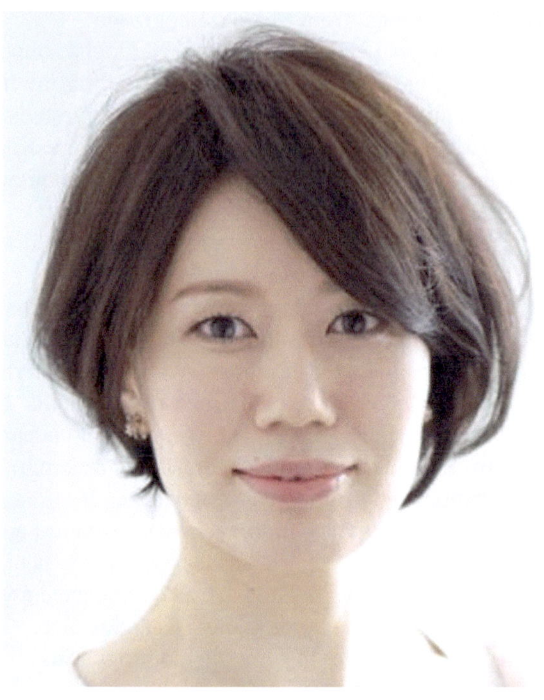

Fig. 23.17 Emiko Morimoto, MD, PhD

She has received research grants from the Japan Society for the Promotion of Science (JSPS) for her work in this field.

Representative Papers

- Yokota H, Uetani H, Tatekawa H, Morimoto E, et al. Focal cortical dysplasia imaging discrepancies between MRI and FDG-PET: Unique association with temporal lobe location. *Seizure.* 81: 180–185, 2020.
- Mori-Yoshimura M, Mizuno Y, Yoshida S, Morimoto E, et al. Psychiatric and neurodevelopmental aspects of Becker muscular dystrophy. *Neuromuscul Disord.* 29(12): 930–939, 2019.
- Chien A, Xu M, Yokota H, Morimoto E, et al. Nonsphericity Index and Size Ratio Identify Morphologic Differences between Growing and Stable Aneurysms in a Longitudinal Study of 93 Cases. *AJNR Am J Neuroradiol.* 39(3): 500–506, 2018.
- Morimoto E, Kanagaki M, Okada T, et al. Anterior temporal lobe white matter abnormal signal (ATLAS) as an indicator of seizure focus laterality in temporal lobe epilepsy: comparison of double inversion recovery, FLAIR and T2W MR imaging. *Eur Radiol.* 23(1): 3–11, 2013.
- Morimoto E, et al. Evaluation of focus laterality in temporal lobe epilepsy: A quantitative study comparing double inversion-recovery MR imaging at 3T with FDG-PET. *Epilepsia.* 54(12): 2174–83, 2013.

Here is a message from Emiko Morimoto

Neuroradiology can be daunting for general radiologists, and the imaging diagnosis of refractory epilepsy is particularly challenging, even for specialists.

Epilepsy is one of the most prevalent intractable diseases, affects 0.5–1% of the population, with about one-third considered for surgery. However, there is still a lack of epilepsy specialists and facilities that can provide appropriate treatment, including surgery, for intractable epilepsy in Japan. Many clinicians are hesitant to pursue a specialized role in managing refractory epilepsy due to its high level of specialization. Additionally, despite the essential role of imaging for epilepsy surgery, there are very few trained neuroradiologists to perform presurgical evaluations for refractory epilepsy. Imaging peculiarities of epilepsy, such as unreproducibility of nuclear medicine results due to fluctuations in epileptic hyperactivity of the brain, makes it difficult for radiologists to understand the diagnostic imaging in epilepsy. Identifying an epileptogenic lesion by combining multiple imaging is highly time-consuming, making it difficult to incorporate into the regular workload of radiologists who are already handling a large volume of tasks. Currently, diagnostic imaging for refractory epilepsy relies heavily on the voluntary efforts of a small number of neuroradiologists who have a specific interest in epilepsy. How to increase support in this area is a key challenge for radiology and the medical field moving forward.

Epileptologists hope more neuroradiologists will take an interest in epilepsy, but the situation is challenging. Increasing education and understanding about diagnostic imaging of refractory epilepsy is necessary to attract more neuroradiologists. Improved reimbursement and support systems are also needed. My goal is to continue working to provide better preoperative diagnoses for more refractory epilepsy patients and to increase radiology's role in epilepsy care.

Junko Kikuta, MD, PhD

After graduating from Saitama Medical University in 2005 and subsequently working at Nippon Medical School, Junko Kikuta is currently an Assistant Professor in the Department of Radiology at Juntendo University (Fig. 23.18). She also serves as a councilor for the Japanese Society of Magnetic Resonance in Medicine and the Japanese Society of Neuroradiology, where she is particularly dedicated to bridging the gender gap. She is a mother of two and has successfully balanced her professional and personal life.

She has published numerous papers using advanced MRI techniques, such as DWI and diffusion tensor imaging, and has received awards at both domestic and international conferences, including the AOCR. Some of her recent papers are as follows:

- Hara S, Kikuta J, Takabayashi K, et al. Decreased diffusivity along the perivascular space and cerebral hemodynamic disturbance in adult moyamoya disease. *Journal of Cerebral Blood Flow & Metabolism*. 2024. Online ahead of print.
- Kikuta J, Kamagata K, Abe M, et al. Effects of arterial stiffness on cerebral WM integrity in older adults: A neurite orientation dispersion and density imaging

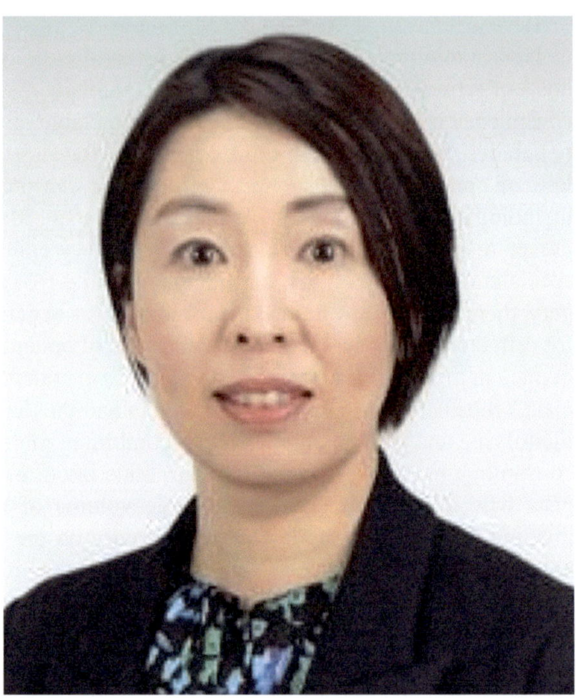

Fig. 23.18 Junko Kikuta, MD, PhD

and magnetization transfer saturation imaging study. *American Journal of Neuroradiology*. 2022; 43(12): 1706.

- Kikuta J, Kamagata K, Taoka T, et al. Water diffusivity changes along the perivascular space after lumboperitoneal shunt surgery in idiopathic normal pressure hydrocephalus. *Front Neurol*. 2022; 13: 843883.
- Kikuta J, Kamagata K, Takabayashi K, et al. An investigation of water diffusivity changes along the perivascular space in elderly subjects with hypertension. *American Journal of Neuroradiology*. 2022; 43(1): 48.
- Wada A, Shizukuishi T, Kikuta J, et al. Altered structural connectivity of pain-related brain network in burning mouth syndrome—investigation by graph analysis of probabilistic tractography. *Neuroradiology*. 2017; 59(5): 525–532.

Here is a message from Junko Kikuta:

One of the most notable experiences in my career was participating in the Japanese Society of Neuroradiology, where I had the opportunity to meet many specialists in the field. Neuroradiology imaging diagnosis can be quite challenging, but seeing doctors who are passionate about discussing imaging, almost as if it were a hobby, left a strong impression on me. As AI in imaging diagnostics becomes more prevalent, I realize that radiologists mastering their sub-specialties and accumulating valuable experience is a significant strength and a source of fulfillment. During my doctoral studies, I learned about brain image analysis, which allows for evaluating morphological and functional changes in the brain associated with various diseases. This is an area I find highly intriguing.

I aim to continue refining my skills as a radiologist to provide imaging diagnoses that contribute to clinical diagnosis and treatment. I also plan to pursue research in neuroradiology and aim to present at conferences and publish papers. In Japan, only about 20% of physicians are women, and their representation in hospitals, academic societies, and other organizations remains low, making it difficult for their opinions to be reflected. While work styles for physicians have diversified significantly since my early years in child-rearing, many still find it challenging to continue their careers due to childcare or caregiving responsibilities. I believe it is important to collectively consider what measures and systems would allow them to maintain their careers and thrive in their roles.

Maki Umino, MD, PhD.
After graduating from Mie University School of Medicine in 2006, Maki Umino joined the Department of Radiology, where she has consistently published research papers in the field of neuroradiology. Her research is notable for its meticulous approach to each case, carefully identifying new imaging findings that are immediately useful for clinical practice. She is also a mother of two and has experienced the challenges of returning to work after maternity leave. Despite these challenges, she has published 27 original research papers and has been actively involved in mentoring junior colleagues.

Her representative papers are listed below. Amazingly, the first one was finalized right after the birth of her second child, with the newborn being cared for at the nurse station while she worked on the final draft:

- Umino M, Maeda M, Kogue R, et al. Evaluation of cortical superficial siderosis in patients with cognitive dysfunction using 3D FLAIR and 3D DIR. Eur Radiol. 31: 6411–6418, 2021.
- Umino M, Maeda M, Ii Y, Tomimoto H, et al. 3D double inversion recovery MR imaging: Clinical applications and usefulness in a wide spectrum of central nervous system diseases. J Neuroradiol. 46: 107–116, 2019.
- Umino M, Maeda M, Ii Y, et al. Low-signal-intensity rim on susceptibility-weighted imaging is not a specific finding to progressive multifocal leukoencephalopathy. J Neurol Sci. 362: 155–159, 2016.
- Umino M, Maeda M, Matsushima N, et al. High-signal-intensity abnormalities evaluated by 3D fluid-attenuated inversion recovery imaging within the drainage territory of developmental venous anomalies identified by susceptibility-weighted imaging at 3 T. Jpn J Radiol. 32: 397–404, 2014.

Here is a message from Maki Umino:

Participating in international and domestic conferences has been very inspiring and has allowed me to exchange ideas with doctors from other institutions, providing valuable insights beyond my own institution. Seeing the success of my peers, especially those of my generation, has been a great source of encouragement and has motivated me to keep striving in my work.

After returning from maternity leave, it was difficult to resume research activities due to the gap created during my absence.

To continue engaging in neuroradiology in some capacity.

Even if women temporarily step away from their careers for maternity leave, childcare leave, or fertility treatments, it is important to stay connected with the field, even if only through online study sessions. If possible, occasionally attending in-person meetings can be stimulating. By doing so, I aim to stay up-to-date with neuroradiology practices and avoid being left behind.

Minako Azuma, MD, PhD

After graduating from Kagoshima University School of Medicine in 2008, Dr Minako Azuma trained as a radiologist at Kumamoto University, where there were many great neuroradiologists, including Prof. Mutsumasa Takahashi, who hosted SNR XV (1994). She is currently Professor and Chairman of the Department of Radiology, Faculty of Medicine, Miyazaki University. She is also a board member of the Japan Radiological Society (JRS) and the Japanese Society for Magnetic Resonance in Medicine (JSMRM), and a council member of the Japanese Society of Neuroradiology (JSNR). She will serve as Program Chair for SNR XXIV (2030) in Sapporo, Japan.

She has published papers using advanced MRI techniques such as QSM and 3DFLAIR.

Her representative papers are listed below:

- Azuma M, et al. Characterization of carotid plaque components by quantitative susceptibility mapping. AJNR Am J Neuroradiol. 41: 310–317, 2020.
- Azuma M, et al. Usefulness of contrast-enhanced 3D-FLAIR MR imaging for differentiating Rathke cleft cyst from cystic craniopharyngioma. AJNR Am J Neuroradiol. 41: 106–110, 2020.
- Azuma M, et al. Lateral asymmetry and spatial difference of iron deposition in the substantia nigra of patients with Parkinson disease measured with quantitative susceptibility mapping. AJNR Am J Neuroradiol. 37: 782–8, 2016.

Here is a message from Minako Azuma:

I was a student in the science department of Kyushu University studying marine biology before entering medical school. My background was unusual compared to other Japanese doctors, and I thought it might be difficult to get an academic position because of my age.

However, my mentors gave me many opportunities, and I gained experience in presenting at conferences and writing papers. I became more confident and eager to advance my career.

Although I was privileged to be trained as a neuroradiologist, not every young radiologist can be in such a desirable environment. After the COVID-19 pandemic, we had access to web meetings/conferences where we could easily connect with specialists around the world. These systems can be invaluable in providing young physicians with opportunities to engage in a wide range of academic activities and to connect with potential mentors.

One of my missions is to send a message to the community that anyone can be a successful radiologist and scientist. I believe that SNR XXIV will be an important opportunity for us to expand the capacity of this movement. I would like to create more opportunities for young Japanese neuroradiologists to present their work at international meetings and nurture the young leaders to become bright stars of the future.

Shoko Hara, MD, PhD.
Dr Shoko Hara graduated from the Faculty of Medicine at Tokyo Medical and Dental University (TMDU) in April 2010 and joined the Department of Neurosurgery at the same university (which has been renamed the Institute of Science Tokyo as of October 2024) (Fig. 23.19). She is responsible for the clinical management and research of all patients with moyamoya disease at her institute and has published numerous papers in the field of Neuroradiology. Alongside her husband working a full-time job, she is raising two school-age children and has busy life. Dr Hara currently serves as a Junior Associate Professor in her institute, a member of the ISMRM Annual Meeting Program Committee, a board member of the Japanese Society for Magnetic Resonance in Medicine, and a councilor of the Japanese Society of Neuroradiology.

Her representative papers are listed below:

- Hara S, Kikuta J, Takabayashi K, et al. Decreased diffusivity along the perivascular space and cerebral hemodynamic disturbance in adult moyamoya disease. J Cereb Blood Flow Metab. 2024. Online ahead of print.

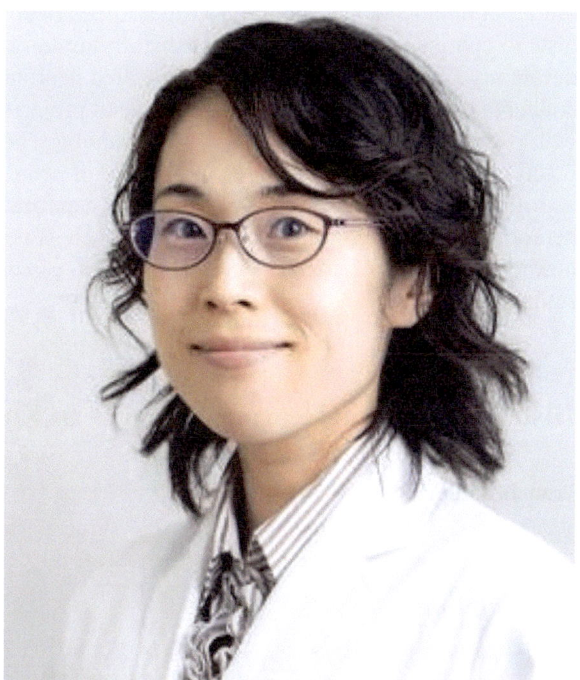

Fig. 23.19 Shoko Hara, MD, PhD.

- Hara S, Hori M, Murata S, et al. Microstructural damage in normal-appearing brain parenchyma and neurocognitive dysfunction in adult moyamoya disease. Stroke. 49: 2504–2507, 2019.
- Hara S, Tanaka Y, Ueda Y, et al. Noninvasive evaluation of CBF and perfusion delay of moyamoya disease using arterial spin-labeling MRI with multiple post-labeling delays: comparison with 15O-gas PET and DSC-MRI. AJNR Am J Neuroradiol. 38: 696–702, 2017.

Here is a message from Dr Shoko Hara:

As a young neurosurgeon, I began my research on ASL-MRI in moyamoya disease. I was captivated by the beautiful images and the academic, open atmosphere of the Japanese Society of Neuroradiology and AOCNR. Since then, I have conducted various studies on MR perfusion, diffusion MRI of brain microstructures, and nuclear medicine studies (^{123}I-IMP-SPECT and ^{15}O-PET) in cerebrovascular diseases such as moyamoya disease.

After becoming pregnant early in my career, I was unable to work overtime for several years. Neuroradiology research allows me to perform data analysis at home, making it easier to balance research with childcare. These accomplishments led to my current position, despite having fewer night shifts, less overtime and less surgical experience compared to my male peers for more than 10 years due to pregnancy, childbirth, and childcare.

My clinical and administrative duties have increased every year, leaving me with little time for the neuroradiology research that I truly love. To balance my responsibilities at home and in the hospital, I feel I need to collaborate with neuroradiologists to continue my research, rather than trying to do everything myself as I did during my PhD. I am fortunate to have skilled neuroradiologists with whom I can collaborate, and I am currently running several projects.

I love continuing my research in neuroradiology because it can benefit clinical practice in patient care. Compared to my field of neurosurgery, many women serve as role models in various workplaces within neuroradiology. I hope that women neuroradiologists will influence other fields such as neurosurgery and demonstrate how to achieve a work-life balance, advance their careers, and lead fulfilling professional lives.

History of Women Neuroradiologists In Korea

Won-Jin Moon

Introduction

The Korean Society of Neuroradiology (KSNR), founded in 1980 as a platform for discussing clinical problems and advancing research in neuroradiology, initially saw limited participation from female physicians. In the early 1990s, women accounted for only 2 out of less than 30 neuroradiologists in Korea. However, the landscape has transformed dramatically over the past few decades. By 2020, the proportion of female neuroradiologists had surged to an impressive 57%.

This remarkable increase in female representation is not just about numbers. Women in neuroradiology have consistently demonstrated exceptional expertise across various subspecialties (brain imaging, head and neck imaging, and neurointervention), contributing tremendously to the field's advancement. Today, they are actively engaged in research, clinical practice, and even hospital administration, playing a pivotal role in shaping the future of neuroradiology in Korea.

This chapter explores the evolving role of women in the KSNR, highlighting their invaluable contributions, the challenges they have overcome, and the future prospects with the coming generation of young women neuroradiologists.

Gradual Change

Until the early 1990s, most female neuroradiologists in South Korea specialized in breast, chest, or abdominal imaging. The field of neuroradiology itself—along with related specialties like neurosurgery, neurology, or otolaryngology—is male-dominated in academia and professional societies. In the early 1990s, two female radiologists, *Dr Hye Young Choi* of Ewha Woman's University Hospital and *Dr Eun Kyung Yun* of Kangbuk Samsung Hospital, joined the Korean Society of Neuroradiology (KSNR). Dr Eun Kyung Yun focused on head and neck imaging. Although Dr Hye Young Choi initially participated in the neuroradiology society, she later shifted her professional focus to breast imaging.

Around 2000, several young female radiologists began neuroradiology fellowship training at major academic hospitals, beginning to contribute to the diversity of KSNR.

In 2005, *Dr Hyun-Sook Kim* of Eulji Hospital became the first female to join the KSNR executive board as a chair of the public communication committee, marking the beginning of female leadership within the society.

The ninth executive board of the KSNR, led by Dr Sang Joon Kim from Asan Medical Center, marked a significant shift in 2011 by appointing four female neuroradiologists. *Dr So Lyung Jung* (Yeouido St Mary's Hospital), *Dr Won-Jin Moon* (Konkuk University Medical Center), *Dr Jeong Hyun Lee* (Asan Medical Center), and Dr *Young Hen Lee* (Korea University Ansan Hospital) joined the 14-member executive board. Since then, the participation of female neuroradiologists on the board has steadily increased, and currently, approximately 40% (10 out of 24) of the executive board members are women.

Furthermore, at the end of 2020, two out of the four research study groups within the KSNR were led by women (*Dr Won-Jin Moon* for Aging and NeuroDegeneration Imaging (ANDI) Study Group and *Dr Sun Won Park* [SNU-SMG Boramae Medical Center] for Head and Neck Radiology Study Group), demonstrating the remarkable participation in terms of society leadership and achievements of female neuroradiologists in academic research. These then-young female neuroradiologists played a crucial role in publishing a multicenter study on the diagnosis of thyroid cancer in the head and neck [1].

Current Leaders

While the primary focus of female neuroradiologists was mainly in the head and neck area, especially in the early 2000s, more recently, a growing number of women are advancing into other neuroimaging subspecialties such as dementia and brain tumors. Notably, the following individuals have demonstrated exceptional academic achievements and leadership, significantly contributing to the advancement of KSNR.

Dr So Lyung Jung of Yeouido St Mary's Hospital is a distinguished head and neck imaging research scholar and an enthusiastic educator. She expanded her research to include thyroid imaging, where her work analyzing the safety and efficacy of radiofrequency ablation for benign thyroid nodules earned her the Korean Journal of Radiology (KJR) Most Cited Article Award [2] (Fig. 23.20). She served as the chair of the scientific committee of KSNR and is currently the president of the Korean Society of Thyroid Radiology (which branched out from KSNR), where she continues to make significant contributions and dedicate herself to mentoring future generations of radiologists.

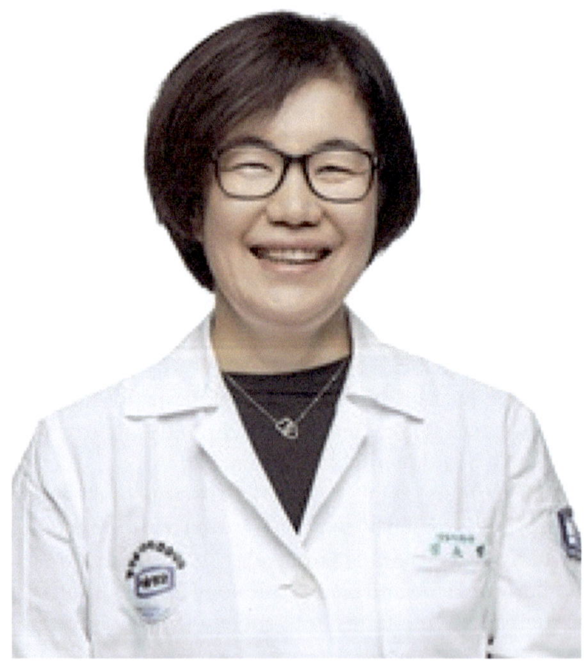

Fig. 23.20 Dr So Lyung Jung

Dr Won-Jin Moon of Konkuk University Medical Center is recognized for her outstanding research achievements in neurodegenerative disease, particularly Alzheimer's disease, as evidenced by the National Research and Development Top 100 Excellence Award [3–7] (Fig. 23.21). She has served as the chair of the scientific committee of KSNR and is currently chair of the international liaison committee, focusing on collaborations with international societies. She is a former section editor for neuroradiology for the KJR and currently serves as a deputy editor for the Journal of Magnetic Resonance Imaging (JMRI).

Dr Jeong Hyun Lee of Asan Medical Center is leading Korea's largest head and neck imaging fellowship program. She has contributed significantly to advancing the field through her research and education in head and neck cancer imaging [8] (Fig. 23.22). Currently, she serves as the president of the Head and Neck Radiology Study Group and is the section editor for head and neck imaging for KJR.

In addition, *Dr Young Hen Lee* of Korea University Ansan Hospital, who previously served as the treasurer of KSNR and is currently serving as the chair of the health policy/practice committee of KSNR, is dedicated to academic research in head and neck and thyroid imaging (Fig. 23.23). *Dr Jinna Kim* of Severance Hospital has also published numerous impactful papers in head and neck imaging [9–11] (Fig. 23.24). She previously served as the treasurer of KSNR and currently holds director at Large of KSNR.

While not as prominent in KSNR leadership roles as some colleagues, four women neuroradiologists deserve recognition for their significant contributions.

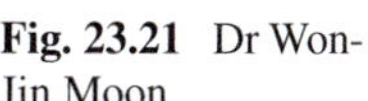
Fig. 23.21 Dr Won-Jin Moon

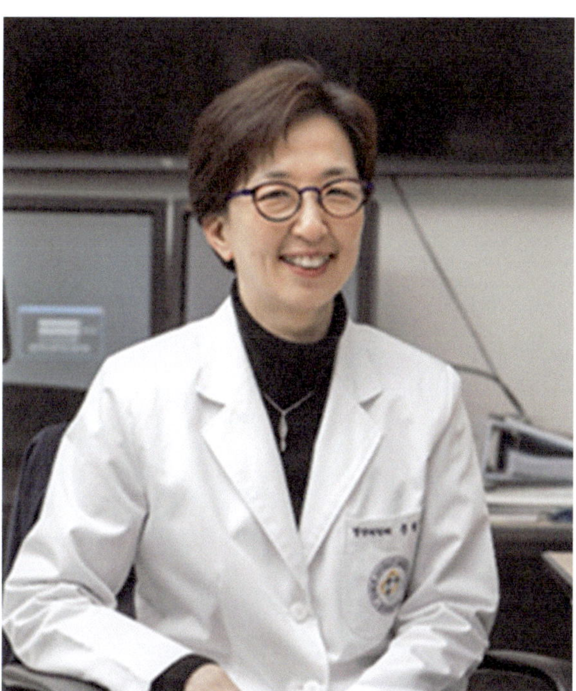

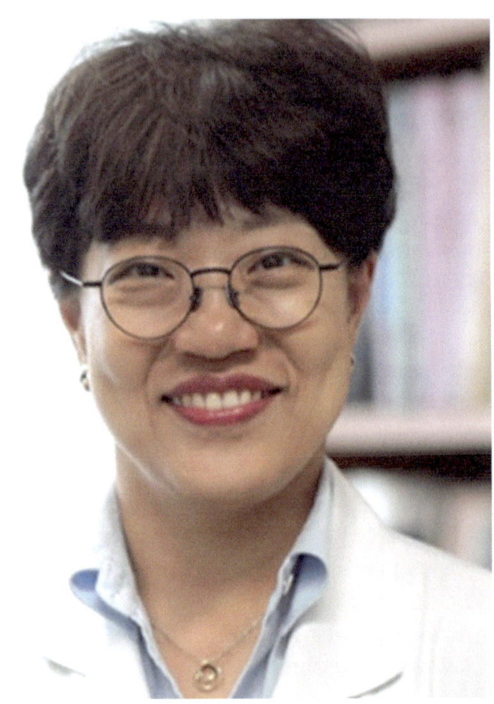

Fig. 23.22 Jeong Hyun Lee

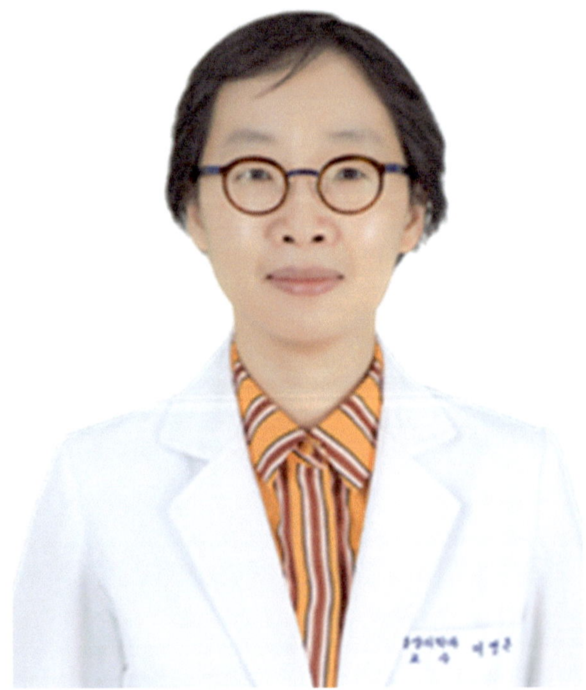

Fig. 23.23 Young Hen Lee

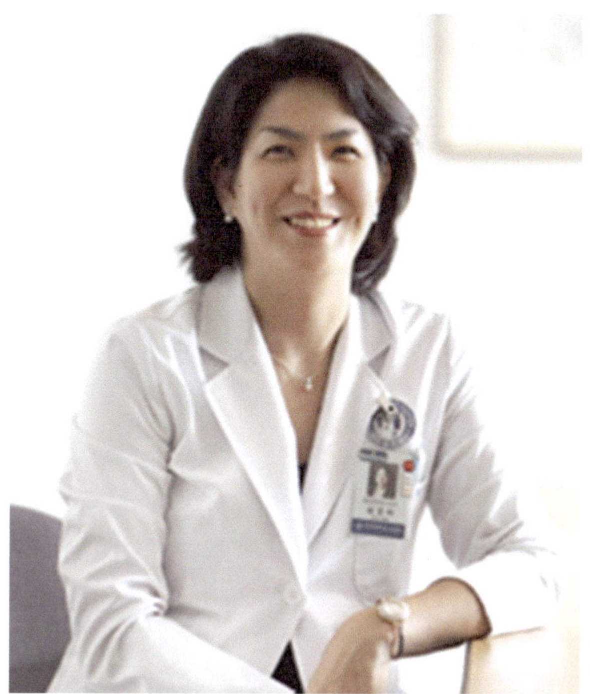

Fig. 23.24 Dr Jinna Kim

Dr Sun Won Park of SNU-SMG Boramae Medical Center is a leading head and neck neuroradiologist (Fig. 23.25). She is a past president of the Head & Neck Radiology Study Group, notably serving as the first woman to hold that position. *Dr Soo Mee Lim*, a skilled neuro-interventional radiologist and hospital administrator at Ewha Womans University Seoul Hospital, served as KSNR Secretary General for 1 year before stepping down to become the hospital director (Fig. 23.26). *Dr Hyun Jung Kim* of Daejeon St. Mary Hospital, who has expertise in stroke intervention, has published impactful papers on acute stroke collateral imaging [12] (Fig. 23.27). Drs. Lim and Kim are rare examples of female neuroradiologists who have transitioned into the neurointervention field. Additionally, *Dr Eun Ja Lee* of Dongguk University Ilsan Hospital is a dedicated educator and the chief neuroradiologist (Fig. 23.28).

Bright Futures

Currently, neuroradiologists in their 30s and 40s actively contribute to the field with outstanding research achievements, serving as editorial board members or higher for renowned international journals and participating as key members in international conferences. The following individuals have demonstrated exceptional academic achievements while exhibiting leadership within KSNR. They are poised to become future leaders of our society.

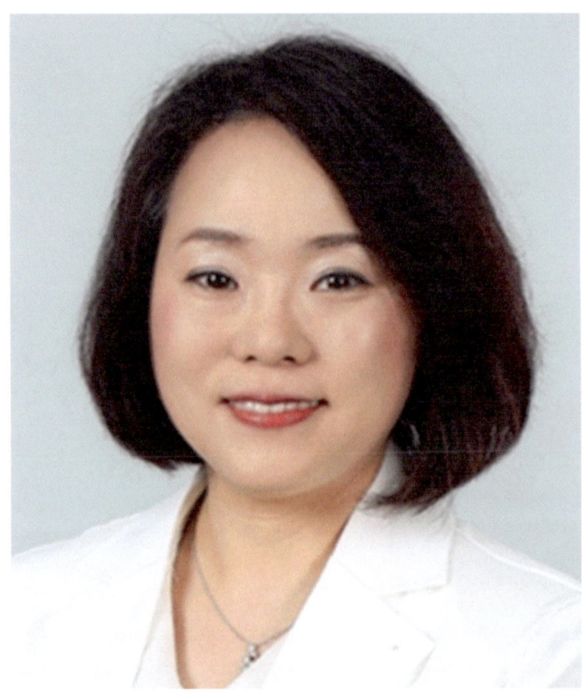

Fig. 23.25 Sun Won

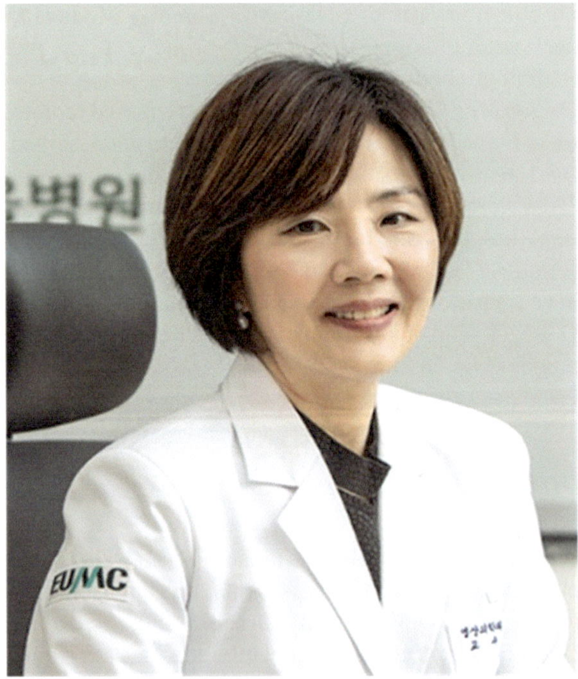

Fig. 23.26 Dr Soo Mee Lim

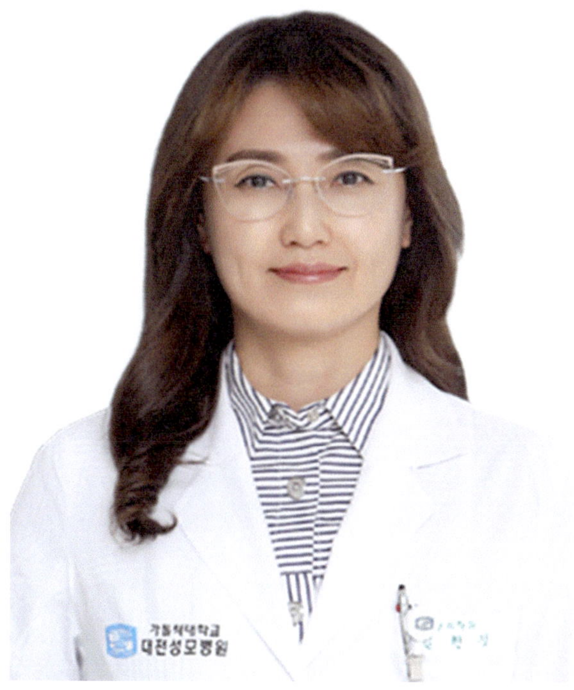

Fig. 23.27 Dr Hyun Jung Kim

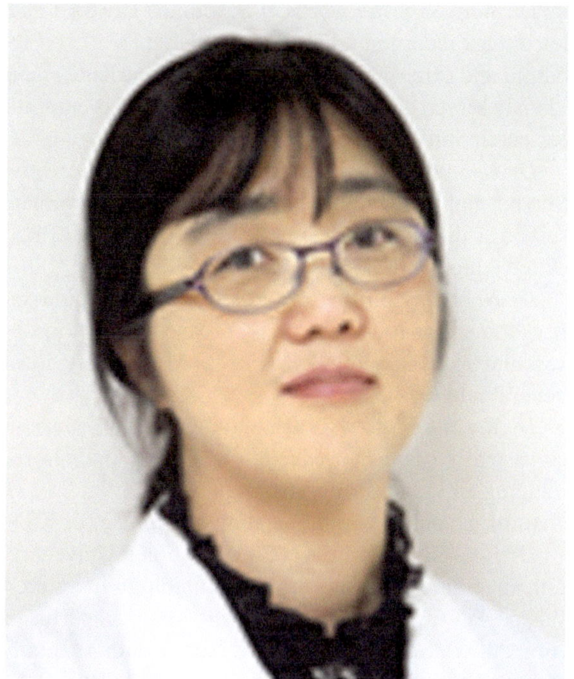

Fig. 23.28 Dr Eun Ja Lee

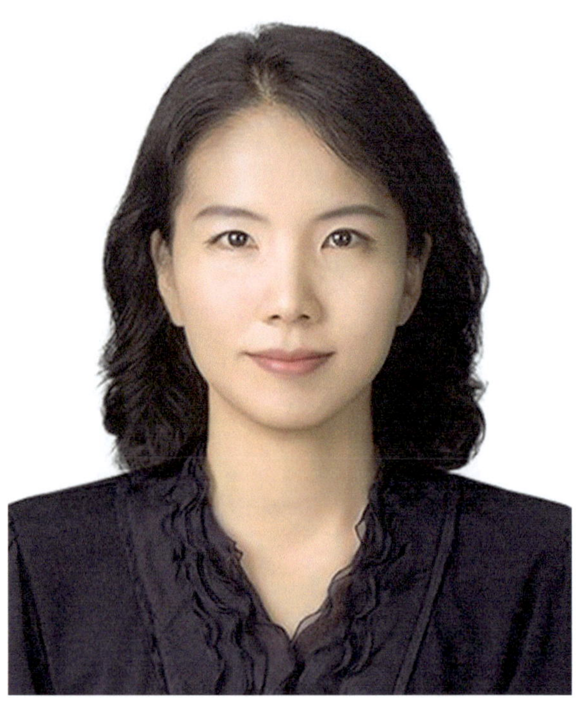

Fig. 23.29 Dr Sung Soo Ahn

Dr Sung Soo Ahn works at Severance Hospital and has established an unparalleled track record in brain tumor research [13–15] (Fig. 23.29). Her robust research output and extensive research network contribute significantly to the field. She previously served as the treasurer of KSNR and is currently leading the Brain Function Research Study Group under KSNR.

Dr Koung Mi Kang works at Seoul National University Hospital (Fig. 23.30). She has published high-quality research in neuroimaging [16–20]. She previously served as the chair of the publication committee of KSNR and is currently an associated editor of the British Journal of Radiology.

Dr Na-Young Shin works at Severance Hospital and has produced high-quality research publications, primarily focused on Parkinson's disease imaging and perivascular space imaging [21] (Fig. 23.31). She previously served as the secretary for general affairs of KSNR.

Dr Yun Jung Bae works at Seoul National University Bundang Hospital and has consistently published excellent research findings related to Parkinson's disease imaging and glymphatic imaging [22–24] (Fig. 23.32). She currently serves as the chair of the public communication committee for KSNR.

Dr Roh-Eul Yoo works at Seoul National University Hospital. She has made significant contributions to the neuroradiology literature with publications in various subspecialties, including glymphatic MRI and perfusion-weighted imaging [25–28] (Fig. 23.33). She is currently a Deputy Editor of European Radiology and serves as the chair of the education committee of KSNR.

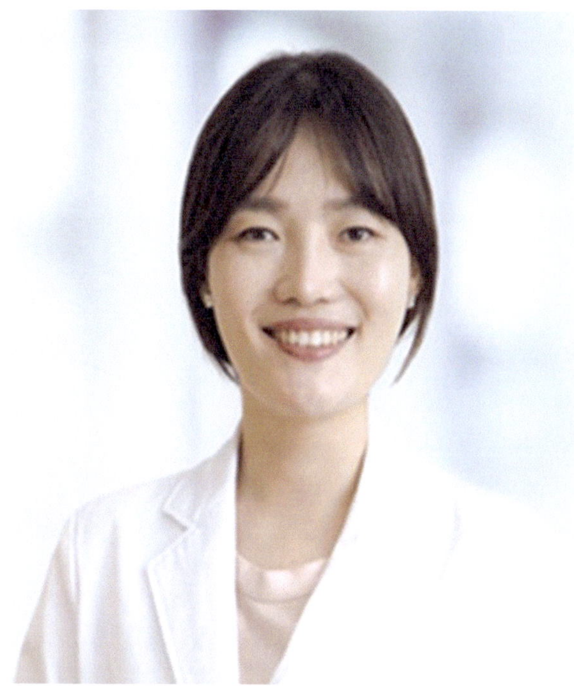

Fig. 23.30 Dr Kyoung Mi Kang

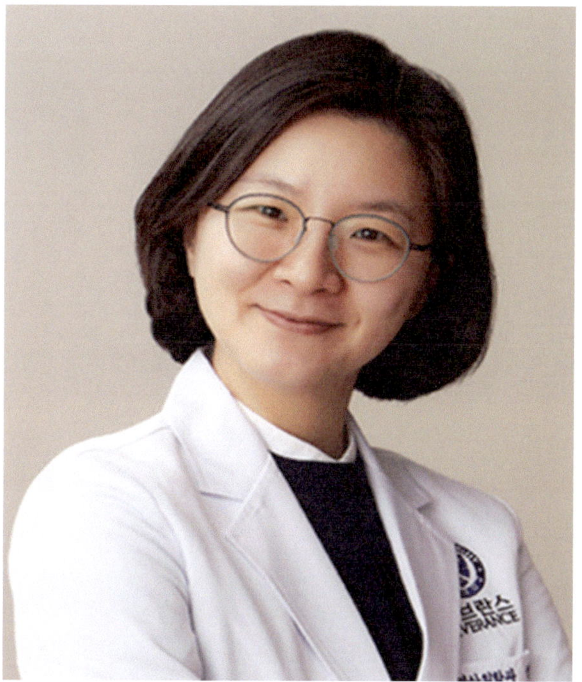

Fig. 23.31 Na-Young Shin

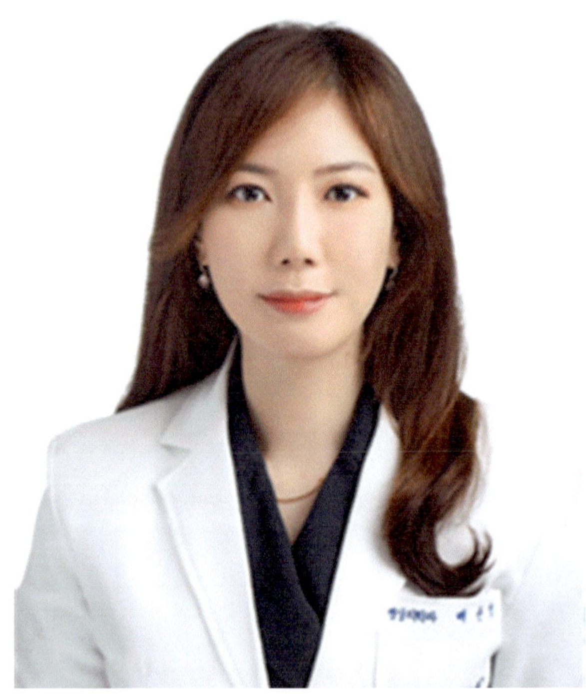

Fig. 23.32 Dr Yun Jung Bae

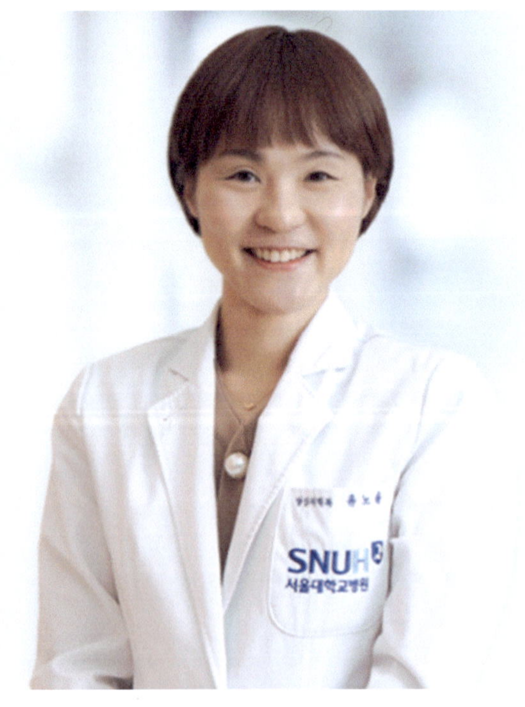

Fig. 23.33 Dr Roh-Eul Yoo

Dr Ji Eun Park works at Asan Medical Center in Seoul and has built an unrivaled research portfolio in brain tumors and artificial intelligence [29–33] (Fig. 23.34). Her exceptional interpersonal skills have made significant contributions to international collaborative networks. She is the deputy editor for neuro-oncology for JMRI and formerly served as the secretary of the research committee for KSNR and the secretary of the scientific program committee for the Korean Congress of Radiology.

Dr Mina Park works at Gangnam Severance Hospital and has conducted important research, mainly on dementia imaging and meningeal lymphatic imaging [34, 35] (Fig. 23.35). She serves on the Journal of Neuroradiology editorial board and is currently the secretary of the Brain Function Research Study Group under KSNR.

This new generation of talented female neuroradiologists is making significant contribution to the field, both in Korea and internationally. They are expanding their roles and influence by pursuing opportunities abroad, with some even relocating to other countries to further their careers. One notable example is *Dr Yoon Sung Choi* at the National University of Singapore, a renowned researcher in radiomics and artificial intelligence applications for neuroimaging [36] (Fig. 23.36). She also serves as an editorial board member for KJR.

Fig. 23.34 Dr Ji Eun Park

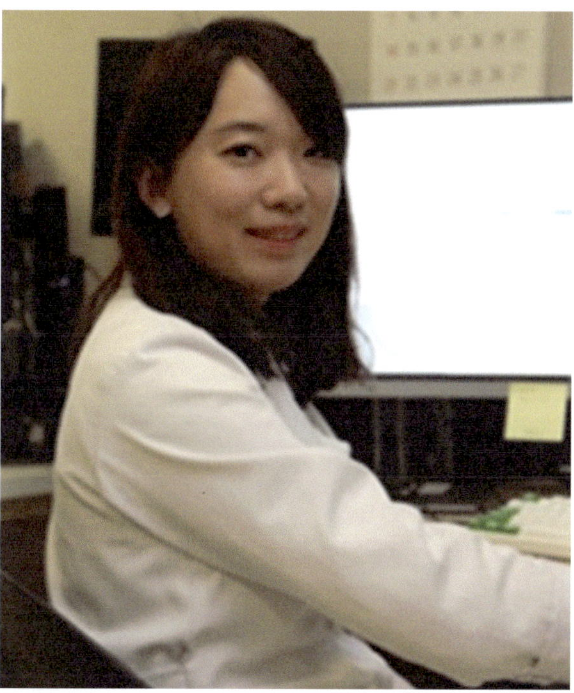

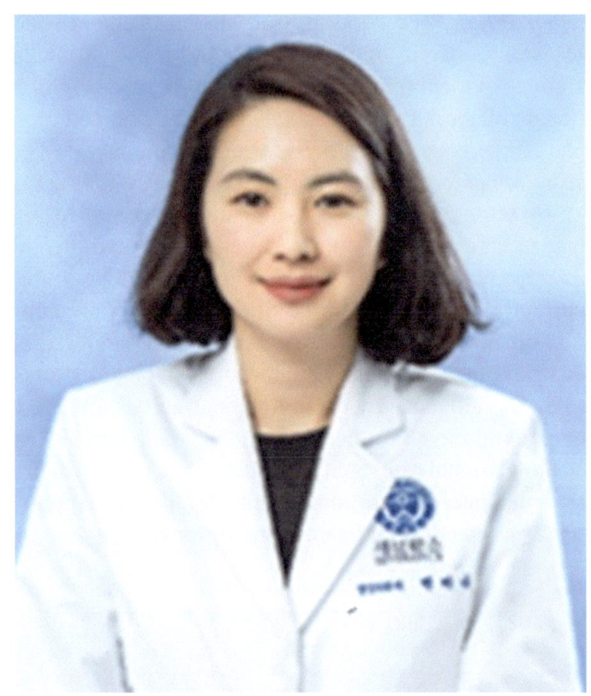

Fig. 23.35 Dr Mina Park

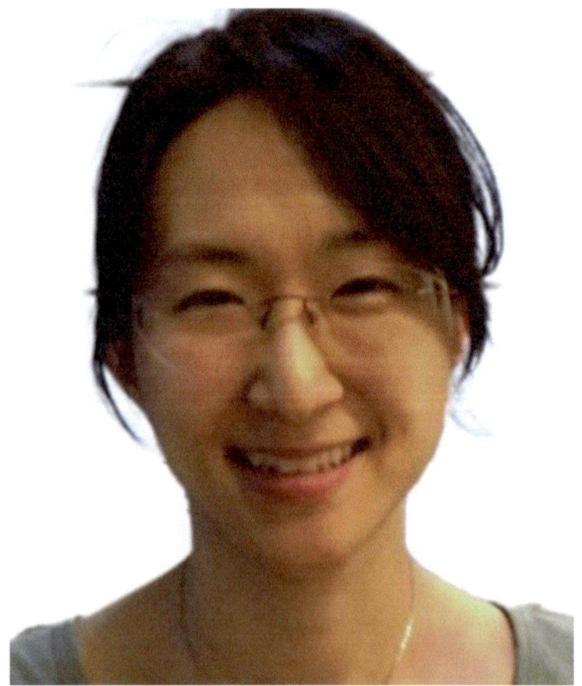

Fig. 23.36 Dr Yoon Sung Choi

Persistent Problems

Despite increased participation of women in neuroradiology research and KSNR societies over the past 30 years and a more favorable socio-cultural climate within medical institutions, female neuroradiologists in Korea still face challenges. These include a severe shortage of radiologists and the demanding work environment prevalent in Korean hospitals due to the increase in radiological examinations [37], which makes work-life balance difficult, coupled with the intense pressure of Korea's education system and challenging childcare environment. Moreover, neuroradiology generally has a higher workload compared to fields like breast imaging, which female radiologists traditionally favor. These factors discourage young radiologists from pursuing neuroradiology.

Conclusion

The history of female participation in neuroradiology in Korea has undergone a dramatic transformation in a relatively short period, with an increasing number of women taking on prominent roles in research and leadership. While the future is somewhat uncertain due to the current shortage of radiologists in Korea and the persistent socio-cultural challenges faced by female physicians, the distinction between male and female radiologists is already diminishing in terms of achievements. In the future, gender will likely become irrelevant, even regarding leadership and governance within the field.

Women in Radiology and Neuroradiology in Malaysia

Norlisah Mohd Ramli

Celebrating Pioneering Women in Neuroradiology: Achievements from the Southeast Asia Region

Let us delve into the past, present, and future prospects of women in neuroradiology in Malaysia and appreciate their significant contributions to the field.

According to the National Specialist Registrar in Malaysia, the subspecialty of neuroradiology remains within a special interest group in Clinical Radiology. However, it does not stop the advancement of subspecialty neuroradiology training and research in this field. The Neuroradiologist training in Malaysia was initially done overseas. The first neuroradiologist in Malaysia was Prof. Dr Norlisah Mohd

Ramli, who received her radiology training at Queens Medical Center in Nottingham in 1996. She further specialized in neuro-interventional radiology at Bicetre Hospital in Paris. She was also working as a consultant Neuroradiologist at Middlesbrough NHS Hospital in the UK before returning to Malaysia in 1999 to continue her post as a Lecturer at the Faculty of Medicine University Malays and as a consultant neuroradiologist at the University Malaya Medical Center, Kuala Lumpur. This robust academic foundation has positioned her as a leading figure in neuroradiology.

Professor Dr Norlisah Mohd Ramli

Professor Dr Norlisah Mohd Ramli's research has made substantial contributions to the field of neuroradiology and neuroimaging (Fig. 23.37). Her work has focused on various aspects of traumatic brain injury (TBI), neurodegenerative disorders, and glioma, significantly advancing understanding and treatment approaches.

In the realm of traumatic brain injury (TBI), Professor Norlisah has provided critical insights into the long-term effects of even mild TBI. Her research, published in journals such as Applied Neuropsychology: Adult and BMJ Open, has highlighted the structural and cognitive impairments associated with mild TBI. Her studies have demonstrated the efficacy of neuropsychological assessments and cognitive rehabilitation for patients suffering from attention deficits following mild TBI. Additionally, her longitudinal research on neuropsychological outcomes and neuro-metabolite changes has further elucidated the enduring impacts of TBI on brain function and structure.

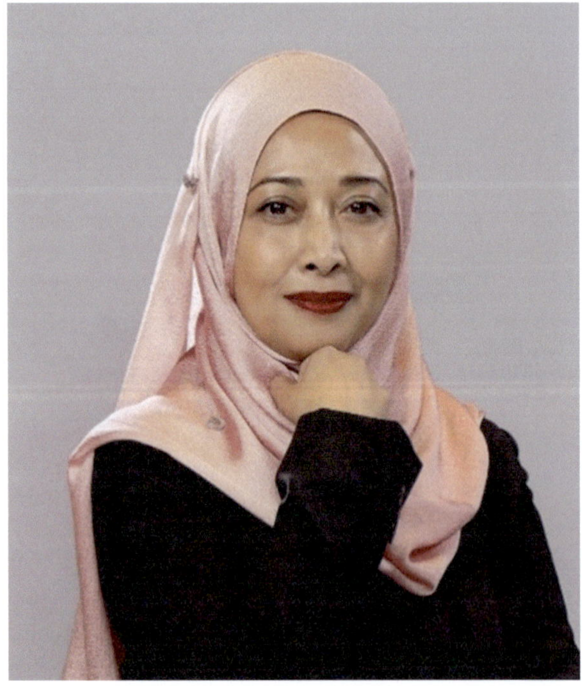

Fig. 23.37 Professor Dr Norlisah Mohd Ramli

Professor Norlisah's contributions to the study of neurodegenerative disorders are equally impactful. Her research on Parkinson's disease, detailed in publications like Neurology Asia and Parkinsonism & Related Disorders, has explored the effects of genetic mutations on disease progression and body composition. This work has implications for early detection and personalized treatment strategies. Furthermore, her development of an automated detection model for Alzheimer's disease, as reported in Pattern Recognition Letters, represents a significant advancement in diagnostic accuracy and early intervention for this debilitating condition.

In the area of glioma research, Professor Norlisah has made notable strides in understanding the role of lipidomics in glioma metabolism and aggressiveness. Her systematic reviews and studies in journals such as Metabolites and Academic Radiology have shed light on lipid alterations in glioma, aiming to identify novel biomarkers and therapeutic targets. Additionally, her investigations into quantitative MRI and radiogenomic biomarkers, as published in NeuroImage: Clinical and The British Journal of Radiology, have enhanced the precision of glioma characterization and treatment strategies. Her research on novel imaging techniques, including chemical shift gradient echo sequences, has also contributed to improved detection and grading of gliomas.

Overall, Professor Dr Norlisah Mohd Ramli's research has significantly advanced the field of neuroimaging, providing valuable insights into TBI, neurodegenerative disorders, and glioma. Her work enriches scientific understanding and has practical implications for enhancing patient diagnosis and treatment.

Professional Roles and Achievements

In her professional capacity, Prof. Dr Norlisah is a Professor in the Department of Biomedical Imaging at the Faculty of Medicine, Universiti Malaya. She is also the President of the College of Radiology, Academy of Medicine of Malaysia, and the Executive Councilor of the Asian Oceanian Society of Radiology. Her leadership roles extend to being the Co-Chair of the Quality, Safety, and Standards Committee. Her contributions to the field have been recognized through numerous awards and honors, including the Merdeka Award in 2008 and several best publication awards from Universiti Malaya. She has published over 100 peer-reviewed papers and has actively organized and directed neuroradiology workshops. She has published over 100 peer-reviewed papers and has actively organized and directed neuroradiology workshops. She has over 2801 citations with an H index of 29 [Google Scholar accessed 16 Sept 2024] and PubMed H index of 21.

In addition to her research and teaching roles, Professor Norlisah is actively involved in professional societies and committees. She has served on the editorial board for several radiology and neuroimaging journals, where she reviews submissions and contributes to advancing scientific knowledge in her field. Her expertise is also sought after in various advisory roles, where she provides guidance on research grants, clinical protocols, and policy development. She has been pivotal in the

Guidelines for Clinical Practice in Radiology (Malaysia) First and Second Edition. Under her tutelage, there are now several outstanding neuroradiologists in Malaysia who are now taking leadership roles. Mention two would be Dr Norzaini Rose, who is now Senior Consultant Neuroradiologist and Head of the Department of Radiology at National Cancer Institute Putrajaya, and Prof Kartini Rahmat, who is Head of the Department of Biomedical Imaging, Universiti Malaya.

In summary, Prof. Dr Norlisah Mohd Ramli's academic background, extensive research contributions, and leadership in radiology underscore her significant impact on the field. Her work continues to advance our understanding of neuroimaging and its applications, while her diverse interests and roles highlight her dedication to her profession and personal growth.

Dr Norzaini Rose Binti Mohd Zain
Dr Norzaini Rose is a Neuroradiologist who graduated with her MBBS degree from the Faculty of Medicine, University of Malaya, in 1995. She subsequently completed her Master's in Radiology from Universiti Kebangsaan Malaysia (UKM) in 2003. She became a Fellow of the Royal College of Radiologists (FRCR, UK) in 2011. She then did her Neuroradiology Fellowship under the Subspecialty Program of the Ministry of Health Malaysia from 2007 to 2009, followed by fellowships at the Royal Melbourne Hospital from 2008 to 2009 and at the Brain Research Institute, Melbourne, Australia, in 2009.

Professional Roles and Achievements

Dr Norzaini Rose is currently a Senior Consultant Neuroradiologist and Head of Department, Radiology, at the National Cancer Institute Putrajaya. She is also the National Head of Radiology Specialties for the Ministry of Health Malaysia. Her leadership extends to coordinating the Neuroradiology Fellowship Program under the Ministry of Health, a program she pioneered. She chairs several committees and is an active participant in multiple local and regional radiological committees.

Dr Norzaini Rose is an Ordinary Member of the Academy of Medicine Malaysia, a Co-opted Council Committee member (National Head of Specialty for Radiology) at the College of Radiology Malaysia, a UK Fellow of the Royal College of Radiologists, and a Registered Specialist on the National Specialist Registry. She also holds membership in the European Society of Radiologists.

In addition to her clinical and leadership roles, Dr Norzaini Rose has contributed to journal publications and clinical management guidelines, including the Malaysian Consensus and Standard Operating Procedures for Neurosciences and Radiology Services. Among the notable ones are Clinical Practice Guidelines in the Management of Multiple Sclerosis and Nasopharyngeal Carcinoma in 2015, Malaysian Consensus Statement on Brain Death 2023, and Handbook on Young Onset Dementia in 2014 and 2018. She is a frequent presenter at local and international conferences and received multiple Excellent Service Awards in 2007, 2015, and 2018. As the National Head of Specialty for Clinical Radiology since 2022, her leadership involves overseeing the Radiology services in 149 public hospitals in Malaysia and developing standards and policies that overarches into the realm of Radiology practice for the entire country.

Her research interests include neuroinflammatory diseases, demyelinating disorders, and neurodegenerative diseases. She has various publications, including studies on multiple sclerosis, neuromyelitis optica, and comparative studies on tumefactive demyelinating lesions and CNS neoplasms.

Dr Norzaini Rose is a dedicated and accomplished neuroradiologist who has made significant contributions to the field. Her expertise, leadership, and research have positively impacted Malaysia's healthcare system and patient care.

Professor Dr Kartini Rahmat

Professor Dr Kartini Binti Rahmat is a Consultant Radiologist and distinguished professor in the Department of Biomedical Imaging at the Faculty of Medicine, Universiti Malaya (UM). She holds an MBBS from UM and a Master of Radiology (UM) and is a Fellowship member of the Royal College of Radiologists (FRCR). She completed subspecialty training in Breast Imaging at the Royal Perth Hospital, Australia (2008). She furthered into diagnostic Neuroradiology fellowship training at the Universiti Malaya Medical Center under the preceptorship of Professor Dr Norlisah Ramli (2010–2012), followed by an Advanced Neuroimaging Fellowship at the Queensquare Hospital London (UK) under the European Society of Magnetic Resonance Imaging (ESMRMB) MRI observership program (2016). Her expertise spans medical diagnostic imaging, focusing on cancer imaging and diagnostic neuroradiology, including advanced modalities such as MRI, mammography, ultrasound, CT scans, and stereotactic-guided breast biopsy.

Professional Roles Professor Kartini has held various administrative positions at UM. She is currently the Head of the Department of Biomedical Imaging and has led the Universiti Malaya Research Imaging Center from January 2018–2024. She has served in several leadership positions, including Chairman of the Scientific Committee and Coordinator of postgraduate programs. She is an Ordinary Member of the Academy of Medicine Malaysia and a Council Committee member at the College of Radiology Malaysia; she has contributed to National clinical guidelines in radiology and coordinated major congresses such as the Asian Association of Radiology and Asian Oceanian Congress of Radiology 2021 (AOCR).

Achievements Professor Kartini is a prominent figure in radiology, with numerous awards to her name. She was a multiple award recipient at the Malaysian Congress of Radiology (MCOR) in 2022 and has been recognized for her research in Automated breast ultrasound and liver fibrosis. Her scientific contributions extend internationally, earning awards at prominent conferences such as the ASEAN Oceanian Congress of Radiology and the College of Radiology Annual Scientific Meetings. Additionally, she holds certifications in clinical MRI teaching from the European Society of Magnetic Resonance in Medicine and Biology. She has been consistently recognized with Excellent Service Awards by UM for her academic and clinical contributions.

Professor Kartini has extensive work and numerous publications, many of which have been featured in WoS-indexed journals. She has published over 120 peer-reviewed articles, with over 2500 citations, an H index of 29 [Google Scholar] and a PubMed H index of 21. Professor Kartini's research in neuroimaging is particularly notable. She has significantly contributed to understanding microstructural changes in neurodegenerative diseases and other neurological conditions. Her studies include investigating persistent postural-perceptual dizziness and examining alterations in the delicate network responsible for maintaining balance. Additionally, she has explored the microstructural integrity of peripheral nerves in Charcot-Marie-Tooth disease, highlighting abnormalities in nerve structures through MRI evaluation.

In neuroimaging for epilepsy, Professor Kartini has delved into current practices and evolving trends, offering insights into MRI imaging techniques for managing refractory epilepsy. Her work also extends to CNS tuberculous and brain tumor research, where vascular and contrasted perfusion-weighted MRI imaging provided crucial findings for assessing brain vascularity, contributing valuable data on brain changes in these conditions. Prof. Kartini's research on pediatric neuroimaging is equally impressive, with studies on white matter maturation in children with developmental delays using diffusion tensor imaging.

Apart from neuroimaging, the range of diagnostic imaging in Professor Kartini's research portfolio is vast. The area of her research entails studies on the diagnosis and detection of breast cancer, including the evaluation of advanced breast MRI techniques, mammographic density, automated breast ultrasound, and the applications of machine learning Artificial Intelligence. Her research also covers novel imaging techniques, such as fusion imaging for detecting axillary lymph node metastasis and exploring the role of single necleotide polymorphism (SNPs) in mammographic density. Professor Kartini's diverse contributions underscore her expertise and impact across multiple medical imaging domains.

Professor Kartini's expertise, leadership, and research have profoundly impacted the biomedical imaging field. Her contributions have advanced our understanding of various diseases and improved patient care. She is a role model for aspiring radiologists and a valuable asset to the medical community.

Future Directions and Conclusion

As the field of neuroradiology continues to evolve, female neuroradiologists have a unique opportunity to shape its future. They can contribute to research, clinical practice, and education advancements by leveraging their skills, expertise, and perspectives.

One potential direction for female neuroradiologists is to embrace emerging technologies and methodologies to investigate novel areas in neuroradiology. This could involve exploring the applications of artificial intelligence, machine learning, and advanced imaging techniques to improve diagnosis, treatment planning, and patient outcomes. Additionally, female neuroradiologists can play a crucial role in mentoring and supporting younger female colleagues, creating a more inclusive and supportive environment within the field. By sharing their experiences, providing guidance, and advocating for their advancement, they can help to inspire the next generation of female neuroradiologists.

The contributions of women in neuroradiology have been transformative, shaping both the practice and research of the field across Southeast Asia. Pioneering figures like Professor Dr Norlisah Ramli, Dr Norzaini Rose, and Professor Dr Kartini Rahmat have made significant strides in neuroimaging, revolutionizing the early detection of neurodegenerative diseases and brain tumors. Their work highlights the exceptional impact of female neuroradiologists and inspires future generations.

This chapter underscores women's evolving representation and leadership in neuroradiology, reflecting a growing recognition of their vital role in advancing diagnostic practices and research innovations. Building on these achievements by fostering collaboration, supporting emerging talents, and promoting diversity is imperative as we look to the future. By doing so, the field of neuroradiology can continue to thrive and evolve, ultimately improving patient outcomes and expanding our understanding of the brain.

Women In Radiology and Neuroradiology in Nepal

Dr Akriti Baral

There are no female neuroradiologists from Nepal; however, there are few general radiologists who have shown excellence in this sector.

Dr Benu Wagle Lohani

One of the influential female radiologists is Professor Benu Wagle Lohani. She completed her MBBS from Chennai University, India in the year 1992 and Post-Graduation in Radiodiagnosis and Imaging from PGIMER, Chandigarh, India in 1998. She joined the Department of Radiology & Imaging of TU Teaching Hospital, IOM from March 1998.

She was the former Head of the Department of Radiology & Imaging at Institute of Medicine, TU Teaching Hospital & also the PG coordinator of MDRD of the institute. She has been actively involved in the academics, research, and services of the department. She practices Diagnostic Radiology with special interest in Women's Imaging.

She was also the coordinator for curriculum development of radiology specialty for National Board of Medical Specialties (NBMS) at Medical Education Commission (MEC) under the Government of Nepal which has started from the year 2021. She was also former General Secretory of Nepal Radiologists' Association (NRA) and organized the first international conference of Radiology (SACOR 2008) in Nepal, has presented a number of papers in national and international conferences, authored and coauthored scientific publications in national and international journals. She is also a resource person, chairperson, & panelist for conferences and CMEs, peer reviewer for journals. She is a member of Ethical Review Board of Nepal Health Research Council.

Dr Akriti Baral

Dr Akriti Baral completed her MBBS at Kathmandu Medical College, Nepal, graduating in 2013. She is currently pursuing her residency in Radiology at the same institution, with a focus on expanding her expertise in this dynamic field. In a country where the number of female neuroradiologists is limited, Dr Baral has developed a strong passion for both Interventional Radiology and Neuroradiology. Her ambition is not only to contribute to these specialized fields but also to inspire more women to take up roles in these underrepresented areas of medicine. Additionally, she is actively involved in research, currently conducting a study titled “Rotterdam CT Severity Index in Predicting Early Outcomes in Traumatic Brain Injury.” Her work aims to enhance the understanding of traumatic brain injury prognosis, ultimately improving patient outcomes in a critical area of medical care.

Women in Neuroradiology in Singapore

Ling Ling Chan

Today, the practice of neuroradiology in public and private institutions on our little red dot is supported in no small part by women who trained locally and/or elsewhere around the world in diagnostic imaging of the brain, head and neck, and spine and neurointerventional radiology. Women neuroradiologists in Singapore have excelled professionally in the field, with many leading in both the clinic and academia. This Chapter celebrates the contributions of women in neuroradiology in Singapore, exemplified by the following individuals in alphabetical order.

Dr Chan Ling Ling, a Professor at the Radiological Sciences and Neuroscience Academic Clinical Programs in Duke-NUS Medical School, is the Academic Vice Chair, Research, Radiological Sciences at the SingHealth Duke-NUS Academic Medical Center; Vice-Chair, Research Training Review Panel, Ministry of Health, Singapore; Research Director, Division of Radiological Sciences and in the Research Executive Committee, Research Office, Singapore General Hospital (SGH) (Fig. 23.38). She is also an Examiner at the Joint MMed (Diagnostic Radiology)—Final FRCR Part B examinations, President of Neuroradiology Subsection, Singapore Radiological Society and was Program Chair of the highly successful 2023 AOCNR-SGCR meeting. She currently leads a SingHealth team evaluating the impact of ultra-high field MRI ownership for research and the clinic.

Dr Chan started radiology training in the SGH after medical school at the National University of Singapore. The mystery of radiological diagnosis intrigued her, and the immense impact Radiology has on patient care drew her in. After FRCR

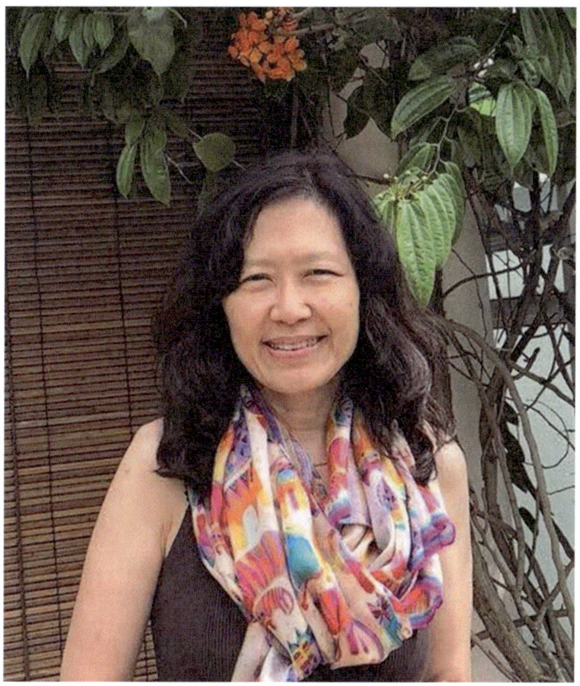

Fig. 23.38 Dr Chan Ling Ling

specialist accreditation, she completed an almost 2-year clinical neuroradiology fellowship stint at the MD Anderson Cancer Center, Texas Children's Hospital and The Methodist Hospital in the Houston Texas Medical Center. This exposed her to state-of-the-art management of brain and head & neck tumors, neurovascular intervention and clinical research. Helming Neurology, Neurosurgery, brain tumor, Neuro-ophthalmology, and Oculoplastic X-Ray rounds for nearly 2-decades as SGH faculty further honed her clinical acumen and helped her build strong rapport with clinicians. She collaborates with MR radiography and physicist teams to translate advanced MRI techniques into service to solve clinical problems. She credits mentors and seniors such as Drs Tan Kim Ping, Wilfred Peh, John Hoe, Vincent Chong, Tan Bien Soo, Winston Lim, Lo Yew Long, Tchoyoson Lim, Tan Eng King, Thng Choon Hua, Andrew Tan, Louis Tan, Tay Kiang Hiong, Chan Lai Peng, Larry Ginsberg, Don Schomer, and Normal Leeds for their inspiration and support, and many opportunities they have availed her to grow professionally in the field.

Dr Chan is a three-time national Clinician Scientist awardee, leading a neuroimaging research program focusing on chronic neurological diseases such as Parkinsonism, gait disorders, traumatic brain injury, aging, and dementia. She has local, international, university, and industry collaborations with centers from Korea, Taiwan, Europe, and USA. Her partnerships have widened the repertoire of advanced MRI and AI tools that her team evaluates and uses to track structural and functional changes in disease and aid in the neuroradiological workflow for diagnosis and prediction of neuropathology. She has 200 peer-reviewed publications, 4940 citations, and an i10-index of 116. As academic faculty of the three Singapore medical schools, Dr Chan has mentored many students in research, presented or co-authored >260 abstracts at local, regional, and international conferences, and received numerous national and international scientific awards and accolades as PI or mentor. She is an invited speaker at numerous international conferences, including the RSNA and ISMRM.

Dr Chan is free spirited and enjoys diversity, swimming, cycling, pushing her limits, and connecting with nature in hiking, imbibing festivities and also checking out the less trodden paths in her travels.

Dr Fan Yoke Fun was a pioneer female neuroradiologist from Singapore. She graduated from the Medical School in the National University of Singapore in 1979 and was among the few from her graduating class to choose to specialize in Diagnostic Radiology. Plain film interpretation was what attracted Dr Fan to Radiology. She underwent training in Diagnostic Radiology locally, and for a year in Guy's Hospital under Drs Hugh Saxton, Sheila Rankin, and John Reidy as part of the training program then. She enjoyed her time in London very much. She was conferred her specialist FRCR certification in Diagnostic Radiology by the Royal College of Radiologists, United Kingdom, in 1984. Thereafter, she joined the Singapore General Hospital, the largest public and teaching hospital in Singapore, as faculty. Among the largely male dominated faculty in Singapore General Hospital, Dr Fan was well known for her attention to detail and good and quick pair of hands. She was the go-to guru for difficult procedures such as lymphangiography. She was interested in patterns and "things" that did not conform to the usual or stereotype. To understand and differentiate what was abnormal from the range of normal and attendant variations, she painstakingly collected many radiological cases for teaching. She put her case collection and sharp eyes to good use in tutorials and was a favorite sought-after tutor among radiology trainees. Singapore General Hospital was also the first to spearhead and lead in subspecialty radiology practice in Singapore.

Even though Dr Fan was an unwilling head and neck radiologist to start off due to limited clinical indications in those early days, her love for and dedication to the unusual and non-stereotypical led her to amass many excellent illustrative imaging cases from clinical reporting. These were featured among her more than 40 pictorial essays published in peer reviewed journals where she described the many facets of local and perineural spread of nasopharyngeal carcinoma, and complications to treatment, in partnership with Dr Vincent Chong, who had a flair for academic writing. This was a massive feat especially as access to publications and journals in Singapore was hard to come by at that time. In 2005, Dr Fan took the courage as a senior female steward neuroradiologist to join Dr James Khoo at the Diagnostic Imaging Department in the Singapore National Cancer Center to help attend to the heavy service load of nasopharyngeal carcinoma and other head and neck cancers seen in the then "young" institution. At the current time, Dr Fan is happily retired, and enjoying life travelling with her better half.

Dr Kheok Si Wei is a Neuroradiologist and Head and Neck Radiologist at Singapore General Hospital. After graduating with a medical degree from the

National University of Singapore, she did her Radiology residency in SingHealth, Singapore. Upon joining the hospital as a certified radiologist, she had the opportunity to take up short visiting fellowships at University Hospital in Frankfurt, Germany and Hospital of the University of Pennsylvania, USA. Under the Singapore Ministry of Health Manpower Development Plan, she furthered her specialist training in Head and Neck Imaging at Massachusetts Eye and Ear Infirmary, USA.

She returned to Singapore at the peak of the Covid pandemic, where apart from reporting unusual presentations of the disease, she helped to re-organize the medical student radiology elective program in the division to adapt to the new requirements. In 2023, the Neuroradiology section became a newly formed department and at the time of writing she serves as Director of Head and Neck Radiology, Director of MRI patient care services, and Deputy Head of Department for Neuroradiology at Singapore General Hospital.

She holds academic appointments at all three medical schools in Singapore and shares her knowledge as an invited conference speaker, as well as through teaching residents and medical students. She is committed to the development of an excellent head and neck radiology unit with the collective efforts of the team. In addition, she oversees the MRI service in the division, which is one of the busiest in the nation, together with a group of dedicated and highly skilled radiographers.

Her current research interests are in multidisciplinary collaborations to develop deep learning models in enhancing patient care, to explore the potential of imaging science in uncovering previously undetected diseases, and to predict difficult head and neck surgeries.

Rain or shine, what motivates her to turn up to work is the meaningfulness she finds in serving a broader population in a government public hospital.

Dr Sumeet Kumar is a Senior Consultant Neuroradiologist at the National Neuroscience Institute (NNI), with over 11 years of experience in advancing the field of neuroradiology. She plays a vital role in academic medicine in Singapore, serving as an Adjunct Assistant Professor at Duke-NUS Medical School and the Director of Advanced Magnetic Resonance Imaging Research within the Radiological Sciences Academic Clinical Program (RADSC ACP) at SingHealth Duke-NUS Academic Medical Center. Additionally, she holds the position of Research Head for the Neuroradiology Department at NNI.

Passionate about educating the next generation of radiologists, Dr Kumar teaches at the European Courses for Neuroradiology, organized by the European Society of Neuroradiology, and has been invited to speak at numerous prestigious local and international conferences, including the European Congress of Radiology, the European Society of Neuroradiology, and the International Society for Magnetic Resonance in Medicine (ISMRM). In 2016, Dr Kumar's contributions to education were recognized with the Residency Education Award.

Dr Kumar's research focuses on dementia and normal pressure hydrocephalus, with several peer-reviewed publications in these areas. A recipient of the RADScience ACP Pitch for Funds grant, she has conducted research on Diffusion Kurtosis Imaging in Alzheimer's disease, a study that earned the SingHealth Publish! 2023 award. Dr Kumar began her medical career in Mumbai, India, and went on to specialize in neuroradiology through fellowships in London, UK. After relocating to Singapore in 2009, she completed advanced specialist training and joined NNI in 2013. In 2015, Dr Kumar obtained the European Diploma in Neuroradiology and completed a fellowship at Leiden University, focusing on dementia and neuropsychiatric lupus research using 7T MRI technology.

Outside of professional achievements, Dr Kumar takes pride in a wide range of experiences that have shaped her emotional intelligence and cross-cultural communication skills. These include teaching radiology in Kenya, hosting a children's TV show, participating in theater and storytelling workshops, and exploring activities like skydiving and paragliding. Driven by a passion for learning, Dr Kumar constantly seeks new skills and challenges.

Dr Lishya Liauw studied Medicine at Leiden University in the Netherlands. For specialist training, she was considering Otolaryngology and as an intended preparation she worked 1 year in General Surgery as a junior doctor not in residency training. The Netherlands does not implement the HO and MO system for junior doctors as in Singapore or the UK. Dutch junior doctors work within a residency training program or do similar work outside a residency training. During her year in General Surgery, she frequently consulted the radiologist for patients presenting with "acute abdomen". She was fascinated by the use of Ultrasonography as a first line diagnostic imaging method and wanted to be able to master Ultrasonography. Since no immediate positions were open for the Radiology residency training, she started off in a junior doctor position not in residency training in the Neuroradiology section of the Diagnostic Radiology department in Leiden University Medical Center (LUMC). One year later, she started the official residency training in LUMC.

For subspecialization within radiology, she considered Interventional Radiology and Neuroradiology/Head Neck radiology and decided on the latter in view of more variety. In the early times that she trained and worked in radiology, there were not many female radiologists, the majority were men. But her batch of trainees started with increasing number of female trainees although the majority were male. She was unaware of the concept of mentorship but in retrospect she would have appreciated help to navigate life in radiology waters, she experienced that the old boys network did not include women. She tried research during her PhD training but decided it was not a perfect fit. Since 2008, she works as a neuroradiologist in Singapore, currently in Singapore General Hospital. She always liked the idea of having an overseas experience and Singapore seemed a good fit with the high quality of healthcare and the English language spoken. Finally, she has moved more into Head and Neck Radiology, which is a challenging field but so much more enjoyable with an improved understanding of the intricate anatomy. In both the Netherlands and Singapore, she has been engaged in administrative positions. She likes to facilitate, simplify and streamline processes. In both the Netherlands and Singapore, she has been engaged in administrative positions, where she enjoys facilitating, simplifying, and streamlining processes. She brings the same strengths to her new role as the team Wellness Advocate. She prefers working in this environment due to the stimulating effect of newbee trainees and need to keep updated in her field.

Dr Ai Peng Tan is a senior consultant at the Department of Diagnostic Imaging, National University Hospital, Singapore, and a clinician-scientist funded by the National Medical Research Council. Dr Tan also has a joint appointment at the A*STAR Institute for Human Development and Potential (A*STAR IHDP) as a Principal Investigator, where she assumes leadership of the Neuroimaging Domain and spearheads neuroimaging research pertaining to GUSTO, the biggest birth cohort study in Singapore. In 2016, Dr Tan was honored with the Academic Medicine Development Award and completed a prestigious Pediatric Neuroradiology Fellowship at Great Ormond Street Hospital for Children, NHS Foundation Trust, which included a pivotal research attachment at the Center for the Developing Brain, King's College London. This experience laid the foundation for a distinguished career in pediatric brain mapping research. Dr Tan possesses in-depth knowledge of various advanced neuroimaging techniques, including diffusion tensor imaging and functional MRI, that form the basis of human brain mapping. Her research focuses on clinical translation of MRI-based brain connectivity profiling, particularly in neurodevelopmental and mental health disorders. She is currently recognized as the sole neuroradiologist in Singapore actively conducting research in the mapping of the developing human brain. This recognition is further highlighted by the recent award of the National Medical Research Council (NMRC) Transition Award for the research proposal "Precision BRAin COnnectivity Profiling of Learning Difficulties for future therapeutic strategy using network-targeted neurostimulation (BRACO-LD)." As the Research Director for the Department of Diagnostic Radiology at NUS and the Department of Diagnostic Imaging at NUH, Dr Tan oversees significant research initiatives and contributes actively to the scientific community through membership on the NHG Domain Specific Review Board (DSRB). Dr Tan is also an established academic writer and speaker, having presented at numerous local and international conferences and published extensively in peer-reviewed journals. Driven by a vision to embed MRI-based brain network profiling into clinical practice for children with neurodevelopmental and neuropsychiatric disorders, Dr Tan is actively engaged in the development of brain-network targeted interventions to further advance this critical field of research. Outside of the professional realm, Dr Tan is passionate about traveling. The combination of solo travel, great coffee, people watching, and music is her idea of a perfect vacation. This balance of exploration and relaxation provides a refreshing complement to a demanding career in neuroimaging research

Dr Judy Tan started her radiology training soon after graduating from medical school, National University of Singapore in 2000. She obtained her postgraduate qualifications from the Royal College of Radiologists, UK and National University of Singapore in 2005. She embarked on her neuroradiology subspecialty training in Singapore General Hospital, which is the largest acute tertiary hospital in Singapore with nearly 1800 beds and over 50 clinical specialties. She chose Neuroradiology as she felt that imaging plays a very important role in this specialty, and often has a strong correlation with patients' clinical signs and symptoms. In 2007, she obtained an MRI visiting fellowship at the New York University Medical Center. This was followed by a SingHealth HMDP fellowship in Diagnostic Radiology to pursue her study in clinical applications in Advanced Neuroradiology and Head and Neck imaging at the University of Washington Medical Center. In 2008, Dr Tan led a study to evaluate how the newer multislice CT machines in the Singapore General Hospital affected radiation doses delivered to the eye lens, the results of which were published in a well-cited paper in the American Journal of Neuroradiology. She entered private practice at the end of 2010, joining Radiology Consultants Pte Ltd, which provides radiological services to Parkway Radiology, a division under IHH Healthcare Singapore – Singapore's largest private healthcare operator. With the benefit of being part of a big radiology group, Dr Tan still enjoys the privilege of devoting at least 70% of her clinical time to her subspecialty of interest, participating in clinical neuroscience meetings and reporting neuroradiological CT and MRI. Her current practice encompasses the entire gamut of neuroradiology from stroke to demyelination, temporal bone pathologies, brain, and head and neck tumors.

Dr Tang Phua Hwee is an Associate Professor at the Duke-NUS Medical School, and Deputy Head and Senior Consultant at the Department of Diagnostic & Interventional Imaging, KK Women's and Children's Hospital. She is a pediatric radiologist who has been doing pediatric neuroimaging for close to two decades and is a recipient of Singapore Health Quality Service Award and SingHealth Long Service Award. She is a graduate of the National University of Singapore. After obtaining her Fellowship of the Royal College of Radiologists (FRCR) and Masters in Diagnostic Radiology, she spent 6 months in University of California San Francisco learning the finer points of pediatric imaging, including pediatric neuroimaging and fetal imaging. This was followed by a mini-fellowship in neuroradiology at Cincinnati Children's Hospital Medical Center and a visiting fellowship at Athinoula A. Martinos Center for Biomedical Imaging. She completed the Khoo Clinical Scholar's Program to improve her research skills and was awarded the Essential Skills in Medical Education (ESME) Certificate in Medical Education on completion of the ESME Course and Report.

With increasing number of children with headache sent for MRI across the years, she was instrumental in implementing an Ultrafast MRI brain protocol for screening such patients with better cooperativeness of children for the shorter, more cost-effective scans. Her randomized control trial to evaluate the effectiveness of videos on cooperativeness of children undergoing MRI won the Ella Preiskel Prize in 2018, the use of a checklist to determine which child undergoing MRI requires general anesthesia won the Ella Preiskel Prize in 2019 and the most useful cranial ultrasound predictor of neurodevelopmental outcomes at 2 years of age for preterm infants won the Ellis Barnett Prize in 2021. "KKH Ultrasound Training Programme for Residents" has also received the RadSci ACP Program Excellence Award in 2022 for application of best practices into a training curriculum.

As Director of Pediatric Imaging of the SingHealth Duke-NUS Radiological Science Academic Clinical Program, she oversees the pediatric imaging service, ensuring value drive care and timely imaging for pediatric patients while optimizing staffing requirements. Being Associate Program Director of SingHealth Diagnostic Radiology Residency Program, Site Director and Core Faculty of National Healthcare Group Residency, she ensures that residents are given adequate training, supported in their learning journeys and have access to databases to capitalize on research and innovation opportunities. For these, she won the Outstanding Faculty (Residency) RADSC ACP Education Award in 2019. She contributes to the local radiology societies such as the Chapter of Diagnostic Radiologists Committee section of the College of Radiologists, Singapore, and is a Neurosection committee member of the Singapore Radiological Society. Dr Tang has given many lectures internationally and locally, the latest ones in 2024 being at American Society of Neuroradiology 62nd Annual Meeting and 57th Singapore-Malaysia Congress of Medicine, respectively.

The brain has always been fascinating for her. As a medical student, she watched in awe how Professor Loong Si Chin demonstrated a neurological examination, which allowed him to pinpoint the location of the stroke patient had suffered. It was absolutely inspiring to be able to have been taught by such an experienced excellent teacher who was so ready to share his knowledge with all. The neuroradiologists mentors she had as a radiology registrar in National Neuroscience Institute, Professors Tchoyoson Lim and Sitoh Yih Yian, were also great role models and instrumental in her exposure to research activities demonstrating how it is possible to maintain great clinical acumen while pushing forth the boundaries of knowledge with research. With Professor David Stringer setting up KK Women's and Children's Hospital's MRI service in 2005, it was a very exciting time building up the pediatric MR neuroimaging service.

Dr Tang enjoys visual arts and finds it highly gratifying to be able to appreciate the internal structures of the human body on a daily basis. She attempts to incorporate regular exercise and stretches into her daily routine to balance the "tech neck" that affect many radiologists.

Dr Joanna Pearly Ti has been fascinated by neuroanatomy since medical school and she has always enjoyed working with her hands, so choosing a career as an interventional neuroradiologist was a no-brainer for her! After graduating from the Royal College of Surgeons, Ireland/Penang Medical College in 2003, she completed radiology training in Dublin, Ireland in 2010. Her 8 years of working in Beaumont Hospital, Dublin, a tertiary neuroscience referral center with passionate and experienced mentors, provided her with a solid foundation upon which to build her career. Following fellowship appointments in both Interventional Neuroradiology at University of Illinois, Chicago and Diagnostic Neuroradiology at Northwestern Memorial Hospital, Chicago, she chose to move to Singapore with her husband, an endocrinologist at the Singapore General Hospital. She is currently a Senior Consultant Neuroradiologist, Department of Neuroradiology, at the National Neuroscience Institute. She has a particular interest in vascular disorders of the brain, including aneurysms and acute stroke. Dr Ti has three wonderful children, the youngest one born in Singapore. She believes Singapore is one of the best countries where women can enjoy both career and family. She loves her work and enjoys a great work-life balance, alongside who she claims is the world's most supportive spouse.

Dr Jocelyn Wong graduated from the Yong Loo Lin School of Medicine at the National University of Singapore and thereafter undertook her radiology training locally. During the first 3 years of the training program, there were general radiology rotations at the Tan Tock Seng Hospital, National University Hospital (NUH), KK Women's and Children's Hospital, and the National Neuroscience Institute. It was during this period of time that she discovered a sense of satisfaction in looking for clues in a brain scan and correlating it with the patient's clinical symptoms, putting everything together to solve a puzzle, which is to arrive at a correct diagnosis for the patient. This budding interest was encouraged by a few neuroradiology mentors, who advised her to pursue a career in this specialty. Hence, for the next 2 years of subspecialty training, she chose to train in Neuroradiology and Head and Neck Imaging at the National University Hospital, the Singapore General Hospital, and the National Cancer Center. These were vital experiences as she got to "learn the trade" from various faculty members in the neuroradiology, head and neck imaging section across the island. Notable faculty members include Professor Vincent Chong, Associate Professor Goh Poh Sun, Dr Eric Ting, Dr Winston Lim, Professor Chan Ling Ling, Dr Tan Tiong Yong, Dr Lim Tch Aun, Associate Professor Francis Hui, Professor Tchoyoson Lim, Dr Sitoh Yih Yian, Dr Lishya Liauw, Dr Patrick Teo, Dr Kei Pin Lin, Dr Julian Goh, and many others, who have all generously shared their time and expertise with her during those years. Memories of walking under the hot sun to nearby coffee shops and cafes for lunch with various faculty members were unforgettable. Her entire subspeciality training concluded with an opportunity to do a visiting neuroradiology fellowship at the Massachusetts General Hospital (MGH), sponsored by the Ministry of Health, under the Health Manpower Development Plan (HMDP). At MGH she attended the training program for the MGH neuroradiology fellows and sat in during their daily reporting sessions, radiology-clinical rounds, and various tutorials. Notable faculty members like Professors Ramon Gonzalez, Otto Rapalino, Bradley Buchbinder, William Copen, Michael Lev, and Pamela Schaefer among others, have taught her generously and shared their expertise on general neuroradiology, brain tumor imaging, stroke imaging, and functional MRI. The MGH fellows were also friendly and welcoming and shared much with her as well.

After completing the HMDP training, Jocelyn returned to Singapore and joined NUH as a neuroradiologist. Over the years she had helped set up a Functional MRI service for pre-operative tumor assessment, worked on parametric brain tumor imaging protocols using MR perfusion, MR spectroscopy and conventional MRI to tackle common diagnostic problems, such as recurrent brain tumor versus radiation necrosis, pseudoprogression and other post treatment complications. She also gained some experience in the fields of pediatric and fetal brain imaging along the way. During this time, she had also served a term as the division head of the neuroradiology section at NUH. She is currently a senior consultant radiologist at NUH and enjoys sharing what she has learnt with enthusiastic residents who rotate through the department.

Jocelyn is thankful for her supportive family, incredible mentors, colleagues, and friends. She enjoys cooking, reading non-radiology books, and listening to music in her free time.

Dr Yu Wai-Yung graduated from St George's Hospital Medical School in 1993 and initially pursued a career in internal medicine. She started training in Radiology as she wanted to be at the forefront of patient diagnosis and to make a difference at an earlier stage. She subspecialized in Neuroradiology and completed a 2-year Neuroradiology fellowship at the National Hospital for Neurology and Neurosurgery (NHNN), Queen Square, UK. She was a Consultant Neuroradiologist at Atkinson Morley Wing, St George's Hospital, UK, for 5 years before moving to Singapore in 2010.

She is passionate about education and her education philosophy is based on constructivism whereby learning is an active process. Dr Yu strives to create a learning environment that is engaging, supportive, and allows the learner to ask questions and make connections to their prior knowledge and experiences. She has received multiple outstanding faculty awards, including the GCEO excellence award for outstanding educator.

Dr Yu was consulted for two high court medical civil litigation cases where she gave key expert witness evidence, exposing her to the process and complexity of civil litigation and medicolegal trials. This ignited her interest in medical law and she embarked on a Masters in Medical Law and Ethics at the University of Edinburgh, graduating with merit in 2022.

Dr Yu is currently a Senior Consultant and Head in the Department of Neuroradiology at the National Neuroscience Institute (NNI), Singapore. She is also Academic Vice Chair, Education, in the Radiological Sciences Academic Clinical Program (RADSc ACP) and she serves at the national level as a member of the Residency Advisory Committee (RAC) for Diagnostic Radiology Training which oversees the three Diagnostic Radiology residency programs in Singapore. She is an examiner for the Structure Oral Exit Exams in Radiology and holds positions at all three medical schools in Singapore.

In addition to clinical, administrative duties and education, Dr Yu is also interested in innovation, particularly for education, and, together with her team, is currently working on serious games for contrast allergy with an industry partner.

Women in Neuroradiology in Taiwan

Chao-Bao Luo

In Taiwan, women neuroradiologists contribute significantly to the field's advancement through their expertise and dedication. The Neuroradiologist Society of Taiwan includes 78 women among its 439 members. Notable figures in this group include Dr Hsiu-Mei Wu, Dr Ya-Fang Chen, Dr Chao-Chun Lin, Dr Hung-Chieh Chen, and Dr Chih-Chun Wu. These professionals, along with their colleagues, play a crucial role in shaping the landscape of neuroimaging in Taiwan.

Dr Hsiu-Mei Wu graduated from National Yang-Ming Medical College (now the School of Medicine at National Yang-Ming Chiao Tung University) in 1988. After

2 years of internal medicine practice at Chiayi Veterans Hospital, she completed her radiology residency at Taipei Veterans General Hospital. She then spent a year in advanced study at Johns Hopkins Hospital in the United States. Currently, Dr Wu is an attending physician in the Department of Radiology at Taipei Veterans General Hospital and an assistant professor at National Yang-Ming Chiao Tung University.

Specializing in neuroradiology, particularly magnetic resonance imaging (MRI), Dr Wu served as the chief of the MRI section in the Department of Radiology at Taipei Veterans General Hospital from 2018 to 2024. Her research and publications primarily focus on neuroimaging changes following Gamma Knife procedures. Dr Wu is an enthusiastic participant in various educational activities of the Neuroradiology Society.

Dr Ya-Fang Chen graduated from the National Taiwan University College of Medicine in 1995 and began her residency training in the Department of Medical Imaging at the National Taiwan University Hospital. She was promoted to attending physician in 1999, specializing in neuroradiology. In 2003, she spent a year as a research scientist at the Functional Oncoimaging Center at UC Irvine in the United States.

Currently, Dr Chen is an associate professor in the Department of Radiology at National Taiwan University College of Medicine and the chief of the Division of Neuroradiology in the Department of Medical Imaging at National Taiwan University Hospital. She has exceptional expertise in neuroradiology, regularly assisting clinical physicians with challenging cases and excelling in teaching both residents within the department and clinicians from other specialties. Dr Chen is a frequent speaker at various clinical department meetings and is actively involved in the educational programs of the Neuroradiology Society. She has published over 100 papers in international peer-reviewed journals. Her research focuses on dementia, cerebral small vessel diseases, and pediatric cerebrovascular diseases such as moyamoya disease. She has also conducted research and published work on brain tumors and head and neck cancer.

Dr Chao-Chun Lin graduated from Kaohsiung Medical University in 2000 and completed her radiology residency at Kaohsiung Medical University Chung-Ho Memorial Hospital. She then pursued a three-year fellowship in neurointervention at Hualien Tzu Chi Hospital from 2004 to 2007. Subsequently, she earned her PhD in Neuroscience from the Graduate Institute of Medical Device and Imaging at National Taiwan University (2008–2013). Currently, Dr Lin serves as an assistant professor of Radiology and a neuroradiologist at China Medical University. She has a strong passion for teaching neuroradiology, with a particular focus on head and neck imaging.

Dr Hung-Chieh Chen graduated with a degree in Medicine from National Yang-Ming University, Taipei, Taiwan, and completed her radiology training at Taipei Veterans General Hospital. She furthered her expertise with overseas training, attending the 2010 ERASMUS Course on MRI—Head and Neck in Brugge, and participating in the 2013 International Fellowship Program in Japan. With 16 years of professional experience in diagnostic radiology and interventional neuroradiology, Dr Chen is now the Director of the Division of MRI, Department of Radiology at Taichung Veterans General Hospital. Dr Chen specializes in using advanced imaging techniques, such as CT, MRI, and angiography, to diagnose and treat various diseases. She has published 53 papers in SCI journals on topics including headaches and neurodegenerative diseases. Actively participating in international radiology conferences, Dr Chen shares and learns about the latest developments and technologies in the field. She also serves as a guest editor for "Diagnostics" and "Frontiers in Neurology." Dr Chen aims to further enhance her expertise in diagnostic radiology and mentor the next generation of physicians, encouraging more talented professionals to join the field of medical imaging. Her long-term goal is to become an internationally recognized radiology expert, driving innovation and improvements in neuroradiology to increase the efficiency and accuracy of diagnosis and treatment.

Dr Chih-Chun Wu graduated from Kaohsiung Medical University in 2004. After completing her residency training at Taipei Veterans General Hospital from 2005 to 2010, she continued her career there and became a key member of the brain tumor board. In 2016, Dr Wu served as a visiting fellow at NYU Langone Hospital and became an Assistant Professor at National Yang Ming Chiao Tung University School of Medicine in 2018. From 2019 to 2022, she held the position of Secretary-General of the Taiwan Society of Neuroradiology. Dr Wu specializes in neuroradiology diagnoses, with notable research on the use of diffusion-weighted imaging for preoperative glioma grading and predicting the response of acoustic neuromas to Gamma Knife treatment. Her work aims to enhance diagnostic accuracy and improve patient outcomes in neuro-oncology.

Together, these women neuroradiologists exemplify leadership, innovation, and excellence in advancing neuroimaging capabilities in Taiwan. Their collective efforts not only enhance patient care but also inspire and mentor aspiring professionals, ensuring continued progress and innovation in neuroradiology.

Women In Neuroradiology and Neurointervention in Thailand

Nitaya Suwanwela

In Thailand, hospitals in modern medicine mode began about 120 years ago and the first radiographic equipment was installed around 1914. Radiological services were covered by general medical doctors, who were mainly male. However, the number of female medical doctors rapidly increased, including radiologists.

Professor Tawan Surawongse Bunnag, who was trained and received Diplomate of the American Board of Radiologists, returned to work at the King Chulalongkorn Memorial Hospital (KCMH), Bangkok, as a fulltime radiologist. Besides general radiological services, she initiated the first cerebral angiography and pneumoencephalography in the country in 1958.

While neurological services started in Thailand much earlier, neurosurgical services were available around 1950s. At that time, neuroradiological procedures were carried out by the neurosurgeons, in cooperation with the radiologists. Associate Professor Kalaya Chienpradit, a female doctor, returned from her training in the United States and practiced inclusively neuroradiology at King Chulalongkorn Memorial Hospital and Chulalongkorn University Medical School, being the first neuroradiologist in Thailand.

The development of neuroradiology thereafter progressed rapidly with many returned from training in neuroradiology abroad, parallel with the expansion of neurology and neurosurgery services. Modern up-to-date neuroradiological equipment was installed as well as procedures initiated. Professor Nitaya Suwanwela returned in 1971 at Chulalongkorn Hospital Medical School and Professor Preeya Kanchanathithi in 1972 at Siriraj Hospital Medical School, both were responsible in the expansion of neuroradiological services, research, and teaching for radiologists and medical students. Associate Professor Wiyada Bhoopat returned in 1979 to Siriraj Hospital Medical School and helped in initiation interventional neuroradiological service. While specialty training in radiology had been offered as early as 1960s, additional training in neuroradiology as a new subspecialty training for both general radiologists and as full-fledged neuroradiologists was officially recognized later by the Royal College of Radiologists of Thailand.

In 1990s, Professor Orasa Chawalparit and Professor Anchalee Churojana joined the Siriraj group. More females, Associate Professor Pacharin Pakanan and Professor Jiraporn Laothamatas, were responsible for the establishment of neuroradiology at the Faculty of Medicine Ramathibodi Hospital, Mahidol University. Neuroradiological services and training centers were also established outside Bangkok, for example Associate Professor Wantana Prapakorn established one at Chiangmai University Medical School in Northern Thailand.

Interventional neuroradiology in Thailand has developed as a branch of neuroradiology by the effort of many neuroradiologists, namely, Professor Sirintara (Pongpech) Singhara Na Ayudhaya at Ramathibodi Hospital Mahidol University, and Professor Anchalee Churojana at Siriraj and the Group. Under the auspices of the Royal College of Radiologists of Thailand, a separate training for interventional neuroradiology has been established. The Association of Thai Interventional Neuroradiology was then set-up. Professor Sirintara (Pongpech) Singhara Na Ayudhaya was the President of World Federation of Interventional and Therapeutic Neuroradiology (WFITN) during 2015–2017. She became Honorary President of WFNRS in 2021.

Notably, neuroradiologists were recognized in the radiologist circle. Professor Jiraporn Laothamatas and Professor Anchalee Churojana were elected to be the President of the Royal Collage of Radiologists in Thailand during 2013–2017 and 2017–2020, respectively.

Professor Nitaya Suwanwela was involved in the formation of the Asian-Oceanian Society of Neuroradiology and Head & Neck Radiology at Kumamoto, Japan. She served as President of the AOCNHNR Congress organized in Bangkok. She together with Professor Sirintara (Pongpech) Singhara Na Ayudhaya and Professor Anchalee Churojana have served on the board of the Society.

In summary, female neuroradiologists have played a major and important role in the development and progress of neuroradiology in Thailand. It is predictable that the specialty of neuroradiology will flourish in Thailand in the future.

Professor Tawan Surawongse Bunnag

Professor Tawan Surawongse Bunnag was the first woman radiologist in Thailand. She graduated in medicine from the University of the Philippines in 1936 (Fig. 23.39). She, at first, served as a surgeon at King Chulalongkorn Memorial Hospital, and then, in 1939, went for training in radiology at Berlin, Germany. After returning to Thailand, she was appointed Head of the Department of Radiology. In 1952, she went to study at the Bellevue Hospital in New York and was awarded as Diplomate of the American Board of Radiology. As Head of the Department for 30 years, she was significantly responsible for the development and progresses in radiological services, education, and research in Thailand. Notably, she also pioneered in the introduction of cerebral angiography and pneumoencephalography. She was also among the founders of the Radiological Society of Thailand.

Professor Nitaya Suwanwela

Professor Nitaya Suwanwela received her medical degree from Chulalongkorn Hospital Medical School in Thailand in 1963 (Fig. 23.40). She completed the residency program in radiology at Chulalongkorn Hospital. She then undertook fellowship in neuroradiology under the supervision of Professor Isadore Meschan at the Wake Forest University, United States. She worked exclusively as a

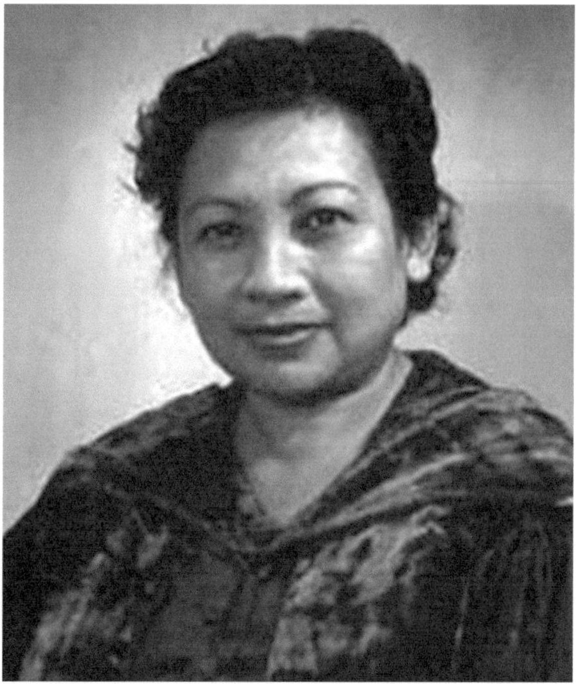

Fig. 23.39 Professor Tawan Surawongse Bunnag

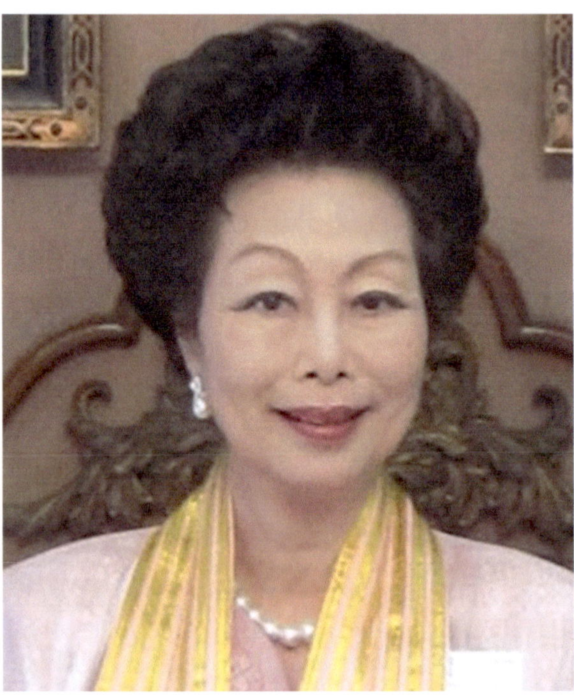

Fig. 23.40 Professor Nitaya Suwanwela

neuroradiologist and pioneered the development of neuroradiology in Thailand. She initiated the training program for residents and fellows in neuroradiology at Chulalongkorn Hospital Medical School. In 1989, she became Chairperson of the Department of Radiology, when CT scan, MRI, and nuclear medicine together with procedures and software expanded the scope of neuroradiology, which was established as a special unit. Research was emphasized and there were widely cited publications in international journals, for example, a morphologic classification of frontoethmoidal encephalomeningocele, arterial narrowing and spasm in acute head injuries, and intracranial mycotic aneurysms from extravascular origins. She served in national and international academic bodies. She was involved in the founding of the AOSNHNR and served as Thai National Delegate as well as Regional Delegate to the World Federation.

Professor Nitaya Suwanwela received many awards, such as Best Research of the Year in Medical Sciences from National Research Council of Thailand, Distinguished Contributor to Nuclear Medicine by Thailand Office of Atoms for Peace, Distinguished Academic Radiologist by the Royal College of Radiologists of Thailand and by the Radiological Society of Thailand, and Most Distinguished Medal in Recognition of Contributions in the Arts and Sciences by the Thai Government.

Professor Preeya Kanchanathiti

Professor Preeya Kanchanathiti was the first neuroradiologist at Siriraj Hospital Medical School, Mahidol University (Fig. 23.41). She was trained in the United States and got her Diploma in Radiology. After returning to Thailand in 1964, she was responsible for neuroradiological services. At that time, neuroradiological procedures were performed by neurosurgeons. She then, in 1972, went for additional training in neuroradiology at Ullevål Hospital University of Oslo, in Norway. She was credited for performing the first transfemoral cerebral angiography at the Siriraj Hospital. She also served for many years as the Head of the Department of Radiology at Siriraj Hospital.

Associate Professor Wiyada Bhoopat

Associate Professor Wiyada Bhoopat graduated in medicine at Siriraj Hospital Medical School, Mahidol University in 1969 (Fig. 23.42). She was a resident at Beth Israel Hospital in Boston, the United States and received the Diplomate of the American Board of Radiology in 1974. She then took up Fellowship in neuroradiology at the Peter Bent Brigham Hospital, in Boston. Upon returning as a neuroradiologist to Siriraj Hospital in Thailand in 1976, she, together with a male neuroradiologist, was responsible for performing the first case of interventional neuroradiology in Thailand.

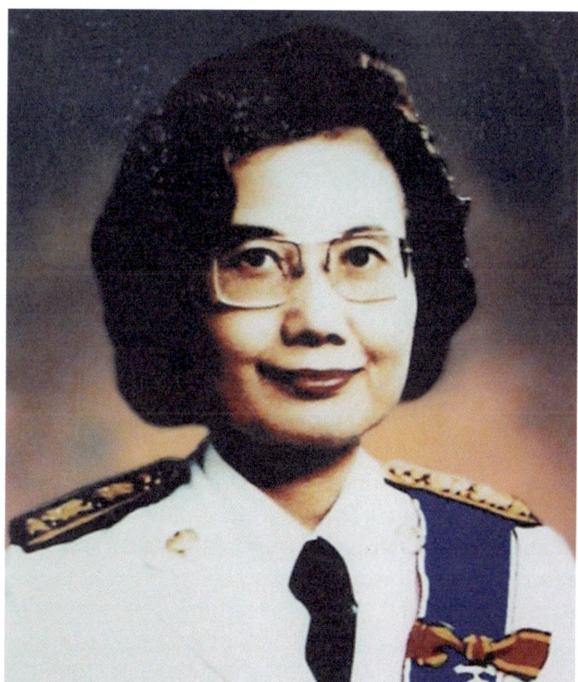

Fig. 23.41 Professor Preeya Kanchanathiti

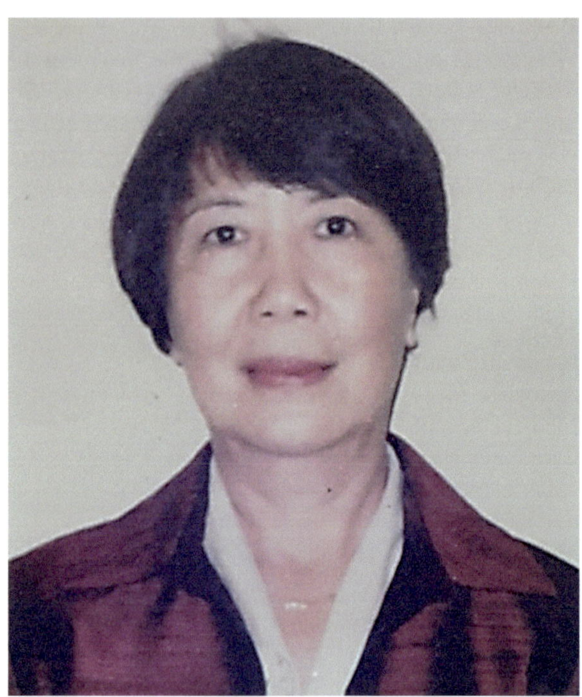

Fig. 23.42 Associate Professor Wiyada Bhoopat

Professor Orasa Chawalparit

Professor Orasa Chawatparit graduated from the Mahidol University in 1983 and completed her radiological residency also at Mahidol University, receiving the Diploma from Thai Board of Diagnostic Radiology in 1989 (Fig. 23.43). She was then a research fellow in neuroimaging at the Massachusetts General Hospital in Boston, United States until 1992. Upon returning to Thailand, she served at Siriraj Hospital Medical School, Mahidol University, in teaching, research, and patient services in radiology as well as neuroradiology. She has also been an examiner for the Thai Board of Diagnostic Radiology and of Neuroradiology.

Professor Anchalee Churojana

Professor Anchalee Churojana graduated in medicine from Siriraj Hospital Medical School, Mahidol University in 1982 (Fig. 23.44). After training in radiology at Siriraj, she was certified by the Board of Radiology of Thailand in 1988. She was, in 1996, a research fellow in interventional neuroradiology at Lahey Hitchcock Medical Center, in Burlington, United States, and then in the following year served as a research fellow in interventional neuroradiology at Bicetre Hospital in France. At Siriraj Hospital, she pioneered the development of interventional neuroradiology, and served as Chief of the Siriraj Center of Interventional Neuroradiology. She received the Diploma of the Thai Subspecialty Board of Diagnostic Neuroradiology as well as the International Diploma in Neurovascular Diseases from Universite Paris XI, Francaise. Professor Anchalee Churojana was the President of the Royal

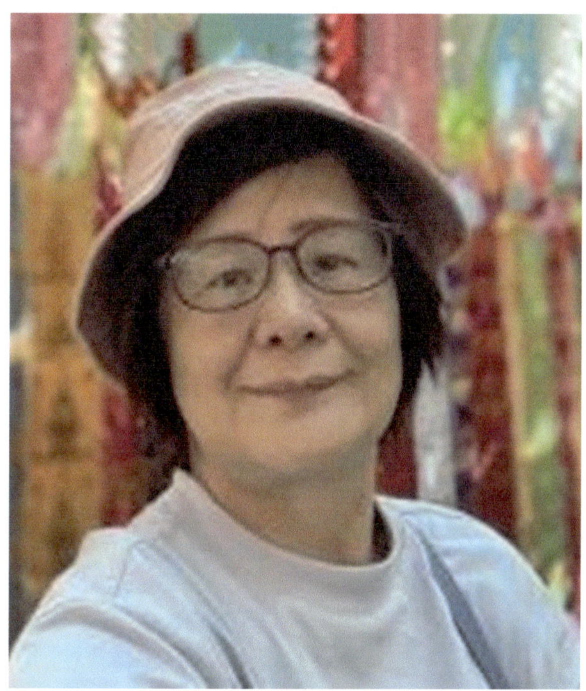

Fig. 23.43 Professor Orasa Chawālparit

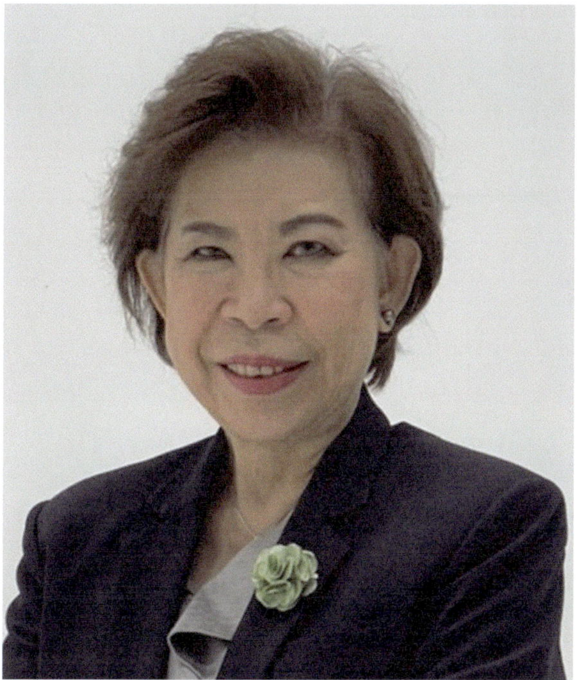

Fig. 23.44 Professor Anchalee Churojana

College of Radiologists of Thailand, and also President of the Association of Thai Interventional Neuroradiology. In 2023, she became Vice-President of AAFITN Council.

Professor Jiraporn Laothamatas

Professor Jiraporn Laothamatas graduated in medicine with honor from the Faculty of Medicine, Chulalongkorn University in 1981 (Fig. 23.45). She completed her residency at the College of Physicians and Surgeons, Columbia University in New York, United States and received the Diplomate of the American Board in Diagnostic Radiology in 1989. She also received Fellowship Certificate in diagnostic neuroradiology from Nahnemann University Hospital in Philadelphia, United States. Upon returning to Thailand, she pioneered the founding of diagnostic neuroradiological services at the Faculty of Medicine Ramathibodi Hospital, Mahidol University. She also served in many professional works, namely, Director of Advanced Diagnostic Image Center of the Faculty of Medicine, President of the Royal College of Radiologists of Thailand, President of the Radiological Society of Thailand as well as Chair of the Subcommittee on Medical Nuclear Energy Utilization of the Thailand Office of Atoms for Peace.

Professor Jiraporn Laothamatas received many awards, and since 2018 has been Dean of the Faculty of Health Science Technology, Chulabhorn Royal Academy, Thailand.

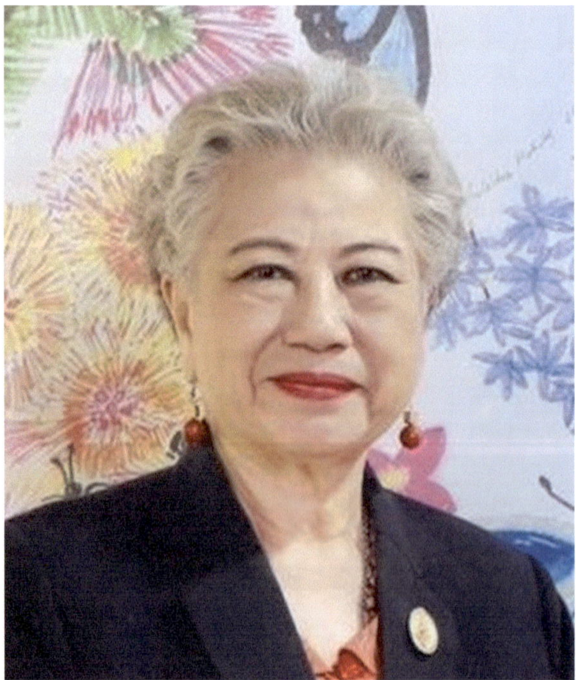

Fig. 23.45 Professor Jiraporn Laothamatas

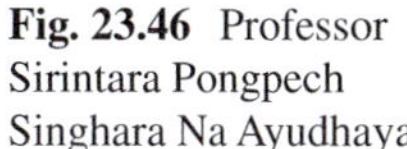

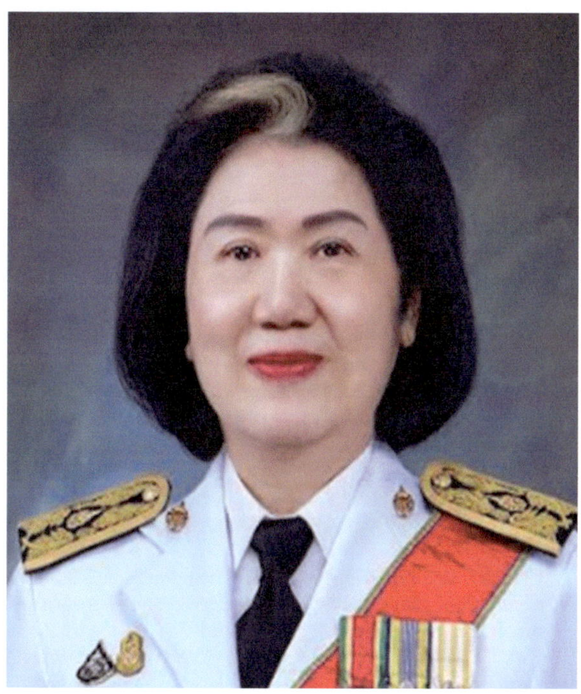

Fig. 23.46 Professor Sirintara Pongpech Singhara Na Ayudhaya

Professor Sirintara Pongpech Singhara Na Ayudhaya

Professor Sirintara Pongpech Singhara Na Ayudhaya graduated as doctor of medicine with honor from Mahidol University in 1983 and after training, received the Certificate of the Thai Board of Radiology (Fig. 23.46). She also was certified by Thai Board of Neuroimaging and Interventional Neuroradiology in 2006. She spent her time under the supervision of Professor Pierre Lasjaunias, and in 1995, received the Certificate in Interventional Neuroradiology from Bicetre Hospital, Paris-Sud University, France. At the Ramathibodi Hospital, Mahidol University, she was active in pioneering teaching, research and patient services, both as neuroradiologist and neurointerventionist. She has also been active in the regional activities, namely, being Honorary Visiting Professor at the University of Medicine and Pharmacy, HCMC, Vietnam, Co-Director of the so called “PLANET” International MSc Course in Neurovascular Diseases, a collaborative effort between Paris-Sud and Mahidol Universities for teaching and training in interventional neuroradiology.

Professor Sirintara Pongpech Singhara Na Ayudhaya received many national and international awards. She was Honorary President of SNRXXII under WFNRS (World Federation of Neuroradiological Societies), and President of AAFITN (Asian-Australasian Federation of Interventional and Therapeutic Neuroradiology.

Readers are suggested to contact the corresponding author for figures if needed.

References

1. Moon WJ, Jung SL, Lee JH, et al. Benign and malignant thyroid nodules: US differentiation – multicenter retrospective study. Radiology. 2008;247:762–70.
2. Jung SL, Baek JH, Lee JH, et al. Efficacy and safety of radiofrequency ablation for benign thyroid nodules: a prospective multicenter study. Korean J Radiol. 2018;19:167–74.
3. Choi JD, Moon Y, Kim HJ, Yim Y, Lee S, Moon WJ. Choroid plexus volume and permeability at brain MRI within the Alzheimer disease clinical spectrum. Radiology. 2022;304:635–45.
4. Kim HW, Lee S, Yang JH, Moon Y, Lee J, Moon WJ. Cortical iron accumulation as an imaging marker for neurodegeneration in clinical cognitive impairment spectrum: a quantitative susceptibility mapping study. Korean J Radiol. 2023;24:1131–41.
5. Moon Y, Jeon HJ, Han SH, et al. Blood-brain barrier breakdown is linked to tau pathology and neuronal injury in a differential manner according to amyloid deposition. J Cereb Blood Flow Metab. 2023;43:1813–25.
6. Oh G, Moon Y, Moon WJ, Ye JC. Unpaired deep learning for pharmacokinetic parameter estimation from dynamic contrast-enhanced MRI without AIF measurements. Neuroimage. 2024;291:120571.
7. Moon WJ, Lim C, Ha IH, et al. Hippocampal blood-brain barrier permeability is related to the APOE4 mutation status of elderly individuals without dementia. J Cereb Blood Flow Metab. 2021;41:1351–61.
8. Choi YJ, Lee JH, Kim HO, et al. Histogram analysis of apparent diffusion coefficients for occult tonsil cancer in patients with cervical nodal metastasis from an unknown primary site at presentation. Radiology. 2016;278:146–55.
9. Park CJ, Kim JH, Ahn SS, Lee SK, Koh YW, Kim J. Preoperative MRI evaluation of thyroid cartilage invasion in patients with laryngohypopharyngeal cancer: comparison of contrast-enhanced 2D spin-echo and 3D T1-weighted radial gradient recalled-echo techniques. AJNR Am J Neuroradiol. 2021;42:1690–4.
10. Bae S, Lee HJ, Nam W, Koh YW, Choi EC, Kim J. MR lymphography for sentinel lymph node detection in patients with oral cavity cancer: preliminary clinical study. Head Neck. 2018;40:1483–8.
11. Shin NY, Lee JH, Kang WJ, Koh YW, Sohn B, Kim J. Clinical usefulness of [18F]FDG PET-CT and CT/MRI for detecting nodal metastasis in patients with hypopharyngeal squamous cell carcinoma. Ann Surg Oncol. 2015;22:994–9.
12. Kim HJ, Lee SB, Choi JW, et al. Multiphase MR angiography collateral map: functional outcome after acute anterior circulation ischemic stroke. Radiology. 2020;295:192–201.
13. Lee JO, Ahn SS, Choi KS, et al. Added prognostic value of 3D deep learning-derived features from preoperative MRI for adult-type diffuse gliomas. Neuro Oncol. 2024;26:571–80.
14. Park YW, Choi KS, Foltyn-Dumitru M, et al. Incorporating supramaximal resection into survival stratification of IDH-wildtype glioblastoma: a refined multi-institutional recursive partitioning analysis. Clin Cancer Res. 2024; https://doi.org/10.1158/1078-0432.CCR-23-3845.
15. Park YW, Jang G, Kim SB, et al. Leptomeningeal metastases in isocitrate dehydrogenase-wildtype glioblastomas revisited: comprehensive analysis of incidence, risk factors, and prognosis based on post-contrast fluid-attenuated inversion recovery. Neuro Oncol. 2024;26:1921–32.
16. Kang KM, Song J, Choi Y, et al. MRI scoring systems for predicting isocitrate dehydrogenase mutation and chromosome 1p/19q codeletion in adult-type diffuse glioma lacking contrast enhancement. Radiology. 2024;311:e233120.
17. Kang KM, Kim KM, Kim IS, et al. Functional magnetic resonance imaging and diffusion tensor imaging for language mapping in brain tumor surgery: validation with direct cortical stimulation and cortico-cortical evoked potential. Korean J Radiol. 2023;24:553–63.
18. Kang KM, Byun MS, Yi D, et al. Enlarged perivascular spaces are associated with decreased brain tau deposition. CNS Neurosci Ther. 2023;29:577–86.

19. Kang KM, Choi SH, Chul-Kee P, et al. Differentiation between glioblastoma and primary CNS lymphoma: application of DCE-MRI parameters based on arterial input function obtained from DSC-MRI. Eur Radiol. 2021;31:9098–109.
20. Kang KM, Byun MS, Lee JH, et al. Association of carotid and intracranial stenosis with Alzheimer's disease biomarkers. Alzheimers Res Ther. 2020;12:106.
21. Shin NY, Bang M, Yoo SW, et al. Cortical thickness from MRI to predict conversion from mild cognitive impairment to dementia in Parkinson disease: a machine learning-based model. Radiology. 2021;300:390–9.
22. Bae YJ, Kim JM, Choi BS, et al. Altered brain glymphatic flow at diffusion-tensor MRI in rapid eye movement sleep behavior disorder. Radiology. 2023;307:e221848.
23. Bae YJ, Kim JM, Sohn CH, et al. Imaging the substantia Nigra in Parkinson disease and other Parkinsonian syndromes. Radiology. 2021;300:260–78.
24. Bae YJ, Kim JM, Kim KJ, et al. Loss of substantia Nigra hyperintensity at 3.0-T MR imaging in idiopathic REM sleep behavior disorder: comparison with (123)I-FP-CIT SPECT. Radiology. 2018;287:285–93.
25. Lee S, Yoo RE, Choi SH, et al. Contrast-enhanced MRI T1 mapping for quantitative evaluation of putative dynamic glymphatic activity in the human brain in sleep-wake states. Radiology. 2021;300:661–8.
26. Ji SH, Yoo RE, Choi SH, et al. Dynamic contrast-enhanced MRI quantification of altered vascular permeability in autoimmune encephalitis. Radiology. 2024;310:e230701.
27. Yoo RE, Yun TJ, Cho YD, et al. Utility of arterial spin labeling perfusion magnetic resonance imaging in prediction of angiographic vascularity of meningiomas. J Neurosurg. 2016;125:536–43.
28. Yoo RE, Yun TJ, Rhim JH, et al. Bright vessel appearance on arterial spin labeling MRI for localizing arterial occlusion in acute ischemic stroke. Stroke. 2015;46:564–7.
29. Park JE, Kim HS, Park SY, Jung SC, Kim JH, Heo HY. Identification of early response to anti-angiogenic therapy in recurrent glioblastoma: amide proton transfer-weighted and perfusion-weighted MRI compared with diffusion-weighted MRI. Radiology. 2020;295:397–406.
30. Joo L, Park JE, Park SY, et al. Extensive peritumoral edema and brain-to-tumor interface MRI features enable prediction of brain invasion in meningioma: development and validation. Neuro Oncol. 2021;23:324–33.
31. Park JE, Kim HS, Kim N, Park SY, Kim YH, Kim JH. Spatiotemporal heterogeneity in multiparametric physiologic MRI is associated with patient outcomes in IDH-wildtype glioblastoma. Clin Cancer Res. 2021;27:237–45.
32. Moon HH, Jeong J, Park JE, et al. Generative AI in glioma: ensuring diversity in training image phenotypes to improve diagnostic performance for IDH mutation prediction. Neuro Oncol. 2024;26:1124–35.
33. Park JE, Oh JY, Park DH, et al. Mapping tumor habitats in IDH-wild type glioblastoma: integrating MR imaging, pathologic, and RNA data from Ivy glioblastoma Atlas Project. Neuro Oncol. 2024; https://doi.org/10.1093/neuonc/noae161.
34. Joo B, Park M, Ahn SJ, Suh SH. Assessment of meningeal lymphatics in the parasagittal dural space: a prospective feasibility study using dynamic contrast-enhanced magnetic resonance imaging. Korean J Radiol. 2023;24:444–53.
35. Park M, Moon Y, Han SH, Kim HK, Moon WJ. Myelin loss in white matter hyperintensities and normal-appearing white matter of cognitively impaired patients: a quantitative synthetic magnetic resonance imaging study. Eur Radiol. 2019;29:4914–21.
36. Choi YS, Bae S, Chang JH, et al. Fully automated hybrid approach to predict the IDH mutation status of gliomas via deep learning and radiomics. Neuro Oncol. 2021;23:304–13.
37. Do KH, Beck KS, Lee JM. The growing problem of radiologist shortages: korean perspective. Korean J Radiol. 2023;24:1173–5.

Chapter 24
Women's Contribution to the World History of Neuroradiology: Europa Chapter

María Isabel Vargas, Sofie Van Cauter, Zulejha Merhemic, Primarius Martina Špero, Jennifer Linn, Chiara Zini, Nicoletta Emanuela Anzalone, Anna Zimny, Marta Drake-Perez, Pia C. Sundgren, Kees J. Simon, Frans W. Zonneveld, Aysenur Cila, and Isil Saatci

M. I. Vargas (✉)
Clinique des Grangettes, Hirslanden, Chêne Bougeries, Geneva, Switzerland
e-mail: maria-isabel.vargas@hirslanden.ch

S. Van Cauter
Department of Medical Imaging, East-Limburg Hospital Genk, Genk, Belgium
e-mail: sofie.vancauter@zol.be

Z. Merhemic
Faculty of Health Care and Pharmacology, University Travnik, Travnik, Bosnia and Herzegovina

P. M. Špero
Department of Radiology, Affidea, Zagreb, Croatia

J. Linn
Institute for Diagnostic and Interventional Neuroradiology, University Hospital Carl Gustav Carus, Dresden, Germany

Medical Faculty of the Technical University Dresden, Dresden, Germany
e-mail: Jennifer.linn@ukdd.de

C. Zini
Department of Radiology, USL Toscana Centro, Firenze, Italy

N. E. Anzalone
Neuroradiology Department, IRCCS San Raffaele Scientific Institute, Milan, Italy

Vita-Salute San Raffaele University, Milan, Italy
e-mail: anzalone.nicoletta@hsr.it

A. Zimny
Department of General and Interventional Radiology and Neuroradiology, Wroclaw Medical University, Wroclaw, Poland
e-mail: anna.zimny@umed.wroc.pl

M. Drake-Perez
Department of Radiology—Neuroradiology, Hospital Universitario Marqués de Valdecilla and IDIVAL, Santander, Spain

D. Birchall (ed.), *A World History of Neuroradiology*,
https://doi.org/10.1007/978-3-032-16653-1_24

Women in Neuroradiology: Belgium

Sofie Van Cauter

Introduction

Neuroradiology in Belgium was established in the 1960s by a group of radiologists and neurologists, and good friends in the different Belgian University Hospitals: professor Louis Jeanmart (Brussels), professor Lucien Appel (Antwerp), professor Georges Cornelis (Brussels), professor André Thibault (Liège), professor Eric VandeVelde (Ghent), and later prof Roland Potvliege (Brussels).

In Belgium, as in many other countries in the 1960s, radiology and neuroradiology were in a period of significant development and transformation with multiple new emerging techniques such as pneumoencephalography, cerebral angiography, X-ray, and later computer tomography.

In the generation after the founding group, there was one notable female neuroradiologist, who still has an impact today, particularly known for her contributions to the development and advancement of neuroradiological techniques and education in Belgium. Let me introduce Professor Danielle Balériaux.

It should be emphasized that neuroradiology in Belgium has been a male-dominated domain since its inception. It has only been a decade since multiple female colleagues have taken up positions in neuroradiology departments in University Hospitals and large tertiary centers, which makes the career of Professor Balériaux even more noteworthy.

P. C. Sundgren
Department of Radiology, Institution of Clinical Sciences/Lund, Lund University, Lund, Sweden
e-mail: Pia.Sundgren@med.lu.se

K. J. Simon · F. W. Zonneveld
Historical Section of the Dutch Society of Radiology, Domus Medica, Utrecht, The Netherlands
e-mail: kjsimon@molenbocht.nl; nvvr@radiologen.nl

A. Cila
Radiology Department, Medipol University, Istanbul, Turkey
e-mail: acila@medipol.edu.tr

I. Saatci
Private Koru Hospitals, Interventional Neuroradiology Department, Ankara, Turkey

A Summary of the Career of Professor Danielle Balériaux

Danielle Balériaux was born in Ostend, at the Belgian seaside. Her father was an engineer and taught her to reason without prejudice. She will take this advice as one of the most important lessons throughout her life.

After obtaining her medical degree *cum magna lauda* at the Université Libre de Bruxelles (ULB, Free University of Brussels), she applied for a position as a neurologist but was refused and therefore applied for a residency in radiology at the Bordet Institute in Brussels, a specialized general hospital and research institute of the ULB specializing in oncology, and today a renowned Belgian hospital. The university's Neurosurgical department was also located in this hospital.

She was recruited by the head of the Department of Radiology, Professor Georgette Melot, who herself had a special interest in neurology and neuroradiology. Georgette Melot had ordered new equipment specifically devoted to neuroradiological procedures but unfortunately passed away suddenly due to a subarachnoid hemorrhage during a congress in London. As Danielle Balériaux had a special interest in neurology, she was asked to install and develop the new neuroradiological procedures foreseen by Professor Melot. She completed at the same time her training in radiology successfully and was appointed staff radiologist in the same hospital.

At the beginning of her career, Danielle Balériaux visited multiple neuroradiology departments throughout Europe to obtain knowledge about the different developing techniques in neuroradiology. She developed successfully pneumoencephalography, cerebral angiography, and computed tomography at the radiology department of the Bordet Hospital.

In 1976, she worked with one of the first CT scanners in Belgium. Her research was conducted to compare brain slices obtained by autopsy with the CT images obtained before death, to better understand neuropathology. At that time, no dedicated brain atlas was available, and specimens of histopathologists only comprised coronal sections.

She collaborated on the first book on neuro-anatomico-pathology together with Professor Auguste Wackenheim (Strasbourg, France), also one of the founders of ESNR.

In 1980, she changed hospitals to the newly opened Hôpital Erasme (Erasmus Hospital), the academic teaching hospital of the ULB. She successfully built a section of neuroradiology, with an excellent reputation for clinical practice and scientific research. In recognition of her academic and scientific achievements, she was appointed in 1981 as professor of neuroradiology at the ULB. In 1992, she became vice-chairman of the department of radiology at Hôpital Erasme. This would be her main workplace until 2006 when she retired.

In the early 1980s, Danielle Balériaux was a pioneer in the use of magnetic resonance imaging (MRI) in neuroradiology. She visited the first MRI research facilities in Europe and especially in the United States and attended the very first MR meetings. At the same time, she established a close collaboration with Philips Medical Systems in Best, the Netherlands, to develop the first neuroradiological applications for MRI, developing and evaluating MR sequences together with scientists. From early 1983, she traveled weekly to the Philips factory in Best to scan selected patients, which led to an early evaluation of MR images and to the installation of one of the first MRI units in a Belgian academic center in 1984. Her work helped to establish MRI as a vital tool for non-invasive and detailed imaging of the brain and spinal cord.

Professor Balériaux has accumulated an impressive scientific curriculum vitae. She has (co-) authored more than 214 peer-reviewed scientific papers and written 36 book chapters. She successfully introduced several important innovations in the organization of clinically oriented scientific research and teaching. She was the editor of a series of educational CD-ROMs on neuroradiology. She trained numerous radiologists and neuroradiologists, of whom many have become notable international neuroradiologists.

She was one of the co-founders of the European Course of Neuroradiology (ECNR) of the European Society of Neuroradiology (ESNR), together with Professor Pierre Lasjaunias (Paris, France), Professor Claude Manelfe (Toulouse, France), and Professor Ugo Salvolini (Ancona, Italy). From 1993 to 1996, she was vice president of ESNR. Since 1990, she has also been involved in the Erasmus Course on Magnetic Resonance Imaging (EMRI). In 1993, she organized together with Brigitte Appel, the annual meeting of ESNR in Bruges. In 1994, she developed a partnership with Rui Jin Hospital affiliated with Shanghai Medical University, where she was a visiting professor. Her leadership roles in these organizations helped to advance the field both in Belgium and internationally.

Throughout her career, she received numerous awards and honors in recognition of her contributions to neuroradiology. In 1995, she was awarded the Torgny Greitz lecturer prize (Karolinska Hospital, Stockholm, Sweden). She became a member of the prestigious Royal Academy of Medicine of Belgium and a corresponding member of the Académie Nationale de Médecine Française. She is an honorary member of the European Society of Neuroradiology, the Japanese Society of Neuroradiology, and the French Society of Radiology. She is a fellow of the International Society of Magnetic Resonance in Medicine (ISMRM). In 2006, in recognition of her international efforts and service to the country of Belgium, she was appointed "Grand Officier de l'Ordre de Léopold" (Belgium's highest civilian honor). These accolades underscore her impact on the field and her commitment to advancing medical science.

Danielle Balériaux's legacy in neuroradiology is marked by her dedication to clinical excellence, research, and education. Her work has had a lasting impact on the field, influencing both the practice of neuroradiology and the training of future specialists.

About the Author

Sofie Van Cauter (Fig. 24.1) is a Belgian neuro- and head and neck radiologist since 2015. She followed her radiology training at the University Hospitals of Leuven in Belgium with additional fellowships at the University of Florida, USA, with professor Anthony Mancuso, Sick Kids Hospital in Toronto, and Erasmus University Medical Centre in the Netherlands. In 2013, she obtained an awarded PhD on advanced MR imaging techniques in gliomas. Since 2015, she has been a staff radiologist at East Limburg Hospital in Genk and a professor of neuroanatomy at Hasselt University. She is a member of multiple working groups on neuro- and head and neck radiology in the College of Oncology in Belgium, the European Society of Neuroradiology (ESNR), the European Society of Radiology (ESR), and the World Federation of Neuroradiological Societies (WFNRS), and regularly gives lectures at national and international conferences. She has been the president of the neuroradiology section of the Belgian Society of Radiology in 2021–2022. Currently, she is the Section Editor of AI and Advanced Imaging in Neuroradiology. Her current research interests are artificial intelligence and neurovascular imaging.

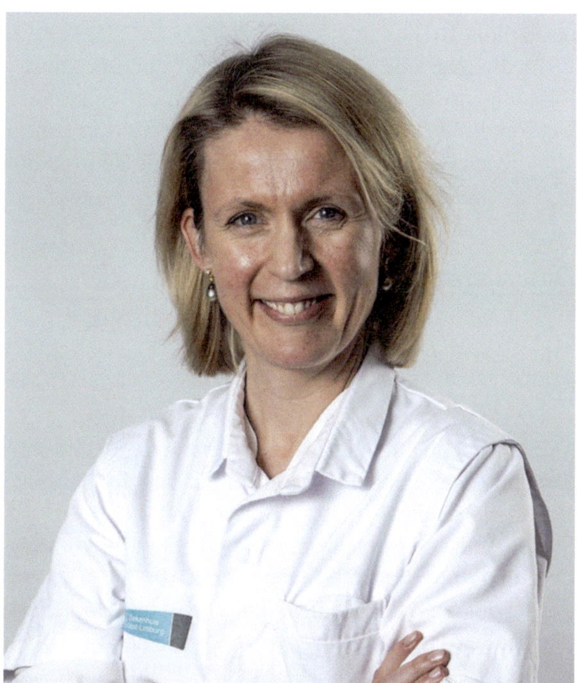

Fig. 24.1 Sofie Van Cauter

Women in Neuroradiology: Bosnia and Herzegovina

Zulejha Merhemic

Introduction

Radiology in Bosnia and Herzegovina has a long history, which begins with the installation of the first X-ray machine in the State Hospital—Koševo in 1899, where Dr. Preisberger, Head of Surgery, demonstrated the use of this machine.

In 1920, a special Radiology Department of the Sarajevo State Hospital was founded. It was a rather neglected department until the appointment of Prof. Dr. Lovrinčević as Head of Radiology in 1974. Prof. Lovrinčević reorganized the radiology by departments and the Neuroradiology Department was thus created. In 1978, we got a CT (the first in the former Yugoslavia), and in 1989, the Magnetic Resonance Imaging machine was also the first in Yugoslavia.

Although there were more than half of female radiologists at the Institute of Radiology, the Department of Neuroradiology was somehow male-dominated, and only at the end of the twentieth century women took the lead in Neuroradiology throughout BiH.

In Bosnia and Herzegovina, all doctors must complete specialization in Radiodiagnostics, which lasts 5 years, and since there is no subspecialization in Neuroradiology, all doctors acquire the right to bear the name of neuroradiologist after 5 years of work in the Department of Neuroradiology.

Description

Marijana Karlović-Vidaković, MD, General radiologist, Subspecialist Neuroradiologist

Dr. Marijana Karlović-Vidaković was born in Sarajevo, graduated from the Medical Faculty at the University Sarajevo, Bosnia and Herzegovina. She worked as a Family Medicine Physician, after which she specialized in Radiology at the University Clinical Centre in Sarajevo (2003).

She finished subspecialization in Neuroradiology at the University Clinical Centre in Split, Croatia, in the year 2010.

She obtained her Medical diploma in the Medical Faculty of Zagreb in 2013 and finished her PhD studies at the Medical Faculty in Split, Croatia.

She worked at the University Clinical Hospital in Mostar, Bosnia and Herzegovina. Since 2015–2019, she worked as the Head of Neuroradiology Department, 2019–2020 as the Deputy Head of Clinic for Radiology, and 2020–2021 as Head of Clinic for Radiology, Mostar, Bosnia and Herzegovina. She worked as a teaching assistant at the Medical Faculty, University of Mostar (2004–2021).

Currently works as a Deputy Head of Radiology Department in Medikol Polyclinic, Split, Croatia.

She has been full Member of European Society of Radiology since 2003 and Member of POC, Quality, Safety and Standards Committee Delegate (2011–2015), Member of Research Committee of the ESR (2015–2019); Full Member of Balkan Society of Radiology since 2012 and Member of Bylaws Committee of BCR since 2016; Vice president of the Association of Radiology of Bosnia and Herzegovina (2018–2024); Full member of European Society of Neuroradiology and European Society for Magnetic Resonance in Medicine and Biology. She is a full member of Croatian Society of Neuroradiology.

She has presented papers (published abstracts and papers), participated as an invited speaker on National Congresses and Magnetic Resonance Schools, and as an invited speaker at the Balkan Congress of Radiology since 2012 on topics in the fields of neuroradiology, head and neck and emergency radiology.

She speaks Croatian, Bosnian, Serbian, English, and German languages.

Svjetlana Jefić, MD was born in Banja Luka, Bosnia and Herzegovina. She obtained her medical degree from the University of Novi Sad, Serbia, subsequently undertaking a Course of family medicine offered by the Queens University, Toronto, Canada, in collaboration with the University of Banja Luka, Bosnia and Herzegovina, and obtained the title of Family Medicine Physician. She specialized in general radiology at the University of Banja Luka, and subspecialized in neuroradiology at the University of Novi Sad. Svjetlana has worked on cross-sectional and body imaging, with a strong focus on neuroradiological imaging, skull base pathology, and head and neck radiology. Besides attending numerous courses and conferences, she obtained certificates from the European Society of Neuroradiology by completing the European Course of Head and Neck Radiology (EDiHNNR), as well as the European Course of Neuroradiology (EDiNR). She worked as a teaching assistant at the Medical Faculty, University of Foča, Bosnia and Herzegovina. While obtaining extensive experience working at the University Clinical Centre of the Republic of Srpska, Svjetlana is currently employed at private practice. She has been an EPOS reviewer for the ECR, Head and Neck section, as well as the Neuro section, and has been invited to speak at many national conferences, as well as the BCR. She is a member on national Radiological Association, ECR, ESNR, ESHNR.

Daliborka Maric was born in 1980 in Derventa, and finished high school and the Faculty of Medicine in Banja Luka, Bosnia and Herzegovina, where she still lives and works today.

In 2006, she obtained the title of Doctor of Medicine at the Faculty of Medicine of the University of Banjaluka.

Since 2007, she has been employed at the Department of Clinical Radiology at the University Clinical Center of the Republic of Srpska.

In 2010, she began doctoral studies at the University of Nis, Serbia and since 2015, she has been a teaching assistant at the Department of Radiology at the Faculty of Medicine in Banja Luka.

While she was a radiology resident in 2011, thanks to the ESOR scholarship, she had the opportunity to spend 3 months training in Antwerp at UZA Hospital, Belgium.

She has been a general radiologist since 2012 with a strong interest in neuroradiology and musculoskeletal radiology.

In 2019, she obtained the European Diploma in Neuroradiology (EdiNR) in Oslo, which enabled her to participate much more daily in the field of neuroradiology.

She thinks that it is a big challenge to solve the pathology of the musculoskeletal and nervous system, considering that the spine and peripheral nerves are the links between the brain and the muscles on the periphery.

Prof. Dr. Zulejha Merhemic (Fig. 24.2) was born in Sarajevo in 1955, graduated from the Medical Faculty and specialized Radiology in Sarajevo, and from 1988 to 2012 worked at Clinical Center University Sarajevo, since 1996 at the Department of Neuroradiology. Three semesters were spent on University of Vienna, Austria, where she passed 10 exams and received a diploma of the Medical Faculty in Vienna. She worked in the MRI Department, AKH Vienna, and wrote a dissertation with Prof Imhof. She finished subspecialization in angiology in Sarajevo, and got an EU diploma with subspecialization in Neuroradiology. She wrote her dissertation and got a PhD at the University Sarajevo. She is Honorary Member of Slovenian

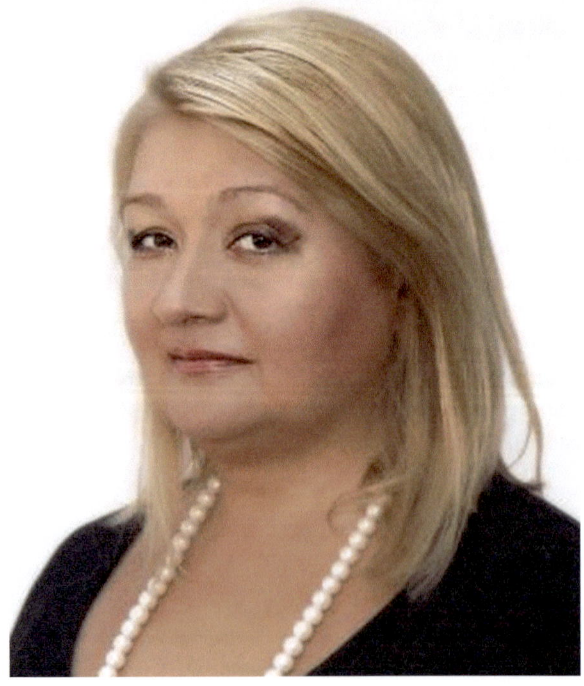

Fig. 24.2 Prof. Dr. Zulejha Merhemic, MD, PhD

Society of Neuroradiology, Serbian Society of Radiology, Serbian Society of Neuroradiology, Member of European Society of Radiology and member of scientific committee (2011–2013) and Scientific Committee Chairman in Neuro 2017; Executive committee member of Balkan Society of Radiology; Full member of European Society of Neuroradiology; and member of the Education Board and Examiner for EDiNR since 2013; Member of Association of Radiology of Bosnia & Herzegovina (and President 2010–2018); Associate Professor of Radiology, Faculty of Health Care and Pharmacology, University Travnik. She has presented papers and participated as an invited speaker at national and international congresses and schools. (more than 100 invited lectures, more than 130 published abstracts, 27 published papers, and 6 chapters in books).

She speaks Bosnian, Croatian, Serbian, English, and German languages.

Women in Neuroradiology: Croatia

Primarius Martina Špero

Description

In the Croatian language, the word "neuroradiology" is a feminine noun, which in a symbolic way reflects the strength of women, medical doctors in this important field of Croatian radiology.

Neuroradiology in Croatia officially begins with the foundation of the Section of Neuroradiology of the Croatian Society of Radiology in 1993, with its first president, Professor Nada Bešenski, who was the first woman neuroradiologist in Croatia [1].

From the very beginning of her professional life, Professor Bešenski was dedicated to neuroradiology and during the years she became a well-known and distinguished neuroradiologist at home and abroad, across Europe and in the United States of America (USA).

Nada Bešenski was born in 1943 in Krapina, a small town in the hilly Zagorje region in northern Croatia. In 1968, she graduated from the University of Zagreb School of Medicine. In 1971, she started residency in radiology at the "University Hospital Centre Zagreb" and became a certified radiologist after passing the radiology board exam in October 1974.

She continued her education in the field of neuroradiology at the University Klinik J.W. Goethe in Frankfurt, Germany, where she spent 2 months each year from 1974 to 1976. Professor Bešenski received a master's degree in 1976 and the PhD in 1979 in the field of neuroradiology.

From 1974 till 1980, she worked as a general radiologist, but mainly as a neuroradiologist. From 1980, she worked exclusively as a neuroradiologist at the

"University Hospital Centre Zagreb". In 1985, she became an associate professor at the Department of Radiology, University of Zagreb School of Medicine, and in 1988, she became a professor of radiology at the same University. In 2002, professor Bešenski left Croatia and worked as a neuroradiologist at the Medical University South Carolina (MUSC) in Charleston, USA. In 2007, she received an official license as a professor of neuroradiology by the European Board of Neuroradiology. In 2008, Professor Bešenski returned to Croatia and worked as the professor of neuroradiology at the University of Split School of Medicine until her retirement in 2013.

During her rich career, Professor Bešenski was dedicated to teaching and clinical work, brain injury, brain tumors, and white matter diseases representing special fields of interest in her research work. In her teaching career, she was devoted to graduate and postgraduate students, radiology residents, and residents of neurology, ophthalmology, and neurosurgery.

In her productive professional career, Professor Bešenski has organized many teaching courses in Croatia on the topic of neurotraumatology, brain tumors, CT and MRI in neuroradiology for radiology residents, radiologists, and neuroradiologists.

Professor Bešenski was also an invited speaker at many courses, professional meetings, symposia, and congresses at home and abroad in Austria (European Congress of Radiology) Hungary, Poland, Czech Republic, Bosnia & Herzegovina, Romania, Slovenia, and Slovakia. She is cited in the "Contribution a l'histoire de la neuroradiologie europeenne, ESNR XVI Congress—XX Anniversaire, Paris 2–6 Juliet 1989, page 92", due to her first lecture given in Europe at the XI Symposium Neuroradiologicum held in Wiesbaden 1978, titled "A Comparative study of computerized tomography and ventriculography with water soluble contrast medium".

Nada Bešenski is the author of more than 120 papers published mostly in international peer-reviewed journals, the author of the textbooks "Clinical neuroradiology of the brain" and "Clinical neuroradiology of the spine and spinal cord", and co-author of 26 chapters in different textbooks. During her professional life, she was awarded with a number of awards in the country and abroad for her scientific and teaching work with students and residents. At the Medical University of South Carolina, she was awarded with the Golden Apple Award for excellence in teaching in 2003 and with the Appreciation for enthusiastic commitment to education in Neurology in 2007.

Professor Bešenski is a member and honorary member of many professional and scientific domestic and international radiology and neuroradiology societies. She was the president of the Croatian Society of Radiology from 1996 to 2000, and was re-elected in 2000 to 2004. Professor Bešenski is a very open-minded person, highly professional with high standards. Among colleagues, she will always be considered a person who unselfishly transfers the knowledge and rich experience to younger colleagues, students and residents.

During her rich professional life Professor Bešenski had an opportunity to witness the development of neuroradiology at home and abroad, and to be a part of it. In 1992, the Croatian Society of Radiology (CSR) was founded as the professional society of the Croatian Medical Association (CMA) [1]. Foundation of the Section of Neuroradiology of the CSR followed in 1993 with Nada Bešenski as the first president and national delegate of Croatia in the ESNR.

The Section of Neuroradiology was dissolved in October 2022 and the Croatian Neuroradiological Society—Diagnostic and Interventional was founded in June 2023 under the CMA, as the legal successor of the Section of Neuroradiology of the CSR.

In 1994, the Ministry of Health of the Republic of Croatia officially recognized neuroradiology as a subspeciality in the field of radiology. For more than a decade in Croatia, the residency in radiology lasts for 5 years and is completed by the radiology board exam in front of the three-member board of radiologists appointed by the Ministry of Health. After becoming a board-certificated radiologist, one can begin a formal training in the field of neuroradiology under the supervision of a mentor who is a board-certified radiologist and neuroradiologist with at least 5 years of experience in the field of neuroradiology, officially appointed by the Ministry of Health. Board exam in front of the board consisting of a three neuroradiologists appointed by the Ministry of Health follows 2 years of fellowship in neuroradiology, including both diagnostic and interventional. For less than a decade, the European Diploma in Neuroradiology, issued by the ESNR, is formally recognized by the Ministry of Health of the Republic of Croatia as an equivalent of neuroradiology board certificate for radiologists in Croatia.

Currently, there are about 80 board-certificated neuroradiologists working in Croatia. About half of that number are women neuroradiologists. Nine neuroradiologists have since completed education and passed exams in front of the ESNR board receiving the European Diploma in Neuroradiology—about half of them are women neuroradiologists as well.

Women neuroradiologists in Croatia mainly deal with diagnostic neuroradiology, including pediatric neuroradiology and dental radiology as well. We try to leave our mark by publishing our work in peer-reviewed journals, writing textbooks and chapters in different books, lecturing to students and at courses, professional meetings, and congresses. Women neuroradiologists are also active in the Croatian Neuroradiological Society—Diagnostic and Interventional in the roles of a secretary general and treasurer, members of the Society's Executive Committee, and national delegate in the Institutional Council of the ESNR. We are also participating in organization of courses and congresses of the Croatian Neuroradiological Society—Diagnostic and Interventional where we also act as speakers.

I also have to mention the second Croatian woman neuroradiologist, Professor Majda M. Thurnher. Professor Thurnher was born in Croatia, in the beautiful ancient town named Pula on the Istrian part of the Adriatic coast. She graduated from the University of Rijeka Faculty of Medicine in 1989. After the graduation, life took her to Austria's capital Vienna, where she continued her medical career in radiology and neuroradiology and became one of the well-known and distinguished neuroradiologists in Europe and in the world. She has never forgotten her origins and over the past two decades she selflessly helped many young Croatian radiologists and neuroradiologists by teaching and supporting them in their education.

Short biography of the author of the text.

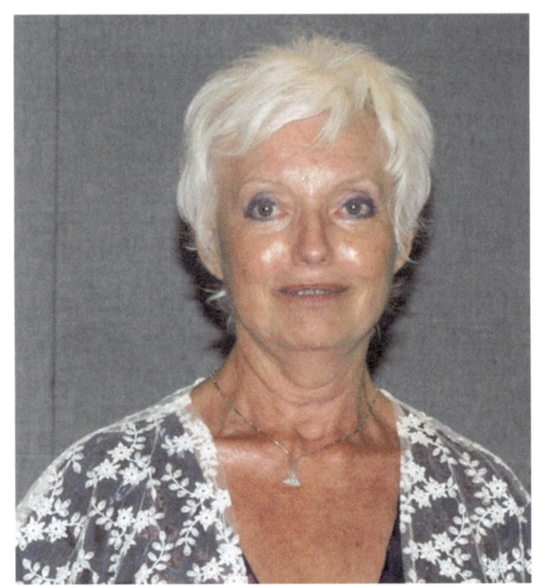

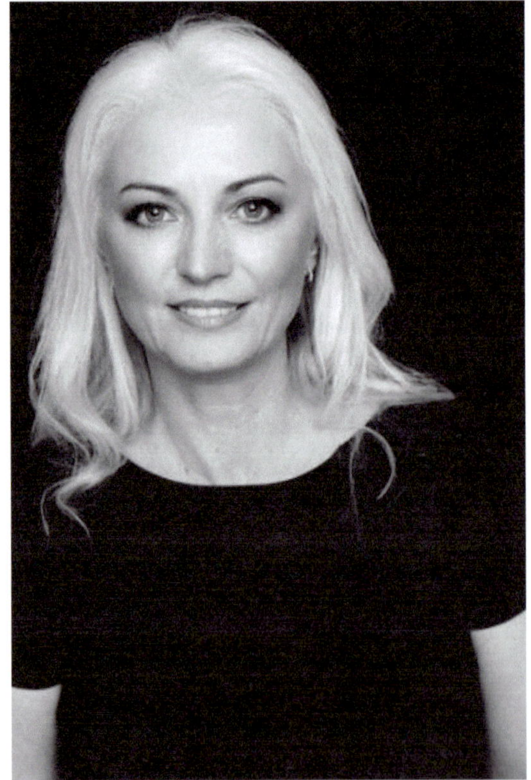

Martina Špero (Fig. 24.3) was born in 1972 in Zagreb, the capital of Croatia. In 1997, she graduated from the University of Zagreb School of Medicine. In May 2004, she became board-certified radiologist and in December 2010, board-certificated neuroradiologist. In 2011, she received a European Diploma in Neuroradiology, and in November, the PhD in the field of Biomedicine and Health Sciences at the University of Zagreb School of Medicine. She is the co-author of two textbooks issued by Springer, "Neuroradiology: Expect the Unexpected" and "Neuroradiology: Images vs Symptoms", author and co-author of several chapters in different textbooks, and author and co-author of several articles published in domestic and international journals. Currently, she serves as the Secretary General of the Croatian Neuroradiological Society—Diagnostic and Interventional and is a national delegate in the Institutional Council of the ESNR. She often participates in the organization of domestic courses and congresses with international participation and is often an invited speaker at many professional meetings, courses, and congresses at home and abroad.

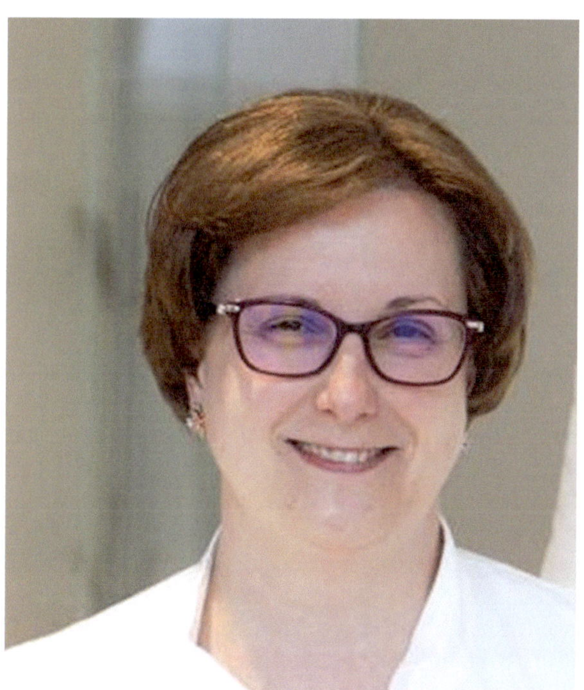

Fig. 24.3 Martina Špero

Women in Neuroradiology: Germany

Jennifer Linn

Description

Prof. Dr. med. Helga Gräfin von Einsiedel (*1938, †2018) was one of the female pioneers in German neuroradiology. After completing her residency in Neurology and Psychiatry—including intensive training in Neuropathology and (Neuro-) Radiology—at the *Nervenklinik* of the University Munich and at the *Röntgeninstitut und Strahlenklinik* of the municipal hospital of Köln-Merheim, she led the Department of Neuroradiology at the *Röntgeninstitut und Strahlenklinik* of the latter hospital in the early 1970s. Simultaneously, she performed a postdoctoral fellowship at the *Max-Planck-Institut für Hirnforschung* in Köln-Merheim. From 1976 until 2003, Helga Gräfin von Einsiedel was head of the Department of Neuroradiology at the *Institut für Röntgendiagnostik* of the *Klinikum Rechts der Isar* at the Technical University Munich. She was the secretary of the German Society of Neuroradiology from the very beginning and for over a decade (from 1971 to 1983) and its first female president in 1982/1983. In this position, she also organized and chaired the Annual Meeting of the society in Munich in 1983. Besides her commitment to our subspeciality, she was appointed as a member of the *Bundesgesundheitsrat* by the German government in 1985.

Prof. Dr. med. Monika Warmuth-Metz is internationally recognized as the founder and head of the German reference center for imaging of pediatric brain tumors at the University Hospital Würzburg. After her training in pathology, general radiology, and radiotherapy, she specialized in neuroradiology and started a close collaboration with the delegates for brain tumors of the *Gesellschaft für pädiatrische Hämatologie und Onkologie (GPOH)*. She established the above-mentioned reference center, initially on a voluntary basis and later on in a full-time function. At the beginning, Monika Warmuth-Metz was responsible for the central imaging review for the HIT trials on malignant pediatric brain tumors, while later on, the central review became mandatory for all German pediatric brain tumor trials. On account of this, the founding of the reference center by the *Deutsche Kinderkrebsstiftung* was extended, and a working group could be established by Prof. Warmuth-Metz. The nationwide reference center in collaboration with the study centers allowed for a state-of-the-art treatment of affected children. As a reference radiologist of the brain tumor group of the European Society of Pediatric Oncology (SIOP-E) and member of the RAPNO (Response Assessment in Pediatric Neuro-Oncology) committee for medulloblastoma and leptomeningeal seeding tumors, Prof. Warmuth-Metz contributed significantly to the standardization of imaging in children with brain tumors. Her major achievements in this regard refer to the correct interpretation of early-postoperative MR images, in particular, the differentiation of the very frequently found unspecific subdural enhancement on spinal imaging from pathological changes. With Prof. Warmuth-Metz´ retirement in 2017, she handed over the leadership of the German reference center for imaging of pediatric brain tumors to her colleague, Dr. med. Brigitte Bison, who later moved to the University Hospital Augsburg.

Prof. Dr. med. Ulrike Ernemann was appointed Chair of the Department of Diagnostic and Interventional Neuroradiology at the University Hospital Tübingen in 2008, as the first appointed female head of an independent neuroradiological department at a German university hospital. After completing her residency at the University Hospital Würzburg, the Zentralklinikum Augsburg and the University Hospital Tübingen, she specialized in neuroradiology in 2000. During her postgraduate training, she completed several internships at the Department of Interventional Neuroradiology of the Hôpital Lariboisière and at the Hôpital Fondation Rothschild in Paris, France. Her clinical as well as her research focus lies on the diagnosis and interventional therapy of vascular malformations. She is a member of the board of directors and speaker of the Centre for Vascular Abnormalities (ZVA) at the University Hospital Tübingen. She organized and chaired the 49th Annual Meeting of the German Society of Neuroradiology in Cologne in 2014 as the second female congress president in the history of the DGNR. Since 2023, Ulrike Ernemann has been appointed Vice Medical Director of the University Hospital Tübingen.

Prof. Dr. med. Isabel Wanke is one of the most experienced German neurointerventionalists. She completed her residency at the Massachusetts General Hospital, Boston, USA (Radiological Department) and the University Hospital Essen (Departments of Radiology, Neurology and Neuroradiology). Already at a very early stage of her career, she focused on interventional neuroradiology with a special clinical and scientific interest in endovascular treatment of intracranial aneurysms. In 2008, she was appointed Professor of Interventional Neuroradiology at the University Hospital Essen, thus being the first appointed Professor for this subspeciality in Germany. In parallel, she started her clinical activities at the Centre for Neuroradiology of the Hirslanden Hospital in Zürich, Switzerland, and established the Swiss Neuro Radiology Institute (SNRI) in Zürich together with Prof. Daniel Rüfenacht. Isabel Wanke was very much involved in the foundation of the European Society of Minimal Invasive Neurological Therapy (ESMINT), led the Education Committee of the society, organized the "Advanced Neurointerventional Course" (ANIC) for several years and was ESMINT treasurer from 2011 to 2014. Since 2022, Isabel Wanke is president of the Swiss Society of Neuroradiology (SGNR).

Prof. Dr. med. Elke Hattingen is an internationally renowned specialist for advanced, multi-parametric neuroradiological magnetic resonance imaging. Her particular research focus lies on proton and phosphorus MR spectroscopy, MR perfusion and quantitative MRI in brain tumors, epilepsy, neurodegenerative, as well as inflammatory diseases. After completing her residency and her postgraduate specialization in neuroradiology, Prof. Hattingen was clinically active as consultant of Neuroradiology at the Department of Neuroradiology at the University Hospital Frankfurt and—in parallel—chaired the MRI research group at the Brain Imaging Center of the latter institution. In 2014, she was appointed Professor of Neuroradiology at the University Hospital Bonn and since 2018, she is Chair of the Department of Neuroradiology at the University Hospital Frankfurt. Since 2022, Elke Hattingen is a board member of the committee for scientific equipment and information technology of the *Deutsche Forschungsgemeinschaft* (DFG). She is DGNR delegate for several interdisciplinary, national guidelines, member of the DGNR guideline commission, as well as neuroradiological delegate in The German working group for the scientific medical societies (*AWMF*). Prof. Hattingen is a member of the executive committee of the German Society of Neuroradiology (treasurer) and was congress president of the 58th Annual Meeting of the DGNR. Currently, she is president elect of the German Society of Neuroradiology for the legislative period from 2026 to 2028, and thus will be the first "regularly" elected female DGNR president in the society's history.

Prof. Dr. med. Elke Gizewski completed her postgraduate clinical training in radiology, neuroradiology, and nuclear medicine at the University Hospital Essen. As board-certified neuroradiologist and consultant at the Department of Diagnostic and Interventional Radiology and Neuroradiology at the latter institution, she was also nominated head of the ultra-high field 7 Tesla MRI neuroscience research group at the Erwin L. Hahn Institute in Essen. In 2009, she was appointed Associate Professor for Neuroradiology at the University Duisburg-Essen, followed by an Professorship for Diagnostic and Interventional Neuroradiology at the Justus-Liebig University Gießen from 2010 to 2012. In 2012, she was appointed Professor for Neuroradiology at the Medical University Innsbruck (MUI) and director of the university´s Core Facility for Imaging in Neuroscience. Her current scientific portfolio covers a wide range of both diagnostic and interventional neuroradiological research questions. From 2014 to 2023, she was executive director of the Radiology Department at the MUI. Since 2024, Elke Gizewski is appointed director of the University Hospital for Radiology at the Medical University Innsbruck. She organized and chaired several large neuroradiological congresses, including the Joint Annual Meeting of the German and Austrian Societies of Neuroradiology in 2016 in Cologne and the Annual Meeting of the Austrian Society of Neuroradiology in 2022 in Innsbruck. In addition, she is very dedicated to teaching and trained a lot of young colleagues in interventional neuroradiology, among them eight women within the last 15 years.

Currently, Elke Gizewski is president of the Austrian Society of Neuroradiology (ÖGNR).

Prof. Dr. med. Franziska Dorn currently is one of the most experienced interventional neuroradiologists in Germany. She started her neurointerventional training already during her residency at the Departments of Neuroradiology and Radiology at the Klinikum Rechts der Isar at the Technical University Munich. Her research focuses on endovascular treatment of ischemic stroke (mechanical thrombectomy) as well as on advanced-techniques for endovascular aneurysm treatment. She was consultant neuroradiologist at the University Hospital Cologne and consultant and head of the neurointerventional section of the Department of Neuroradiology at the University Hospital of the Ludwigs-Maximilians-University, Munich. Since 2020, Franziska Dorn is Director of Neurointervention and Deputy Director of the Department of Diagnostic and Interventional Neuroradiology at the University Hospital Bonn. She was founding member of the task force "Work and family" of the German Society of Neuroradiology and she currently chairs the ESMINT "Women in Neurointervention" (WIN) working group.

Finally, I would like to introduce myself, *Prof. Dr. med. Jennifer Linn* (Fig. 24.4). I started my scientific work doing basic research at the Institute of Neurophysiology at the Technical University Munich for my doctoral thesis on *Spontaneous Network Oscillations in the Necortex of Newborn Rodents*. During my residency at the Departments of Radiology and Neuroradiology of the Ludwig-Maximilians-University Munich (*LMU*, *Klinikum Großhadern*), my scientific interest switched to more clinically based research questions, with a particular focus on cerebral amyloid angiopathy and other cerebral small vessel diseases as well as hemorrhagic stroke. Besides my clinical work as neuroradiological consultant, I was head of the MR-based research group of the Department of Neuroradiology of the LMU from

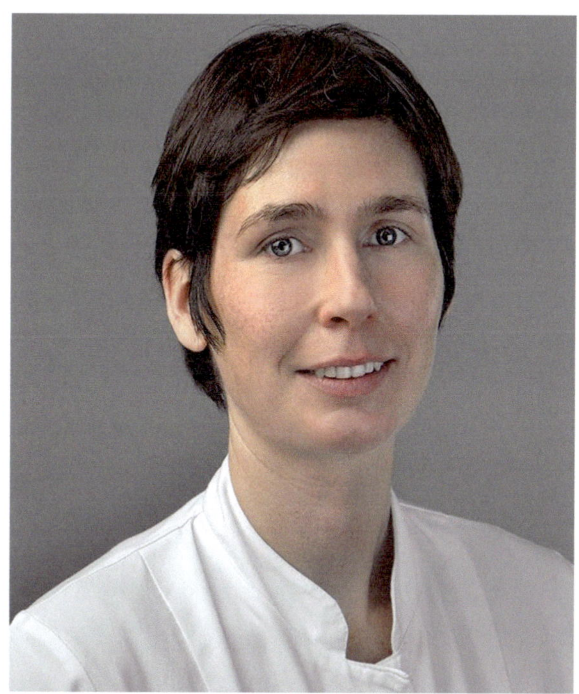

Fig. 24.4 Prof. Dr. med. Jennifer Linn, Chair of Diagnostic and Interventional Neuroradiology at the University Hospital Carl Gustav Carus at the Technical University Dresden

2009 to 2014. For my work on superficial siderosis as a new MR-marker of cerebral amyloid angiopathy, I was awarded the Marc-Dünzl-Preis (2006) and the Kurt-Decker-Preis (2011) of the German Society of Neuroradiology, the Perovitch Grant for European Neuroradiologists at Johns Hopkins University (2011), and the Founders Award for Diagnostic Neuroradiology of the European Society of Neuroradiology (ESNR, 2015).

Since 2014, I am appointed Chair for Neuroradiology at the Technical University and Director of the Institute for Diagnostic and Interventional Neuroradiology of the University Hospital Carl Gustav Carus, Dresden. In 2017, I initialized the Dresdner Neurovascular Centre (DNVC) at the latter institution and prepared and realized the initial certification of the East-Saxonian Neurovascular Network (SOS-NET) according to the Guidelines of the German Stroke Society.

Women in Neuroradiology: Italy

Chiara Zini and Nicoletta Emanuela Anzalone

Introduction

Neuroradiology in Italy formally began in 1910 in Milan with the establishment of the Istituto Neurologico Vittorio Emanuele III. However, it was not until 1924 that neurologist Carlo Besta performed the first pneumoencephalography, and the institute was later renamed the Istituto C. Besta in his honor for his commitment.

During the same period, Mario Bertolotti, a neuroradiologist, became the first full professor of neuroradiology in 1920.

Historically, neuroradiology in Italy has been closely linked to neurology, with the earliest neuroradiologists being neurologists who had a special interest in imaging.

In the Forties and Fifties, Italian neuroradiologists trained abroad, first in Sweden (where Di Chiro and Ruggiero specialized in invasive procedures) and later in France. This era led to the emergence of a new generation of professionals qualified as neuroradiologists. However, it was not until 1969 that new legislation officially recognized neuroradiology as an independent hospital specialty in Italy.

The first dedicated neuroradiology department in Italy was not established until 1964, when Prof. Alberto Calabro founded the Department of Neuroradiology at Ospedale Cardarelli in Naples.

Today, there are 30 neuroradiology departments (Unità Operative Complesse, UOC) in Italy. Of these, eight are headed by women, with one of these women specializing in interventional neuroradiology (Bracco in Siena) [17].

A 2022 report by the Italian Society of Medical and Interventional Radiology (SIRM) revealed that only 17% of neuroradiology department chiefs are women, even though 52.3% of radiology residents are female [18].

The situation in academia mirrors this trend. According to the SIRM report, women constitute 26% of radiology faculty, but only 11% hold full professorships. In neuroradiology (scientific and academic fields code MED37), there are 20 full professors, including four women (Granata, Pantano, Picecchio, and Splendiani), and 20 associate professors, of whom six are women (Anzalone, Caramia, Castellano, Conforti, Pizzini, and Ukmar).

However, outside Italy, several distinguished Italian female neuroradiologists hold prominent positions across Europe and the Americas. Notable figures include Biondi in France and Tampieri in Canada. They represent Italian excellence in leading neuroradiology roles worldwide, highlighting a significant shift from the past, when Italian professionals had to leave the country to pursue neuroradiology training.

In 2023, the Italian Association of Neuroradiology (AINR) had 290 female members out of a total of 722. Notably, women occupy two positions on the Executive Committee, serving as Vice President (Anzalone) and Secretary (Gerevini). Additionally, the subcommittees feature 2 female representatives (Bracco, Castellano) out of 11, including one on the Interventional Radiology Committee (Bracco).

Of the 326 Italian members of the European Society of Neuroradiology (ESNR), 153 are female, with 25 not disclosing their gender. Notably, an Italian female member has served as Chairperson of the Spine Neuroradiology Committee (Zini, Fig. 24.5b).

These numbers are quite interesting, and we hope to close the gap between male and female representation both in academia and hospitals.

Competence is essential, but a strong, supportive system that helps women achieve fulfillment in both their personal and professional lives is also crucial.

To offer a more detailed view of the state of Italian neuroradiology, I decided to explore the field through the story of Nicoletta Anzalone, who served as an inspiration during my MD thesis.

Description

Prof. Nicoletta Anzalone (Fig. 24.5a) is a highly esteemed neuroradiologist with over 25 years of experience in her field. She earned her medical degree from Università degli Studi di Milano and completed her residency in both neurology and radiology at the same institution. Her deep interest in the complexities of the brain and nervous system led her to transition from clinical practice to a focus on neuro-

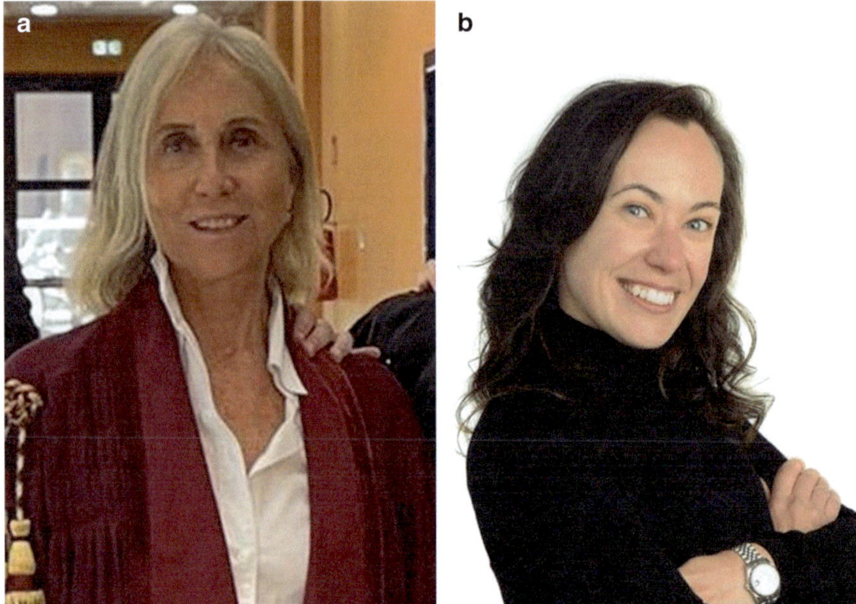

Fig. 24.5 (**a**, **b**) On the left of the image Prof Nicoletta Emanuela Anzalone and on the right Dr Chiara Zini

radiology. Currently, Prof. Anzalone is a leading authority at Vita e Salute University, Scientific Institute HS San Raffaele in Milan, where she has made notable advancements in neuroimaging techniques. Additionally, she is a committed mentor, actively shaping the future of aspiring neuroradiologists.

Inspiration and Career Path

During my neurology residency, CT was the main diagnostic tool for brain diseases, and MRI was just beginning to emerge. I was particularly captivated by how significantly imaging improved the evaluation of neurological patients. This was especially evident in emergency situations where CT was invaluable, as well as in more complex and challenging neurological cases. It was during these critical moments, both at the bedside and in emergency settings, that I discovered my passion for the diagnostic aspect of the process. Imaging greatly simplified the often-challenging task of neurological assessment. Over time, MRI has become central to diagnosing neurological conditions, frequently preceding clinical evaluations. As a result, our role as neuroradiologists has become crucial in diagnosing neurological diseases.

Type of Work

For the reasons I mentioned above, and possibly due to my neurological background, I have a deep love for clinical work. I enjoy being involved in the diagnostic process and discussing cases with various clinical professionals, including neurologists, neurosurgeons, and oncologists. This interdisciplinary collaboration is another wonderful aspect of my job. Additionally, as an academic, I have the privilege of teaching neuroradiology to students and residents. This is a rewarding part of my work because young people are curious and constantly challenge me with their expectations. After so many years in this field, I never imagined my job could be so fulfilling.

Challenges and Gaps

Looking back, I realize that my hard work was driven by a strong sense of responsibility, a trait that comes from being the eldest daughter. Being a passionate working woman with a family definitely enriches your life, but it can also be challenging and expose you to prejudices. Many people assume that if you are a woman with a family, you won't be able to dedicate enough time and effort to your job. Consequently, they often exclude you from potential opportunities without even giving you a chance to prove yourself.

Advantages of Being a Neuroradiologist

As I mentioned, neuroradiology is essential to the diagnostic process. Additionally, this field is closely tied to technology, which is continually evolving and improving. This job will never become outdated, and you'll never grow tired of it. You must stay updated and constantly aware of all the latest technical advancements.

Mentorship

I don't see myself as a mentor, but I was pleasantly surprised to realize that young people—students, residents, and even young radiologists—looked up to me, not only for my work and achievements but also for how I approached my job. As time goes on, I find myself increasingly focused on supporting young people. I hope to convey a positive message about the rewarding nature of being a neuroradiologist and to show young women that they can succeed in this field without sacrificing their personal lives.

Advice for Aspiring Radiologists

Building on what I mentioned earlier, I highly recommend the field of neuroradiology. If you have an interest in neurology and neuroscience, you'll find a vast and exciting world awaiting you. This field encompasses clinical neuroradiology, research applications, and therapeutic neuroradiology—each playing a crucial role in patient care.

For young individuals interested in neuroradiology, my primary advice is to approach the subject with enthusiasm and curiosity. Begin by understanding the clinical needs and strive to address them both in clinical practice and through research.

Acknowledgement I would like to thank Prof. Scotti for his guidance and support in preparing and reviewing this chapter, Prof. Luca Maria Sconfienza for his continual support and crucial help with data collection, and Prof. Caranci for his considerate assistance in reviewing the manuscript.

Women in Neuroradiology: Poland

Anna Zimny

Introduction

The history of radiology in Poland started a few weeks after Wilhelm Roentgen had discovered X-rays and published his work in January 1896. Plain radiograms of the skull were the first neuroradiological examinations and remained the main neuroimaging method till 1950s. The first Polish woman in those pioneering years, dominated by men, was Maria Skłodowska-Curie (1867–1934), who during World War I developed mobile radiography units to provide X-ray services to field hospitals; they were used, among others, for the localization of bullets in the skull. In Poland, the first woman-pioneer in the field of radiology was Dr. Bronisława Korabczyńska (1881–1949)—head of the Radiology Department in Łazarz Hospital in Kraków in 1913–1949. After the Second World War, the strongest neuroradiology center in Poland was based in the Medical University Hospital in Kraków, in the Department of Radiology, which was chaired by professor Stanisława Janczyszyn-Spettowa. She initiated Polish School of Neuroradiology and thus is named the Mother of Polish Neuroradiology. It was her together with her team, who introduced brain angiography to a routine clinical practice and started new procedures such as pneumocephalography and myelography in the 1950s. Medical University of Łódź was another Polish center very strongly involved in those neuroradiological procedures with doctor Bronisława Wygodzka-Lipska (1922–1996) working there.

A new era in neuroradiology started with an introduction of CT and later MRI scanners into clinical practice. The first CT unit in Poland was installed in 1979 in Poznań and an MRI scanner in 1991 in Warsaw. The first MR spectroscopic examinations were initiated in 1997 by professor Maria Sokół from the Department of Medical Physics in Gliwice and the first functional MRI studies in 1998 in Kraków and Łódź by professors Bożena Góraj and Agata Majos. At the same time, interventional neuroradiology started to rapidly develop in several centers in Poland, including Warsaw, Katowice, Łódź, and Lublin. In the 1990s, professor Małgorzata Szczerbo-Trojanowska became the head of the Department of Interventional Radiology and Neuroradiology in Lublin. She is one of the most prominent radiologists in Poland of all time and has been widely recognized in Europe. She was the President of the European Congress of Radiology in 2010. In those years, there were also other women in different centers in Poland who were getting more and more involved in CT and MR imaging and interventional neuroradiology, among them professor Zdzisława Bem (1932–2018) in Wrocław and professor Romana Bogusławska-Walecka (born 1953) in Warsaw, while in Kraków, former students of prof. Janczyszyn-Spettowa, doctors: Barbara Sikorska, Barbara Jedlińska, Barbara Kamieniecka, and Henryka Uhl.
The Division of Neuroradiology of the Polish Society of Radiology was established in 1963. Since 2000, it has been chaired exclusively by women: in 2010–2013, president prof. Barbara Bobek-Billewicz, vice president prof. Elżbieta Jurkiewicz, in 2013–2016, president prof. Barbara Bobek-Billewicz, secretary Dr. Aleksandra Kiełtyka, in 2016–2023: president prof. Agata Majos, vice president prof. Anna Zimny, secretary Dr. Edyta Maj and from 2023 till now, president prof. Joanna Bladowska, vice president Dr. Edyta Maj, secretary Dr. Jagoda Jaców-Nowicka.

The most prominent women in neuroradiology after 1990 in Poland are summarized below.

Prof. Bożena Góraj, MD, PhD (born 15.07.1956)—Head of the Section of Neuroradiology at the Radboud University Medical Center Nijmegen in the Netherlands since 2004. She was appointed to this position in recognition of her previous work and achievements. She was born and graduated in Łódź, Poland, where in 1993 she became a Head of CT and MRI Division of the "Institute of Polish Mothers" Health Center, Chair of the Department of Radiology of Medical University of Łodź and a Director of the Institute of Radiology and Nuclear Medicine of the same University. Her early scientific interest in the late 1980s was focused on neurosonography in neonates as a novel technique, and later on transcranial doppler in adults. In the late 1990s, she developed a strong interest in new advanced MRI techniques such as MRS and fMRI in pediatric and adult patients. She is an ESNR-certified neuroradiologist and a lecturer on many ESR, ESNR, and Erasmus courses. She chaired the ECR Neuroradiology Committee and was its member for several years. Within ESNR, she held the position of Membership Committee Chairperson. To create awareness of the importance and advances in neuroradiology, she organized Seminars of the Neuroradiology Division of the Polish Medical Society of Radiology, of which she served as a vice president (1998–2001).

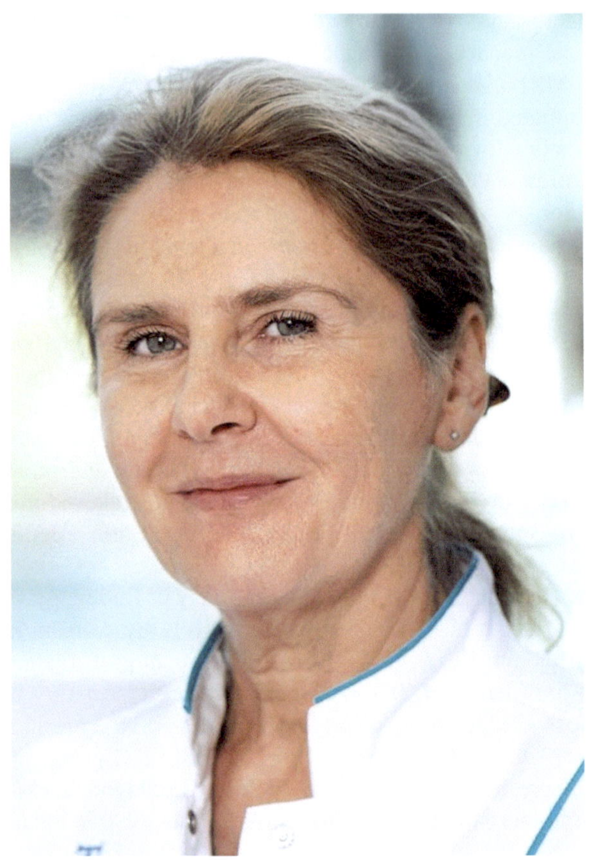

Prof. Barbara Bobek-Billewicz, MD, PhD, MBA (born 25.04.1955)—Head of Maria Skłodowska-Curie National Research Institute of Oncology in Gliwice in Poland, since 2004. She is a neuroradiologist and a specialist in nuclear medicine. Her main interests have been head and neck imaging as well as neuro-oncology and imaging of neurological complications of oncological treatment. She was one of the first in Poland to start performing preoperative fMRI and DTI in patients with brain tumors, which resulted in the first brain tumor removal surgery in Poland using fMRI and DTI performed in January 2007 at the Silesian Medical University. She is an author/co-author of 94 scientific publications and 37 chapters in textbooks. She has been a teacher and lecturer at the Medical College in Krakow and the Medical University in Gdansk. She has been a lecturer on numerous postgraduate courses for radiologists, neurosurgeons, and oncologists in Poland and also on European courses and congresses, including ESNR. She is a co-founder and lecturer of the best-known postgraduate school of radiology in Poland, called Entomografia, established in 2007, which up till now has conducted 154 courses with over 8400 participants, mainly on neuroradiology and head and neck radiology. She is the former president of the Neuroradiology Division of the Polish Medical Society of Radiology in the years 2010–2016.

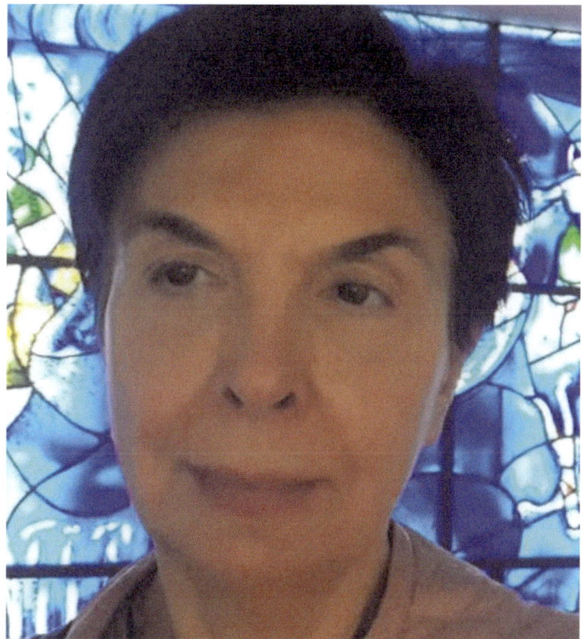

Prof. Elżbieta Jurkiewicz, MD, PhD (born 23.01.1956)—Head of Department of Radiology at the Children's Memorial Health Institute in Warsaw since 2010. She is a pediatric radiologist and neuroradiologist. Her early interest in the 1990s focused on interventional radiology and MRI in the pediatric population. She started performing new procedures of embolizations of complex vascular malformations in children, including vein of Galen malformations and spinal malformations. Later, she got involved in MRI and neuroimaging with the main focus on tuberous sclerosis, white matter diseases, including MS, vanishing white matter disease, and spinal tumors. She also introduced a new method of intra-arterial chemotherapy of retinoblastoma. She is an author of many chapters in Polish and international textbooks and the chief editor of the Polish textbook entitled Diagnostic Imaging in Pediatrics, published in 2017.

She is a lecturer at many Polish courses and congresses. She is a former vice president of the Neuroradiology Division of the Polish Medical Society of Radiology in the years 2010–2013.

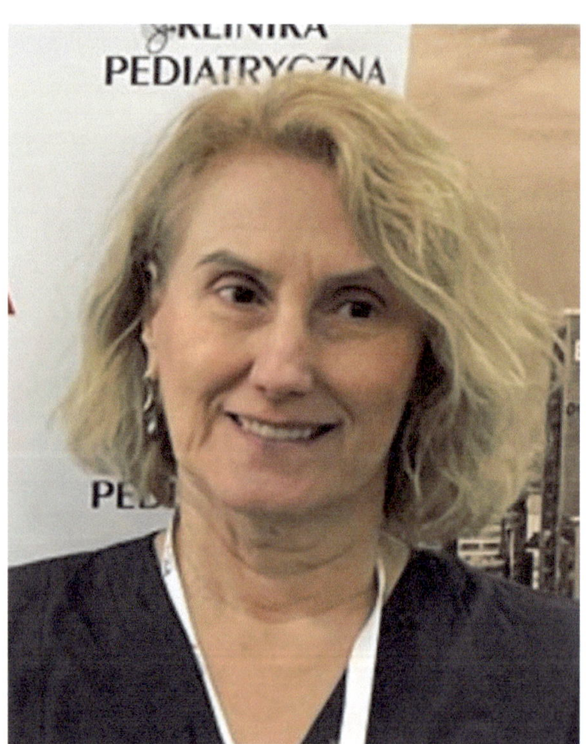

Prof. Agata Majos, MD, PhD (born 09.08.1964)—Head of the II Department of Radiology and Diagnostic Imaging, Medical University of Lodz since 2010. Leading topics of her scientific work were related to the field of fMRI research, in which she was a pioneer in Poland and Europe, and even in the world regarding fMRI with the use of contrast agents. It resulted in an EAR Research Grant in 2001 and participation in Neuro Imaging Expert Panels since 2008. She has also been a pioneer in the use of different computer applications. At present, she is involved in the application of artificial intelligence in Graves' disease, tumor vascularization, and multiple sclerosis. Since 2017, she has served as Neuroradiology Section Editor of the Polish Journal of Radiology. She has given numerous lectures during Polish and international courses and congresses, including ECR and Erasmus, which she organized in Warsaw in 2019. In addition, she has played a variety of leading roles such as President of Neuroradiology Division of the Polish Medical Society of Radiology (2016–2023), Vice President of Polish Medical Society of Radiology (2019–2023), a member of several ECR Committees: Research (2018–2022), Structural Reporting (2018–2022), Quality, Safety and Standards (2017–2018), and Neuroradiology Committee (2020–2024). She has been a Polish delegate for the UEMS Division of Radiology since 2018.

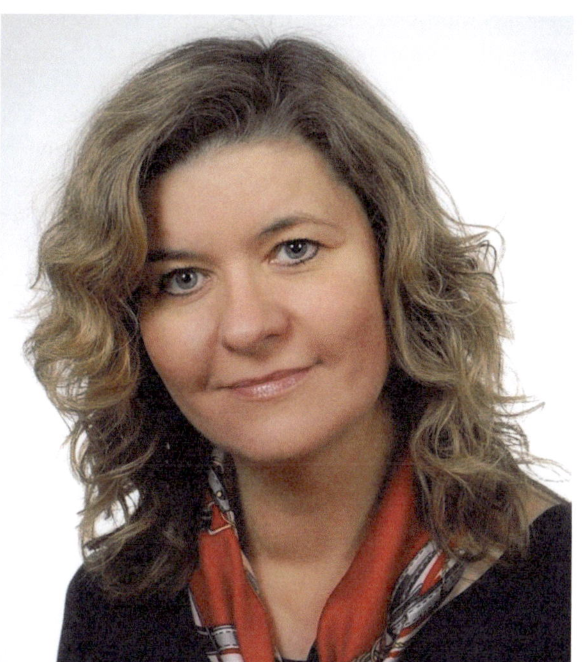

Prof. Monika Bekiesińska-Figatowska, MD, PhD (born 22.04.1966)—Head of Department of Diagnostic Imaging of the Institute of Mother and Child in Warsaw since 2006. She has been involved in MRI since the beginning of this method in Poland in 1991 at the Central Railway Hospital in Warsaw, where she was performing the first MR examinations in Poland. As a pioneer in MRI in Poland, she is a recognized expert in the field of white matter diseases, congenital malformations of the central nervous system, neurological rare diseases, neonatal brain imaging, and fetal MRI. She is an author/co-author of 199 scientific publications and 30 chapters in textbooks. She has been regularly lecturing at courses on neuroradiology in Poland since 1993, and also at European courses and congresses, including ESNR meetings, Erasmus and Galen courses. Since 2004, she has been actively involved in ECR and, since 2017, in the European Diploma in Radiology as a member of the Written Evaluation Committee. Since 2019, she has been on the Board of Directors of the Polish Medical Society of Radiology, acting as Chair of the Scientific Affairs Committee. She is an organizer and chairwoman of the Scientific Committee of the Autumn Scientific Meetings in Poland (15 editions, 2006–2023).

Prof. Joanna Bladowska, MD, PhD (01.04.1976)—Head of the Radiology Course at the Faculty of Medicine at the Wroclaw University of Science and Technology, head of the Department of Neuroradiology at Wroclaw 4th Military Clinical Hospital, as well as Neuroradiology Consultant in Emergency Medicine Center at Marciniak Lower Silesian Specialist Hospital since 2023. She is a former deputy head of the Department of General and Interventional Radiology and Neuroradiology at Wroclaw Medical University in the years 2016–2023. She is a radiologist and a certified neuroradiologist with an ESNR Diploma in neuroradiology (2015). Her main scientific interest has been focused on pituitary gland imaging and the use of advanced MRI techniques in white matter diseases and infectious diseases of the brain. In recognition of her work, she was awarded many awards, including, among others an ESNR Award in Diagnostic Neuroradiology for the best scientific paper in 2013. She is an author/co-author of many scientific papers and chapters in textbooks, including The Clinical Neuroradiology published by ESNR. She is a lecturer on many Polish and international courses and congresses such as ECR, ESNR, and Erasmus courses. She is the President of the Neuroradiology Division of the Polish Medical Society of Radiology since 2023 and a President of the Scientific Society of the Lower Silesia branch of the Polish Medical Society of Radiology since 2019.

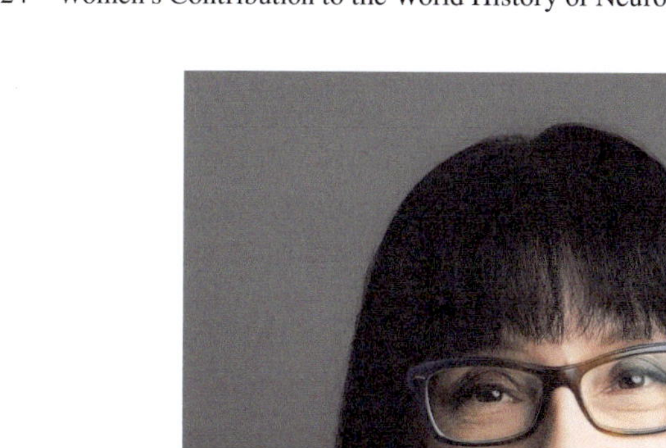

Prof. Anna Zimny, MD, PhD (born 04.11.1976) (Fig. 24.6)—Head of the Department of General and Interventional Radiology and Neuroradiology at Wroclaw Medical University since 2024, former head of the MRI Department in the same institution since 2015. She is a radiologist and a certified neuroradiologist with ESNR Diploma in neuroradiology (2015). Her main scientific interest has been focused on the use of advanced MRI techniques in brain tumors and dementia. She has been involved in several international scientific projects and grants including PURE-Mind and ERANET. She is an author/co-author of many scientific papers and chapters in textbooks, including The Clinical Neuroradiology published by ESNR. She is a lecturer on many Polish and international courses and congresses, including ECR, ESNR, and Erasmus courses. She has been twice awarded the Best Scientific Presentation Award in the field of neuroradiology at ECR (2010, 2013). She is a former vice president of the Neuroradiology Division of the Polish Medical Society of Radiology from 2016 to 2023 and a Polish delegate for the UEMS Division of Neuroradiology since 2018. Since 2021, she has been acting as an examiner at the ESNR diploma examination.

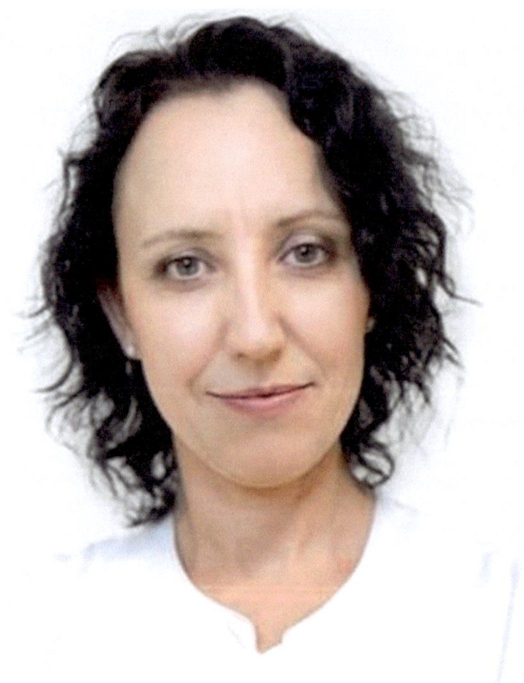

Fig. 24.6 Prof. Anna Zimny, Head of Department of General and Interventional Radiology and Neuroradiology at Wroclaw Medical University

The Role of Women in Spanish Neuroradiology

Marta Drake-Perez

Introduction: A Brief Review of the Role of Women in the History of Spanish Medicine and Radiology

The integration of women into medicine in Spain was late, and their incorporation into the speciality of radiology was even later. Although women's rights movements reached their peak in the nineteenth century, it was not until the second half of the twentieth century that the presence of female doctors in Spain became widespread.

In the speciality of radiology, there are few references from the first half of the twentieth century regarding women in radiology. Perhaps, one of the pioneers in the speciality (and one of the few references we have) is Maria Lluïsa Quadras-Bordes, who founded in 1920 the Institute of Electrology, Radiology and Gynaecology in Barcelona (3). The first woman to belong to the Spanish Society of Radiology (SERAM) was Encarnación Ramírez Pérez, who joined the Society in 1966, although its foundation was in 1916 (there are official records of the Minutes of the Board of Directors since 1945).

Currently, the number of women in medicine, and specifically in the speciality of Radiology, is equal or even slightly higher than the number of men, and growing.

As a representation of the current situation in our country, in 2021, the SERAM secretariat had a total of 5528 registered members, 53% of whom were women. In the same year, 58.1% of the radiology residents were women, which reflects a certain upward trend in the future.

The Role of Women in Spanish Neuroradiology

The Spanish Society of Neuroradiology (SENR) originated as a working group within the Spanish Society of Neurology (SEN) in 1963, promoted by the interest in the radiology of the neurological system of some members, such as Dr. Mariano Rovira Molist, Dr. M. Subirana Cantarell, Dr. I. Pascual Castroviejo, and Dr. Joan Solé Llenas. In 1970, the need to set up a society independent of the SEN was considered, even though a link with that society was maintained, and joint annual meetings were held. In 1971, the new society (SENR) was officially constituted, and a year later the first general assembly was organized.

In Spain, the radiological subspecialties with the highest percentage of women have traditionally been pediatric radiology or breast imaging. Neuroradiology has been considered a markedly male section, perhaps because of its relationship with interventional radiology. However, in recent years, there has been an increase in the percentage of female radiologists in this subspecialty.

In 2022, the percentage of women members of SENR was 38%. However, it is striking that it is one of the radiology subspecialties in which the percentage of women on the National Society board exceeds the percentage of women members in the society. In 2022, women accounted for 66% of the board, and since the year of its creation there have been two women presidents. As of today in 2024, the SENR board is composed of eight members, five of whom are women, including the current President, Dr. Nuria Bargalló, Dra. Sofía González Ortiz, and Dra. Teresa Cabada Giadas as the Secretary and Vice Secretary, Dra. Eloísa Santos as the Treasurer, and Dra. Amaya Hilario as a Member of the Scientific Committee.

Prominent Female Neuroradiologists in Spain

Dr. Ana Ramos, MD, PhD, is the current Head of Neuroradiology at University Hospital 12 de Octubre in Madrid, one of the largest hospitals in the city. She also works at the Clara Campal Oncology Center, part of the HM Hospital group in Madrid.

Her work is primarily focused on cranial and spinal trauma, as well as neuro-oncological pathology. Hospital 12 de Octubre is the busiest Level 1 trauma Center in Madrid and a leading Neuro Oncology center in Spain.

Dr. Ramos was the first woman to be appointed as the President of the Spanish Society of Neuroradiology and continues to play an active role in the Society. She also serves on the Executive Council of the Sociedad Ibero-Latino Americana de Neuroradiología (SILAN), where she is responsible for promoting and teaching neuroradiology, as well as providing mentorship and scholarships to support professionals in Latin American countries.

In addition, Dr. Ramos participates in the European Society of Neuroradiology as a member of the Diagnostic Committee, which is chaired by Prof. Meike Vernooij from the Netherlands.

In the near future, Dr. Ramos will serve as the Chair of the Scientific Subcommittee of Neuroradiology for the European Congress of Radiology (ECR) in 2026. She is also going to be appointed as the President of the ESNR Congress, which will be held in Madrid in 2027.

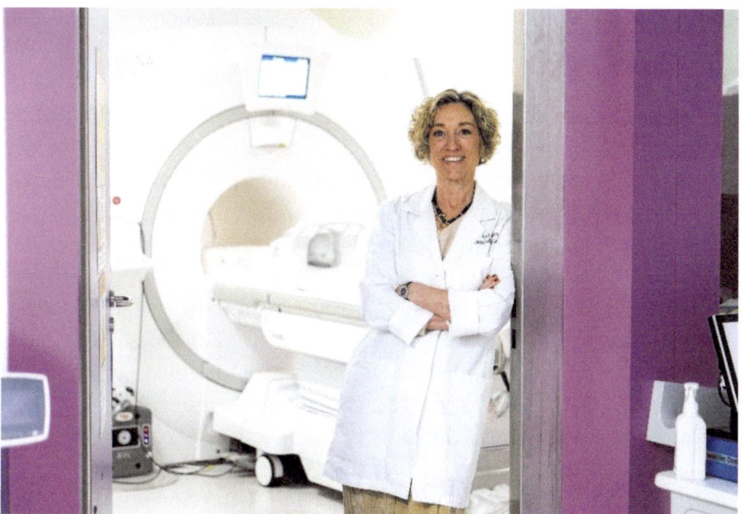

Dr. Laura Oleaga, MD, PhD, received her medical degree from the School of Medicine of the Autonomous University of Madrid. She completed her training in radiology at the Hospital Donostia in San Sebastian. She trained as a Research Fellow in Magnetic Resonance Imaging at the University of Pennsylvania in the Department of Radiology. She served as a staff member specialist in Magnetic Resonance Imaging in the Hospital of Basurto (Bilbao). She earned a PhD degree in medicine from the University of the Basque Country (Spain) in 1998. Dr Laura Oleaga was appointed Chair of the Radiology Department of the Hospital Clínic in Barcelona in 2009. Since 2008, she has also worked as Neuroradiologist at the Hospital Clínic of Barcelona and has served as Professor of Radiology at the University of Barcelona. In 2022, she stepped down as the Chair of the Hospital Clinic. She now continues working as a clinical neuroradiologist, while also serving as the Director of the Core Lab at the Monclinic Foundation.

Prof. Laura Oleaga is an active member of many scientific societies and organizations. She served as the vice president of the Spanish Radiological Society (SERAM) from 2002 to 2006, and as the Chair of the Scientific Committee of SERAM from 2006 to 2008. She was appointed as the Chair of the Education Committee of the European Society of Radiology (ESR) from 2015 to 2018. She has served as the Scientific Director of the European Diploma in Radiology from 2018 to the present.

She has been actively involved in educational activities in neuroradiology and head and neck imaging, with a primary focus on brain and head, and neck tumors. Her work has been dedicated to advancing education in radiology.

She has authored and co-authored more than 100 peer-reviewed scientific papers and 10 book chapters.

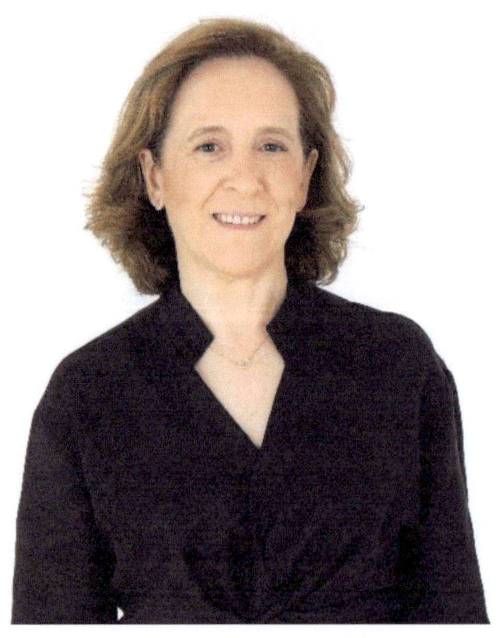

Dr. Núria Bargalló, MD, PhD, is the current President of the SENR and Head of Neuroradiology Section at the Hospital Clinic, in Barcelona. She is also an Assistant Professor of Radiology at the University of Barcelona, and the Strategic Director of the Magnetic Resonance Image Core Facility at the IDIBAPS, Barcelona, Spain. Previously she has served as the Chair of the Subspecialities and Allied Science Committee and the Chair of the Quality, Safety and Standard of the European Society of Radiology. She has led a European working group on functional MR in epilepsy within the European Society of Neuroradiology, and she was a member of the diagnostic committee of this society from 2014 to 2020.

Dr. Bargalló received her medical degree from the School of Medicine of the Autonomous University of Barcelona. She completed her training in radiology at the Hospital Clínic in the same city. She earned a PhD degree in Medicine and Surgery from the University of Barcelona (Spain) in 2004. She has done several training stays in different hospitals in the United States and the United Kingdom to learn new imaging techniques in neuroradiology.

She has focused on the study of advanced imaging of degenerative diseases, psychiatric diseases and epilepsy. She has co-authored 11 chapters in books, and edited two textbooks in radiology. She has published 362 articles as an author/co-author in international peer-reviewed journals, with a H-index of 59. She has obtained 39 research project competitive grants (national and international), and five research grants as principal investigation. She has supervised five PhD thesis.

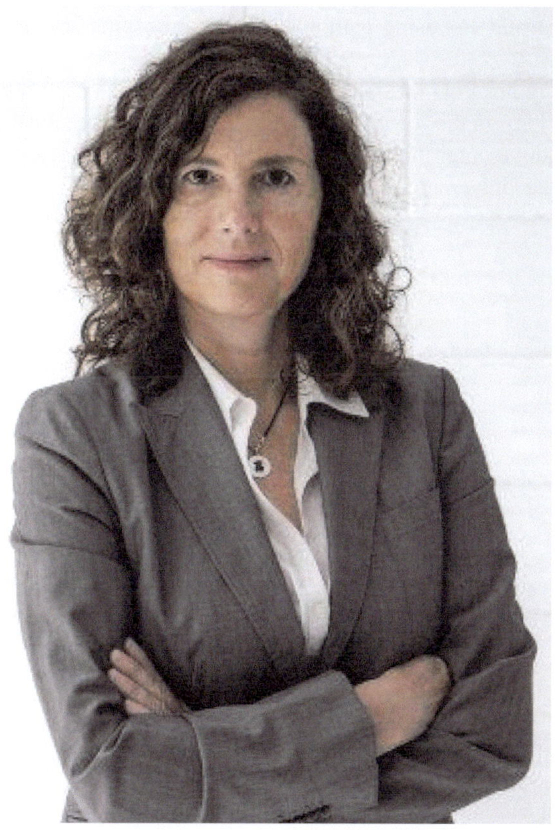

Dr María Rosario Barrena Caballo is one of Spain's pioneering women in interventional neuroradiology.

She took her first steps in diagnostic neuroradiology in 1989, at the Miguel Servet Hospital in Zaragoza, when she was in her fourth year of radiology residency. Subsequently, the hospital hired her to work in the Neuroradiology Section, combining diagnostic and interventional vascular care for the first 5 years.

In those years there were few women who were committed to interventional radiology; Dr. de Miguel, Dr. Frutos and Dr. Sola, who also share a good friendship with each other, cooperated in this field.

Dr Barrena has spent periods of training in France, with Dr Casasco at Lariboisière Hospital and La Pitié Salpêtrière Hospital, and instructive stays in Essen (Dr Chapot), Limoges (Dr Mounayer), Geneva (Dr Mendes), Stuttgart (Dr Henkes), Bern (Dr Gralla) and Stockholm (Dr Andersson). In this way, she has been able to learn different approaches of understanding vascular pathologies and their therapeutic approaches.

During her professional life, she has written and collaborated in 59 national and international publications and 150 oral communications. She has served as a member of the board of the SENR and also the GENI (Spanish group of Interventional Neuroradiology), and is currently a member of the Societies of Diagnostic and Interventional Neuroradiology (SENR, ESNR, GENI, ESMINT, SILAN). She is a member of the stroke and carotid pathology and complex cerebral vascular pathology committees, and has participated in the development of protocols for SAH, treatment of carotid stenosing pathology, and the hospital stroke code of Aragon (Spain).

After reading her PhD thesis "Radiological evolutionary study of patients with cerebral aneurysms in the reference area of the Miguel Servet Hospital in Zaragoza, treated by endovascular therapy", Dr. Barrena has joined the Department of Radiology at the University of Zaragoza as an Associate Professor.

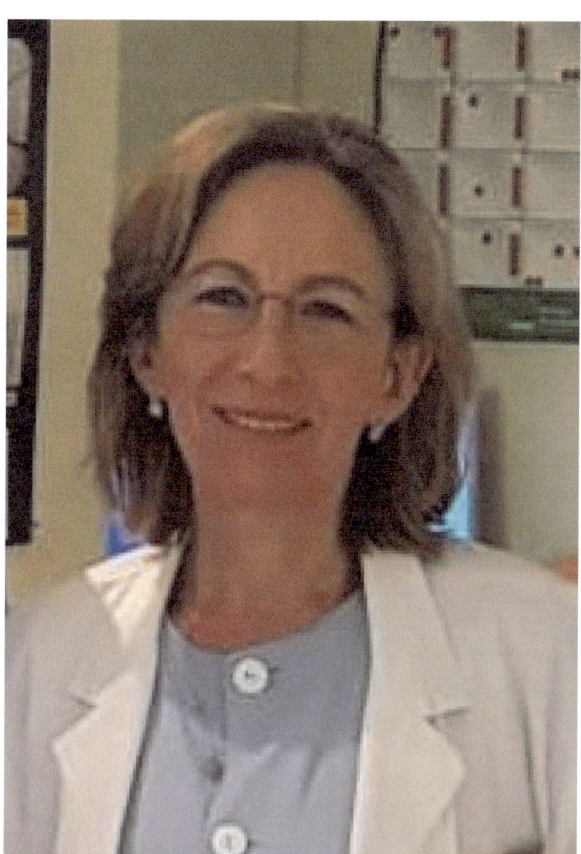

Women in Neuroradiology: Sweden

Pia C. Sundgren

Introduction

The history of women in neuroradiology in Sweden is marked by the contributions of several female neuroradiologists, who dedicated their careers to advancing the field of neuroradiology in Sweden. Their participation in local radiological departments, in radiological societies, and their scientific and technical contributions have brought Swedish neuroradiology forward. This chapter presents some of the most influential Swedish female neuroradiologists and their contribution to Swedish neuroradiology. Neuroradiology has been a subspecialty in Sweden for many years. Female neuroradiologists have constantly increased over the past years. Latest statistics from 2021 show that Sweden had 150 certified neuroradiologists of whom 58 were women. Several female neuroradiologists have or currently hold positions as professors and academic leaders at their institutes/universities. Both Raili Raininko and Elna-Marie Larsson were pioneers in MR research already in the early era of the first MR scanners. They as well as Pia Sundgren, Isabella Björkman-Burtscher, Maria Wiberg, Ida Blystad, and Anna Falk Delgado have focused on imaging techniques, advanced MR applications in brain imaging research and implementation in clinical practice. Female neuroradiologists have been incremental for the development of interventional neuroradiology in Sweden. Presently, Birgitta Ramgren and Åsa Kuntze Söderqvist are well-known national and international interventional neuroradiologists.

Raili Raininko, MD, PhD, received her MD degree (1970) and PhD degree in Medical Sciences (1978) from the University of Turku, Finland. She received specialist degrees in radiology (1975) and in neuroradiology (1980) in Finland. After working at the University hospitals of Turku and Helsinki in Finland, she worked at the University of Michigan in 1992–1993. In 1994, she moved to Sweden as a professor of Neuroradiology at Uppsala University. After the official retirement 2012, she continued her scientific work. She has published about 170 original articles in peer-reviewed scientific journals and 43 review articles and book chapters. She has been a supervisor for 11 PhD students. She started working with MR imaging as early as 1984. Diagnostic utility of new methods and description of the normal structures in the brain and spine in different age groups with different techniques have been main areas in her research. Rare hereditary neurological diseases in children and adults have been a special object of her interest. She developed the education of medical students by integrating neuroradiology in teaching of anatomy. She has organized radiological and neuroradiological courses at different levels, nationally and internationally. She has been chief of the neuroradiological unit at the Meilahti Hospital, Helsinki University Hospital, Finland, and at the Uppsala University Hospital, Sweden.

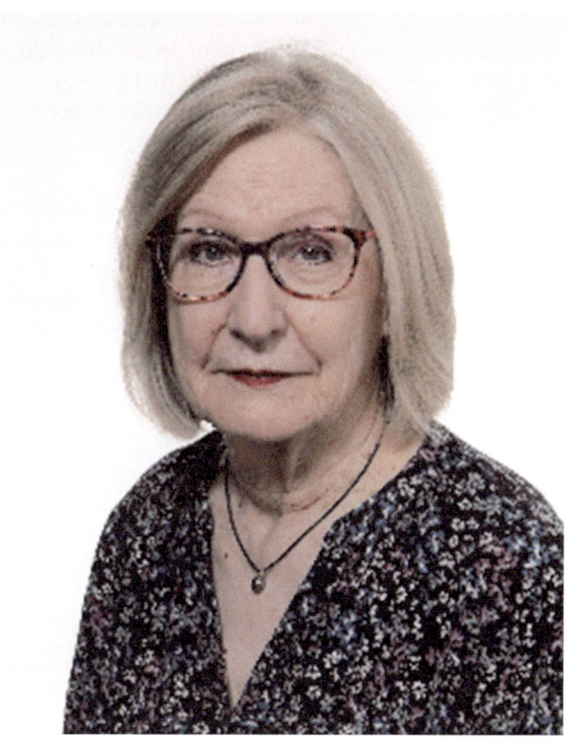

Elna-Marie Larsson, MD, PhD, received her medical degree from Lund University (1977), Sweden, and her doctoral degree (PhD) in diagnostic radiology from the same university (1989). This was followed by a post-doc for one year at the University of Texas Health Science Center, San Antonio, Texas, USA. During 2006–2009, she had a position as professor of radiology at Aarhus University, Denmark. In 2009, she moved back to Sweden and became appointed as professor of neuroradiology at Uppsala University and from 2010, also visiting professor of neuroradiology at Linkoping University, both until retirement in 2018. She has published more than 200 papers in peer-reviewed scientific journals and 30 descriptive articles and textbook chapters. She has been the main supervisor of 14 PhD and co-supervisor for 14 PhD students. Her research has been focused on advanced cerebral MR imaging of the brain with applications in dementia, brain tumors, and normal pressure hydrocephalus. Her clinical activity has included CT and MRI of the brain, spine, and head&neck. She has been the director of neuroradiology and of MRI at the department of radiology, Lund University Hospital and at the department of radiology, Uppsala University Hospital, Sweden. She has vast experience in teaching (national and international) with emphasis on MRI and neuroradiology and has organized several MRI and neuroradiology courses, including European Society of Magnetic Resonance in Medicine and Biology (ESMRMB) courses. She has been president of ESMRMB, the Swedish Society of Neuroradiology (SFNR), the Nordic Society of Neuroradiology (NSNR), and the Danish Society for Medical Magnetic Resonance (DSMMR).

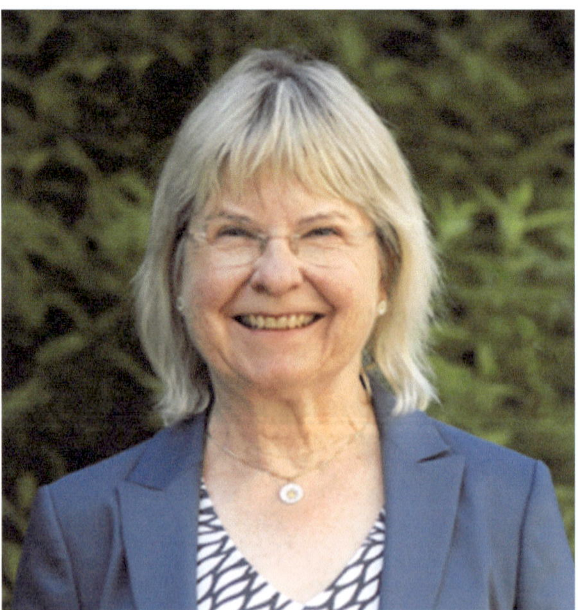

Maria Kristoffersen Wiberg MD, PhD, received her medical degree at the medical school in Umeå 1981, received her specialization in radiology 1992, in neuroradiology 2005, and her doctoral degree (PhD) in diagnostic radiology 2002. She has been a senior lecturer since 1998 at Karolinska University Hospital (KS) Huddinge. She was the head of the MRI-unit at the Department of Radiology at KS Huddinge (1998–2010) and Head of Department of Radiology at KS Huddinge (2011–2016). She became professor in Radiology at Linköping University 2017 and is present professor emeritus at Linköping University since 2022. Her contribution to the field of radiology and neuroradiology is broad but with a focus on MR methods both in neuroradiology and musculoskeletal radiology. She set up the first MR unit in Sundsvall 1992, implemented the method in clinical routine, and implemented breast MR in clinical routine in 2002. She moved to KS in 1994, responsible for the installation and clinical start-up of the new MR-equipment at KS and was involved in the planning and installation of the new building for the radiological department and operation theaters at KS Huddinge (2010–2020). Her research focus has been in the diagnosis of neuroinflammation and neurodegeneration in cooperation with clinical specialists with, for example, the start of a longitudinal still ongoing standardized collection of MRI in multiple sclerosis and imaging for volumetric assessments in dementia with established standardized evaluations. She participated in the start of the Swedish MS-registry. Since 1994, she has participated in teaching in areas such as MRI in general, as a method, and specifically in diagnosis of neuroinflammation and neurodegeneration. She has supervised several master students and four PhD students as mains supervisor and five as co-supervisor.

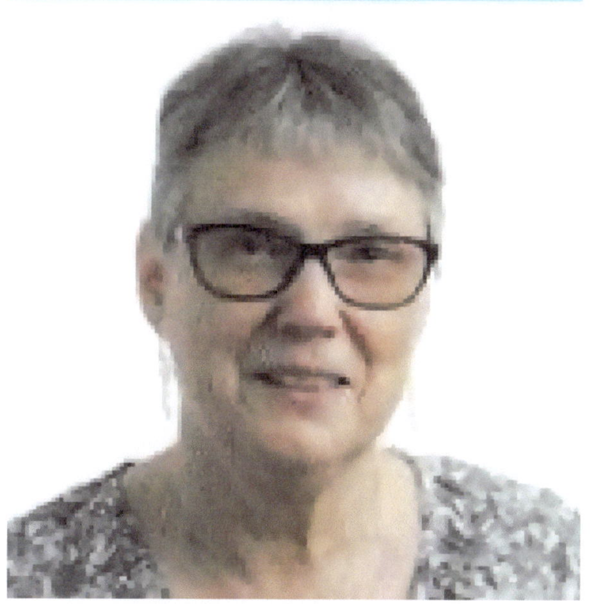

Pia C. Maly Sundgren MD, PhD, received her medical degree from Lund University (LU), Sweden (1986), and her doctoral degree (PhD) in diagnostic radiology (1991), followed by specialization in radiology (1993) and subspecialization in neuroradiology (1997), and associate professor (1995) at the same institution. After working as a neuroradiologist with special focus on adult and pediatric neuroradiology, she went to the Department of Radiology at the University of Michigan, USA, 2001, where she became a full professor in 2006. In 2009, she returned to Sweden as appointed Professor of Diagnostic Radiology at LU and, as of 2016, also Co-Director for Lund University BioImaging Centre. She has published over 210 papers and reviews in peer reviewed scientific journals, and 22 textbook chapters. Her supervision covers ongoing and concluded PhD projects as main supervisor for eight PhD students and as co-supervisor for three PhD students, 14 master students, and over 20 undergraduate and graduate students in research. Her main area of research is advanced MR imaging of the brain with applications in brain tumors and autoimmune diseases in which she collaborates nationally and internationally. She has been the president of the International Society of Magnetic resonance imaging in Medicine (ISMRM), president of European Society of Neuroradiology (ESNR), and is presently General Secretary of the World Federation of Neuroradiology Societies (WFNRS) and Deputy Chair of the European Board of Neuroradiology. She is a well-recognized faculty at congresses and courses with over 400 internationally invited lectures and workshops. Prof. Sundgren has been awarded, among others, the MICHR Michigan Clinical and Translational Research Distinguished Mentor Award, the Minerva Leadership Award from the Medical Faculty of Lund University, and the Nelson Mandela Gold medal for unique contribution to the South African Radiology, South Africa. She is a Senior ISMRM Fellow.

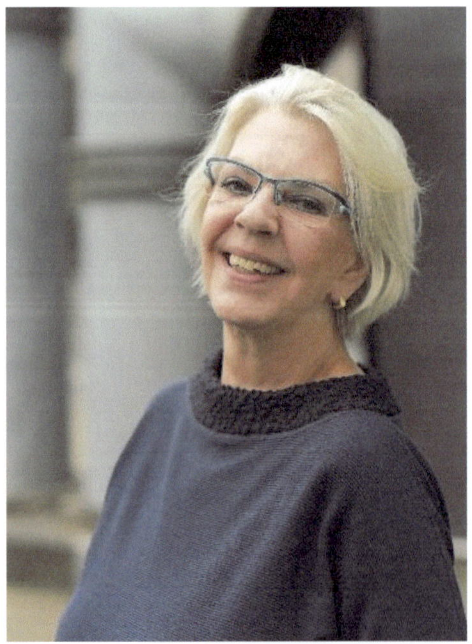

Isabella Björkman-Burtscher MD, PhD, received her medical degree and doctoral degree (PhD) from the Leopold-Franzens-University (1995), Innsbruck, Austria. After moving to Sweden in 1995, she enrolled in a PhD program at Lund University (LU) and received her PhD in diagnostic radiology in 1999 with a thesis on MRS in brain tumors. She specialized in radiology and neuroradiology at Skåne University Hospital (SUS), where she worked as a senior consultant, pediatric neuroradiologist, and senior lecturer at LU until 2018. She was appointed as the professor of neuroradiology at the University of Gothenburg and a senior consultant at Sahlgrenska University Hospital (SU) in 2018, where she is currently working. Enabling PhD students to follow their interests, research projects spanned from lung tomosynthesis and experimental pig models to MR safety issues at 7T and advanced MR neuroimaging encompassing MRS, diffusion-based techniques, and currently also sodium MR. She has introduced MRS as a clinical tool at SUS, introduced clinical 7T MRI to Sweden as co-director of the first 7T MR facility in Sweden, and is currently introducing sodium MR to the clinical imaging arsenal at SU in Gothenburg. Her own research has focused on advanced MR methods and their application to brain diseases such as epilepsy and brain tumors. She has held committee appointments within the European Congress of Radiology (ECR), the International Society of Magnetic Resonance in Medicine (ISMRM), the Swedish Society of Neuroradiology (SFNR), and the Swedish Society of Radiology (SFMR) and is a board member of the latter two. She has published 100 scientific original papers; review articles and book chapters and supervision cover ongoing and concluded PhD projects as main supervisor for nine and as co-supervisor for eight PhD students.

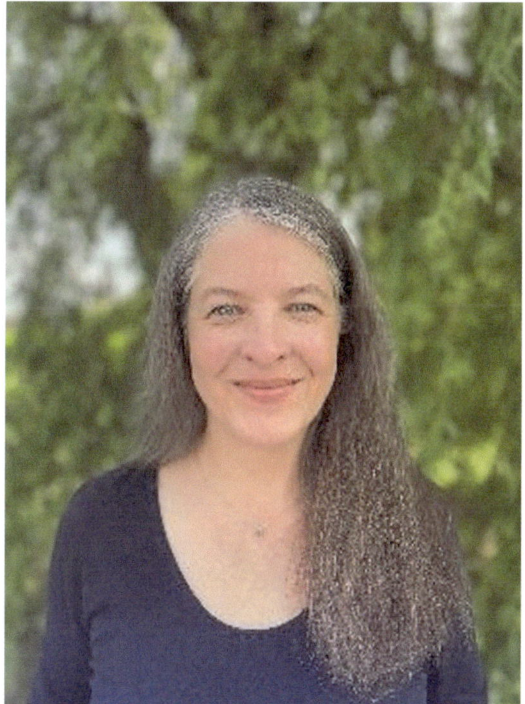

Ida Blystad MD, PhD, received her medical degree 2002 at Linköping University, followed a specialization in radiology (2010) and a subspecialization in neuroradiology (2013) at the same institution and the European Diploma in Neuroradiology in 2016. In parallel with the neuroradiology fellowship, she enrolled as a PhD student with focus on syntactic MR in brain tumors and received her PhD in 2017. Her main supervisor was Prof Elna-Marie Larsson. Dr Blystad has continued to engage in multidisciplinary research projects, where neuroradiology is situated in the intersection between clinical specialties and the technical faculty, always with a focus on imaging of the brain and is mentor for PhD students and master students. She was a board member of the Swedish Society for Radiology between 2011 and 2020 acting as secretary between 2015 and 2020. She is since 2023, president of the Swedish Society of Neuroradiology.

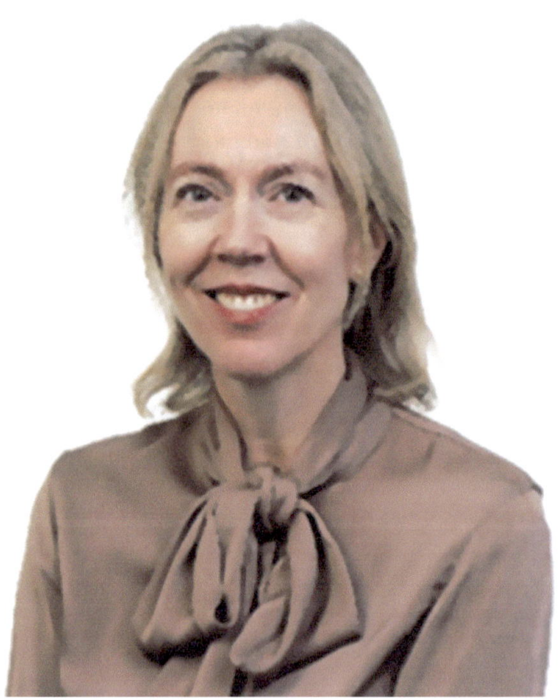

Anna Falk Delgado MD, PhD, received her medical degree in 2009 at Karolinska Institute (KI) in Stockholm. Her focus was early on radiology/neuroradiology partly related to studying for 2 months at the University of Southern California (USC) in Los Angeles, where she encountered patients with a wide range of neurosurgical and neurological conditions as well as the thrill experience of attending radiology rounds during her internship. During her residency training in Radiology at Uppsala University (UU) Hospital in Sweden, she became part of an interesting project investigating patients with suspected low-grade gliomas by PET and MRI together with her main supervisor Professor Elna-Marie Larsson. This became the focus of her PhD studies, which she defended in 2016 at UU. She later continued her residency and neuroradiology training at the Department of Neuroradiology in Stockholm. In 2021, she became an Associate Professor and founded her research group "Clinical Brain Imaging Methods" at KI. Reconnecting to her PhD studies, she recently had the opportunity to train as a resident physician at the Department of Nuclear Medicine at Karolinska University Hospital, to deepen her knowledge in hybrid imaging methods of the brain. Clinically, the focus of primary brain tumors and multidisciplinary rounds has continued to evoke her desire to evolve and cooperate with other specialties. She sees great future potential in the rapidly evolving field of Neuroradiology that has never ceased to intrigue her.

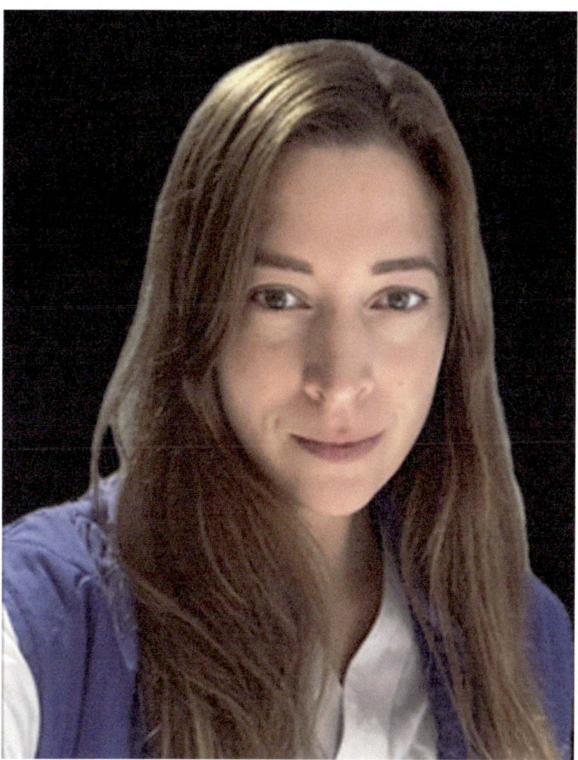

Birgitta Ramgren, MD, PhD, received her medical degree at Lund University in 1987. She received her specialty in Diagnostic Radiology, 1995, and in Neuroradiology, 1998, and received her PhD, 2014. She was early recruited to the Neuroradiology Department, which she remained loyal to throughout her professional career. A collaboration between neurosurgeons/neuroradiologists in Lund and the interventional neuroradiologist Prof. Jacques Moret, Paris, had started 1993 to set up interventional neuroradiology in Lund. Dr Ramgren went, after initial training in Lund by Dr. Mats Cronquist and prof Jaques Moret, to Paris for additional training in neurointervention. Together with radiographers, anesthesiologists, and neurosurgeons, a neurointerventional team was established at Lund University Hospital in 1996. She was head of the Dept. of Neuroradiology (2004–2013), and head of the section of interventional neuroradiology (2019–2022). She has mentored many diagnostic and interventional neuroradiologists, personnel, and medical students locally, nationally, and internationally. She has been lecturer at both national and international courses/conferences, and a member of several steering committees. She is certified by the European Society of Neuroradiology (ESNR) with European Certificate of Neuroradiology and by the European Board of Neuroradiology (EBNR) with European Diploma in Interventional Neuroradiology (EDiINR). She was the secretary and treasurer of the Nordic Society of Neuroradiology (NSNR) 2003–2009, vice president 2009–2010, and president 2011–2012 of the Swedish Society of Neuroradiology (SFNR). She has been in the steering committee of the Swedish National quality registry for patients that underwent endovascular treatment for stroke (EVAS) (2012–2024). Recently retired from her clinical profession, she still does research in co-operation with the Lund Stroke Imaging Group and co-supervises three PhD students.

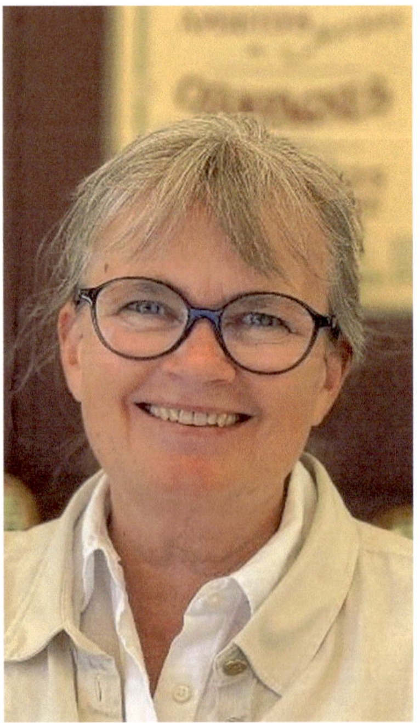

Åsa Kuntze Söderqvist MD, PhD, received her medical degree (1994) at Karolinska institute, Stockholm, followed by specialization in radiology at Danderyds Hospital in Stockholm and received her PhD in 2016. Since 2004, she has been working at the Department of Neuroradiology at Karolinska University Hospital and as interventional neuroradiologist since 2008. Her career has been significantly marked by her contributions to the development and refinement of mechanical thrombectomy for acute ischemic stroke. Her work highlights the importance of this technique in cases of large cerebral artery occlusions and basilar artery occlusion, demonstrating superior results compared to traditional thrombolysis methods. She also has an interest in and has practiced spinal interventions for both diagnosis and treatment. In addition to her clinical practice, she is actively involved in education and training, offering courses designed to enhance the skills of residents and specialists in acute stroke care. These courses emphasize the latest advancements in radiological diagnostics and reperfusion therapy, contributing to the overall improvement of stroke treatment.

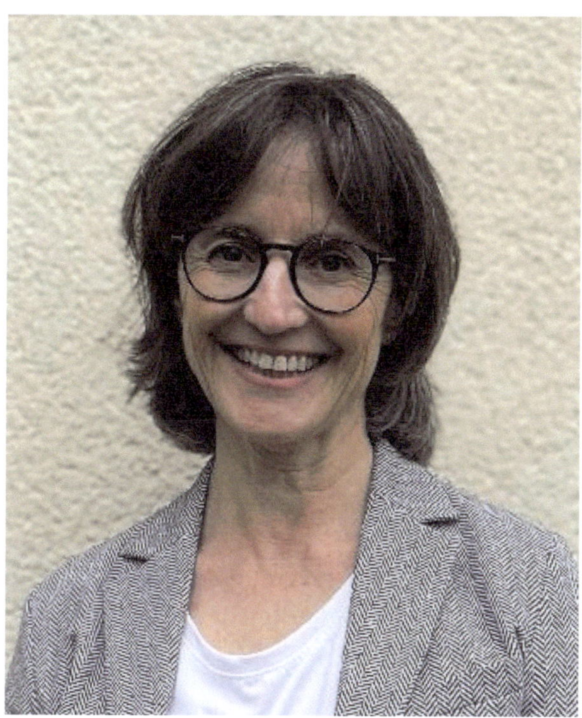

Women in Neuroradiology: Switzerland

María Isabel Vargas

Introduction

In Switzerland, neuroradiology is a subspeciality of radiology.

We have a system of board certification in neuroradiology, in which training is performed in centers accredited with a clear curriculum guided by a log book and two examinations, one in diagnostic and one in interventional neuroradiology.

Switzerland is one of the rare countries in Europe that have this title of subspecialty.

The subtitle for neuroradiology was established in 1991, 2 years after the foundation of the Swiss Society of Neuroradiology in 1989. The foundation members of the Swiss Society of Neuroradiology were Anton Valavanis from Zurich, Peter Huber from Bern, Ernst-Wilhelm Radü from Basel, and Othmar Schubiger from Zurich.

The currently president of the SSNR is a women Prof. Isabel Wanke (see detailed biography in German Chapter).

Currently, there are 78 women working as diagnostic neuroradiologist and 6 as interventional neuroradiologist in our country.

Prominent Woman Neuroradiologists in Switzerland

Dr. Marcelle Megret She is a French national born in Algeria. She studied neuroradiology in Strasbourg with Prof. A Wackenheim. In 1972, she moved to Geneva, where she worked in the neurology department. Then, she moved to radiology, where she became Head of diagnostic neuroradiology. She worked there for more than 20 years.

She was a diagnostic and interventional neuroradiologist. In 1986, she wrote one of the first books showing images with CT scans, Computed Tomography of the Cranial Skeleton (Face and Skull): 58 Radiological Exercises for Students and Practitioners (Exercises in Radiological Diagnosis). This was the first book she wrote as a neuroradiologist and one of the first with very demonstrative schemas done by the author herself. The book also provided a series of high-quality images.

She was a pioneer. Have you heard Megret's line? She described it, and it is a landmark in recognizing the choroidal arteries of the fourth ventricle, branches of the posterior inferior cerebellar artery.

Dr. Jacqueline Delavelle (1945–2024) She was born in Poitiers-France; she received her title as a Medical Doctor in Paris in 1973, and after she moved to Evian les Bains.

She was the head of the diagnostic neuroradiology unit at the Geneva University Hospital.

Dr Delavelle was a very enthusiastic teacher who was most appreciated by the students.

She was a prolific author, with around 90 papers published in esteemed international journals.

The predilection subjects were pediatric neuroradiology and epilepsy.

Her infectious enthusiasm for new technologies and their application in neuroradiology sparked excitement for the future of the field, inspiring many students to follow in her innovative footsteps.

She retired in 2010.

Prof. Dr. MD María Isabel Vargas (author of the chapter) (Fig. 24.7).

She was born in Ecuador and received her title as a Medical Doctor in 1994. She moved to Switzerland, where she studied first Radiology (1996–2001) and then Neuroradiology (2001–2004). She was board-certified as a diagnostic neuroradiologist in 2006, Head of Diagnostic Neuroradiology in 2013, and Professor of neuroradiology in 2016.

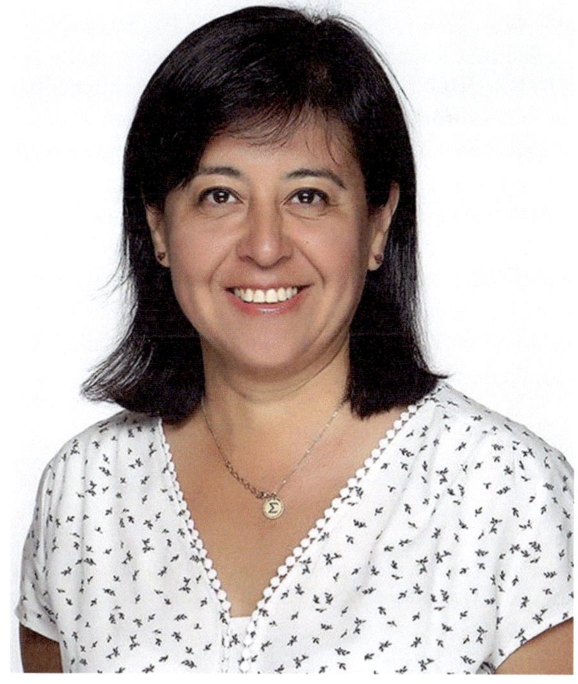

Fig. 24.7 Prof. María Isabel Vargas

She has been writing more than 200 papers, two books, and several chapters.

She was a pioneer in using advanced techniques to study peripheral nerves.

Her centers of interest are not just limited to the conventional imaging, but also extend to new and advanced techniques for neurological diseases such as epilepsy, tumors, vascular diseases, the spine, and peripheral nerves, reflecting her enthusiasm for progress and innovation.

Her other passion is teaching and finding playful methods of teaching.

Women in Neuroradiology: The Netherlands

Kees J. Simon and Frans W. Zonneveld

The Rise of Female Neuroradiologists in the Netherlands

Introduction

In the Netherlands, the movement for women's emancipation emerged in the second half of the nineteenth century. In 1878, Aletta Henriette Jacobs (1854–1929) was the first female medical graduate. A year later, she defended her thesis on a then-and-now current neurological topic: the theory of localization. (1) She became the epitome of women's empowerment in the Netherlands.

The first female professor in medicine was the pediatrician Cornelia de Lange (1871–1950). She was appointed in 1927 (University of Amsterdam) and is known for the syndrome named after her, a condition with neuroradiological features (2).[1]

But it was not until 1998 that the first female professor of diagnostic radiology was appointed (Erasmus University Rotterdam): Myriam G.M. Hunink (born 1958), known for her expertise in medical decision-making and technology assessment.

In our country, medicine was a male-dominated world, and this was even more true in radiology.[2] Over the past century, women remained significantly underrepresented in radiology, less than 10%. But at the beginning of this century, ±30% of radiologists in training were women. As a result, the percentage of women among radiologists is currently 36%.

[1] The very first female professor in the Netherlands was the botanist Johanna Westerdijk (1883–1961), appointed in 1917, in Utrecht. She was the daughter of radiologist Bernard Westerdijk (1853–1927).

[2] On January 1, 2024, an overrepresentation of female physicians was found: 58% (see BIG-registration).

A Brief History of Neuroradiology in the Netherlands

The development of neuroradiology can be roughly divided into two periods: before and after the 1970s. For both periods, we list the names of radiologists who were important for the development of the field in the Netherlands.

Before the 1970s, the era of classical radiology. Hendrik W. Stenvers (1889–1973), Bernard G. Ziedses des Plantes (1902–1993), and Lourens Penning (1922–2006) can be mentioned.

Stenvers is the founder of neuroradiology in our country and is known for the projection of the petrous bone named after him. Ziedses des Plantes is world-famous for his discoveries of tomography and subtraction. Lourens Penning held the first chair in neuroradiology in 1970 (Groningen). For his merits, the Lourens Penning Prize was created, an award for young researchers in neuroradiology.

After the 1970s, the modern era of radiology (computers, CT, and MRI). Neuroradiologists Jaap Valk (1929–2024) and Johannes Th. (Jan) Wilmink (1943–2021) came to the fore. Both were professors of neuroradiology and honorary members of the European Society of Neuroradiology. The driven Valk was (co) author of various standard works in the MRI field with many awards (including honorary member of the Radiological Society of North America). He was the supervisor of *two women* who have done important work in the field of neuroradiology: Marjo S. van der Knaap and Ragnhild G.M. de Slegte. The biographical details of Van der Knaap are listed below, together with the current generation of women at the top of the field.

Dutch Society of Neuroradiology

The Dutch Society for Neuroradiology (DSNR) started in the 1950s as an informal meeting of neuroradiologists on the initiative of Ziedses des Plantes and Penning. In 1993, it became an official subsection of the Dutch Society of Radiology, with Valk as chairman and Wilmink as vice chairman. Membership was subject to conditions, including balloting. Around 2000, it had about 25 members, including a few women. It now has 256 members, including 117 women (45%).

Prominent Female Neuroradiologists in the Netherlands

Prof. Dr. M.S. (Marjo) van der Knaap (born 1958)

Although not a neuroradiologist by profession, she has done very important work in this field. In the early days of MRI, she brought order to the abnormalities of the white matter in the brain, in close collaboration with her supervisor Jaap Valk, professor of neuroradiology. There is even a disease named after her: *Van der Knaap disease* or megalencephalic leukoencephalopathy with subcortical cysts. Her book, *Magnetic resonance of myelination and myelin disorders*, is a standard work. For this, she received the *Gold Award of the International Society of Magnetic Resonance in Medicine*. She is an internationally recognized authority.

Since 1999, she has been the professor of child neurology at the VU in Amsterdam. She integrates radiology, neurology, and genetics in her research. She received three *TOP grants (ZonMw)* for excellent research, received the *Sidney Carter Award* from the American Academy of Neurology and was a *Spinoza laureate* in 2008. She is an *Honorary Member* of the American Society of Neuroradiology (2001) and received the *Gold Medal* of the American Society for Pediatric Neuroradiology in 2014. She has been a *member of the KNAW* (Royal Dutch Academy of Sciences) since 2006.

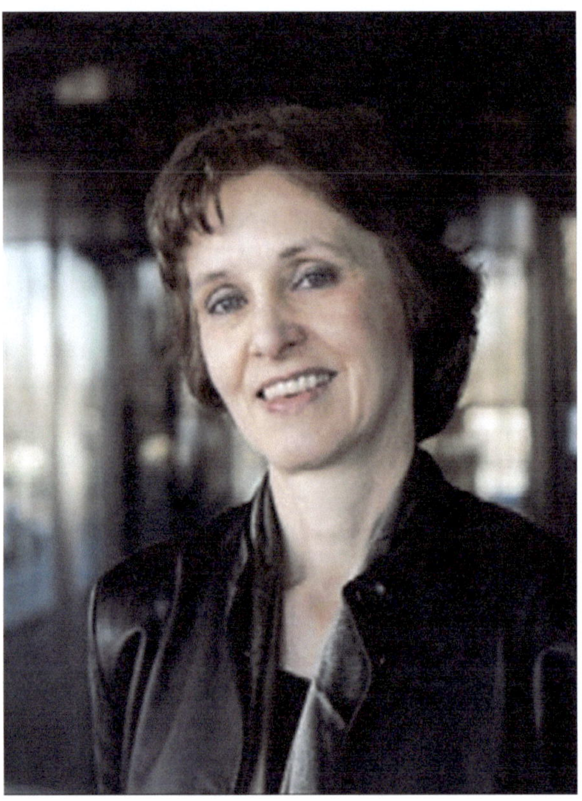

Prof. Dr. M.W. (Meike) Vernooij (born 1978)

Neuroradiologist Meike Vernooij has been using population imaging, the acquisition of medical images in large cohorts, since 2005, to study the development of brain and vascular diseases. She is responsible for the Population Imaging in the important Rotterdam Study. A specific focus of her work is on imaging markers that can be used as preclinical markers for cerebrovascular and neurodegenerative diseases, including dementia.

Her work has been recognized with the European Prize for Neuroradiology (*Lucien Appel Prize* 2014), the *Stroke Innovation Prize* of the Journal *Stroke* and the *Lourens Penning Prize* of the Dutch Society for Radiology. She has received many grants for her research.

Meike is professor of Population Imaging since 2017 and Medical Delta professor (Erasmus MC and TU Delft) since 2023. She is also involved as a neuroradiologist and a board member at the Alzheimer Center Erasmus MC. Meike is chair of the Diagnostic Committee and member of the Executive Committee of the European Society of Neuroradiology, and chair of the European Diploma in Radiology (EDiR) Written Evaluation Committee.

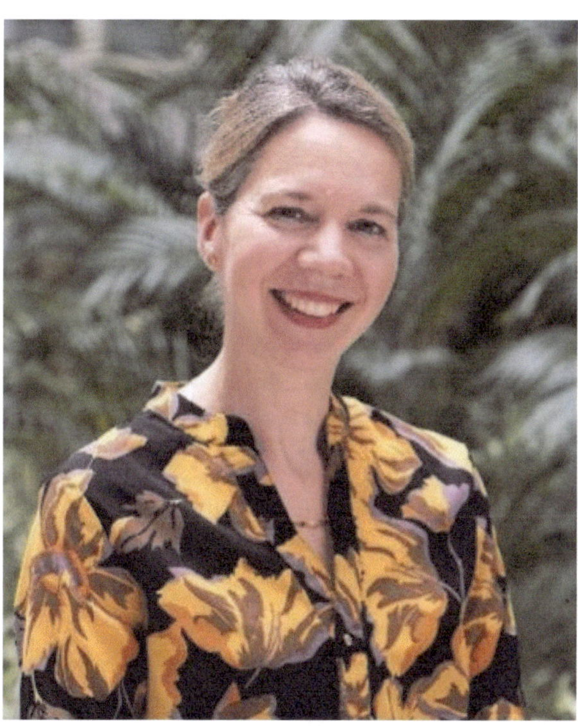

Prof. Dr. M. (Marion) Smits (born 1972)

Marion Smits is a professor and head of neuroradiology at Erasmus MC—University Medical Center Rotterdam (NL). She combines research with clinical work with a particular focus on neuro-oncology at the Brain Tumor Center of the Erasmus MC Cancer Institute, Rotterdam (NL). In addition, Marion has an honorary appointment as professor of Neuroradiology at the Faculty of Applied Sciences of Delft University of Technology (TU Delft) and a Medical Delta Professorship with the aim of advancing technological innovations in healthcare. Marion is chairman of the Research Committee and a member of the Executive Council of the European Society of Radiology, chairman of Research and International Relations, and a board member of the Radiological Society of the Netherlands, former chairman of the Brain Tumor Group Imaging Committee and of the Imaging Group of the European Organization for Research and Treatment of Cancer (EORTC). She is a former president of the European Society for Magnetic Resonance in Medicine and Biology (ESMRMB) (2020) and of the Dutch Society of Neuroradiology (2018–2021).

She received *honorary membership* in the American Society of Neuroradiology in recognition of her outstanding contributions to the field of neuroradiology. In 2021, she was named "*most influential radiology researcher*" by AuntMinnie Europe. In 2022, she received a *senior fellowship* from both the ESMRMB and the International Society of Magnetic Resonance in Medicine (ISMRM) in London for her groundbreaking work at the intersection of technical innovation and clinical neuroradiology. She received many awards and grants. In 2007, she received the *Lourens Penning Prize* and in 2023 *a Vici personal grant* from ZonMw.

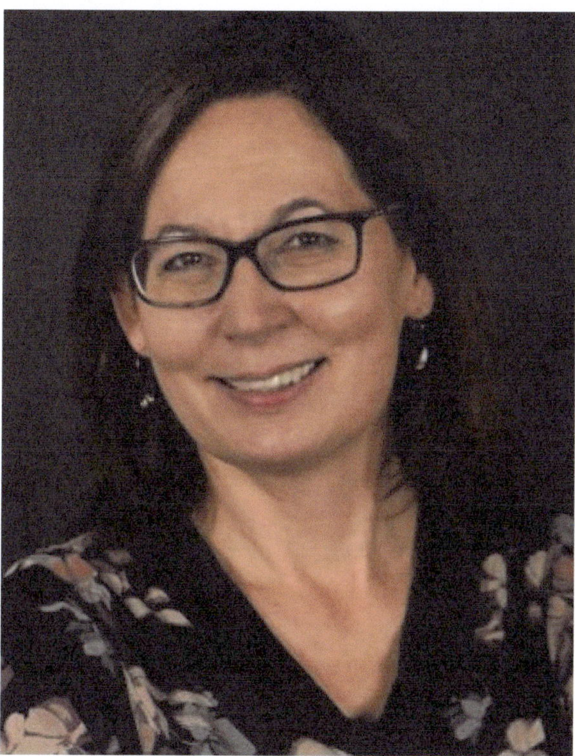

Prof. Dr. L. (Liesbeth) Reneman (born 1968)

Liesbeth Reneman is Professor of Translational Neuroradiology and Neuroradiologist at the Amsterdam University Medical Center, location AMC in Amsterdam (NL). She worked as a post-doctoral research fellow at top universities and laboratories abroad (including Johns Hopkins Medical Institution and Imperial College) and currently heads the "Translational Neuroradiology" research group. Examining the effects of drugs and medications (such as ecstasy, amphetamine, chemotherapy, methylphenidate, and antidepressants) on the brain and behavior using a highly multidisciplinary and translational approach is at the heart of her work. Her innovative work provides critical insights into the benefits and risks of psychotropic drugs on the brain (in development), with applications in personalized medicine and the novel field of psychoradiology. She is a former program leader of the Brain Imaging research program within the Amsterdam Neuroscience research organization. Her work has received many grants and prizes, including the *Hersenstichting Trofee voor de Wetenschap*, the European *Marie Curie Award* (Society of Nuclear Medicine) and several *personal grants*, including a *Fullbright OiO Grant*.

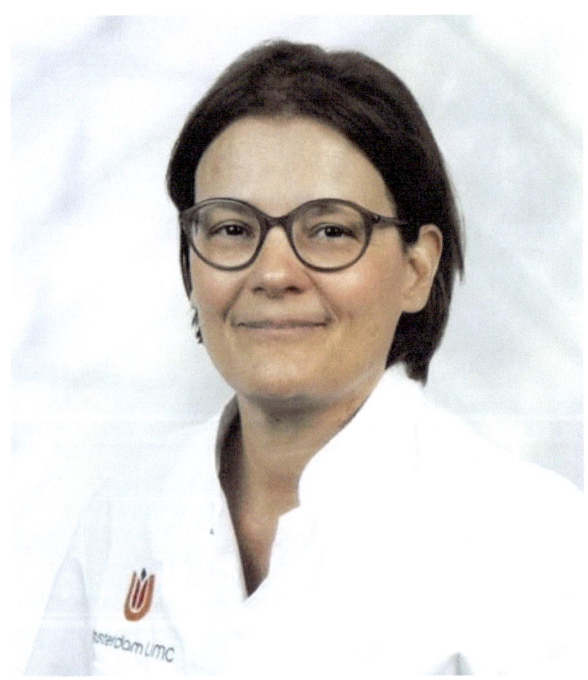

Women in Neuroradiology: Turkey

Aysenur Cila and Isil Saatci

Women in Neuroradiology in Turkey

Even though the first use of an X-Ray device dates back to the Ottoman Crimean War in 1895, the use of X-Ray-based radiology only became widespread at the end of the 1950s in the modern Turkish Republic. Unfortunately, there exists no comprehensive or published record detailing the initiation and evolution of neuroradiology in Turkey. The first CT was installed in 1976, whereas the first MRI machine was set up in 1988.

Until the 1980s, neurologists and neurosurgeons took the lead in the performance of X-Ray-related neuroradiological examinations, such as air ventriculography and percutaneous cerebral angiography, among whom female neurologists, Dr. Hayrünnisa Denktaş from Istanbul University Cerrahpaşa Medical Faculty and Dr. Sara Bahar from Istanbul University Capa Medical Faculty, took part along with their male counterparts. In 1980, Istanbul University published the first angiography book in Turkish, authored by Prof. Dr. Hayrünnisa Denktaş and Prof. Dr. Sabahattin Kerimoğlu. Around this time, very few female radiologists were in this male-dominated field. With the second generation of CT devices becoming available in the early 1980s, many residents—including several women—were attracted to the field of radiology.

Zerrin Yetkin from Ege University in İzmir and Canan Erzen from Ankara University took on pioneering roles in neuroradiology. In their residencies, they started working primarily with CT, but their close collaboration with neurosurgeons led them to take up neuroradiology, turning them into experts in their field. Professor Yetkin has spearheaded the functional MRI and resting-state functional MRI at the Medical College of Wisconsin, and still works at the University of Texas Southwestern Medical Center. Professor Erzen worked in Hacettepe University (Ankara) and Marmara University (Istanbul), where she contributed heavily to both research and the education of new generations of neuroradiologists till her retirement.

Following in these footsteps were Aysenur Cila from Hacettepe University and Nilgun Yunten from the Ege University. Both women became leaders in the field through their research productivity, lively teaching styles, and incredible work ethic. Their passion for neuroradiology and its education attracted many brilliant medical residents to the field, who have gone on to advance the area through their inventions and research contributions. After her training on MRI in Rotterdam in 1991, Aysenur Cila focused on MRI and she has always been very influential in establishing contemporary MR Imaging and a mentor in this field. Another female neuroradiologist in the same period was Emel Ada, who had one year of diagnostic and interventional neuroradiology training in France under the mentorship of

Prof. Manelfe in University of Toulouse in 1991. When she was back home in Izmir, she started to work as a diagnostic and interventional neuroradiologist at Dokuz Eylul University, where she has been working as a diagnostic neuroradiologist since 2002.

Isil Saatci (Fig. 24.8), who did her neuroradiology fellowship at Georgetown University, USA, in 1991–1992, was the first female to do a formal neuroradiology fellowship and continued her career in Turkey. In Hacettepe University, where she had graduated from Medical School and had done her residency, she first started to work both in interventional and diagnostic neuroradiology, pediatric neuroradiology in particular, and had many publications. With the increasing workload of interventional neuroradiology, she became dedicated to interventional neuroradiology and created advanced endovascular treatment techniques. International workshops were organized in her institution in which she trained many physicians in these treatment techniques. For many years, she has been travelling worldwide to train neurointerventionists in advanced cerebral aneurysm and AVM treatments. After several years of international live case workshops (Anatolian Course of Interventional Neuroradiology between 2006 and 2008; co-partner with LINNC 2009–2011), she and her colleagues started the World Live Neurovascular Conference (WLNC) in 2013, which rotates around the world, being held in a different continent every year to serve for the education and training in the field of interventional neuroradiology. She is among the founders of CREF (Cerebrovascular Research and Education Foundation), which supports neurointerventionists with limited financial resources. She took part in

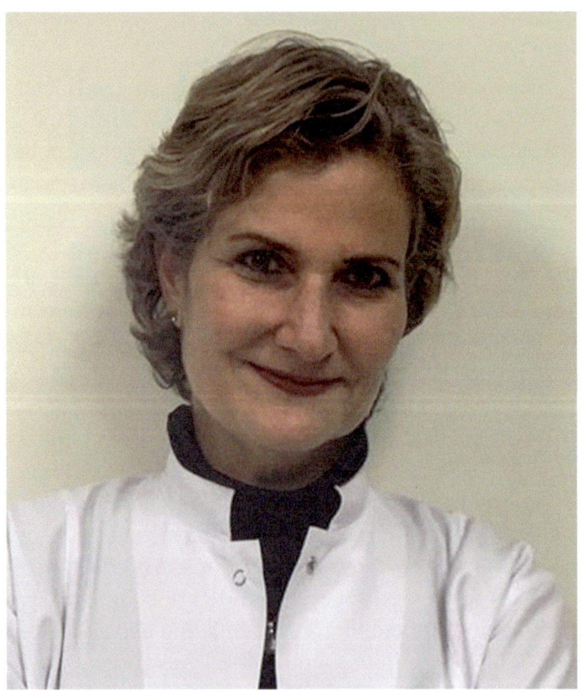

Fig. 24.8 Dr. Isil Saatci

several international studies and worked as the Section Editor of Interventional Neuroradiology in the NEURORADIOLOGY for several years. Currently, she is an Associate Editor of Journal of Neurointerventional Surgery (JNIS). She is the Chair of Interventional Neuroradiology in European Society of Neuroradiology (ESNR) executive committee. She is organizing courses, webinars worldwide and participating in international meetings, serving to the purpose of INR training.

There are several female neuroradiologists, namely Kader Karlı Oğuz and Burce Ozgen from Hacettepe University, Yelda Ozsunar from Aydin Menderes University, Serra Sencer from Çapa University-Istanbul, and many others in the next generation to follow, who are subspecialized and very actively working in their academic environments. Professor Karlı Oğuz, doing a fellowship at University of John Hopkins in 2001, focusing on functional MRI, conducted multidisciplinary research on MRI studies, surgery, and neuroscience; worked as an adjunct professor at the National Magnetic Resonance Research Center along with Hacettepe University for several years. Currently, she continues her work at UC Davis Medical Center in Sacramento, California. Burce Ozgen who had her fellowships in Neuroradiology in Harvard University and in Head and Neck Radiology, currently works in University of Illinois at Chicago.

There are currently 132 female members of the Turkish Society of Neuroradiology, which was founded in 1991, 50 of whom are in an academic environment. Two of them, Prof. Ozlem Alkan and Prof. Gülgün Yılmaz Ovalı, are currently in the Executive Committee of the Society, working very actively to advance the subspeciality of neuroradiology further. We owe a great deal to all the above-mentioned women and many others for establishing and advancing the field of neuroradiology in our country and contributing to our field worldwide.

Readers are suggested to contact the corresponding author for figures if needed.

Further Reading

Croatia

1. Simunic S, Glavina K, Besenski N, Klaric-Custovic R. Croatian Society of Radiology (1928-2008), the Croatian Medical Association – 80 years of existence and activity. Radiol Oncol. 2011;45(2):147–58.

Germany

2. Zanella FE. Geschichte der Neuroradiologie in Deutschland. Clin Neuroradiol. 2015;25(Suppl 2):97–100. https://doi.org/10.1007/s00062-015-0456-1.
3. URL: https://www.hpk.uni-hamburg.de/resolve/id/cph_person_00001134. Downloaded on 02.08.2024.

4. Warmuth-Metz M, Kuhl J, Krauss J, Solymosi L. Subdural enhancement on postoperative spinal MRI after resection of posterior cranial fossa tumours. Neuroradiology. 2004;46:219–23.
5. URL: https://scholar.google.de/scholar?hl=de&as_sdt=0%2C5&q=Ulrike+Ernemann&btnG=.
6. URL: https://www.medizin.uni-tuebingen.de/de/dasklinikum/einrichtungen/zentren/zentrum-fuer-vaskulaere-anomalien.
7. URL: https://scholar.google.de/citations?hl=de&user=kDXPRHIAAAAJ.
8. URL: https://www.snri.ch/.
9. URL: https://scholar.google.de/citations?hl=de&user=BV5PGX4AAAAJ.
10. URL: https://www.dgnr.org/de-DE/37/vorstand-und-ausschuesse.
11. URL: https://www.hahn-institut.de/de.
12. URL: https://scholar.google.de/scholar?hl=de&as_sdt=0,5&q=Elke+Gizewski.
13. URL: https://scholar.google.de/citations?hl=de&user=g91VDEQAAAAJ.
14. URL: https://www.esmint.eu/about/women-in-neurointervention/.
15. URL: https://scholar.google.de/citations?hl=de&user=aADB2tAAAAAJ.
16. Linn J, Halpin A, Demaerel P, Ruhland J, Giese AD, Dichgans M, van Buchem MA, Bruckmann H, Greenberg SM. Prevalence of superficial siderosis in patients with cerebral amyloid angiopathy. Neurology. 2010;74:1346–50. https://doi.org/10.1212/WNL.0b013e3181dad605.

Italy

17. https://www.dati.salute.gov.it/it/dataset/elenco-nazionale-direttori/.
18. Giovagnoni A, Gandolfo N, Miele V. Women in radiology: the SIRM believes in equal opportunity. Radiol Med. 2022;127(3):225–7. https://doi.org/10.1007/s11547-022-01474-9. Epub 2022 Mar 23. PMID: 35320463; PMCID: PMC8940974.
19. https://cercauniversita.mur.gov.it/php5/docenti/cerca.php.

Spain

20. Martinez C, Pastor R, de la Pascua M, Tavera S. Mujeres en la historia de España: enciclopedia biográfica. Barcelona: Planeta; 2007.
21. Gallar P. Sobre las radiólogas españolas. Madrid: L&C Diseño; 2005.
22. Consejo General de Colegios Oficiales de Médicos de España. Mujeres pioneras en la medicina española. 2022. Disponible en: https://www.cgcom.es/sites/main/files/minisite/static/4b479141-9304-47e1-82c9-73b5685e234b/Mujeres-pionerasen-la-Medicina/index.html. Consultado 17 Mar 2022.
23. Hasebrook J, Hahnenkamp K, Buhre WFFA, de Korte-de Boer D, Hamaekers AEW, Metelmann B, et al. Medicine goes female: Protocol for improving career options of females and working conditions for researching physicians in clinical medical research by organizational transformation and participatory design. JMIR Res Protoc. 2017;6:e152. https://doi.org/10.2196/resprot.7632.
24. Gallar P. El feliz viaje de las radiólogas españolas. Radiología. 2021;63:385–90. https://doi.org/10.1016/j.rx.2021.04.001.
25. Cayón Somacarrera S, Alonso Rodríguez C, Del Campo Del Val L, Oleaga Zufiría L, Rodríguez Carnero P. Women in radiology: a perspective from Spain. Radiologia (Engl Ed). 2024;66(2):121–31. https://doi.org/10.1016/j.rxeng.2023.04.009. Epub 2024 Apr 4. PMID: 38614529.
26. Guàrdia Mas E, Solé Llenas J. Breve historia de la neurorradiología española [A brief history of neuroradiology in Spain]. Radiologia. 2010;52 Suppl 2:3–9. https://doi.org/10.1016/j.rx.2010.03.015. Epub 2010 May 20. PMID: 20493503. Spanish.

Switzerland

27. Mégret M. Computed tomography of the cranial skeleton (face and skull): 58 radiological exercises for students and practitioners (exercises in radiological diagnosis). Berlin Heidelberg: Springer; 1986.
28. Megret M. A landmark for the choroidal arteries of the fourth ventricle--branches of the posteriorinferior cerebellar artery. Neuroradiology. 1973;5(2):85–90. https://doi.org/10.1007/BF00337489.

The Netherlands

29. Jacobs AH. Over localisatie van physiologische en pathologische verschijnselen in de groote herdenen. Thesis, 1879.
30. de Lange C. Sur und type nouveau de degeneration (typus Amstelodamensis). Arch Med Enfants. 1933;36:713–9.
31. Stenvers HW. Roentgenography of the os petrosum. Acta Otolaryngol. 1921;3(1):266–81.
32. Ziedses des Plantes BG. Planigraphie en subtractie. Rontgenographische differentiatiemethoden. Thesis, 1934.
33. Valk J, Knaap MSVD. Magnetic resonance of myelin, myelination, and myelin disorders. Berlin: Springer-Verlag; 1989.
34. Valk J, Barkhof F, Scheltens P. Magnetic resonance in dementia. Berlin/London: Springer; 2002.
35. de Slegte RGM. Cisternographic anatomy of the posterior cranial fossa (high resolution CT and MRI study). Thesis, 1986.

Chapter 25
The History of Women in Neuroradiology in Latin America

Maria de Fátima Viana Vasco Aragao, Carolina Tramontini, Katiuzka Casares, Jose Alejandro Bacalla, Carolina Mejias Soto, Carlos Rugilo, Eduardo Gonzalez, Carolina Servin, Janeth Bu, Valeria Schoenstedit, Maria Honrado, and Jorge Boschi

M. d. F. V. V. Aragao (✉)
Department of Radiology, Clinica Diagnostika Endoscopia e Radiologia, LTDA, Recife, Brazil

Department of Surgery and Postgraduate Department of Neuropsychiatry and Behavioral Sciences at UFPE, Centro de Ciencias Medicas da Universidade Federal de Pernambuco (UFPE), Recife, Brazil

C. Tramontini
Radiologia Departmente, Clínica Universitaria Colombia, Clinicas Colsanitas, Bogota, Colombia

K. Casares
Department of Neuroimaging, National Institute of Neurology and Neurosurgery, Mexico City, Mexico

J. A. Bacalla
Department of Diagnostic Imaging, Instituto Nacional De Ciencias Neurologicas, Lima, Peru
e-mail: jose.bacalla.v@upch.pe

C. M. Soto
Centro Nacional de Imágenes Médicas, Caja Costarricense del Seguro Social, Alajuela, Costa Rica

C. Rugilo
Diagnostic Imaging, Hospital Garrahan, Buenos Aires, Argentina

E. Gonzalez
Radiología-Radiology, Hospital Universitario CEMIC. CEMIC University Hospital, Caba, Argentina

C. Servin
Medical Imaging, Centro Medico La Costa, Asunción, Paraguay

J. Bu
Department of Radiology, hospital de especialidades instituto honduras, Comayagua, Honduras

V. Schoenstedit
Department of Radiologia, Clínica Alemana De Santiago, Santiago, Chile

D. Birchall (ed.), *A World History of Neuroradiology*,
https://doi.org/10.1007/978-3-032-16653-1_25

History of Women Neuroradiologists in Brazil

Most Influential Brazilian Female Neuroradiologist Doctors

Dr. Maria Lúcia Soares MD (Fig. 25.1) is a Brazilian neuroradiologist. She was one of the first female neuroradiologists in Brazil. She graduated in medicine in the state of São Paulo (Faculty of Medicine of Jundiaí) in 1979, followed by a residency in Radiology at Instituto de Assistência Médica ao Servidor Público Estadual de São Paulo (IAMSPE-SP) (1980–1982). Her neuroradiology fellowship was done at Med Imagem Hospital de Beneficência Portuguesa de São Paulo, where she trained with Dr. Sérgio Santos Lima, Dr. Enio Cesar Viera Pereira, and Dr. Renato Adam Mendonça, becoming part of the Neuroradiology staff from then on. In 1989, she started a new Fellowship at the Foundation Ophtalmologique Adolph Rothschild, Paris/France, working with MRI, as an emergent technology, with Dr. Jacqueline Vignaud. In 1998, she obtained the title of Specialist in Diagnostic Neuroradiology

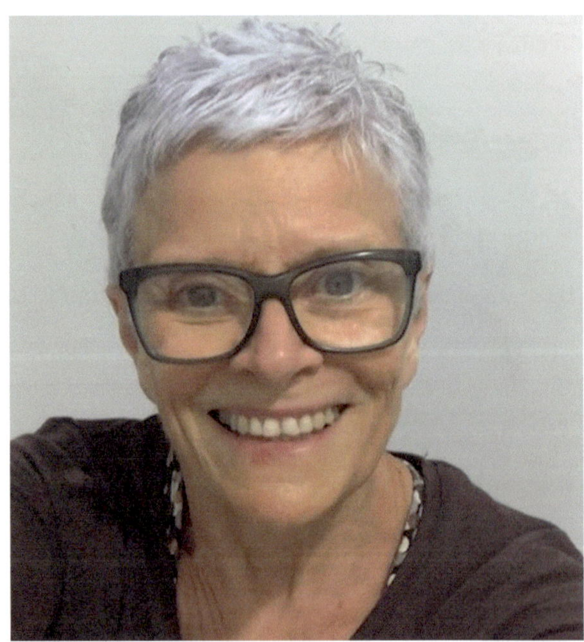

Fig. 25.1 Dr. Maria Lúcia Soares

M. Honrado
Department of Nueroradiology, CIMEN S.A.S, Santiago, Dominican Republic

J. Boschi
Departement of Radiology, Medica Uruguaya, Montevideo, Uruguay

from the SBNRDT. She was part of the Medimagem team from 1982 until 2005. From 2008, she started working as a professor of radiology at the Faculty of Medicine at UFAL (Alagoas).

Edla Chadrycki MD graduated with a degree in medicine from the Federal University of Rio de Janeiro in 1979, followed by a medical residency at the same university in 1982. With a career spanning from 1983 to the present, she brings extensive experience and expertise to her role. Her work focuses on the medical field, particularly in medical radiology, with a dedication to cancer research and treatment. As a public servant, she holds a position at the National Cancer Institute, contributing to the advancement of knowledge and treatment in the field of oncology.

Dr. Maria de Fátima Viana Vasco Aragao MD PhD (Fig. 25.2) was also one of the first female neuroradiologists in Brazil. She graduated in Medicine from the Federal University of Pernambuco (UFPE) in her hometown of Recife in 1987, followed by a Radiology Residency in the Hospital das Clínicas da Universidade de São Paulo (USP) at Ribeirão Preto (1991). She did fellowships in CT, MRI and in neuroradiology in Brazil at Med Imagem Hospital de Beneficência Portuguesa de São Paulo and also had the great opportunity to learn and be part of this group of neuroradiologists at Med Imagem (1991–1993) with Dr. Sergio Santos Lima, Dra. Maria Lucia Soares, Dr. Renato Mendonça, and Dr. Lazaro Amaral. Later, she completed a research fellowship at Mount Sinai Hospital Center in New York in 1996

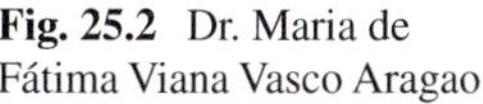

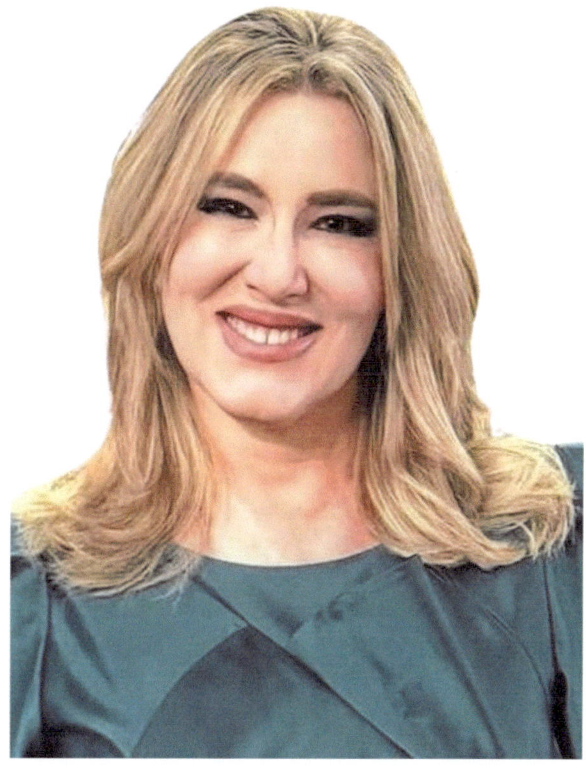

Fig. 25.2 Dr. Maria de Fátima Viana Vasco Aragao

and 2008 with Drs Scott Atlas, Peter Som, Meng Law, and Thomas Naidich. In 2010, she completed her PhD in neuroscience at UFPE in Recife. She is a founding member of the Brazilian Society of Neuroradiology (SBNR). She served as President of the Pernambuco Radiology Society for two terms from 2014 to 2018, and as Secretary of the Brazilian Society of Neuroradiology (SBNR) also for two terms (2008–2010 and 2012–2014). She served as Second Secretary of the Executive Board of the Brazilian College of Radiology (2019–2020). She was elected to the position of Member at Large of the World Federation of Neuroradiological Societies (WFNRS) for the 2018–2022 term and was subsequently re-elected to the same position for the 2022–2026 term. Currently, she is an Adjunct professor of Radiology in the Surgery Department and Permanent Professor in the Department of Post-Graduation in Neuropsychiatry and Behavioral Sciences at the Center for Medical Sciences UFPE, Brazil. In 2016, Dr. Aragao led a group of researchers in their study of Congenital Zika Virus Syndrome. Several articles were published including the first article in Magnetic Resonance Imaging describing this disease of which she was the first author, published in the British Medical Journal (BMJ 2016;353:i1901). Dr. Aragao received recognition for her work in the European Congress of Radiology in Vienna (2017). She was also recognized during the 57th Annual Meeting of the American Society of Neuroradiology (ASNR 2019), in Boston, among the ASNR neuroradiologists' highlights (ASNR Member Spotlight). She and her research group also described the injury found in the olfactory bulbs of COVID-19 patients detected by MRI (2020) that was published in the American Journal of Neuroradiology (Setembro de 2020, 41 (9) 1703-1706). She is member of many International Societies and has lectured at many Radiology Meetings in Brazil as well as in Vienna (European Congress of Radiology in 2017 and in 2018), Canada (ASNR 2018), Colombia, Bolivia, Cuba, Portugal, Uruguay, Dominican Republic, Porto Rico, Chile (SILAN), and Taiwan (XXI Symposium Neuroradiologicum-WFNRS, 2018). Since 2024, she has been a member of the RSNA Educational Exhibits Awards Committee Reviewer, as well as the RSNA Regional Committee for Latin America (RCLA). Dr. Aragao's maternal grandmother, her mother (Janete, biologist), and almost all of his aunts had higher education degrees and worked in their respective fields. Her great-aunt (Isaura Lemos Mesquita) was the first female doctor from Pernambuco state (Brazil), graduating from the Pernambuco School of Medicine in 1935. Dr. Aragao is married to a doctor (Maurício) and is the mother of two beloved sons, Lucas and João Pedro, and have the daugther-in-law Julia (Lucas's wife) who are all young doctors. She is also the doting grandmother of a beloved baby boy (Luiz).

Dr. Fabiane Lorenzoni Sesti, MD, graduated from the Faculty of Medicine of the Pontifical Catholic University of RGS in 1984. She is a specialist in radiology, having completed Medical Residency in 1987 at the Hospital São Lucas of the Catholic University of Rio Grande do Sul (RGS). She earned the title of Specialist in

Neuroradiology and Imaging Diagnosis from the Brazilian College of Radiology. In 1991, she took a Fellowship at Med Imagem/Hosp Beneficiencia Portuguesa de SP with Dr. Sérgio Santos Lima and Renato Mendonça as mentors. In 1996, she took a Research Fellowship in Neuroradiology at Mount Sinai Hospital in New York with Dr. Scott Atlas and in Diagnosis with Head and Neck Image with Dr. Peter Som. She is a Founding Member of the Brazilian Society of Neuroradiology, Associate of the American Society of Neuroradiology, with Master's Degree at the Catholic University of RGS. She was Preceptor of the Radiology Medical Residency at the Santa Casa De Misericórdia Hospital in Porto Alegre and in the Porto Alegre Municipal Emergency Hospital, with an emphasis on teaching and research.

She is the Manager and Head of the Imaging Diagnostic Service at the Hospital Dom Vicente Scherer da Santa Casa de Misericórdia, and Coordinator of the Telemedicine Research Project in medical imaging, developed in partnership with the Fraunhofer Institute in Germany and the European Union. She implemented and coordinated the RUTE Project (University Telemedicine Network) at the Telemedicine Center of the Santa Casa Hospital in Porto Alegre. She is the author of articles published in indexed medical journals, and the English/Portuguese translator of several radiology books published by Art Med. She was Medical Director and Head of the Imaging Diagnostic Service at the Municipal Emergency Hospital of Porto Alegre, where she works as a radiologist to this day, as well as a neuroradiologist in Unimed RS's own services.

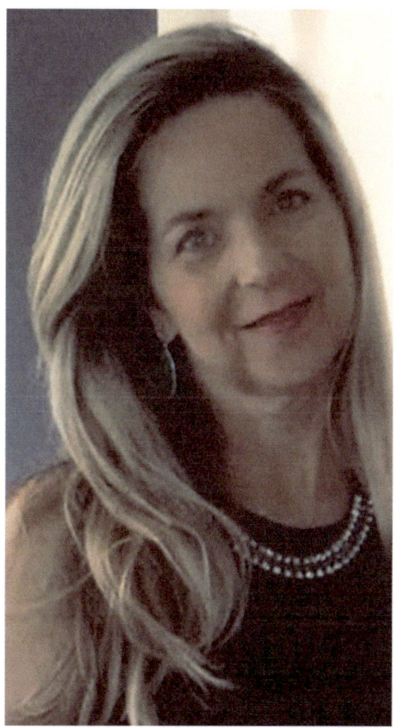

Dr. Claudia Costa Leite MD PhD had her undergraduate medical degree from Faculdade de Medicina da Universidade de São Paulo (FMUSP) in 1989, Brazil, followed by a Radiology Residency in the Hospital das Clínicas from the same university and 1 year as chief of the Radiology residency. She was a Neuroradiology research fellow at the University of Texas at San Antonio from 1994 to 1996, supervised by Dr. Randy Jinkins. Dr. Leite went back to Brazil in 1997 to be a Radiology attending at the Inrad of Hospital das Clínicas at FMUSP. In 1998, she finished and presented her PhD thesis at FMUSP, and she became a professor at the Radiology Department. Dr. Leite was the first woman in the Radiology Discipline of that University. From 2013 to 2016, she was also an associate professor at UNC at Chapel Hill, North Carolina. She has supervised many undergraduate, postgraduate and Radiology residents, has published 13 books and 27 book chapters, and has more than 300 published articles. In 2020, she received the RSNA educator award. Nowadays, she is an associate professor at the Department of Radiology and Oncology at FMUSP, and furthermore, she is the chief of Research and Education at Inrad of Hospital das Clínicas at FMUSP, Chief of Research of the Radiology Residents at Hospital Sirio Libanes, and is a master Radiologist at Grupo Fleury. Besides her career, she is a dedicated mother of two children, a wife, and a daughter.

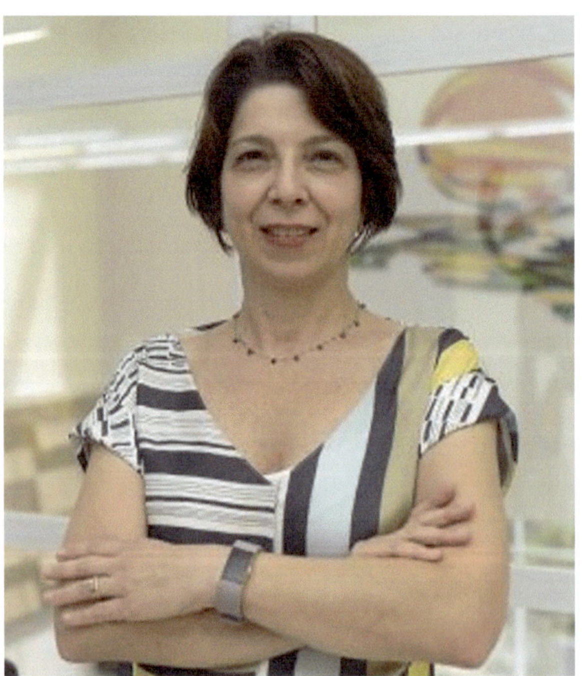

Dr. Christiane Monteiro de Siqueira Campos MD (Fig. 25.3) graduated in Medicine from the Federal University of Pernambuco (Recife, Brazil) in 1990. She completed her Medical Residency in Radiology at the Brasilia Radiologic Center in Brasilia in 1992. Dr. Campos started her fellowship in interventional peripheral and interventional Neuroradiology at Med Imagem-Beneficência Portuguesa de São Paulo in 1993 and 1994, under the supervision program done by Dr. Renan Uflacker and Dr. Ronie Leo Piske, respectively. She was later invited to join the staff group as a medical assistant at the same institution. In 1998, she spent 6 months in France at the Hospital Le Kremlin Bicêtre working under the supervision of Professor Pierre Lasjaunias. During this time, she published two papers on basilar tip anatomy and basilar tip aneurysms. Dr. Campos obtained a Master's Degree in Neurovascular Disease from the University of Paris in 2002. In 2008, she began working in the Neuroradiology diagnostic area at Med Imagem—Hospital da Beneficencia Portuguesa de São Paulo after completing a 1-year diagnostic neuroradiology fellowship at the same institution (Med Imagem), where she continues to practice. She currently serves as the scientific coordinator of the Interventional Neuroradiology Department at Beneficência Portuguesa de Sao Paulo. Dr. Campos is a member of several specialty societies, including the Sociedade Brasileira de Neuroradiologia (SBNR), Sociedade Paulista de Radiologia (SPR), and the Brazilian College of Radiology. In 2021, she received her Diploma in Diagnostic Neuroradiology from the European Society of Neuroradiology (EDiNR). She has authored more than 50 scientific papers in peer-reviewed journals and contributed to various book chapters dedicated to radiology and neuroradiology. Dr. Campos has

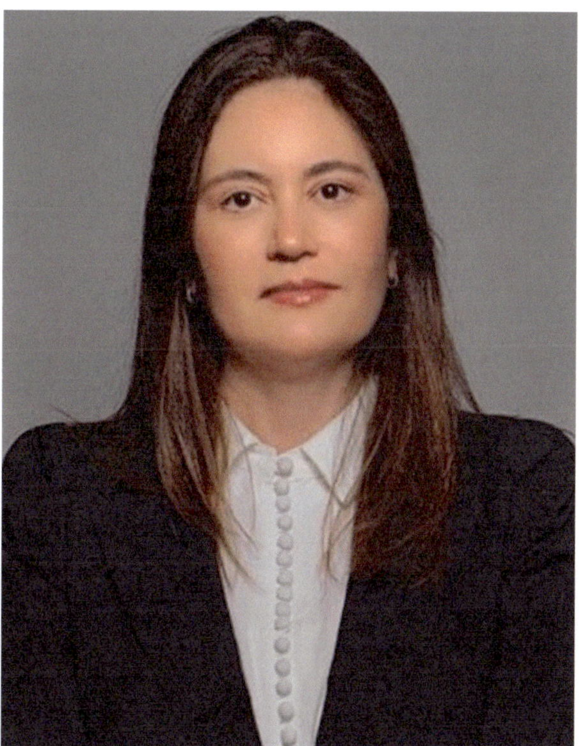

Fig. 25.3 Dr. Christiane Monteiro de Siqueira Campos

delivered over 100 lectures at international and national meetings in the fields of radiology, neurology, neurosurgery, and oncology.

Dr Lara Brandão MD (Fig. 25.4) went to medical school at the Fluminense Federal University in Niteroi (Rio de Janeiro, Brazil)—the city in which she was born. She did her residency in radiology at the Federal University of Rio De Janeiro (UFRJ). A year after finishing her residency, she spent a month at the UCLA in the Neuroradiology Department as a visiting fellow. At that time, Dr. Benson was the chairman of the Department. A year later, she did another Fellowship in Neuroradiology at the Massachusetts General Hospital in Boston, USA, where she spent 3 months. Dr. Gilberto Gonzalez was then the chairman of the department. That was a great experience for her. She attended every American Society of Neuroradiology (ASNR) meeting from 1999 to 2019. She also spoke at that meeting three times and became a member of the ASNR. In 2022, she was successful in the exam to become a member of the European Society of Neuroradiology that was held in Lisbon—qualifying her to be a member of the ESNR. Dr. Lara is a former president of the Brazilian Society of Neuroradiology. She was also the neuroradiologist responsible for the Neuroradiology Scientific Program for the Brazilian College of Radiology, meeting for four consecutive years. She directed a yearly neuroimaging course in Rio De Janeiro from 2004 to 2019, inviting many distinguished speakers to share the podium with her, such as Dr. James Barkovich, Dr. James Smirniotopoulos, Dr. David Yousem, Dr. Ellen Grant, and Dr. Aaron Field. She has written a book entitled "MR Spectroscopy of the Brain," published by Lippincott Raven and translated into three languages: Portuguese, English, and Chinese. She has also been the guest editor for some issues of the Magnetic Resonance Imaging (MRI) Clinics of North America and Neuroimaging Clinics (NIC) of North America, having published many articles in both. Dr. Lara Brandão

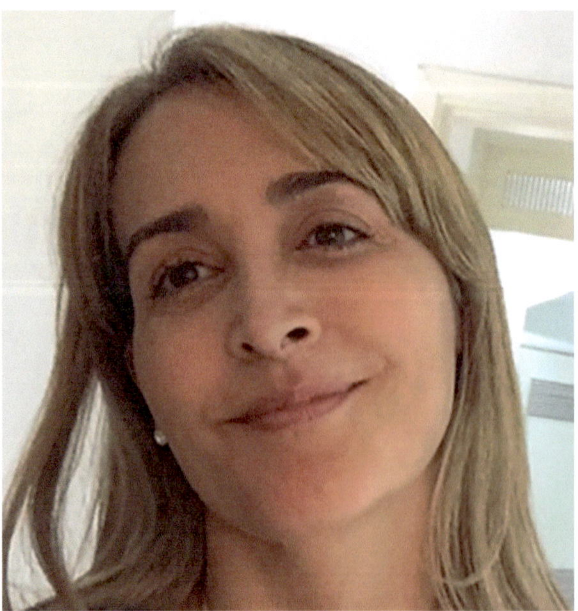

Fig. 25.4 Dr Lara Brandão

has given lectures in many radiologic meetings in Brazil as well as in the US, Mexico, Aruba, Peru, and Prague. She is now Chief of Neuroradiology at the clinic Magnetic Resonance Institute, DR Lara Brandão in Rio De Janeiro, Brazil.

Dr. Alessandra Mertens Brainer Lima MD PhD (Fig. 25.5) graduated in Medicine from the University of Pernambuco (UPE), completing a Medical residency in General Radiology at the Barão de Lucena Public Hospital/SUS/Pernambuco, followed by obtaining a specialist title in Radiology and Diagnostic Imaging from the Brazilian College of Radiology (CBR). She expanded my knowledge through internships in neuroradiology at the University of Campinas (UNICAMP) and at the Santa Casa de Misericórdia Hospital in São Paulo, earning a specialist certification in Neuroradiology, endorsed by the Brazilian Society of Neuroradiology (SBNR) and the Brazilian Medical Association (AMB). Her academic journey continued with a Master's degree from the Oswaldo Cruz Foundation in Pernambuco (FIOCRUZ/PE) with the thesis 'Analysis of the Association Between the Presence of Structural Brain Lesions and the Occurrence of Epileptic Seizures and Epilepsy'. She achieved international recognition in neuroradiology by passing the exams for the European Diploma in Neuroradiology (EDiNR), granted by the European Board of Neuroradiology. In her scientific trajectory, she highlights the collaboration with Dr. Maria de Fatima Aragão's group in the analysis of images of children with Zika virus-related microcephaly at the start of the epidemic in Northeast Brazil, she joined the Microcephaly Epidemic Research Group (MERG), a team of scientists dedicated to the study of Congenital Zika Syndrome. She developed the doctoral thesis "MRI in children with Zika-related microcephaly at the end of the myelination period: association between structural lesions and neurological findings," through which she completed her PhD at UPE.

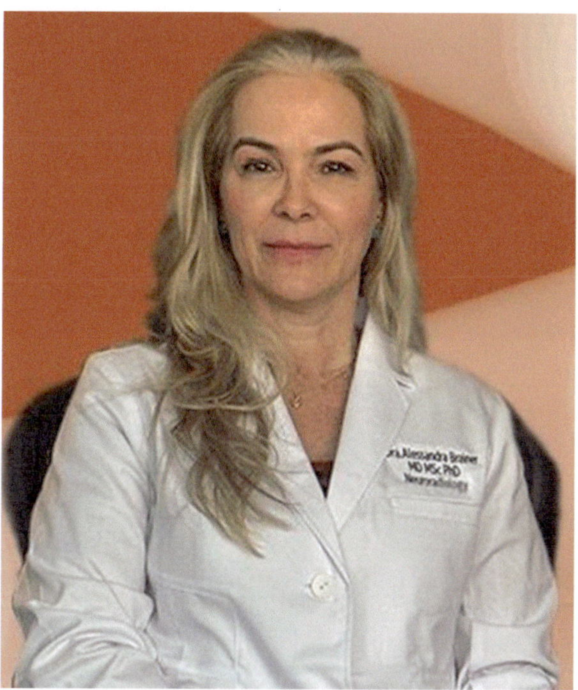

Fig. 25.5 Dr. Alessandra Mertens Brainer Lima

Dr. Natacha Calheiros de Lima Petribu MD PhD (Fig. 25.6) born in Recife (28/November/1973–8/August/2025), Brazil, was a radiologist dedicated to public service, teaching, and research. A graduate of Federal University of Pernambuco, she trained and mentored many young radiologists as coordinator of the Radiology Residency Program at Barão de Lucena Hospital. She earned her MSc and PhD at IMIP (Instituto de Medicina Integral Professor Fernando Figueira), contributed to the Pernambuco Radiology Society and RSNA, and published pioneering work on congenital microcephaly during the Zika virus epidemic. The results of her study were presented at the RSNA Conference in 2014, in Chicago, IL, and later published in the British Medical Journal in 2017 (BMJ 2017; 359: j4188| doi:10.1136/bmj.j4188), reporting her observations on the behavior and evolution of intracranial calcifications in affected patients. Despite a long battle against cancer, she lived with resilience and creativity, expressing her passion for dance and creating “Infinity by Naty” handcrafted candles. Since her passing in August 2025, she has been remembered for her devotion to medicine, her students, and her family, leaving a legacy of faith, strength, and inspiration. An unfulfilled dream of Natacha’s, which friends and family will try to embrace, is a social project to support children and adolescents with disabilities, especially those with after-effects of the Zika virus. The loving memory and the nurturing faith of Natacha will remain as a strong flame to warm and illuminate the lives of her husband André, her children Vinícius (23), Sofia (17), Liz (7), and the countless friends whose hearts she touches.

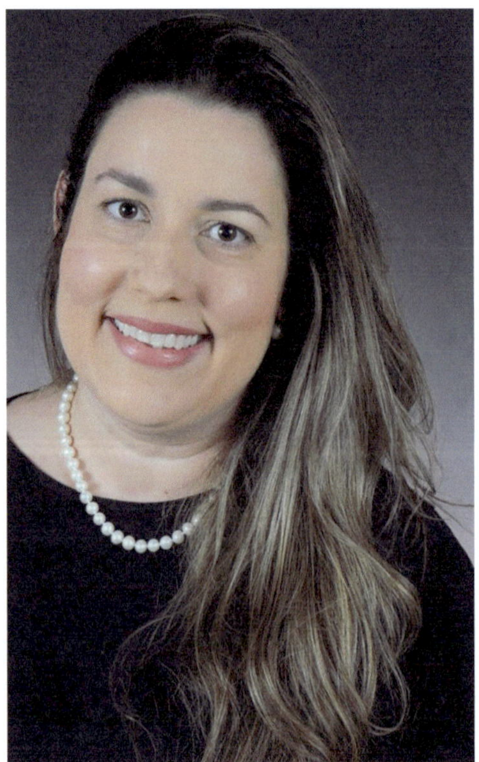

Fig. 25.6 Dr. Natacha Calheiros de Lima Petribu

History of Women Neuroradiologists in Peru

Most Influential Female Peruvian Neuroradiologist Doctors

The history and advancement of neurological, radiological, and neurosurgical sciences are closely related to that of neuroradiology. In the following paragraphs, we intend to recapitulate and acknowledge female doctors whose dedication and contribution to the field have led to its advancement and recognition.

Dr. Raquel del Carpio O'Donovan, who was born in Lima and graduated from Universidad Peruana Cayetano Heredia, is undoubtedly one of the most renowned and influential Peruvian Neuroradiologists. After training in the USA and moving to Canada, she settled in McGill University, where she established a very prosperous practice in Academic Neuroradiology. She has helped a significant number of medical professionals to advance in their radiological careers providing both mentorship and sponsorship. In 2022, she was elected Honorary President by the World Federation of Neuroradiological Societies during the AJNR annual meeting and XXIII WFNRS Symposium Neuroradiologicum, held in New York. In 2024, Dr. Del Carpio was awarded the Order of Canada, which is the highest civil honor and cornerstone of the Canadian Honours System. It recognizes outstanding achievement, dedication to the community and service to the nation.

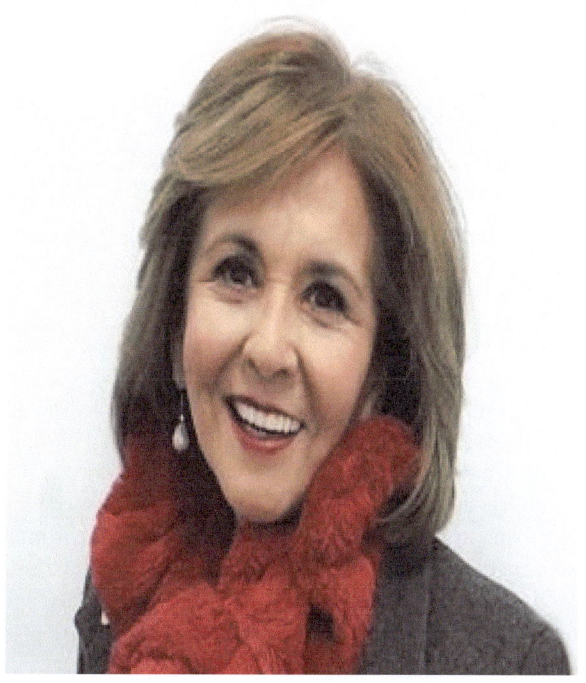

Dr. María Elizabeth Morón Cabrera graduated from the Universidad Nacional San Luis Gonzaga de Ica and pursued further training in radiology at the Hospital Nacional Edgardo Rebagliati under the Universidad Nacional Mayor de San Marcos Residency Program. She is currently working at this institution, the largest tertiary medical center in Lima. For the last 20 years, she has extensively taught medical residents not only from the field of radiology but from many other clinical and surgical programs. She has shaped the careers of many young residents and doctors and always has a teaching case to share. In her free time, she enjoys cooking and spending time with her husband and two daughters.

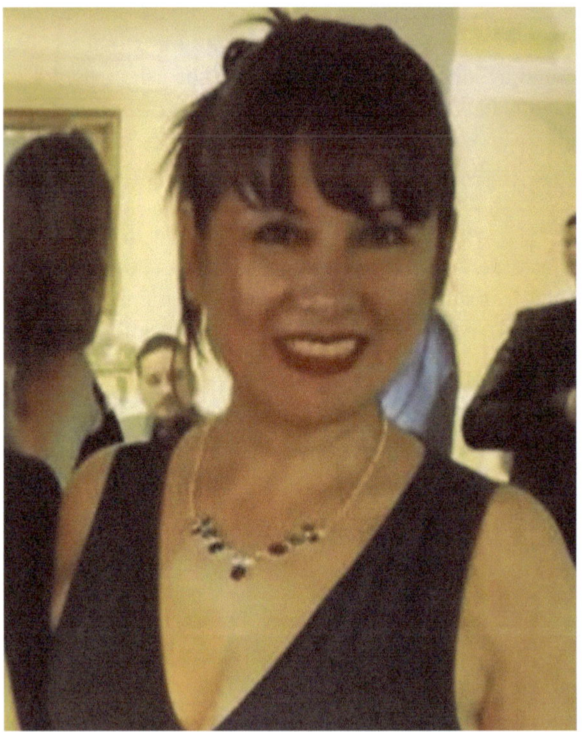

Dr. Romy Ames (Fig. 25.7) was born in Huancayo-Perú. She graduated from Medicine at the Universidad Peruana Los Andes (UPLA) and completed her medical residency at the Universidad Nacional Mayor de San Marcos (UNMSM), specializing in radiology at the Instituto Nacional de Enfermedades Neoplasicas (INEN), the largest oncologic center in Peru. Her interest in neuroimaging soon led her to look for an institution where she could continue specializing, and she successfully obtained a research fellowship degree at the UNC Hospital located in North Carolina, USA. On completion, she returned to Peru to apply what she had learned. Additionally, she obtained a Master's Degree in Clinical Epidemiology at Universidad Peruana Cayetano Heredia and a Master's Degree in Health Management at ESAN Graduate School of Business. She is committed to the

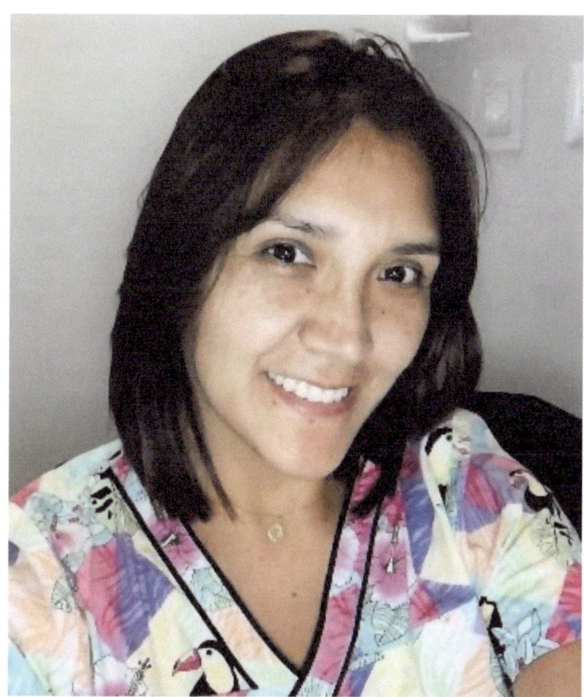

Fig. 25.7 Dr. Romy Ames

academic training of future doctors, which is why she directs the medical residency program at the institutions where she works. She actively participates in multidisciplinary meetings of oncological patients with tumors of the CNS. She is a recurrent lecturer at local and national meetings. She likes spending time with her family, exercising, and eating Italian food. She shares her time between her passion, neuroradiology, and being the mother of two young girls.

Dr. Lourdes Simbron Ribbeck (Fig. 25.8) graduated from Universidad Nacional Mayor de San Marcos, the most ancient Latin American University, where she obtained both her MD and Radiologist Diploma after completing her training in Hospital Nacional Edgardo Rebagliati Martins. During residency, she was awarded the SILAN MCG Visiting Scholarship and trained under Dr. Ramon Figueroa at Augusta University. Her passion toward the field and lack of opportunities for further specialization in Peru made her move to Mexico City, where she trained for 2 years in the Instituto Nacional de Neurologia y Neurocirugia "Manuel Velasco Suarez." Coming back to Peru, she settled in the Instituto Nacional de Ciencias Neurologicas (INCN), the oldest neurological and neurosurgical institute of the country, where people from the nation come seeking treatment and relief. Dr. Simbron serves as Head of the MRI Unit and has established a very active academic practice working with residents from Radiology, Neurology, and Neurological Surgery as well as active participation in the case boards of the Neurovascular and Neuroinfectious working groups. She is a recurrent lecturer both at local and national meetings. Her passion includes traveling and coffee tasting.

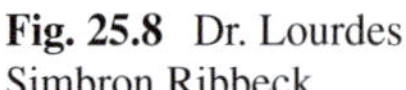

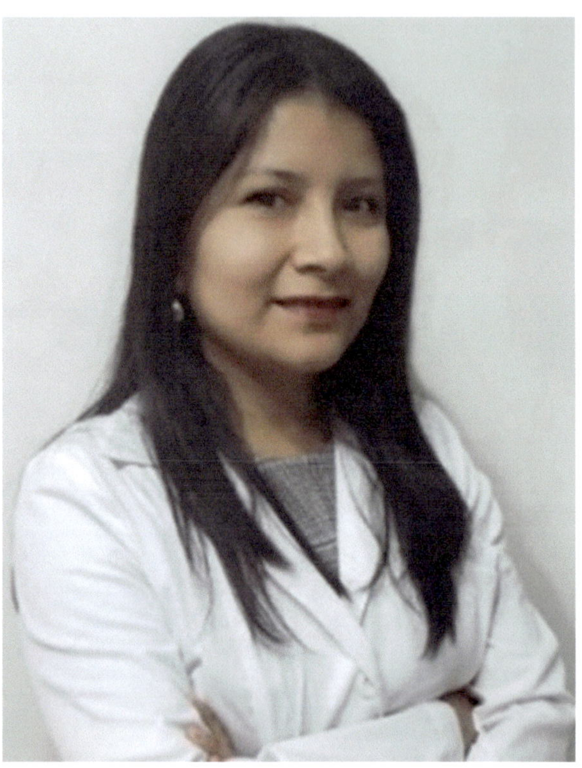

Fig. 25.8 Dr. Lourdes Simbron Ribbeck

History of Women Neuroradiologists in Colombia

Most Influential Female Colombian Neuroradiologist Doctors

The first radiology equipment arrived in Medellin, Colombia, in 1901, and the first radiography (a hand) was taken in June 1902 by Juan Bautista Montoya y Flórez, who had trained in Paris.

The first radiology residency started in 1928 at the Hospital San Juan de Dios in Bogotá, with Gonzalo Esguerra as the Head of the Radiology Department. On July 12, 1945, Gonzalo Esguerra also founded the Sociedad Colombiana de Radiología, one of the first scientific medical societies in the country. The first Colombian Radiology Congress was held in March 1950 (Jornadas Radiológicas Colombianas), and even though the photographs from the Congress show some women, they were the wives of the radiologists. So up to that time, no women appeared in the history of Colombian Radiology. Women started to appear in the field of radiology in the 1970s. Though it is not completely documented, the first woman radiologist in Colombia appears to have been Ms. Ana Elvira Prada from Medellin.

Women in neuroradiology appear later, one of the first being *Ms Aleyda Rodríguez*, who was trained at the Military Hospital and later worked as a neuroradiologist at the Instituto Neurológico de Colombia in the late 1980s. Ms. Sonia Bermudez, also a neuroradiologist, was part of the Editorial Board of the Revista Colombiana de Radiología since its foundation and has been directing the journal since 1996. As there was no formal neuroradiology training in Colombia, in the 1990s, some of our colleagues went to the USA to train, and some took up residence there *(Esperanza Pacheco, Martha Ballesteros, Maria Olga Patiño)*, while some trained in the USA and Canada and came back *(Ana María Granados, María Teresa Mantilla). Elcy Medina* was the first woman neuroradiologist trained formally in Colombia, at the Hospital Universitario Medellin. Later, many of us followed their example and dedicated our studies and our work to neuroradiology. Now, even though we have no neuroradiological society in Colombia, three women of the neuroradiology committee of the Asociación Colombiana de Radiologia (*Feliza Restrepo, Ana Maria Granados, Carolina Tramontini*), with help and support from many other members of the Society, are on our way to creating a Neuroradiology Chapter.

The European Society of Neuroradiology had a great influence on neuroradiology in Colombia, especially on us women. The first three Colombian radiologists, all women, who received the European Neuroradiology Diploma in 2013 were *Carolina Tramontini, Sonia Bermúdez, and Sara Nuñez* . Since then, there has been a close collaboration between the ESNR and the Asociación Colombiana de Radiologia. The European course, ECNR, held in Colombia since 2017, influenced many of our younger colleagues to take the path of neuroradiology. In 2023, *Carolina Tramontini* (Fig. 25.9) was granted Honorary Membership of the ESNR,

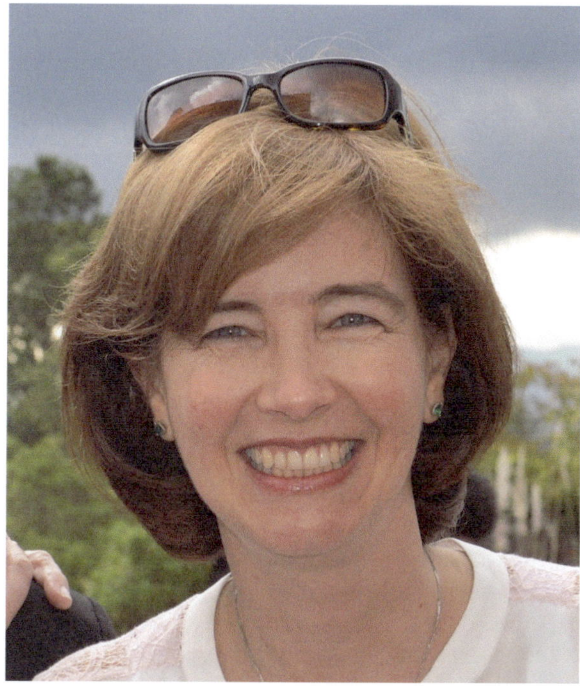

Fig. 25.9 Dr. Carolina Tramontini

being the first Colombian or Latin American neuroradiologist to be awarded this honor. Currently, there are approximately 30–40 women neuroradiologists working in Colombia, and many more are working abroad, mainly in the USA, Canada, and Spain.

History of Women Neuroradiologists in Costa Rica

Most Influential Female Costa Rican Neuroradiologist Doctors

The first doctor of African descent and first radiologist in Costa Rica was *Dr. Grace Curling Rodriguez,* who later pursued her subspecialty in neuroradiology, becoming a pioneer in that area in the country. It should be noted that Dr. Curling, during the 1990s, served as Head of Service at one of the country's National Social Security Hospitals until her retirement. Subsequently, in 2015, *Dr. Carolina Mejías Soto* returned from Mexico as a subspecialist, becoming the second female neuroradiologist in Costa Rica. Currently, Dr. Mejías Soto serves as Director of the National Center for Medical Imaging of the Costa Rican Social Security. These are the only two neuroradiologists that Costa Rica has, leaving evidence that not only for this area but for many other subspecialties of radiology, it is necessary to continue promoting subspecialized training among colleagues, which allows facilitating development and gender equity, as well as to optimize adequate and timely patient care.

History of Women Neuroradiologists in Argentina

Most Influential Female Argentinian Neuroradiologist Doctors

In Argentina, as in the rest of the world, there has been an increasing number of women with a major role in neuroradiology. One early and prominent member of this group was *Professor Dr. Gloria E. Díaz* (1930–2011), who, after a period of specialization in Paris during the sixties, performed over a period of 15 years as Chief of Radiodiagnostics at the Hospital Ramos Mejía, in Buenos Aires. She was also an Associate Professor of Diagnostic Imaging at Buenos Aires University and stood out in the interventional neuroradiological field, being a professor to many undergraduates who have never forgotten her. More recently, there is a group of prominent figures in the field who have achieved important positions in several private centers in Argentina. Such are the cases of *Claudia Cejas MD*, (chief of Imaging Diagnostic at FLENI and vice-president of the Argentine Radiological Society), *Adriana Ojeda, MD* (head of Neuroradiology at Oroño Institute in Rosario and recently designated co-editor of the Argentine Radiological Magazine), *Inés Tamer MD* (neuroradiologist of the SWISS medical group), and *Cristina Besada, MD* (Chief of Neuroradiology at the Hospital Italiano in Buenos Aires). In the field of

Pediatric Neuroradiology, we must mention *Susana Persico, MD,* who, after a training period in France, has been performing as a neuroradiologist at the Hospital Garrahan in Buenos Aires. Last, but not least, there are some outstanding contemporary interventional neuroradiologists, such as *Silvia Garbullino MD.* and *Roxana Ceratto MD*, who are working in the Hospital Británico and ENERI, respectively.

Juan M. Taveras (1919–2002) was a Dominican neuroradiologist who is remembered chiefly for his work in establishing neuroradiology as a separate subspecialty in the United States. He was the principal mover behind the founding of the American Society of Neuroradiology and its primary publication, the American Journal of Neuroradiology as well as SILAN (Ibero Latin American Society of Neuroradiology), in which one of the authors (GT) was a President. In 1964, Juan Taveras and Ernest Wood co-authored the textbook Diagnostic Neuroradiology, the first American textbook on neuroradiology, which became a reference book in the specialty. When you analyze the contents of this book, you find out that the modalities listed were plain films, intracranial pneumography, angiography, and ventriculography. General radiologists were reading the plain films, but the remainder of the procedures were performed by neurosurgeons.

Many women neurosurgeons used those procedures, some of them with multiple publications in the field of neuroradiology:

Dr. Maria Luisa Morete de Pardal (Chair of Neurosurgery-Costa Buero Neurosurgical Institute) published an update on iodoventriculogram in the prestigious journal *Acta Radiologica* from Sweden in 1958.

Dr. Alejandra Teresa Rabadán was a prominent neurosurgeon, researcher, teacher, and scholar in Argentina. She graduated from the Faculty of Medicine of the University of Buenos Aires in 1977 with honors. She was head of the Neurosurgery Division of the A. Lanari Medical Research Institute of the University of Buenos Aires and former head of the Neurosurgery Service of the Italian Hospital of Buenos Aires. She was also an associate professor of Neurosurgery at the School of Medicine of the University of Buenos Aires and head of the Neurosurgery Service at the Juan P. Garrahan Pediatric Hospital.

Dr. Graciela Noemi Zuccaro grew up in La Ciudad de la Plata, Buenos Aires, Argentina, obtaining her degree in medicine with honors at the Universidad de la Plata in August of 1973. In 1974, Dr. Zuccaro moved to the city of Buenos Aires and initiated her first steps in pediatric neurosurgery under the tutorial of Dr. Raul Carrea at the Children's Hospital Ricardo Gutierrez. She graduated as a pediatric neurosurgeon in 1978. Upon finishing her residency, Dr. Zuccaro did a fellowship in microsurgery in 1985 at the Henry Ford Institute in Detroit and continued her formation with base of skull surgery training at the University of Cincinnati and at the University of Virginia. She then became a fellow at the Children's Hospital of Philadelphia under the guidance of Professor Luis Schut. Later on, in 2000, she specialized in neuroendoscopy under the tutelage of Professor Fernando Rueda Franco at the National Institute of Pediatrics in Mexico City. Dr. Zuccaro assumed her first faculty position in 1979 at the Children's Hospital "Ricardo Gutiérrez" in Buenos Aires, a position she maintained until 1987 when she transferred to the National Pediatric Hospital "Prof. Dr. Juan P. Garrahan" where Dr. Zuccaro was appointed Chief of Neurosurgery from 2003 to 2014; simultaneously, she was a professor of pediatric neurosurgery at the Faculty of Medicine of the University of Buenos Aires, where she continues to be an honorary faculty. Dr. Zuccaro has been part of the editorial board of multiple scientific publications; they include La Revista Argentina de Neurocirugía, Child's Nervous System, Journal Brasileiro de Neurocirugía, Surgical Neurology, and Journal of Hydrocephalus. She was the first President of the International Society of Pediatric Neurosurgery.

Dr. Silvia Berner and Beatriz Pazos were also neurosurgeons performing invasive procedures.

Silvia Berner received her MD from the University of La Plata. She is a Board-Certified Neurosurgeon and was the Neurosurgery Chair at Ophthalmologic Hospital Santa Lucia, playing a key role in preserving that hospital. She was Head of Neurosurgery at Sanatorio Santa Isabel. She published important papers related to molecular analysis of pituitary pathology. Dr. Berner is a member of numerous Neurosurgical Associations: Asociación Argentina de Neurocirugía, Sociedad de Neurocirugía de la Provincia de Buenos Aires, Sociedad de Neurocirugía del Cono Sur, Federación Latinoamericana de Neurocirugía, Federación Mundial de Neurocirugía. She is a past president of the Asociación Civil de Neurocirujanos de la Ciudad de Buenos Aires, Sociedad Argentina de Neurocirugía, Sociedad Argentina de Neurociencias. She received a fellowship in Berlin (Grant) University Hospital Klinikum Steglitz under Professor Mario Brock and a fellowship in Zurich under Professor G. Yasargil. She is the recipient of numerous awards including the Annual Prize of The National Academy of Medicine. She has 194 peer-reviewed papers and has participated in 193 national and international meetings.

Dr. Beatriz Pazos was the Head of Neurosurgery at the Hospital Alejandro Posadas.

When digital imaging started, new radiologists took over neuroradiology. Invasive methods were handled by interventional neuroradiologists, and diagnostic methods were managed by diagnostic neuroradiologists. In this stage, many important names surfaced:

Dr. Cristina Besada graduated from the University of Buenos Aires School of Medicine. She completed a Diagnostic Imaging Residency Program at Hospital Frances in Buenos Aires and the Superior Course in Diagnostic Imaging at the Argentine Society of Radiology (SAR). She completed a fellowship in Magnetic Resonance Imaging at Centre Hospitalier Universitaire Robert Debre in Reims, France, and the Superior Course in Diagnostic Imaging at Hôpital Bicêtre in Paris, France. She was an attending physician at the Neurological Center, Hospital Frances Buenos Aires, Head of the Neuroimaging Section at Hospital Italiano Buenos Aires, and Professor of Diagnostic Neuroradiology at Universidad de Ciencias Empresariales y Sociales, Sociedad Argentina de Radiología, and Universidad del Hospital Italiano. She was the Director of the Neuroradiology Chapter at Sociedad Argentina de Radiología. Dr. Besada is a member of the Sociedad Argentina de Radiología, American Society of Neuroradiology, European Society of Radiology, and Société Française de Radiologie. She is the author of many peer-reviewed papers and has contributed to many national and international meetings as a guest speaker and moderator in workshops. She was the first Chair of the Neuroradiology Section at Sociedad Argentina de Radiología.

Dr. Claudia Cejas is a graduate of the Faculty of Medicine at the University of Buenos Aires. She completed her residency in Diagnostic Imaging at Htal. Mariano Castex for 4 years and a Fellowship in Neuroradiology and Head and Neck for 1 year at Hôpital Civil, Université de Strasbourg, France, under the mentorship of Prof. Jean Louis Dietemann. Currently, she is the President of the Argentinian Society of Radiology (SAR). Among her awards, she is an Honorary Member of the American Society of Neuroradiology (ASNR) in 2022. She is a member of the French Society of Radiology (SFR) and the European Society of Radiology (ECR). Her credentials in medical journalism are impressive: she received a scholarship from the American Roentgen Ray Association (ARRS) as the "2016 Lee F. Rogers International Fellow in Radiology Journalism." She excels in teaching and was the Editor-in-Chief of the Revista Argentina de Radiología (RAR) from 2010 to 2018. She is a Professor of Pre-graduate Training at Buenos Aires University, Director of the Radiology Specialist Course at Buenos Aires University, and Director of the Radiology Specialist Course in the Argentinian Society of Radiology (SAR). She serves as a Scientific Consultant for prestigious radiology journals such as Radiology (USA), Radiología (Spain), Stroke (USA), Muscle & Nerve, and Revista Uruguaya de Radiología. To date, she has won 14 awards, given over 100 lectures at national and international courses and conferences, presented over 100 papers (poster-free topic) at national and international conferences, written 48 scientific papers on specialty topics in national and international journals, published a book as the first author, authored chapters in four specialty books, and written over 30 editorials. She chairs the Imaging Department at FLENI, a prestigious neurological center in Argentina. Currently, her area of interest is Magnetic Resonance Imaging in the study of neuromuscular diseases, having developed Nerve and Plexus Magnetic Resonance Neurography at FLENI.

Dr. Adriana Ojeda received her Medical Degree from the University of Buenos Aires. She is a Specialist in Diagnostic Imaging in Santa Fe Province, as well as certified by the National Academy of Medicine and recertified with honors (Argentine Board Certification). She has a Diplome d'Université Radiologie et Imagerie Diagnostique du Système Nerveux from Université Paris IV, Unité de Formation et de Recherche de Médecine Pierre et Marie Curie–France, and Formation Spécialisée en Radiodiagnostique et Imagerie Médicale from CHU Amiens, France. She also has a Diplôme d'Université d'Imagerie par Résonance Magnétique from Faculté de Médecine Paris Sud—Université de Paris XI, France. Dr. Ojeda is a Professor of Neuroradiology for the Argentine Federation of Radiological Societies and a Professor of Neuroradiology in the Chair of Psychiatry at the National University of Rosario. She was Editor-in-Chief of Revista Argentina de Radiología. She was active in 100 national courses and meetings, 29 international meetings, 22 peer-reviewed national publications, and five international publications. She was awarded Magna cum Laude at the RSNA meeting for her work on percutaneous vertebroplasty with methyl-methacrylate. Dr. Ojeda was the pioneer of percutaneous vertebroplasty in Argentina.

Dr. Ines del Valle Tamer is a Diagnostic Imaging specialist from the University of Buenos Aires. She trained in neuroradiology as an Assistant étrangère at Hôpital Lariboisière, Paris, France. She is a neuroradiologist at many institutions in Buenos Aires, Argentina, including Instituto Argentino de Diagnóstico y Tratamiento and Swiss Medical Group. She was in charge of the Neuroradiology Specialists Course at Universidad de Ciencias Sociales y Empresariales. She is very active in SILAN (Iberolatinoamerican Society of Neuroradiology), lecturing and contributing articles, one of which was awarded the Taveras Award for Diagnostic Radiology excellence.

Dr. Rosana Salvatico is a diagnostic radiologist with a medical degree from the School of Medicine, University of Buenos Aires. She is a Diagnostic Imaging Specialist from the Ministry of Health through her residence at Hospital Durand. She has a fellowship and certification in Diagnostic Imaging from SAR (Argentine Radiological Society) and was the first Neuroradiologist in Argentina from the European Society of Neuroradiology. She is an Associate Professor of Diagnostic Imaging and Psychiatry at USAL (University of Salvador, Argentina). She works as a staff radiologist in the most important Neuroradiological Centers: ENERI-FLENI, Clínica La Sagrada Familia (under Prof. Pedro Lylyk MD), and Centro de Diagnóstico Dr. Enrique Rossi. She is also a Consultant at INOVA Center in Bahia Blanca (Buenos Aires Province). She is very active in teaching and is a member of the Neuroradiology staff at SAR. Among her publications, "Diffusion tensor MRI: clinical applications" is in the International Nuclear Information System.

Dr. Gloria Efigenia Diaz was a pioneer in catheter angiography. She started at the Instituto Modelo de Clínica Médica, Hospital Rawson. One of the authors (GT), working in the Nuclear Medicine Department at the same institute, witnessed her working late into the night. She was a Professor of Radiology at the School of Medicine (UBA). She joined the exchange program chaired by one of the authors (GT) with the Faculty of the University of California, Los Angeles, and Clínica Modelo de Lanús as Chair of Radiology. She served as President of SAR (Sociedad Argentina de Radiología), being the first woman to hold that position.

Dr. Silvia Garbugino received her MD from the University of Buenos Aires, School of Medicine. She was a resident of neurosurgery at the prestigious Hospital de Clínicas. She is a member of the Argentinian Neurosurgical Association and founder of the Argentinian College of Neurointerventionism, where she served as President. She is also a member of the World Federation of Interventional and Therapeutic Neuroradiology.

Dr. Rosana Ceratto is an interventional neuroradiologist and a pioneer in the field of diagnostic and interventional neuroradiology. She was a staff member at ENERI, the leading institution in Argentina, where interventional neuroradiology started. She taught neuroradiologists from all over the world. Her vast experience is reflected in articles in national and international peer-reviewed journals.

These women neuroradiologists in Argentina published more than 70 important scientific articles around the world.

History of Women Neuroradiologists in Paraguay

Most Influential Female Paraguayan Neuroradiologist Doctors

In Paraguay, radiology was an exclusively male specialty for many years. The first women radiologists began practicing in the 90 s, dedicating themselves mainly to ultrasound and then to radiology. This trend continues to a certain extent, but currently, there are three women trained in and dedicated to neuroradiology and who are members of the Paraguayan Diagnostic Imaging Society.

Dr. Carolina Servin Zardini (Fig. 25.10), a student at the National University of Asuncion and a resident at the Hospital de Clínicas, received her neuroradiology training first with a SILAN scholarship at MCG USA in 2003 with Professor R. Figueroa, where she fell under the charm of this subspecialty. She was then studying at the CHU Limoges, France. She continued her training in subsequent years with the European Neuroradiology course in Cartagena, Colombia, being a member of the European Society of Neuroradiology. She works in the private sector in the Centro Medico La Costa, in Asunción.

Dr. Rosanna Meza Lopez is also from the National University of Asunción. She originally opted for the specialty of pediatrics and then, in 2009, finally specialized

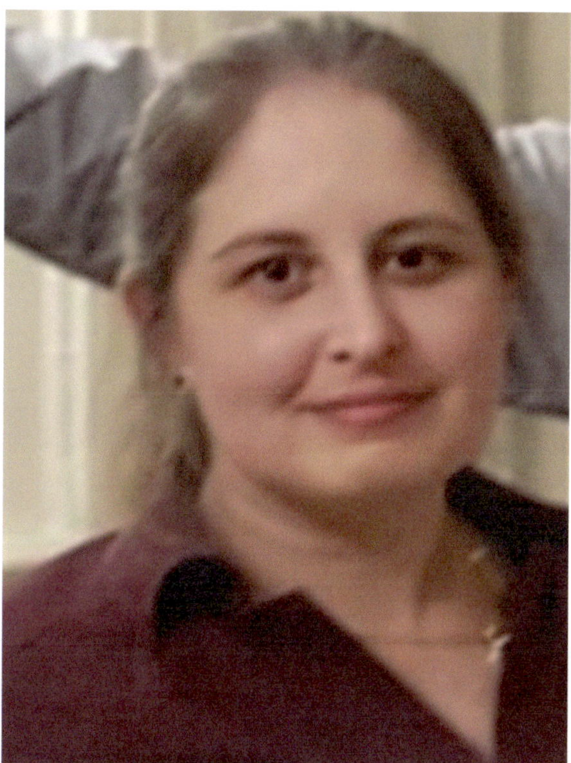

Fig. 25.10 Dr. Carolina Servin Zardini

in Imaging Medicine, with a postgraduate degree in Argentina from the Hospital Sor Maria Ludovica La Plata. She is a member of the Argentine Society of Diagnostic Imaging. She works in the private sector in the Instituto Codas Thompson and, faithful to her beginnings as a pediatrician, is dedicated to performing radiology and neuroradiology on children.

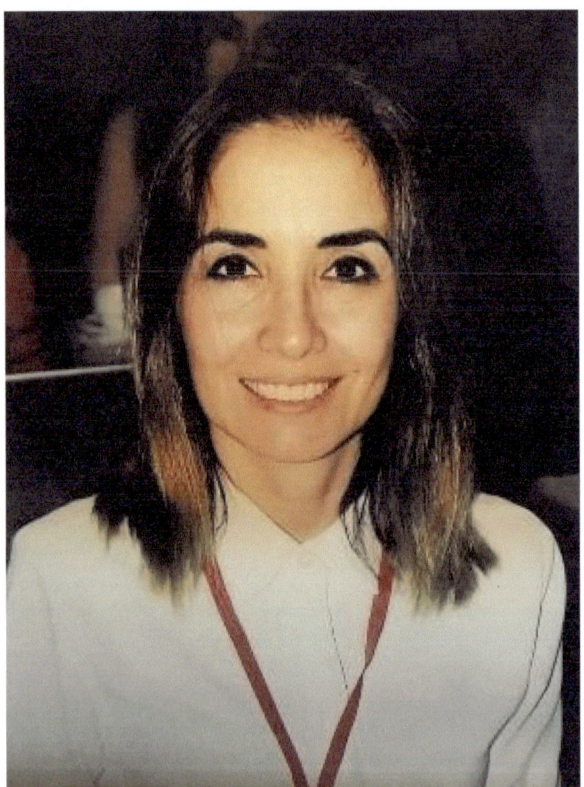

Dr. Barbara Castellano Da Cunha is the youngest of them, and she never thought that her path in the specialty would lead her to dedicate herself to neuroradiology. However, a series of initially fortuitous and then desired events made her a self-made specialist who supported her training through her own dedication, courses abroad, and a multidisciplinary environment. She currently works in the IPS Central in Asuncion, where her work in the Epilepsia Chirurgic Unit is well known, as is her work in the private sector.

These three pioneers also dedicate their time to training young doctors.

History of Women Neuroradiologists in Mexico

Most Influential Female Mexican Neuroradiologist Doctors

Neuroradiology arrived in Mexico in 1959, and for almost 15 years, it was represented by men until the arrival of *Dr. Teresa Olvera in* 1973. She was the first woman to earn a fellowship in neuroradiology. Subsequently, neuroradiology became known among female doctors. Dr. Perla Salgado began her fellowship in 1986. She was the first woman to head the Neuroimaging Department at the National Institute of Neurology and Neurosurgery in 2004. She is a professor who lectures at multiple national and international conferences and is part of the Electronic Work Evaluation Committee at SILAN, and participates with the National Autonomous University of Mexico to evaluate radiology and imaging headquarters nationwide.

Dr. Patricia Silva worked at the National Institute of Neurology and Neurosurgery and was president of the Mexican Society of Radiology and Imaging.

Another internationally recognized Mexican neuroradiologist is Dr. *Katiuzka Casares* (Fig. 25.11), who is an associate professor of neuroradiology at the National Institute of Neurology and Neurosurgery. She was the first woman to be president of the Mexican Society of Diagnostic and Therapeutic Neuroradiology from 2013 to 2015. Currently, she is a professor at the Inter-American College of Radiology, a national and international lecturer, and participates with the Mexican Council of Radiology in evaluating radiologist doctors. Among the ranks of Mexican neuroradiologists who have been pioneers in different areas, we can name doctors Guadalupe Ramirez and Ángeles Gómez, who were the first to have training in endovascular therapy. *Dr. Thalía Moreno* was the first Mexican female neuroradiologist to gain a functional resonance fellowship, training in France in 2004. Dr. Dulce Bonifacio began a highly specialized course in Endovascular Therapy in Mexico City, and Dr. Mariana Garza created a branch in Nuevo León to study neuroradiology with the same academic program as that at the INNN. Currently, in Mexico, we have 40 female neuroradiologists distributed throughout the country, which corresponds to 30% of the total number of neuroradiologists in Mexico. At the National Institute of Neurology and Neurosurgery, 40% of the professors and Fellows in Neuroradiology

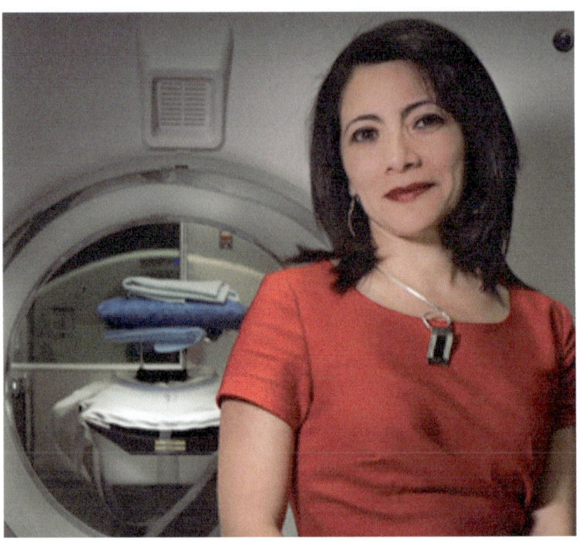

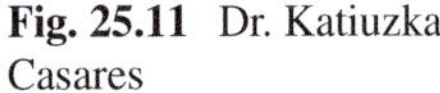

Fig. 25.11 Dr. Katiuzka Casares

are women, training both national and foreign doctors, which makes the institute a fundamental axis in the education of neuroradiology in Latin America.

History of Women Neuroradiologists in Honduras

Most Influential Female Honduran Neuroradiologist Doctors

In the twentieth century, radiology in Honduras was exclusively for men. In the 1980s, *Dr. Martha Cambar* performed x-ray interpretation tasks despite not having had formal training. At the end of the 80 s, *Dr. Virginia Figueroa* entered the country with formal radiology training and worked in her private practice in Tegucigalpa. *Dr Jeaneth Bu Figueroa* becomes the first neuroradiologist in Honduras and Central America. She attended the Faculty of Medicine of the National Autonomous University of Honduras, UNAH. Later in 1989 She studied general radiology at the Mexican Institute of Social Security IMSS and then studied neuroradiology at the National Institute of Neurology and Neurosurgery Dr. Manuel Velazco Suarez, in Mexico City, under the tutelage of Dr. Marco Zenteno. She currently practices at the IHSS and is the teaching coordinator and neuroradiology chair in the postgraduate courses in Radiology, Neurology, Neurosurgery, and Physical Medicine and Rehabilitation.

History of Women Neuroradiologists in Chile

Most Influential Female Chilean Neuroradiologist Doctors

The advancement of women in neuroradiology in Chile has been remarkable. In a historically male-dominated field, the emergence of *Dr. Nelly Rosario Guerrero A.* and *Dr. Ana Pino V.* as the country's first female radiologists in 1959 marked a significant milestone. During the 1980s, the landscape shifted further with the emergence of the first female neuroradiologists. *Dr. Marcia Salinas,* trained in Marseille, along with *Dr. Evelyn Faure and Drs. Steffi Eckhardt,* who brought with them neurology background, led this transformative period. Following this wave, a cadre of talented women, including *Drs. Patricia Orellana, Rosario Rosales, Romina Zunino,* and *Maria Francesca Castoldi*, continued to propel the growth and diversification of neuroradiology in Chile. Their collective contributions solidified the presence and impact of women in this specialized field, shaping its trajectory and inspiring future generations.

Neuroradiology continues to advance with the support of a new generation of young professionals, including *Valeria Schonstedt and Ximena Stecher*, both of whom are specialists in pediatric neuroradiology and epilepsy. They work at Clínica Alemana in Santiago, and their involvement in teaching and strengthening relationships with their Latin American peers enhances development and collaboration in this field.

Latin American women are playing an important role in neuroradiology. May the histories of these Latin American neuroradiologists inspire new generations of young women to choose neuroradiology as a profession and provide excellent patient care, based on humanization and diagnostic accuracy. Furthermore, may the contributions of current women in the field of teaching and science be continued by the upcoming generation.

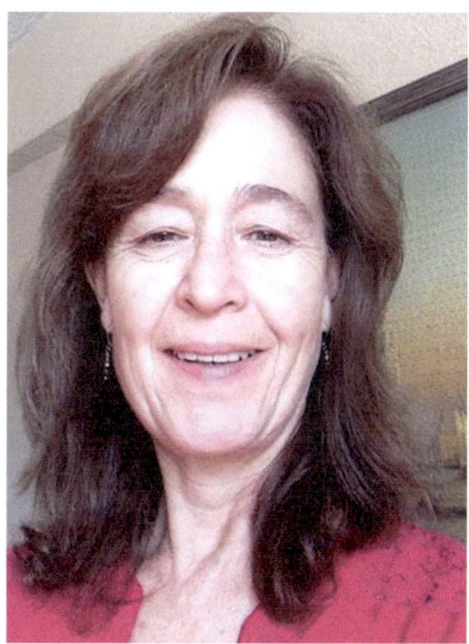

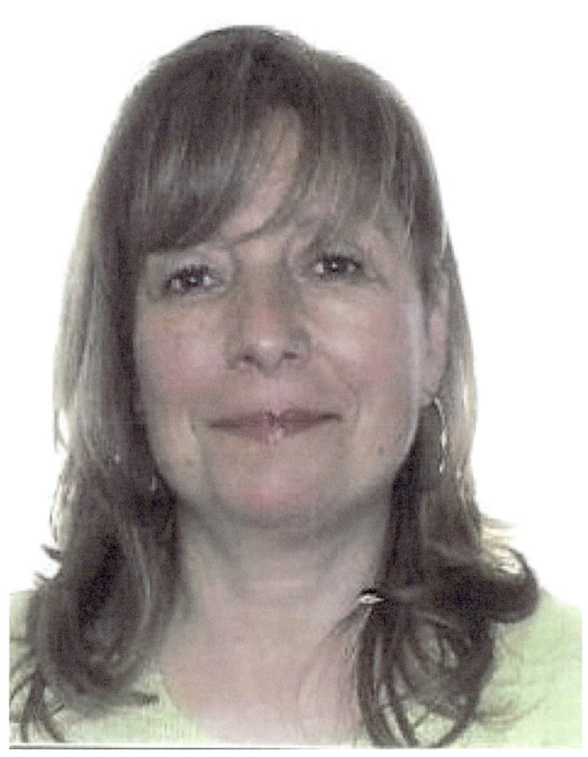

Fig. 25.12 Dr. Salinas

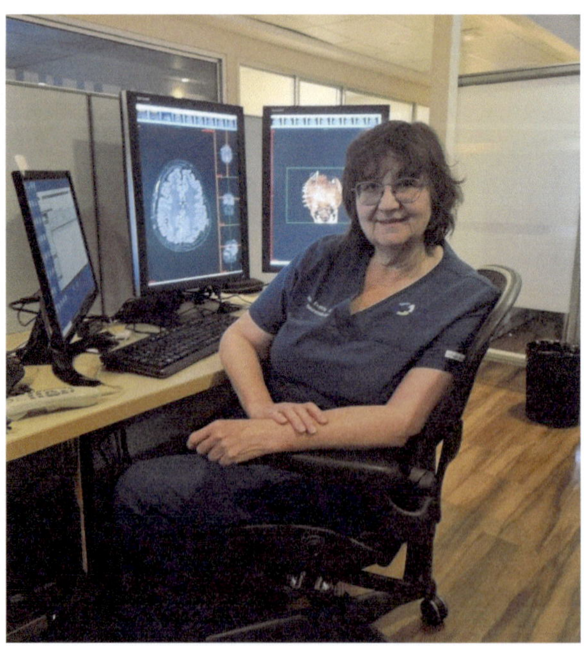

Fig. 25.13 Dr. Faure

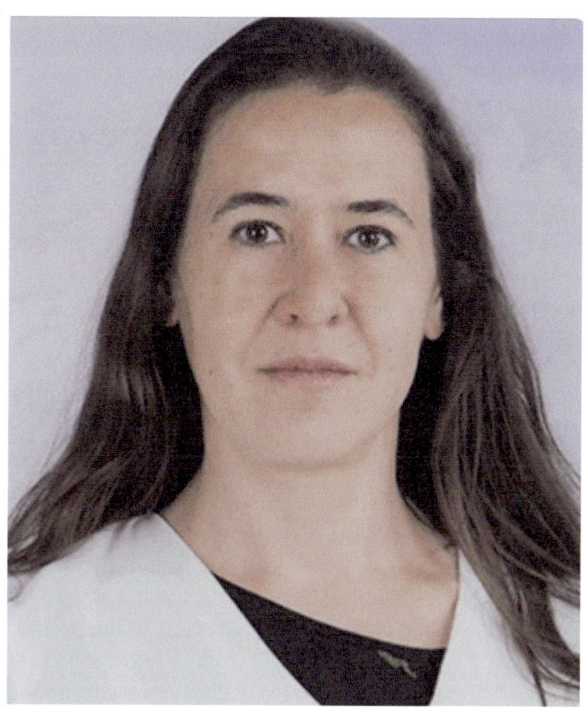

Fig. 25.14 Dr. KValeria Schonstedt

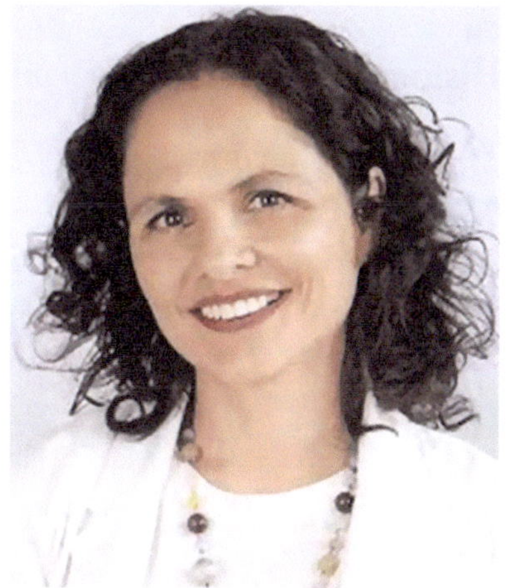

Fig. 25.15 Dr. Ximena Stecher

History of Women Neuroradiologists in the Dominican Republic

Most Influential Female Dominican Neuroradiologist Doctors

The Dominican Republic is proud to have Dr. Juan Manuel Taveras Rodríguez, who was a professor, editor, and Dominican Doctor, born in Moca in 1919, he is considered the Father of modern Neuroradiology, and wrote the first text on the subject and founded both the American Society of Neuroradiology and its scientific journal, of which he was its editor for several years.

The Dominican Republic has few neuroradiologists, predominantly male, the pioneers being Dr. Juan Manuel Taveras, Dr. Miguel Paliza, Dr. Antonio Honrado Castro, Dr. Rafael Fermin, among others. Currently, we have women neuroradiologists, *Dr. Luisa Melo de Jung* as our first neuroradiologist of the country, originally from San Pedro de Macoris, she trained at the Manuel Velasco Suarez Institute of Neurology and Neurosurgery, Mexico, in the period 2014–2016. The second in the country and the first in the Northern region, *Dr. Marian E. Honrado de Lee*, originally from San Francisco de Macorís, trained at the Manuel Velasco Suarez Institute of Neurology and Neurosurgery, Mexico, in the period 2016–2018. Lastly, the third *Dr. Perla M. Almonte Pichardo*, originally from Santiago de los Caballeros, trained at the National Institute of Medical Sciences and Nutrition Salvador Zubiran, Mexico, 2017–2018.

History of Women Neuroradiologists in Uruguay

Most Influential Female Uruguayan Neuroradiologist Doctors

Neuroradiology in Uruguay does not have a fellowship, so if you want to specialize, you have to go to study outside. The first woman in neuroradiology was Angelica Wozniak, who went to study in the USA in the 80's. The first Neurointerventional woman was *Teresa Lin (neurologist),* who studied with Fernanda Viñuela in Canada and UCLA in the 80's.

A new generation of neuroradiologist women started with *Cecilia Purcallas,* who went to study with Dr. Lucato at San Pablo in 2005, *Florencia Birriel,* who studied with Dr. Ramon Figueroa in Augusta medical school in Georgia in 2012, and then Magdalena Pucurull in 2017, who also trained with Dr. Figueroa.

In Neurointerventional Radiology, Dr. Ofelia Marabotto went to France to train, and Mariana Romero and Alejandra Jaume (both originally neurosurgeons) went on to practice with Pedro Lylyk in Argentina.

Conclusion

In summary, as we can see, women neuroradiologists in Latin America have a rich history marked by dedication and innovation. They continue to evolve, doing hard work and playing an essential role in the diagnosis, treatment, and management of neurological disorders, thus improving the lives of patients. They are increasingly having an active voice and thus achieving excellent work in medical education, medical policy, leadership, and science, and serving as an inspiration for future generations.

Readers are suggested to contact the corresponding author for figures if needed.

Acknowledgements We would like to thank Diego Cavalcanti Perrelli and Danilo de Santana Marques for their help in organizing the references and in starting to format the text.

References

1. Historia de la Radiología en Colombia, Asociación Colombiana de Radiologia, 2022.
2. Valente M. Neuroradiology in Brazil. In: Cabanis EA, Iba-Zizen MT, editors. A history of neuroradiology (1895–2002). Paris; 2002. p. 215–6.
3. Piske RL, Raupp E, Freitas M, Maria J, Monteiro Siqueira Campos C, Abath C, da Silva N Jr. History of the neuroradiology in Brazil. In: Cabanis EA, Iba-Zizen MT, editors. A history of neuroradiology (1895–2002). Paris; 2002. p. 217–20.
4. Boletim Colégio Brasileiro de Radiologia e Diagnóstico por Imagem, informativo n°364, 2019;18.
5. Prominent Brazilian radiologist to shed light on Zika virus imaging at ECR 2017, ESR Blog, 2017, disponible in: https://blog.myesr.org/prominent-brazilian-radiologist-to-shed-light-on-zika-virus-imaging-at-ecr-2017/. Access in 08 May 2024.
6. Boletim Colégio Brasileiro de Radiologia e Diagnóstico Por Imagem, informativo n°368, 2019;12, 13.
7. Morete de Pardal ML, Pardal E. Mise au point de l'iodoventriculographie. Acta Radiol. 1958;50(2):34–8. Stockholm, Sweden.

Chapter 26
The History of Women in Neuroradiology in North America from 1990 to the Present

Anne G. Osborn, Patricia Rhyner, Carolyn C. Meltzer, Pamela W. Schaefer, Laurie A. Loevner, Pina C. Sanelli, Tina Young Poussaint, Erin Simon Schwartz, Yvonne W. Lui, Yoshimi Anzai, Donatella Tampieri, Wendy Smoker, Vijay Rao, Michelle Michel, Deborah Shatzkes, Nancy Fischbein, Kristine Mosier, Christine Glastonbury, Jody Tanabe, Jill Hunter, Caroline Robson, Susan Palasis, V. Michelle Silvera, Judy Donovan Post, Alyssa Watanabe, Michelle Johnson, Lubdha Shah, Wende Gibbs, Mary E. Jensen, Raquel Z. del Carpio-O'Donovan, Rona Woldenberg, Tabassum Kennedy, Achala Vagal, Birgit Ertl-Wagner, Tammie Benzinger, Soonme Cha, and Patricia Ellen Grant

---

A. G. Osborn
University of Utah (Retired), Salt Lake City, UT, USA
e-mail: anne.osborn@hsc.utah.edu

P. Rhyner
Mayo Clinic, Jacksonville, FL, USA

C. C. Meltzer
Keck School of Medicine of USC, Los Angeles, CA, USA
e-mail: carolyn.meltzer@med.usc.edu

P. W. Schaefer (✉)
Department of Radiology, Massachusetts General Hospital, Boston, MA, USA

Harvard Medical School, Boston, MA, USA
e-mail: pschaefer@mgb.org

L. A. Loevner
Division of Neuroradiology, University of Pennsylvania Health System, Philadelphia, PA, USA
e-mail: laurie.loevner@pennmedicine.upenn.edu

P. C. Sanelli
Northwell Health, Manhasset, NY, USA
e-mail: psanelli@northwell.edu

T. Y. Poussaint · P. E. Grant
Boston Children's Hospital, Harvard Medical School, Boston, MA, USA
e-mail: tinayoung.poussaint@childrens.harvard.edu; ellen.grant@childrens.harvard.edu

D. Birchall (ed.), *A World History of Neuroradiology*,
https://doi.org/10.1007/978-3-032-16653-1_26

E. S. Schwartz
Division of Neuroradiology, Lurie Family Foundations' MEG Imaging Center, Philadelphia, PA, USA

Perelman School of Medicine, University of Pennsylvania, Philadelphia, PA, USA
e-mail: schwartzes@chop.edu

Y. W. Lui
Department of Radiology, NYU Langone Health/Grossman School of Medicine, New York, NY, USA
e-mail: Yvonne.Lui@nyulangone.org

Y. Anzai · L. Shah
University of Utah Hospital, Salt Lake City, UT, USA
e-mail: yoshimi.anzai@hsc.utah.edu; lubdha.shah@hsc.utah.edu

D. Tampieri
Queen's University Hospital, Kingston, ON, USA
e-mail: donatella.tampieri@kingstonhsc.ca

W. Smoker
University of Iowa Health Care (Retired), Iowa City, IA, USA

V. Rao
Jefferson Health, Sidney Kimmel Medical College, Thomas Jefferson University, Philadelphia, PA, USA
e-mail: vijay.rao@jefferson.edu

M. Michel
Froedtert Hospital and Medical College of Wisconsin, Milwaukee, WI, USA
e-mail: mmichel@mcw.edu

D. Shatzkes
Zucker School of Medicine at Hofstra/Northwell Health, New York, NY, USA

N. Fischbein
Department of Radiology, Center for Academic Medicine, Stanford University, Stanford, CA, USA
e-mail: fischbein@stanford.edu

K. Mosier
Department of Radiology, Section of Neuroradiology and Imaging Sciences, Indiana University School of Medicine, Indianapolis, IN, USA
e-mail: kmosier@iu.edu

C. Glastonbury
University of California, San Francisco, San Francisco, CA, USA
e-mail: christine.glastonbury@ucsf.edu

J. Tanabe
University of Colorado Anschutz, Aurora, CO, USA
e-mail: jody.tanabe@cuanschutz.edu

J. Hunter
Baylor College of Medicine, Houston, TX, USA

Department of Pediatric Radiology, Texas Children's Hospital, Houston, TX, USA
e-mail: jvhunter@texaschildrens.org

C. Robson
Department of Radiology, Department of Otolaryngology, Boston Children's Hospital, Boston, MA, USA
e-mail: caroline.robson@childrens.harvard.edu

S. Palasis
Emory University School of Medicine, Atlanta, GA, USA

Children's Healthcare of Atlanta, Atlanta, GA, USA
e-mail: susan.palasis@emory.edu

V. Michelle Silvera
Mayo Clinic, Rochester, MN, USA

J. D. Post
Boston University Chobanian & Avedisian School of Medicine (Retired), Boston, MA, USA

University of Miami Miller School of Medicine, Miami, FL, USA

A. Watanabe
University of Southern California, Los Angeles, CA, USA

CureMetrix, San Diego, CA, USA

M. Johnson
Yale New Haven Hospital, New Haven, CT, USA
e-mail: michele.h.johnson@yale.edu

W. Gibbs
Department of Neuroradiology, Barrow Neurological Institute, Phoenix, AZ, USA

M. E. Jensen
Department of Radiology and Medical Imaging, University of Virginia Health, Charlottesville, VA, USA

R. Z. del Carpio-O'Donovan
McGill University Health Center, Montreal, QC, Canada
e-mail: raquel.delcarpio.med@ssss.gouv.qc.ca

R. Woldenberg
Zucker School of Medicine at Hofstra/Northwell, Manhasset, NY, USA
e-mail: rwoldenb@northwell.edu

T. Kennedy
University of Wisconsin School of Medicine and Public Health, Madison, WI, USA
e-mail: tkennedy@uwhealth.org

A. Vagal
Department of Radiology, UC College of Medicine, Cincinnati, OH, USA

Center for Clinical and Translational Science and Training (CCTST), University of Cincinnati Medical Center, Cincinnati, OH, USA
e-mail: vagala@ucmail.uc.edu

B. Ertl-Wagner
Department of Diagnostic & Interventional Radiology, The Hospital for Sick Children, Toronto, ON, USA

Department of Medical Imaging University of Toronto, Toronto, ON, USA
e-mail: BirgitBetina.Ertl-Wagner@sickkids.ca

T. Benzinger
Mallinckrodt Institute of Radiology, Neuroradiology Section, Washington University in Saint Louis, St. Louis, MO, USA
e-mail: benzingert@wustl.edu

S. Cha
Department of Radiology & Biomedical Imaging, University of California, San Francisco, San Francisco, CA, USA
e-mail: soonmee.cha@ucsf.edu

Introduction

From 1990 to 2024, women neuroradiologists in North America have made tremendous progress in the areas of leadership, clinical innovation, research, education, diversity, equity and inclusion, and global outreach. In fact, numerous women have made so many important contributions to the advances in neuroradiology in the past several decades that it is impossible to mention every individual and capture every major accomplishment. I have decided to summarize key accomplishments in four domains, followed by short biographical sketches of luminaries organized by leadership roles and areas of expertise, and ending with conclusions and future directions.

Leadership

In the last 34 years, national organizations have developed programs to support the professional advancement of women. In 2012, the ASNR announced the Women in Neuroradiology Leadership Award in partnership with the ACR and AAWR, providing the recipient with funding to attend the ACR Radiology Leadership Institute Summit. The AAWR also currently sponsors two additional RLI Leadership Summit Awards for women radiologists. SCARD developed the LEAD program, a 1-year leadership development program for women, in 2018, for the purpose of increasing the number of women in chair and institutional-level executive positions within their respective organizations. The ASNR Diversity and Inclusion Committee, the RSNA Committee on Diversity, Equity, and Inclusion, and the ACR's Commission for Women and Diversity have all sponsored programs to increase the number of women and other minorities in radiology leadership and research programs.

As a result of these initiatives, as well as an increasing number of women engaged in Neuroradiology, and the help of male champions, the number of women in Neuroradiology Leadership positions has greatly increased. For example, from 1962 to 2004, one woman, Anne Osborn, served as President of the ASNR. From 2005 to 2024, 9 of 19 presidents have been women. Women have, for the first time, also served as President of the Canadian Society of Neuroradiology. Before 1990, two women served as Presidents of the eight affiliated societies of the ASNR. Since then, approximately 45 women have served as Presidents of those societies. As of 2024, approximately 30% of the Division Chiefs in Neuroradiology in the United States are female. Before 1990, no women served as Editor in Chief or as a Senior Editor of the AJNR. Since 1990, approximately 12 women have served as Senior Editors. Women neuroradiologists, for the first time, have served in other prominent radiology leadership positions such as the ASNR representative to the AMA House of Delegates, the Chair of the ACR Board of Chancellors, President of the Association of Academic Radiologists, and the President of the RSNA. Within their own institutions, women in Neuroradiology have also achieved important leadership positions including Deans or Associate Deans of Schools of Medicine, of

Medical School Admissions and of Clinical and Translational Research; Chairs of Departments; Chief or Associate Chief Officers for Quality and Safety and Diversity and Inclusion; and Vice Chairs of Academic Affairs, Education, Quality and Safety, Clinical Operations and Communications. For the first time, women have received Gold Medals from the RSNA, the ASNR, and the CAR, as well as from multiple international Radiology societies. Raquel del Carpio-O'Donovan was appointed a member of the Order of Canada, one of Canada's highest honors, for her extraordinary leadership across multiple domains.

Clinical Innovation and Research

Since 1990, women in Neuroradiology have secured increasing grant funding and have made seminal contributions to advancing clinical care and Neuroradiology Research.

Head and Neck Radiology Since 1990, 11 women have served as Presidents of the ASHNR, and nine have received the gold medal. Collectively, they have advanced our understanding of a wide range of head and neck topics. Several, including Laurie Loevner, Yoshimi Anzai, Christine Glastonbury, and Nancy Fischbein have substantially advanced the field of head and neck cancer imaging, focusing on pathophysiology, genetics, tumor microenvironments, assessing disease progression, and providing prognostic information. Kristine Mosier is a pioneer in the application of functional MR imaging to the head and neck, Wendy Smoker defined imaging of the craniocervical junction and of cranial nerves, and Vijay Rao defined correlative imaging in Otolaryngology. Patricia Rhyner was the first Head and Neck Radiologist to establish a reading room in the ENT outpatient clinic.

Pediatric Neuroradiology Since its establishment in 1993, nine women have served as Presidents of the ASPNR, and four have received the gold medal. Collectively, they have contributed to our understanding of a wide number of pediatric CNS diseases. Tina Poussaint has advanced the field of pediatric brain tumor imaging, with a focus on the correlation of imaging features with molecular subtypes. Dr. Jill Hunter has applied advanced MRI techniques to evaluate traumatic brain injury and complex congenital heart disease. Caroline Robson has defined various aspects of pediatric head and neck imaging, Erin Simon Schwartz has advanced our understanding of magnetoencephalography, Michelle Silvera established imaging criteria for abusive childhood injury, and Susan Blaser focused on inborn errors of metabolism. Ellen Grant is a luminary in the field of neonatal imaging who has developed MRI, MEG, and quantitative Near Infrared Spectroscopy techniques to improve our understanding of normal and abnormal brain physiology. Birgit Ertl-Wagner has performed translational research focused on imaging of pediatric brain tumors, neuroinflammatory and metabolic disorders, neurovascular imaging, and head & neck imaging.

Functional Neuroimaging and Artificial Intelligence Dr. Jodi Tanabe was the first President of the ASFNR. She is renowned for her assessment of DBS, transcranial magnetic stimulation, and focused ultrasound for the assessment of substance and alcohol use disorder. Dr. Yvonne Lui has described the utility of advanced MRI imaging techniques in the assessment of traumatic brain injury and established one of the first radiology programs in machine learning. Dr. Caroline Meltzer used advanced imaging to study the brain's structure and function associated with normal aging, Alzheimer's disease, and neuropsychiatric disorders.

Interventional Neuroradiology Lee Jensen, the only woman radiologist who served as a President of SNIS, co-developed the first percutaneous vertebroplasty and other augmentation techniques in the United States, and Donatella Tampieri performed the first vertebroplasty technique in Canada. Lee and Donatella, as well as Michelle Johnson, have delineated numerous aspects of neurointervention for cerebrovascular diseases.

Spine Imaging and Intervention Since its establishment in 1993, six women have served as Presidents of ASSR, and one has received the gold medal. Lubdha Shah developed noninvasive spine interventional devices using focused ultrasound to treat spine pathologies and developed diffusion imaging sequences to evaluate the spine and spinal cord. Wende Gibbs has defined imaging of spine oncology and pain management, Michele Johnson has mastered neurointerventional techniques for emergent spine pathologies, Judy Donovan Post delineated CT imaging of the spine, Alyssa Watanabe developed several spinal injection procedures, and Erin Simon Schwartz described spinal imaging of congenital anomalies.

Other Brain Pathologies Soonme Cha has defined MR perfusion and other advanced imaging characteristics of brain tumors before and after treatment. Pam Schaefer and Achala Vagal have defined the use of diffusion and perfusion imaging in the evaluation of acute ischemic stroke and other cerebrovascular pathologies. Jacquie Bello performed pivotal research in cerebrovascular disease and epilepsy. Tammie Benzinger has pioneered translational PET and MR imaging techniques to investigate biomarkers for Alzheimer's Disease. Judy Donovan Post elucidated the Neuroimaging of AIDS.

Health Services Research Pina Sanelli and Yoshimi Anzai are experts in comparative effectiveness research. Pina Sanelli received the Radiology Alliance for Health Services Research (RAHSR) Achievement Award for Outstanding Contributions in Research. Yoshimi established the ACQUIRE (Applying Comparative Effectiveness and Quality Improvement in Research and Education) Workshop sponsored by four societies.

Education

The vast majority of North American women neuroradiologists are known for their exceptional teaching. Three have received the ASNR Outstanding Contributions in Neuroradiology Education: Tabassum Kennedy for her development of entirely new ways to engage medical students in the process of learning neuroradiology, Christine Glastonbury for her mentoring programs for neuroradiologists and her exquisite teaching of head and neck pathology and Pam Schaefer for her contributions to setting standards for Neuroradiology fellowships and running education-related committees of multiple societies including the ASNR, the AAR, and the RSNA. Ann Osborne authored numerous best-selling textbooks and established the first online clinical radiology reference system, STATDx, all of which became standards in neuroradiology education. Laurie Loevner served as the neuroradiology editor for *RadioGraphics* and chaired the RSNA Education Committee and refresher course program. Jacquie Bello was the former chair of the AMA Council on Medical Education. Wende Gibbs served as Chair of the ASNR Education Committee and Chair of the Education workgroup for the ACR Neuroradiology Commission. Rona Woldenberg is the Founding Editor of Case in Point, an online daily case presentation sponsored by the ACR. Dr. Ertl-Wagner received the RSNA Honored Educator Award.

Diversity, Equity and Inclusion, and Global Outreach

Carolyn Meltzer served as the Chief of Diversity and Inclusion while she was the Chair of Radiology at Emory University Hospital and established the Women in Neuroradiology Leadership Award while serving as President of ASNR. Erin Simon Schwartz was the founding co-chair of the ASNR's Diversity and Inclusion Committee, which oversaw the revision of numerous society charters to embrace inclusivity. Michele Johnson, as Chair of the ASNR Committee on Diversity and Inclusion, is a tireless champion for equity. She is the Director of the ACR PIER Summer Program, designed to introduce underrepresented medical students to careers in radiology. Yoshimi Anzai is a Past President of the AAWR, a co-director of Women in Health, Medicine, and Sciences at the University of Utah, and internationally renowned for her advocacy for women and underrepresented minorities in Neuroradiology. In honor of Anne Osborn's international collaborations, the ASNR established the Anne G. Osborn International Outreach Professor program, dedicated to delivering neuroradiology education in developing nations.

Biographical Sketches

Presidents of ASNR

Anne G. Osborn, MD, 1988–1989

Anne Osborn (Fig. 26.1) was the first woman president of ASNR. As she states: "The only drawback? It took nearly 20 years for the next one!" Early in her career, following being a distinguished scientist at the AFIP, Anne established a correlation between imaging and pathology. She co-authored 120 scientific articles as well as best-selling textbooks that became standards in neuroradiology. These include *Introduction to Cerebral Angiography* (1980), *Diagnostic Neuroradiology* (1994), a succession of *Diagnostic Imaging: Brain* texts from 2004 to 2021, and *Osborn's Brain*. In 2001, Ric Harnsberger and Anne co-founded Amirsys, Inc., which published numerous textbooks distinguished by bulleted formats and abundant color anatomic/pathologic illustrations. Subsequently, they established the first online clinical radiology reference system, STATDx®, now a standard for training programs around the world.

Among numerous additional accolades, Ann was the Vice-President of the RSNA and Chair of the Board of Trustees of the RSNA's Research and Education Foundation. She was awarded gold medals from the ASNR and RSNA, the first Outstanding Educator Award from the RSNA, and the Marie Curie Award. In 2017,

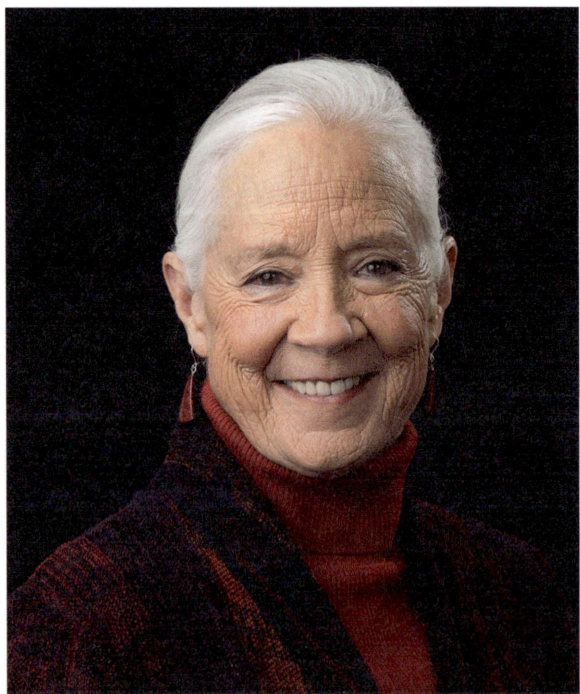

Fig. 26.1 Anne G. Osborn

the ASNR established the Anne G. Osborn International Outreach Professor program, dedicated to delivering neuroradiology education in developing nations. At the University of Utah School of Medicine, she was a distinguished professor and held a Presidential Endowed Chair in Radiology.

Patricia Rhyner, MD, 2005–2006
Pat Rhyner (Fig. 26.2) is a Past President of the ASNR and ASHNR and received the ASNR Gold Medal in 2022. As Pat states, "At one time in the early 2000s, I was both President-elect for the ASHNR (2003) and Secretary for the ASNR when I was asked to run for Vice President of the ASNR. It had been 15 years since Anne Osborne was ASNR president. We joked that she must have done a really bad job, since it took so long to ask another woman to run! I won the election. It was crazy—I was President of the ASHNR, Vice President-elect of the ASNR, and Secretary of the ASNR! The joke in the Ex Comm was that if I was in attendance, we had a quorum." Establishing a Head & Neck radiology reading room in the ENT outpatient clinic at Emory University was the highlight of her career. As Pat states, "Imaging is such a critical part of the ENT surgical specialty, so incorporating CT and MRI in day-to-day patient care made sense. Everyone benefited: ENT and Neuroradiology attendings, trainees, and patients. The surgeons and radiologists collaborated on research, publications, and mutual education. The success of what at the time was truly 'out of the box' thinking was the happiest time of my long career."

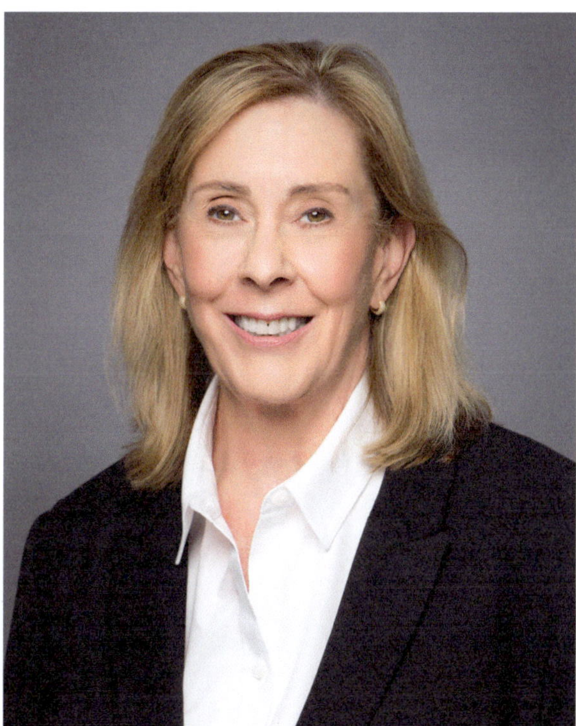

Fig. 26.2 Patricia Rhyner

Carolyn C. Meltzer, MD, FACR, 2010–2011

Carolyn C. Meltzer (Fig. 26.3) has a long history of extraordinary leadership, sponsorship, and mentorship in medicine. She was the third woman president of the ASNR. She is currently the Dean of the Keck School of Medicine of USC and serves on the Council of Deans Administrative Board for the AAMC, Board of Directors of the RSNA, and the Board of the California Institute for Regenerative Medicine (CIRM). Prior to joining USC, Dr. Meltzer served as the Chair of the Department of Radiology and Imaging Sciences at Emory University, where she was also the Executive Associate Dean of Faculty Academic Advancement, Leadership, and Inclusion, and the Chief Diversity and Inclusion Officer. Dr. Meltzer performed landmark research on the brain's structure and function during normal aging, Alzheimer's disease, and neuropsychiatric disorders. She led the clinical evaluation of the world's first human combined PET-CT scanner for cancer staging and treatment. Dr. Meltzer is a fellow of the American Association for the Advancement of Science and received the distinguished service award from the AMA, the gold medal award from the AAR, the outstanding researcher award and gold medal award from the ASNR, and the gold medal award from the Academy for Radiology and Biomedical Imaging Research.

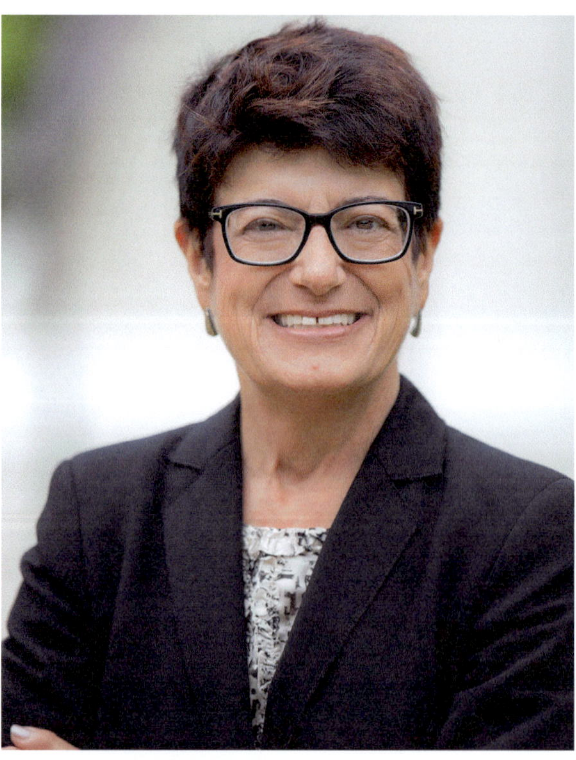

Fig. 26.3 Carolyn C. Meltzer

Pamela W. Schaefer, MD, FAAR, FACR, 2012–2013

Pam Schaefer (Fig. 26.4) is the Vice Chair of Faculty Affairs at MGH, previously serving as the Vice Chair of Education, the Clinical Director of MRI, and the Neuroradiology Fellowship Director. She holds the Theresa McLoud, MD, Endowed Chair in Radiology Education and is Professor of Radiology at Harvard Medical School. She is a past president of the ASNR, the ENRS, and the New England Roentgen Ray Society. Other notable positions include the Chair of the Alliance of Directors and Vice Chairs of Education in Radiology and the Chair of the Education Committee of the AAR, the Chair of the Program Director's Committee of the ASNR, and the Chair of the Scientific Program Committee of the ARRS. She is a fellow of the ACR and AAR, a Deputy Editor for Education of the JACR, and a past Senior Editor of the AJNR. Dr. Schaefer is considered an international expert in diffusion weighted imaging (DWI), stroke imaging, and cerebrovascular imaging. She is a renowned educator and received the 2022 ASNR Outstanding Contributions in Neuroradiology Education Award.

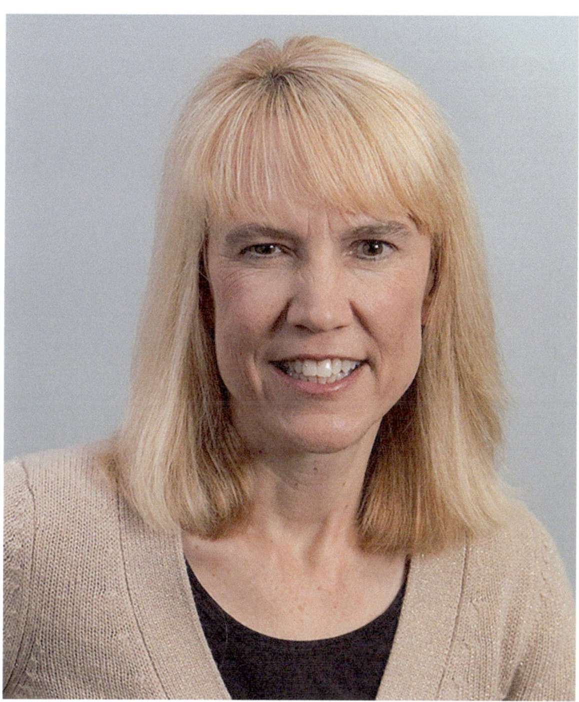

Fig. 26.4 Pamela W. Schaefer

Laurie A. Loevner, MD, 2015–2016

Laurie Loevner (Fig. 26.5) is a Professor of Radiology and the Neuroradiology Division Chief at the University of Pennsylvania. She is a Past-President of the ASNR, the ASHNR, and the ENRS, and has served as the Vice Chair of the Head and Neck/Neuro Oncologic Committee at the ACR Image Network (ACRIN). Dr. Loevner served as the neuroradiology editor for *RadioGraphics* and chaired the RSNA Education Committee and Refresher Course Program. Currently, she is the Co-Chair for the Foundation of the ASNR, having raised over seven million dollars. Dr. Loevner has performed cutting-edge research in head and neck cancer focused on the pathophysiology, genetics, and microenvironments around tumors, assessing disease progression, and providing prognostic information in oncologic patients. Dr. Loevner "takes pride in developing the next generation of radiology investigators and leaders and has mentored too numerous to count trainees and faculty." Dr. Loevner received the IS Ravdin Master Clinician Award, given to one doctor annually throughout the University of Pennsylvania Health system, and is a founding member and Co-Chair of the Academy of Master Clinicians at Penn.

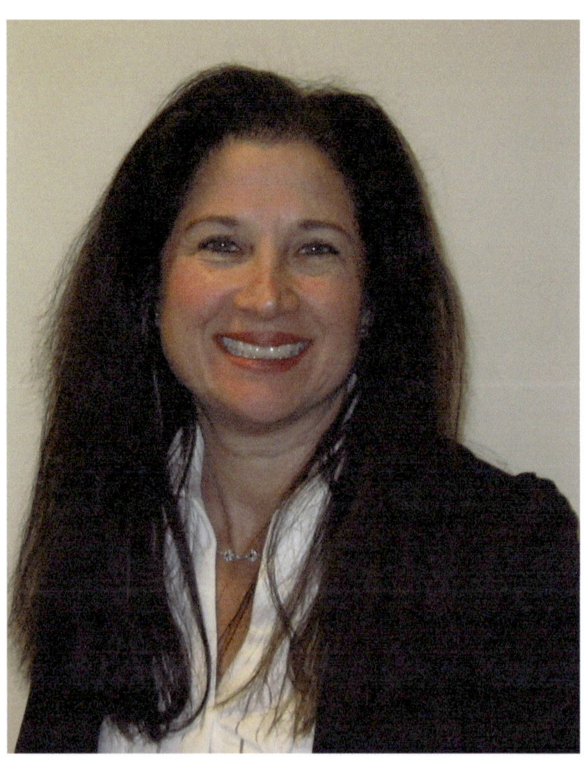

Fig. 26.5 Laurie A. Loevner

Jacquelline A. Bello, MD, FACR, 2017–2018

Jacquie Bello (Fig. 26.6) is the Zimmer-Hardy Professor of Neuroradiology at Montefiore and Professor of Radiology and Neurosurgery at the Albert Einstein College of Medicine. She is a past president of the ASNR and received the ASNR Gold Medal in 2023. She is internationally renowned for her contributions to healthcare policy, quality and safety, medical education, and neuroradiology clinical research. Dr. Bello served as the Chair of the ACR Board of Chancellors and as the Chair of the ACR Commission on Quality and Safety. She is a past president of the AMA Foundation, former chair of the AMA Council on Medical Education, and represents the ASNR in the AMA House of Delegates. Her research has been primarily focused on epilepsy, cerebrovascular diseases, and various head and neck topics. She has shared her acumen for teaching in invited lectures all over the world. She is a Columbia University Alumni Gold Medalist and a past president of the NY Roentgen Society and the NY State Radiological Society.

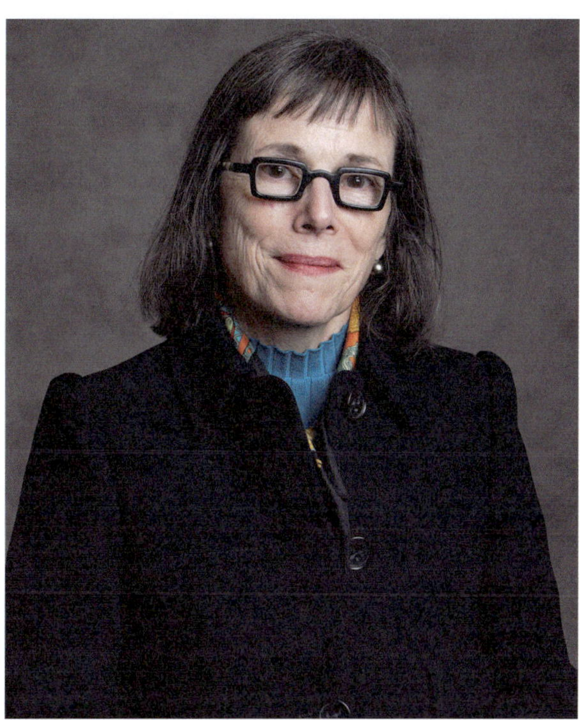

Fig. 26.6 Jacquelline A. Bello

Pina Sanelli, MD, FAAR, FACR, 2018–2019
Pina Sanelli (Fig. 26.7) is a Professor of Radiology at the Donald and Barbara Zucker School of Medicine at Hofstra/Northwell where she serves as the Vice Chair of Research, and Professor in the Institute of Health System Science at the Feinstein Institutes for Medical Research. She is a Past President of the ASNR, the ENRS, and the Alliance for Health Services Research (RAHSR), and served on the Board of Directors for the ASNR, AAR, and ARRS. Dr. Sanelli has performed exceptional technology assessment and clinical effectiveness and outcomes-based research on advanced imaging techniques in patients with cerebrovascular diseases, particularly acute stroke, aneurysmal subarachnoid hemorrhage, and chronic cerebral ischemia. In recognition, she received the Radiology Alliance for Health Services Research (RAHSR) Achievement Award for Outstanding Contributions in Research. Dr. Sanelli is the Co-Founder and Co-Director of the Harvey L. Neiman Health Policy Institute's PRIME (Policy Research and Imaging Effectiveness) Center, sponsored by the ACR. She established the Value of Imaging through Comparative Effectiveness (VOICE) program sponsored by the RSNA and the Comparative Effectiveness Research Training (CERT) program jointly sponsored by the RSNA, ASNR, SIR, and SNMMI.

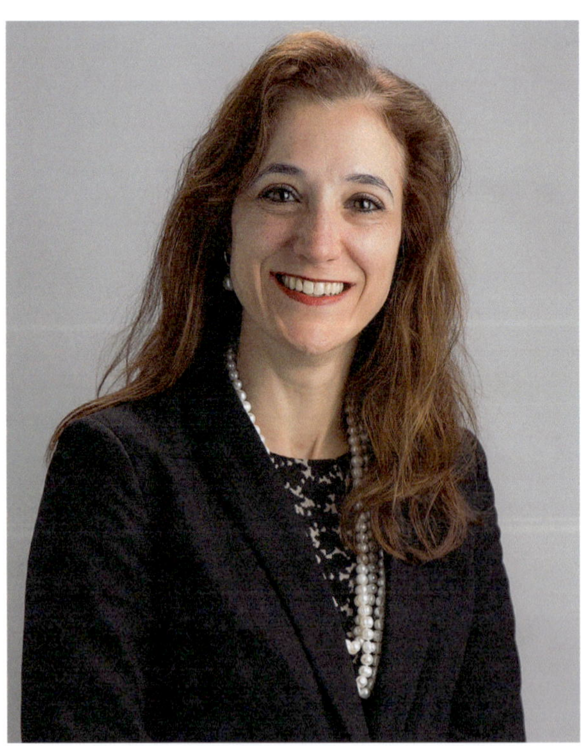

Fig. 26.7 Pina C. Sanelli

Tina Young Poussaint, MD, FACR, 2021–2022

Tina Young Poussaint (Fig. 26.8) is the Radiologist-in-Chief and the Lionel W. Young Chair in Radiology at Boston Children's Hospital and a Professor of Radiology at the Harvard Medical School (HMS). She is a Past President of the ASNR and ASPNR and an ASPNR Gold Medal recipient. She has served as Past Chair of the Radiology Section of the National Medical Association and is also a Fellow of the ASPNR and ACR. Dr. Poussaint is internationally renowned for her research in pediatric brain tumor imaging with a focus on correlation of imaging features with pediatric brain tumor molecular subtypes and the creation and implementation of innovative neuroimaging research protocols for pediatric brain tumor clinical trials. She is Principal Investigator (PI) and Director of the Neuroimaging Center (NIC) of the NIH-funded Pediatric Brain Tumor Consortium (PBTC) and is Director of BCH Neuro-Oncologic Imaging.

Fig. 26.8 Tina Young Poussaint

Erin Simon Schwartz, MD, FACR, FASPNR, 2022–2023

Erin Simon Schwartz (Fig. 26.9) is Chief of the Division of Neuroradiology and Associate Chair for Radiology Diversity, Equity & Inclusion, at Children's Hospital of Philadelphia, as well as a Professor of Radiology at the Perelman School of Medicine, University of Pennsylvania. She holds the Robert A Zimmerman Endowed Chair in Pediatric Neuroradiology and is the Editor in Chief of *Applied Radiology*. She is a Past President of the ASNR, ASPNR, ASSR, and ENRS. These leadership experiences allowed her to promote greater trainee engagement and raise awareness of the crucial role of diagnostic and interventional neuroradiology in patient care. She was the founding Co-Chair of the ASNR's Diversity and Inclusion Committee. As an advocate for women in medicine, she oversaw the revision of numerous society charters to embrace inclusivity, developed succession-planning strategies, streamlined processes to increase sustainability, and reduced overhead to help ensure the future of these vital organizations.

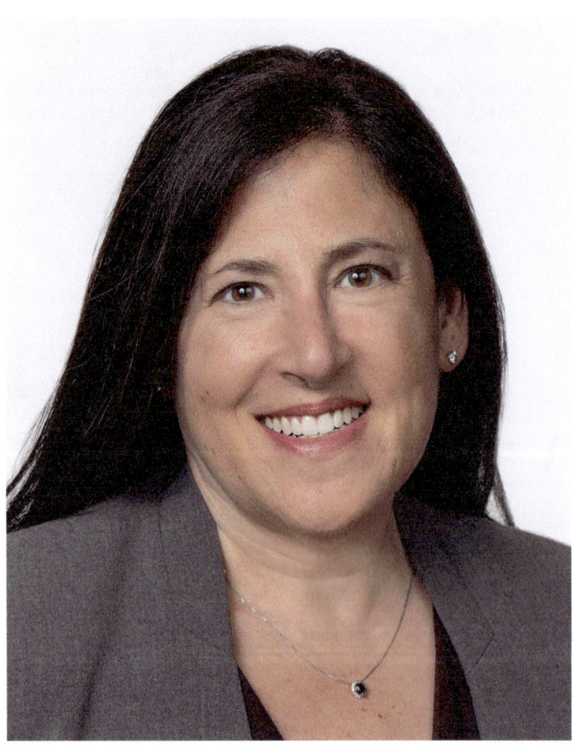

Fig. 26.9 Erin Simon Schwartz

Yvonne W. Lui, MD, FACR, 2023–2024
Yvonne Lui (Fig. 26.10) is Professor and Vice Chair of Research for the Department of Radiology at the NYU Grossman School of Medicine and the Vilcek Institute of Graduate Biomedical Sciences. She is renowned for her research in artificial intelligence and traumatic brain injury. She established deep learning-based MR image reconstruction as a powerful method and oversaw the release of the *fast*MRI dataset, the world's most influential collection of MR images and raw k-space elements. She developed one of the first programs for machine learning in radiology and oversees a leading research program distinguished by cutting-edge imaging technology development and innovative translational research. She is the collaboration lead on major research partnerships, including the NYU Courant Institute and Center for Data Science, Siemens Healthineers, and Facebook AI Research. Dr. Lui is a Past President of the ASNR and of the New York Roentgen Society (NYRS). She was the "voice of the AJNR" as its second podcast editor. She serves on the editorial board of *Frontiers for Young Minds*, mentoring middle and high school students in the peer-review process.

Fig. 26.10 Yvonne W. Lui

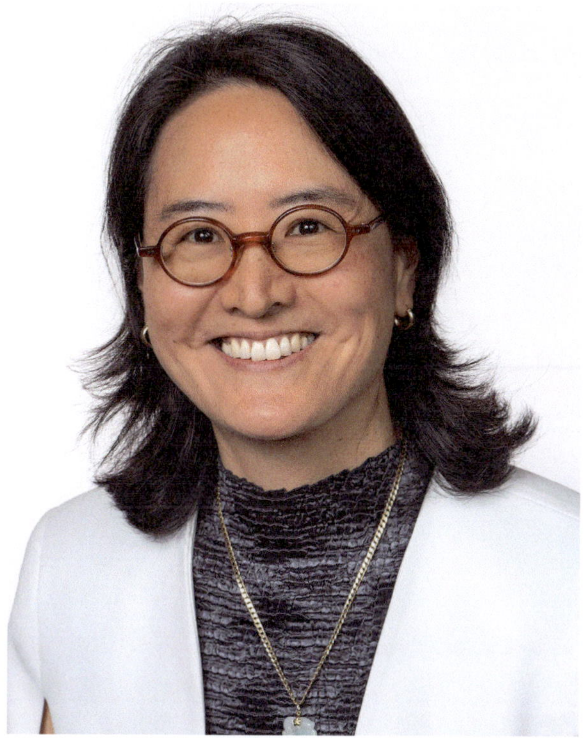

Yoshimi Anzai, MD, MPH, FACR, 2025–2026

Yoshimi Anzai (Fig. 26.11) is a Professor of Radiology and Vice Chair of Quality and Safety in Radiology at the University of Utah, where she previously served as the Associate Chief Medical Quality Officer, as well as the Co-director of the Women in Health, Medicine, and Sciences, and as the School of Medicine Academic Senate representative. She has performed seminal research in head and neck cancer imaging, neurodegenerative disease, and comparative effectiveness of medical imaging. She is the President-Elect of ASNR and a Past President of the AAR and AAWR. She has held many other leadership positions in the ASHNR, RSNA, ACR, AAWR, and WNRS. She is a Deputy Editor for Radiology and a Co-director for the ACQUIRE (Applying Comparative Effectiveness and Quality Improvement in Research and Education) Workshop sponsored by the RSNA, ASNR, SNMMI, and SIR. She has "opened the door" for minority and foreign medical graduate women who pursue neuroradiology. As Dr. Anzai states, "We should keep in mind that we learn and grow most when facing challenges. Enjoy your journeys and bring many friends along the way. The experience you have and the connections you make are the ultimate reward."

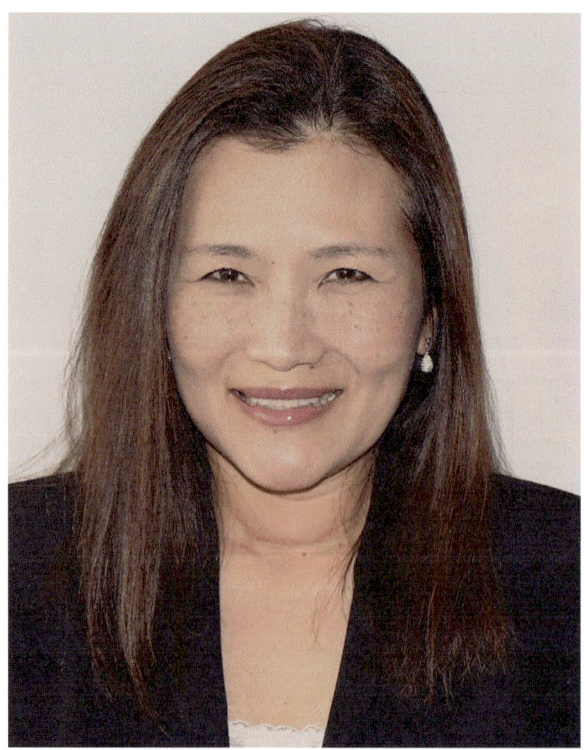

Fig. 26.11 Yoshimi Anzai

President of CSNR

Donatella Tampieri MD, FRCP(C)
Donatella Tampieri (Fig. 26.12) is a Professor of Radiology, Medicine, and Surgery and the Neuroradiology Section Lead at Queen's University in Kingston, Canada. As Chair of the Montreal Neurological Institute for 18 years, she created a cutting-edge Interventional Neuroradiology Section. She was the first Canadian Neuroradiologist to perform vertebroplasty in the mid-1990s, and to use the flow diverter "Silk" for treating brain aneurysms in 2012. She received the Prix d'Excellence en Innovation des Soins de Santé from La Direction du Développement Professionnel Continue (DDPC) of the Fédération des Médecins Spécialistes du Québec (FMSQ) in 2016. She is a Past President of the Canadian Society of Neuroradiology, the ENRS, and the Foundation of the Association of University Radiologists in Quebec. She had "five wonderful mentors in her career—Professors Giovanni Ruggiero, Giuseppe Scotti, Romero Ethier, Denis Melancon, and Karel Terbrugge—who were a true source of inspiration." She could not have accomplished her work without the support and love of her two precious children, Kahile and Paul Jr., and her husband Allen.

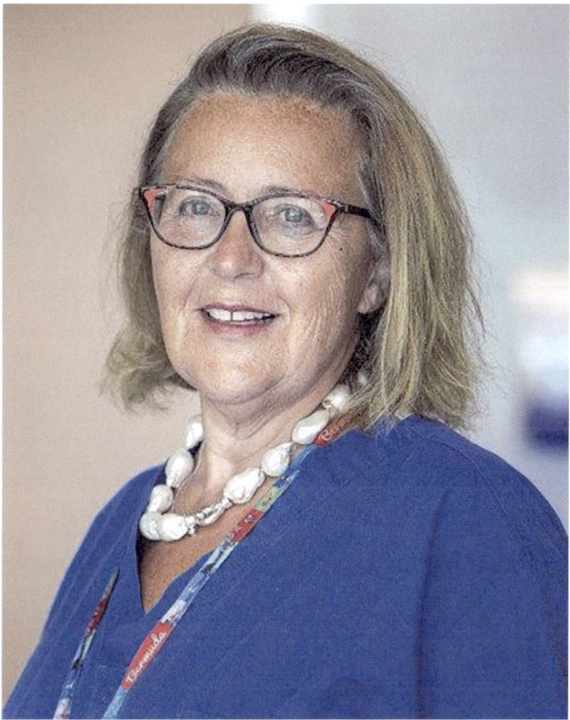

Fig. 26.12 Donatella Tampieri

Additional Presidents and Gold Medalists of ASHNR

Wendy R. K. Smoker, MD, 1998

Wendy Smoker (Fig. 26.13) is a pioneer in head and neck imaging. During her tenure as Professor of Radiology at the University of Iowa, she greatly advanced our ability to diagnose complex head and neck pathologies. She is a Past President of the ASHNR and served with distinction as an AFIP faculty member. Displaying unmatched acumen on the topics of denervation atrophy, granulomatosis with polyangiitis, cranial nerve anatomy and pathology, Horner Syndrome, and the craniocervical junction, Dr. Smoker co-authored over 100 publications and received over 80 scientific exhibit awards. As a dedicated mentor and teacher, her vibrant enthusiasm has launched the careers of several prominent neuroradiologists who will continue to carry her rich legacy of leadership and engagement across generations. She is also known to "sing a mean Carmen."

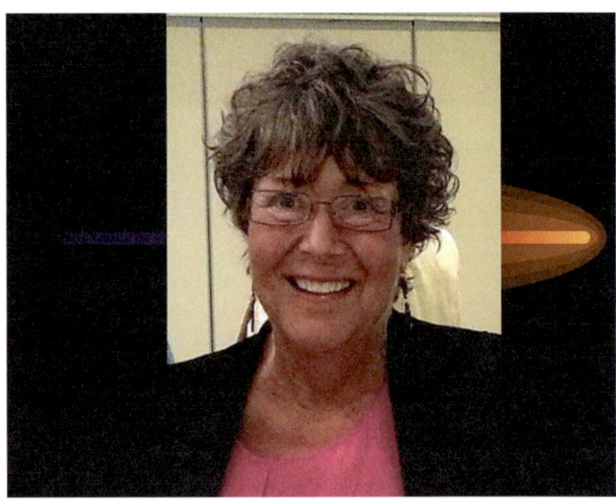

Fig. 26.13 Wendy Smoker

Vijay M. Rao, MD, 2004

Vijay Rao (Fig. 26.14) is the David C. Levin Professor and System Chief of Enterprise Radiology and Imaging at Jefferson Health in Philadelphia. She served as Chair of the Radiology Department at Sidney Kimmel Medical College of Thomas Jefferson University from 2002 to 2022. She is a leading expert in head and neck imaging, health services research in radiology and leadership. She edited the MRI and CT Atlas of Correlative Imaging in Otolaryngology, a treasured resource for trainees. Dr. Rao has held many leadership roles in national organizations, including President of the RSNA, ASHNR, APDR, and AAWR. She is the current RSNA R&E Foundation Board Chair and holds honorary memberships in numerous international societies. Dr. Rao has mentored many residents and fellows who have subsequently become leaders in neuroradiology. She has received numerous awards, including the APDR Achievement Award, the RSNA, AUR, Asian Oceanian Society, and ASHNR Gold Medals, the AAWR Marie Curie Award, and the Jefferson Dean's Lifetime Distinguished Service Award.

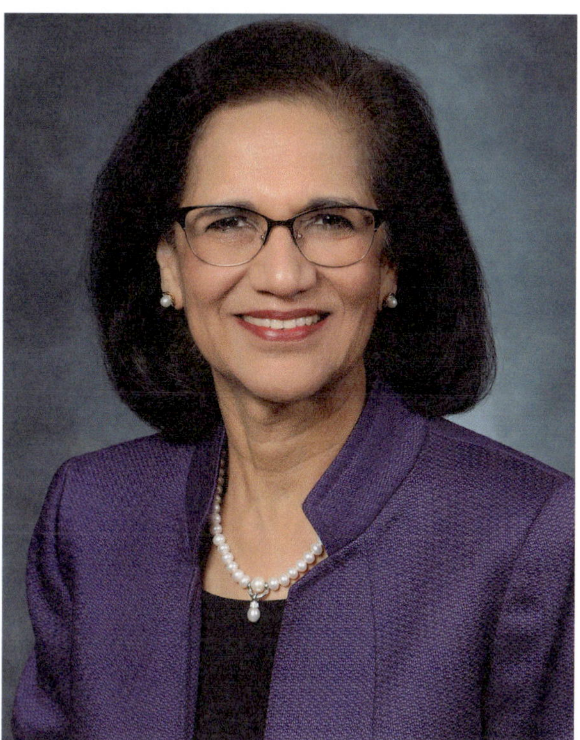

Fig. 26.14 Vijay Rao

Michelle Michel, MD, 2013–2014

Michelle Michel (Fig. 26.15) is a Professor of Radiology and Otolaryngology at the Medical College of Wisconsin. She is a Past President and Gold Medal recipient of the ASHNR. Dr. Michel has also served in leadership roles in the RSNA, ARRS, and ASNR. She co-authored over 100 original articles and book chapters, focused on numerous head and neck topics, and has lectured all over the world, including serving as an RSNA International Visiting Professor in Estonia. She co-edited a number of Amirsys/Elsevier products, including textbooks, StatDx, and RadPrimer. Dr. Michel has been honored with teaching and research awards, including Teacher of the Year at both Vanderbilt University and the Medical College of Wisconsin.

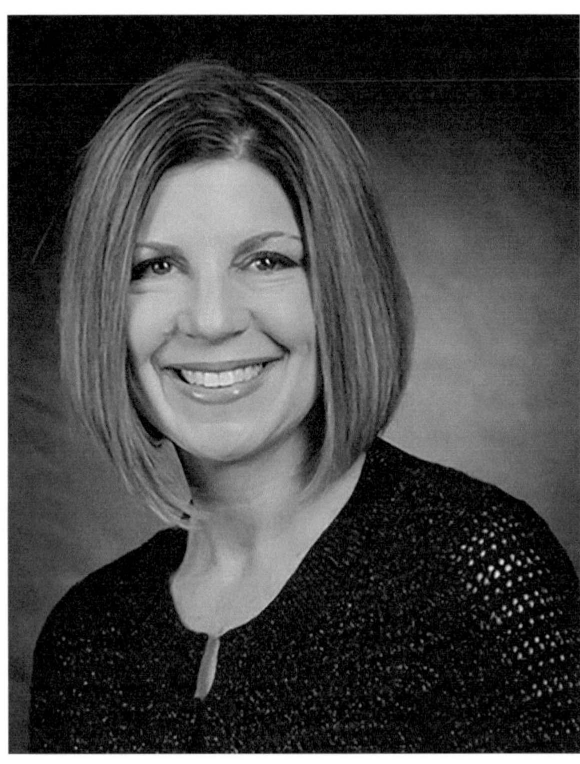

Fig. 26.15 Michelle Michel

Deborah R. Shatzkes, MD, 2018–2019

Deborah Shatzkes (Fig. 26.16) is a Past President and Gold Medal recipient of the ASHNR. As President, she established an agreement between ASHNR and ESHNR that has dramatically increased collaboration between US and European Head and Neck radiologists. She also served as Chair of the RSNA Head and Neck Refresher Course Committee, as an Associate Editor of Radiology, and as Treasurer of the WFNRS. She is most proud of being an exceptional educator who was invited to join the faculty at the ACR Institute of Radiologic Pathology and who has given over 300 national and international lectures, including serving as a Keynote speaker for the Baltic Congress of Radiology in 2022. She served as Chief, Head, and Neck Radiology at Lenox Hill Hospital, as Director of Head and Neck Imaging at the New York Head and Neck Institute, and as a Professor of Radiology at the Zucker School of Medicine at Hofstra/Northwell.

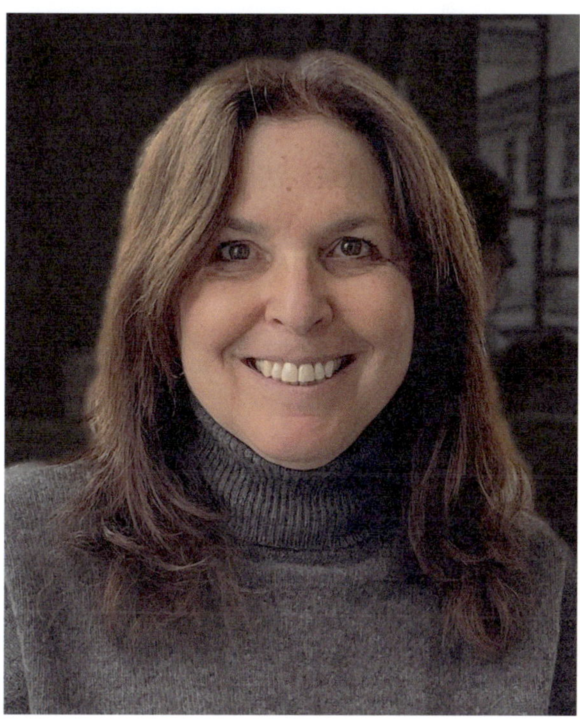

Fig. 26.16 Deborah Shatzkes

Nancy Fischbein, MD, 2021–2022

Nancy Fischbein (Fig. 26.17) is a Professor of Radiology at Stanford University Medical Center, where she has held many leadership roles, including Interim Division Chief and Program Director for the Diagnostic Neuroradiology fellowship. She is a Past President and Executive Committee Member of the ASHNR. She has a particular interest in head and neck cancer and skull base imaging, has co-authored over 180 manuscripts, and has delivered numerous national and international lectures. She is highly dedicated to educating trainees and is proud to have served as the Treasurer of the ASNR and as a Senior Editor for Head and Neck Imaging for the AJNR.

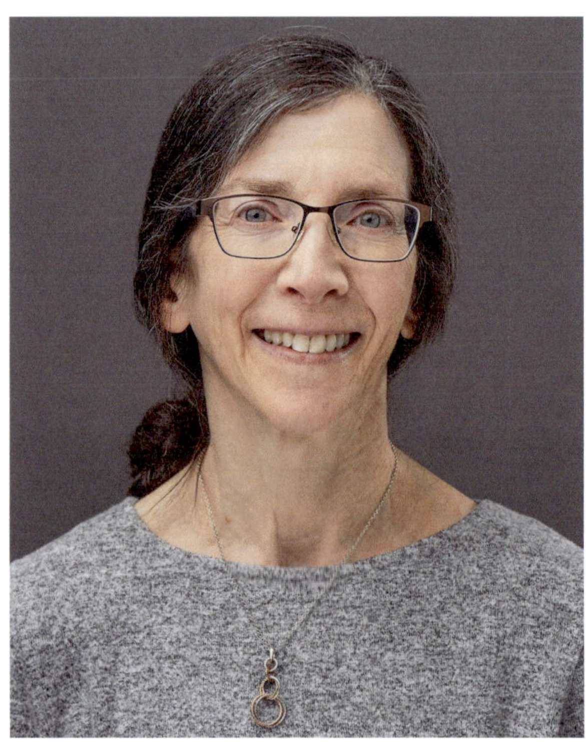

Fig. 26.17 Nancy Fischbein

Kristine Mosier DMD, Ph.D., 2023–2024

Kristine Mosier (Fig. 26.18) is Professor of Radiology and Imaging Sciences, Otolaryngology-Head and Neck Surgery at the Indiana University School of Medicine, where she is Chief, Head and Neck Imaging. She is an internationally recognized expert and lecturer in head and neck imaging and is the immediate Past President of the ASHNR. She has performed ground-breaking research in the application of functional MR imaging to head and neck pathologies. As an exceptional educator, she is the recipient of several research and teaching awards, including the Indiana University Trustee's Teaching Award.

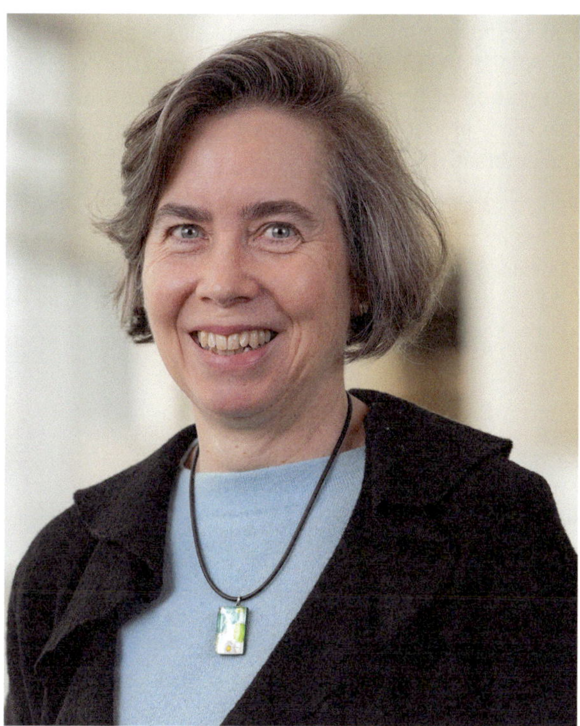

Fig. 26.18 Kristine Mosier

Christine M. Glastonbury, MBBS, 2024–2025

Christine Glastonbury (Fig. 26.19) is a Professor of Radiology & Biomedical Imaging, Otolaryngology-Head & Neck Surgery, and Radiation Oncology at the University of California, San Francisco. She is the Vice Chair for Academic Affairs, having previously served as the Interim Chief of Neuroradiology and the Neuroradiology Fellowship Program Director. As an expert in Head and Neck (HN) Imaging, she works closely with the radiation oncologists and surgeons to optimize HN cancer patient care at UCSF. She is the current President of the ASHNR, a member of the HN Expert Panel for the development of the American Joint Committee on Cancer [AJCC] Staging System, and is the first radiologist member of the National Comprehensive Cancer Networks [NCCN] Head and Neck Cancers Panel. She was the Program President for the WFNRS 2022 meeting and received the ASNR 2024 Outstanding Contributions in Neuroradiology Education Award in recognition of her exceptional commitment to and skill in teaching. She is "proud that she is able to simplify complex Head and Neck imaging so that all radiologists can embrace it."

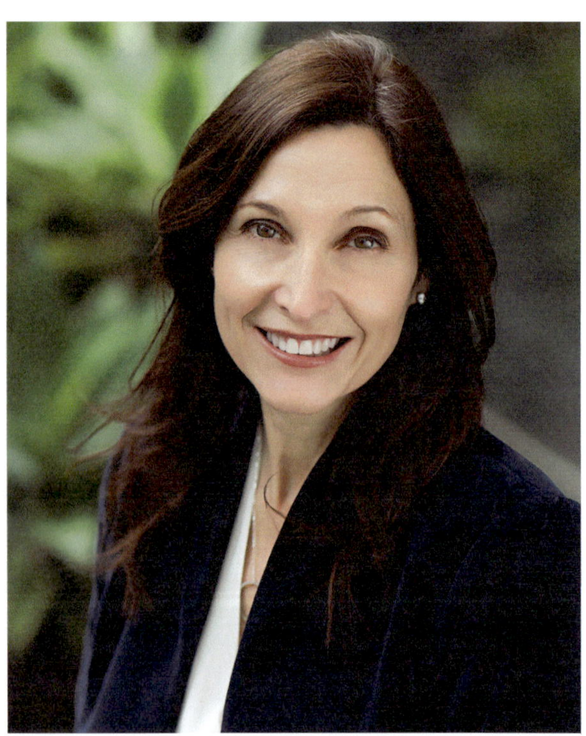

Fig. 26.19 Christine Glastonbury

Presidents of ASFNR

Jody Tanabe, MD, 2024–2025

Jody Tanabe (Fig. 26.20) is a Professor of Radiology at the University of Colorado School of Medicine (UCSOM), where she is the Radiology Vice Chair of Research, previously serving as the Division Chief of Neuroradiology. She is internationally renowned for her research using neuroimaging to study the neural correlates of substance use disorders. With funding from NIH, she has studied DBS for severe methamphetamine use disorder and transcranial magnetic stimulation and focused ultrasound for substance and alcohol use disorder. She was accepted into the prestigious Council of Distinguished Investigators through the Academy for Radiology and Biomedical Imaging Research in 2015. She is currently the first female President of the American Society of Functional Neuroradiology (ASFNR). She is also a Senior Editor of the AJNR, Co-chair of ASNR Corporate Partners, and Co-chair of the Foundation of the ASNR Board of Trustees.

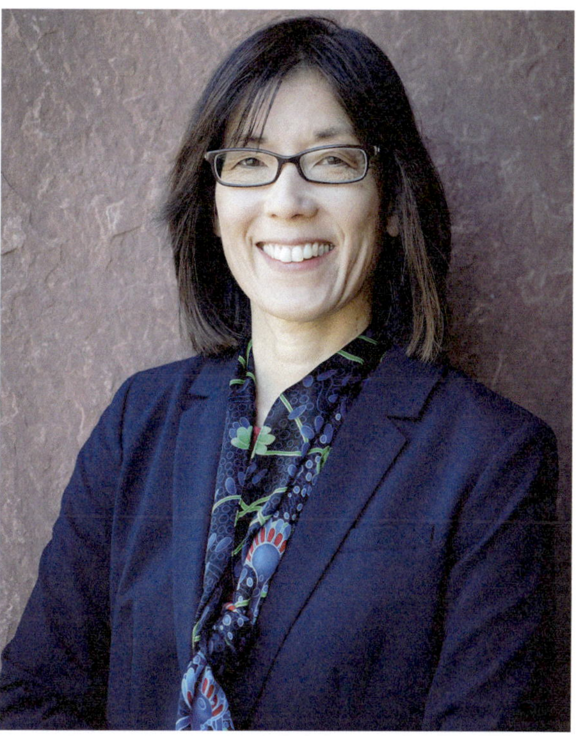

Fig. 26.20 Jody Tanabe

Additional Presidents and Gold Medalists of ASPNR

Jill V. Hunter, MD, 2007–2008

Jill Hunter (Fig. 26.21) is a Professor of Radiology at Baylor College of Medicine and Section Head of Pediatric Neuroradiology at Texas Children's Hospital. She is a Fellow and Past President of the ASPNR and a Past President of the ENRS. She is an outstanding investigator who has performed ground-breaking research. Early in her career, she investigated the rabbit brain lymphatic drainage (a precursor to the more recent description of the glymphatic system), ultrasound in pediatric stroke, and brain pH in children on the ketogenic diet. For the past 20 years, she has focused on applications of MRI to traumatic brain injury and the evaluation of patients with complex congenital heart disease. In recognition of her scholarship, she has been invited to sit on multiple NIH study sections and lecture all over the world. In 2022, she received the lifetime Master Clinician award from Baylor College of Medicine.

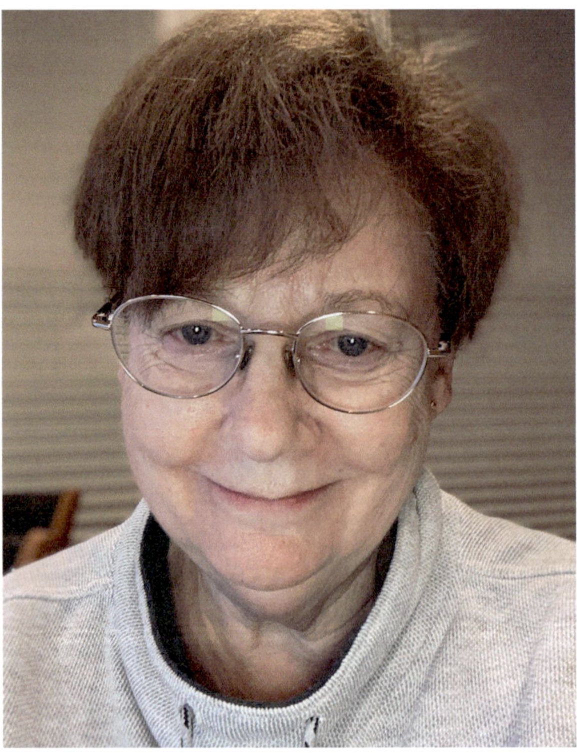

Fig. 26.21 Jill Hunter

Caroline Robson, MD, 2011–2012

Caroline Robson (Fig. 26.22) is the Neuroradiology Division Chief and Director of Head and Neck Imaging at Boston Children's Hospital and is an Associate Professor in Radiology. She is an expert in pediatric head and neck imaging whose research addresses unique imaging features of rarely encountered HN conditions. Important clinical innovations include a program that greatly decreases the number of children who require sedation for imaging, and a rapid MRI exam for patients with hydrocephalus, cysts, and head trauma, thereby eliminating the need for a head CT, which uses radiation. Dr. Robson is a Past President of the ASPNR and of the ASHNR, an honorary lifetime member of the British Society for Head and Neck Imaging, and an AJNR Senior Editor for Pediatric Neuroradiology.

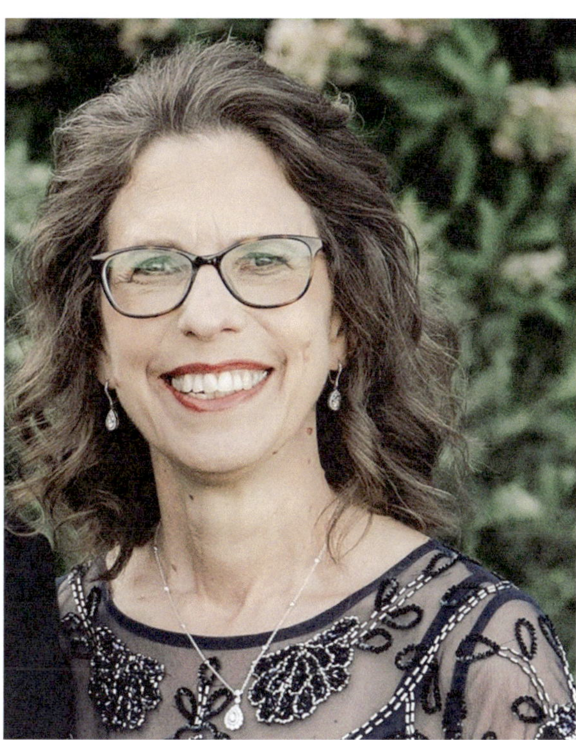

Fig. 26.22 Caroline Robson

Susan Palasis, MD, 2016–2017

Susan Palasis (Fig. 26.23) is a Professor of Radiology, Imaging Sciences and Pediatrics at Emory University School of Medicine and the Director of Pediatric Neuroradiology at Children's Healthcare of Atlanta (CHOA). She was previously Chief of Pediatric Neuroradiology and Vice Chair of Operations at the Ann & Robert H. Lurie Children's Hospital of Chicago. She is an internationally respected leader and educator in the field of Pediatric Neuroradiology. As the President of the ASPNR, Susan implemented the society's first annual scientific meeting. As she acknowledges, "This was a point of inflection for the field of pediatric neuroimaging. It grew the society in a significant way, promoted education, and expanded research in pediatric neuroimaging." She also served on the Executive Board of the SPR.

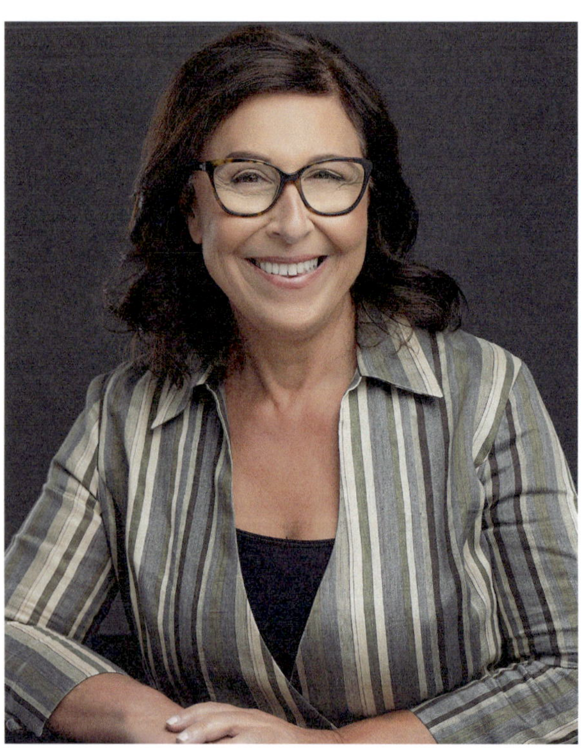

Fig. 26.23 Susan Palasis

V. Michelle Silvera, MD, 2021–2022

Michelle Silvera (Fig. 26.24) is an Associate Professor of Radiology at the Mayo Clinic and Chief of Pediatric Neuroradiology. As President of ASPNR, she was instrumental in launching national pediatric neuroradiology meetings, creating an online educational platform, growing membership, securing financial stability, and establishing key industry partnerships. She is an expert in the imaging of abusive CNS injuries and is an exceptional educator, having developed teaching libraries at prominent institutions and regularly lecturing around the world. As a dedicated mentor, she has guided numerous junior faculty and trainees who now have distinguished careers in pediatric neuroradiology. She is deeply "grateful for the support of her colleagues and finds daily pleasure in the reading room in the enthusiasm, curiosity, and dedication of the trainees."

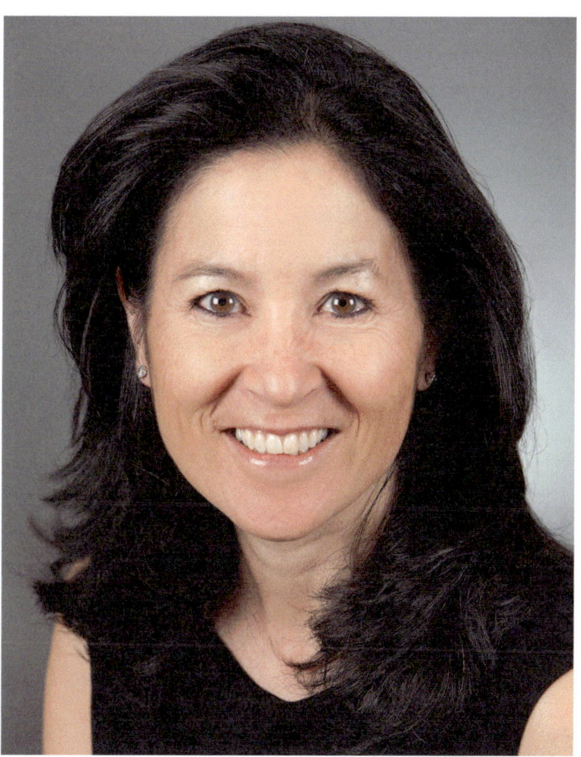

Fig. 26.24 V. Michelle Silvera

Susan Blaser, MD, Gold Medalist 2013
Dr. Blaser (Fig. 26.25) is a Professor Emeritus in the Departments of Neuroradiology and Medical Imaging at the University of Toronto and a Pediatric Neuroradiologist at The Hospital for Sick Children in Toronto. She is widely known for exceptional research focused on congenital diseases of the inner ear, fetal MRI, and inborn errors of metabolism. She co-authored over 200 original articles as well as the Pediatric Neuroradiology issue of the Pocket Radiologist Series, a cherished textbook. She is a well-known international speaker and educator. She received the ASPNR Gold Medal in 2013.

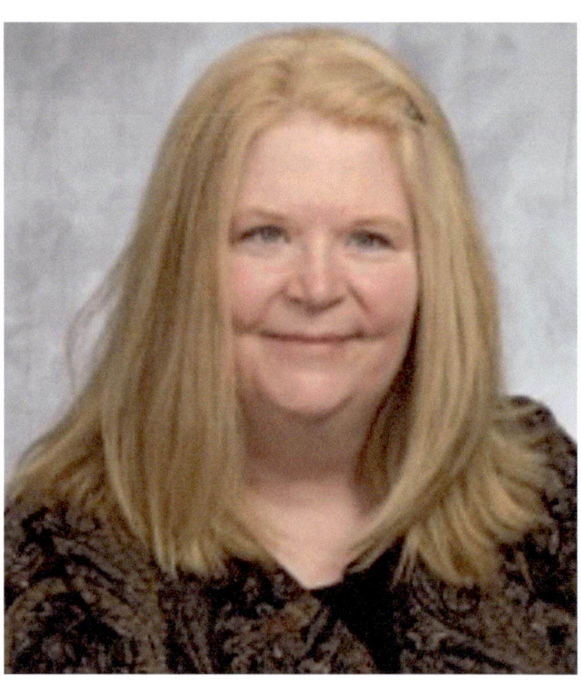

Fig. 26.25 Susan Blaser

Additional Presidents and Gold Medalists of ASSR

M. Judith Donovan Post, MD, 1999–2000

Judy Donovan Post (Fig. 26.26) recently retired. She was a Clinical Professor of Radiology at Boston University School of Medicine and Professor Emeritus at the University of Miami School of Medicine, where she was the Neuroradiology Division Chief. She is a revered expert in imaging of CNS infection, particularly AIDS, and imaging of the spine. She is a Past President and Gold Medal recipient of the ASSR, and a Past President of the SENR. She is a past Treasurer of the ASNR, served on the AJNR Editorial Board, and received the Distinguished Alumnus Award from the University of Kentucky College of Medicine. For decades, Dr. Post was dedicated to taking care of patients by interpreting images, teaching, mentoring, doing research, and collaborating with colleagues around the world. As she states, "Making a positive difference in the lives of patients is what makes it a joy and a privilege to be a neuroradiologist."

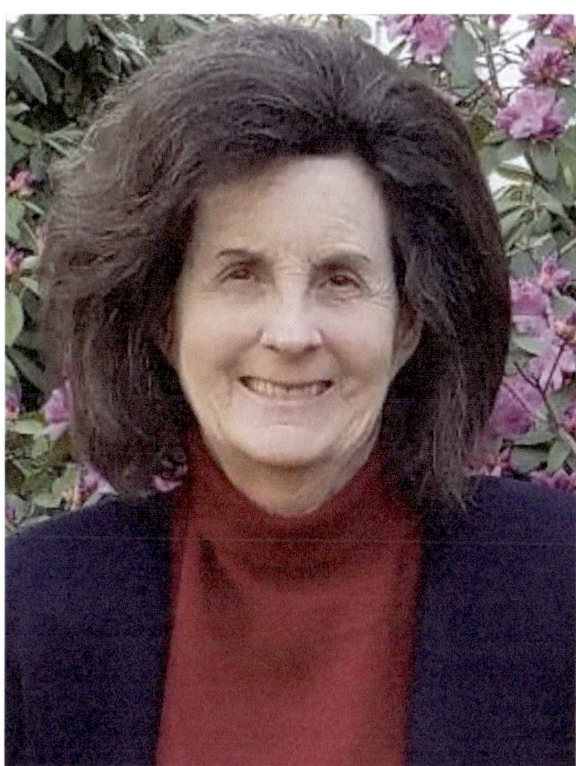

Fig. 26.26 Judy Donovan Post

Alyssa Watanabe, MD, FACR, 2006–2007
Dr. Alyssa Watanabe (Fig. 26.27) is a Clinical Associate Professor of Neuroradiology at USC Keck School of Medicine. She is a Past President of the ASSR and served on the Executive Committees of the ASNR and the California Radiological Society. She is a past recipient of the AAWR Lucy Frank Squire Distinguished Resident Award in Diagnostic Radiology and the ASNR Women in Leadership Award. She was the first and only female interventional neuroradiology fellow at USC. She is an expert in spinal injection procedures, including vertebroplasty and kyphoplasty, as well as in traumatic brain injury imaging, spinal imaging, and artificial intelligence. She is the Principal Investigator of several clinical trials.

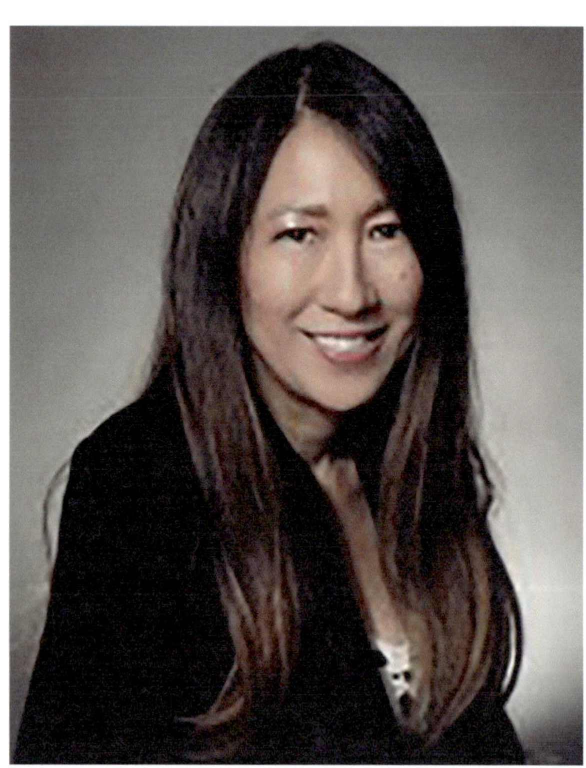

Fig. 26.27 Alyssa Watanabe

Michele H. Johnson, MD, FACR, FASER, 2019–2020

Michele Johnson (Fig. 26.28) is the first African American woman to be appointed full Professor of Radiology and Biomedical Imaging, Neurosurgery, and Surgery at the Yale School of Medicine, where she is the Director of Neurointerventional Radiology. She is an internationally recognized scholar and educator in the neuroimaging and neurointervention of emergent vascular, brain, spine, and head and neck pathologies. She is a Past President of the ASSR, a fellow of the ACR and of ASER, and an ASER Gold Medalist honoree. She received the Distinguished Service Award from the National Medical Association, Section on Radiology and Radiation Oncology. As Chair of the ASNR Committee on Diversity and Inclusion, she is a tireless champion for equity. She is the Director of the ACR Pipeline Initiative for the Enrichment of Radiology (PIER) Summer Program, designed to introduce underrepresented first-year medical students to careers in radiology.

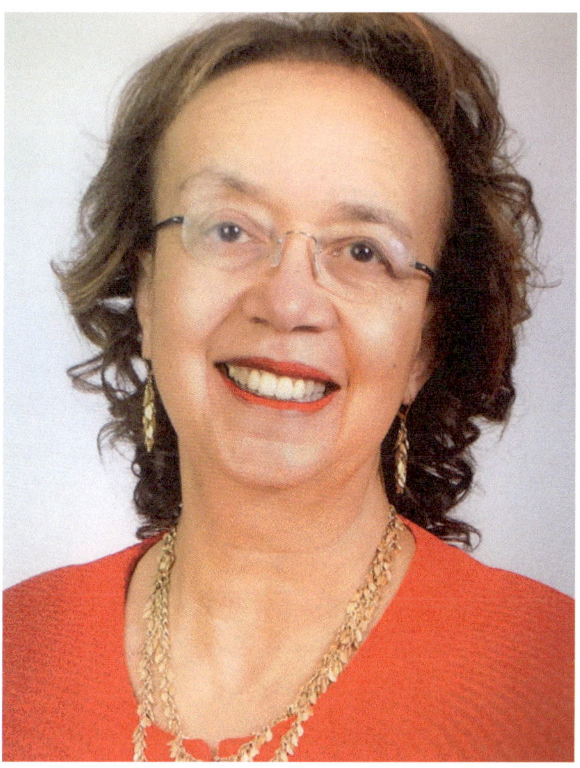

Fig. 26.28 Michelle Johnson

Lubdha Shah, MD, 2021–2022

Lubdha Shah (Fig. 26.29) is a Professor in the Department of Radiology and Imaging Sciences at the University of Utah, where she is the Director of the Spine Imaging, Clinical Functional MRI, and Clinical Focused Ultrasound services. She has co-developed both innovative diffusion imaging sequences to improve diagnosis and noninvasive spine interventional devices using focused ultrasound to treat spine pathologies. Dr. Shah has held numerous national and international leadership positions, including President of the ASSR and Chair of the ACR Practice Parameters Committee, and has served on numerous ASNR committees. She is an AJNR Deputy Editor. As Lubdha acknowledges, “Great mentors have contributed to my accomplishments, and I try to pay it forward by mentoring trainees and junior faculty in their projects and through their career paths.”

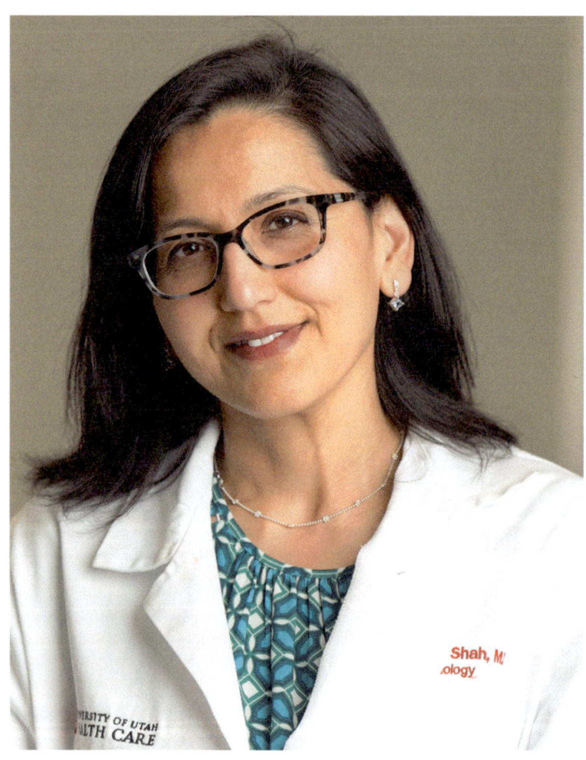

Fig. 26.29 Lubdha Shah

Wende Gibbs, MD, 2023–2024

Wende Gibbs (Fig. 26.30) is the Director of Spine Imaging and Intervention at Barrow Neurological Institute. Her early research focused on Alzheimer's disease, normal pressure hydrocephalus, professionalism, and patient safety. More recently, she has focused on spine intervention, radiology reporting, artificial intelligence, and education. She is the current WNRS President and is a Past president of the ASSR. She has served as Chair of the ASNR Education Committee, Chair of the Education workgroup for the ACR Neuroradiology Commission, the *Radiographics* Podcast Editor, the AJNR Podcast Editor, and as host of the weekly Virtual Global Spine Conference. In her words, "One of my most treasured roles is working to break down specialty silos by representing radiology in multidisciplinary meetings, and by giving invited lectures on communication, reporting, and partnership, in order to advance knowledge and improve our work relationships and lives."

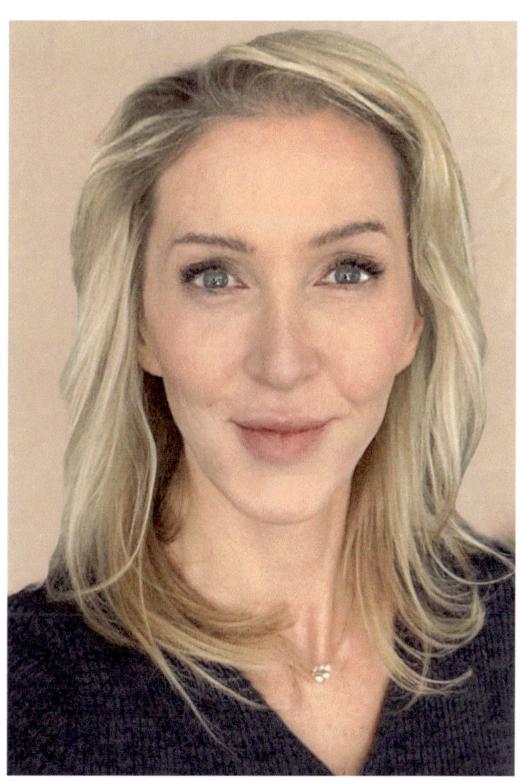

Fig. 26.30 Wende Gibbs

President of SNIS

Mary E. Jensen, MD, FSNIS, 2007–2008

Lee Jensen (Fig. 26.31) is a Professor Emeritus in the Department of Radiology and Medical Imaging at the University of Virginia, where she served as the Director of Neurointerventional Imaging for 21 years. She is a Past President of SNIS, was the first SNIS Foundation Chair, is the SNIS representative to the Brain Attack Coalition, and is the Chairperson of the FDA Neurological Devices panel. Dr. Jensen co-developed the first percutaneous vertebroplasty technique in the United States and later developed multiple additional vertebral augmentation techniques. She is also an internationally recognized expert in minimally invasive procedures for cerebrovascular disease and vascular spinal disorders, and takes pride in having trained numerous fellows who have become leaders in the field of Neurointervention.

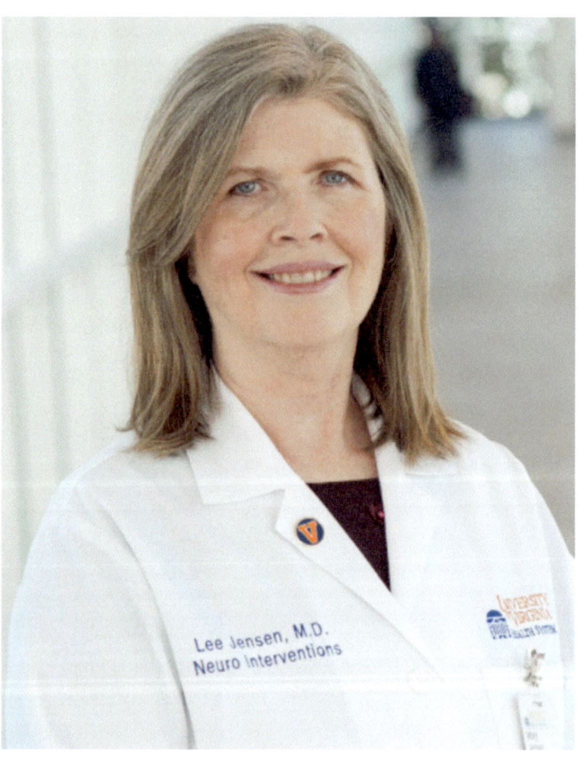

Fig. 26.31 Mary Jensen

Other Notable Luminaries

Raquel del Carpio-O'Donovan, MD

Raquel del Carpio-O'Donovan (Fig. 26.32) is renowned for her leadership, educational initiatives, research, and contributions to international neuroradiology. She has held several prestigious academic and clinical positions, including Professor and Associate Chief of the McGill University Health Center (MUHC) Radiology Department, Vice Chair of the McGill Radiology Department, and Chief Radiologist at Montreal General Hospital. Under the auspices of numerous Canadian and American radiology societies, she has served as an international visiting professor in over 30 countries. She designed the Radiology Resident Program at McGill Hospitals and helped set national standards for residency training. As an Associate Investigator in the Brain Repair and Integrative Neuroscience Program at McGill, she has made significant research contributions. She is a recipient of the Canadian Association of Radiologists Gold Medal and the Prix Albert-Jutras Award from the Societé de Radiologie du Québec. She was elected Honorary President by the WFNS in 2022. In 2024, she was appointed a member of the Order of Canada, one of Canada's highest honors.

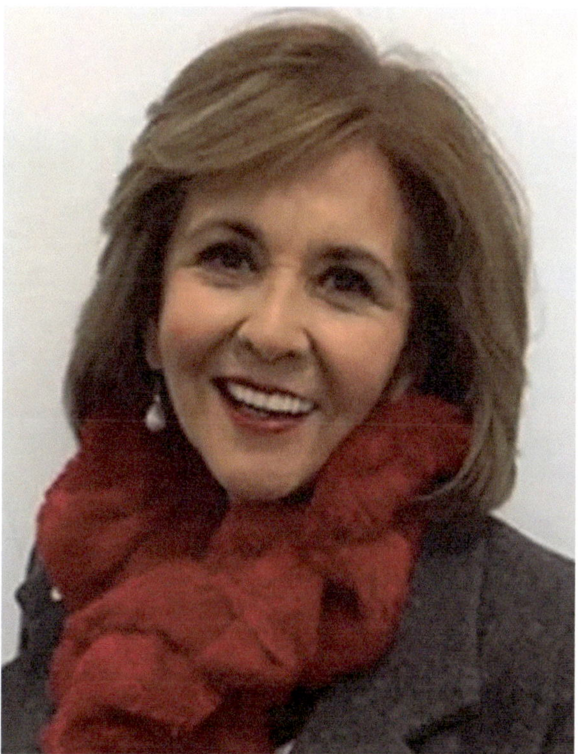

Fig. 26.32 Raquel del Carpio-O'Donovan

Rona Woldenberg, MD, FACR

Rona Woldenberg (Fig. 26.33) is an exceptional leader in radiology education. She is a Professor of Radiology and the inaugural Associate Dean of Admissions at the Zucker School of Medicine at Hofstra Northwell. She is a Fellow of the ACR, is a Past President of the ENRS, and served as a Founding Editor and Editor in Chief of Case in Point, the premier society-sponsored online daily case presentation sponsored by the ACR. She also heads the Neuroradiology section of the ACR-sponsored national radiology in training examination (DIXIT). She serves on the Board of Trustees of the Foundation of the ASNR as well as multiple ASNR committees.

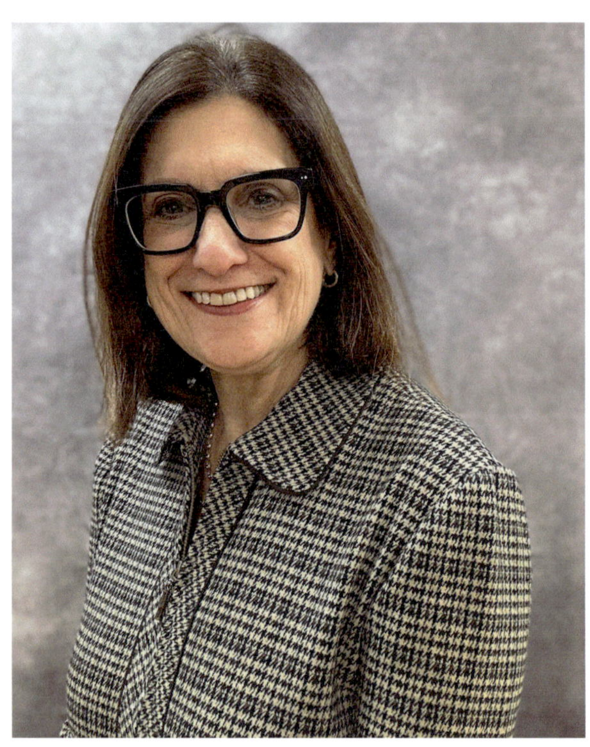

Fig. 26.33 Rona Woldenberg

Tabassum Kennedy, MD

Tabassum Kennedy (Fig. 26.34) is the Joseph Sackett Professor of Radiology at the University of Wisconsin. She is the Vice Chair of Communications and was previously the Neuroradiology Division Chief and Fellowship Program Director. As an exceptional educator, she has invented entirely new ways to engage students in the process of learning radiology. She has received the two most prestigious teaching awards granted at the UW School of Medicine and Public Health. She chaired the ASNR Fellowship Directors Committee, where she directed revision of the ACGME Neuroradiology fellowship requirements. She is an inaugural Co-Chair of the ASNR Section Chiefs' Committee and is a recipient of both the ASNR Women in Neuroradiology Leadership Award and the Outstanding Contributions in Neuroradiology Education Award.

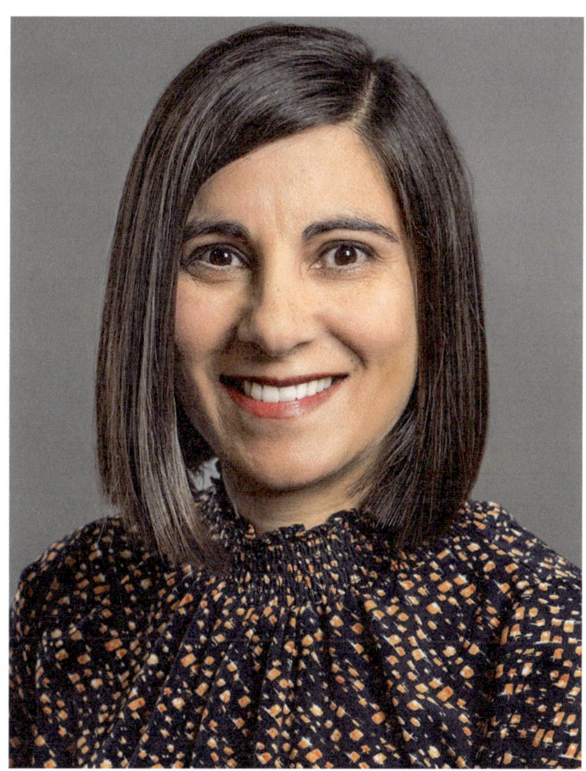

Fig. 26.34 Tabassum Kennedy

Achala Vagal, MD

Achala Vagal (Fig. 26.35) is a Professor of Radiology at the University of Cincinnati College of Medicine, Executive Vice Chair and Vice Chair of Research of the Department of Radiology. She is also the Associate Dean of Clinical and Translational Research and the Co-Director of the Center of Clinical and Translational Science and Training (CCTST), where she strives to "build a diverse, multidisciplinary research workforce." She is internationally recognized for her seminal research in cerebrovascular disease imaging. She is the Director of the NIH StrokeNET Imaging Management Center, overseeing all core imaging activities, and has a leadership role in the NIH/NCATS-funded Clinical and Translational Science Award. She holds multiple national and international leadership positions, including being the current Secretary and a Board member of the ASNR. She received the International Stroke Conference Stroke Innovation Award and the ASNR Women in Neuroradiology Leadership Award in 2019, and has received the RSNA Honored Educator Award twice.

Fig. 26.35 Achala Vagal

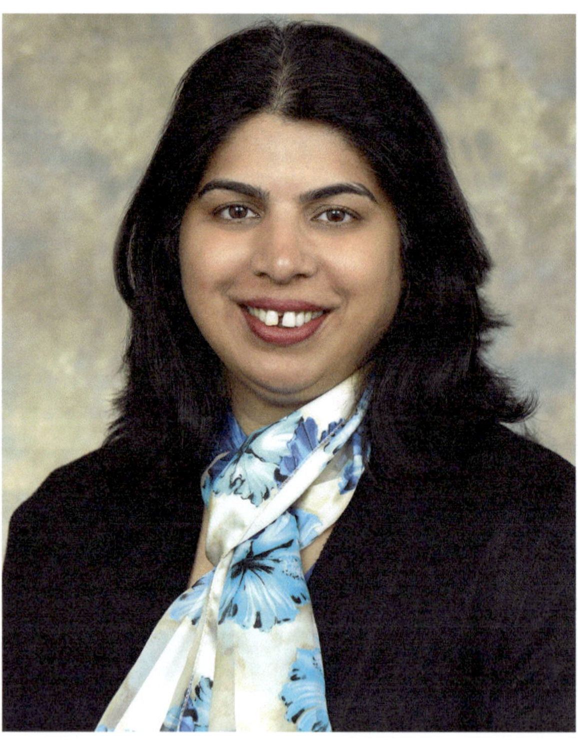

Birgit Ertl-Wagner, MD, PHD, MHBA
Birgit Ertl-Wagner (Fig. 26.36) is renowned for her leadership and contributions to Pediatric Neuroradiology. She is the Radiologist-in-Chief and Derek Harwood-Nash Chair in Medical Imaging at The Hospital for Sick Children (SickKids) in Toronto. She is a Senior Associate Scientist in the Neurosciences & Mental Health Program of the SickKids Research Institute and is a Professor in the Department of Medical Imaging at the University of Toronto. She is a pioneer in translational and imaging-based AI research, employing multiparametric imaging and methods of artificial intelligence/machine learning in research focused on imaging of pediatric brain tumors, neuroinflammatory and metabolic disorders, neurovascular imaging, and head & neck imaging. Dr. Ertl-Wagner is on the editorial board of several renowned scientific journals, including Radiology, AJNR, and Neuro-Oncology, and serves on multiple committees of national and international scientific radiological societies. She has received numerous awards for her research and teaching.

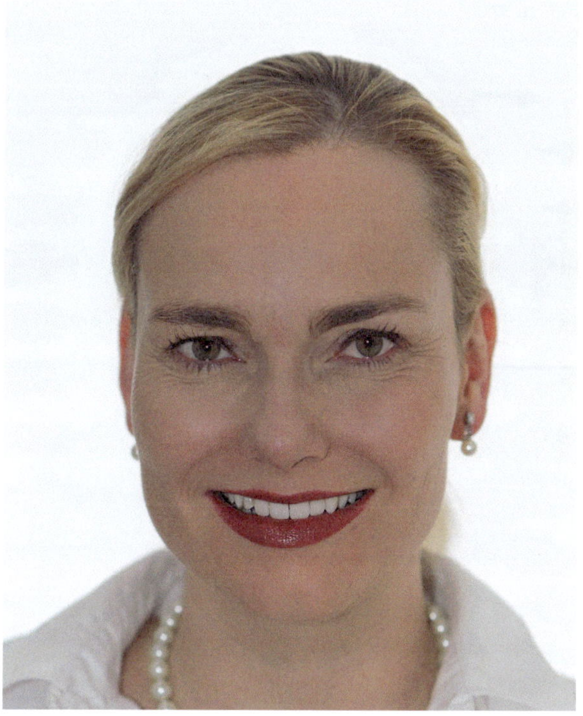

Fig. 26.36 Birgit Ertl-Wagner

Tammie L.S. Benzinger, MD, PhD

Tammie Benzinger (Fig. 26.37) is the Hugh Monroe Wilson Professor of Radiology and Neurological Surgery at Washington University School of Medicine and is the Medical Director for MRI at Mallinckrodt Institute of Radiology and Barnes-Jewish Hospital. Her laboratory has pioneered translational PET and MR imaging techniques to investigate biomarkers for Alzheimer's Disease. Her group serves as the imaging core for the Knight Alzheimer's Disease Research Center as well as for the Dominantly Inherited Alzheimer Network (DIAN) and its clinical trials unit, DIAN-TU. She is a Clarivate/Web of Science Highly Cited Researcher with over 23,000 citations. Dr. Benzinger co-chairs the RSNA Quantitative Imaging Committee and the ASNR Alzheimer's Disease, ARIA, and Dementia Study Group. She is a recipient of the ASNR Scholar Award, the ARRS Scholar Award, and the ASNR Women in Neuroradiology Leadership Award. She is a Fellow of the American Institute for Medical and Biological Engineering (AIMBE), a Fellow of the AAWR, and a Distinguished Investigator of the Academy for Radiology and Biomedical Imaging Research.

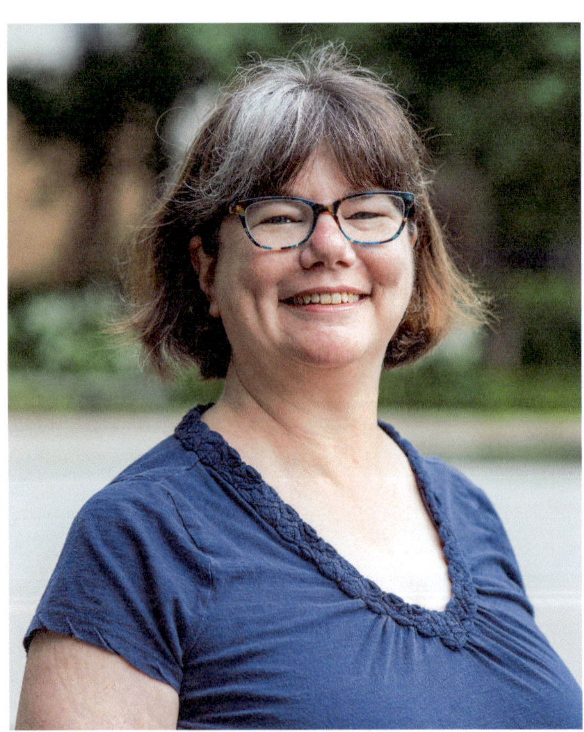

Fig. 26.37 Tammie Benzinger

Soonmee Cha, MD

Dr. Soonmee Cha (Fig. 26.38) is a Professor of Radiology, Vice Chair of Education, and Radiology Residency Program Director at the University of California, San Francisco. She has performed pioneering NIH-funded research in the application of perfusion MR imaging in glioma grading, classification, differentiation between tumor and treatment effect, and surgical planning, and in the evaluation of CNS lymphomas. She has also played a vital role in advancing radiology education internationally and fostering future clinician educators. In her words, she has "championed patient care focused radiology with hands-on clinical training while providing access to a cutting-edge research environment." She is proud that her trainees have gone on to build strong professional reputations, developing innovative radiology training curricula and setting practice standards. Dr. Cha has received numerous research, teaching, and clinical excellence awards and is a highly sought-after national and international speaker.

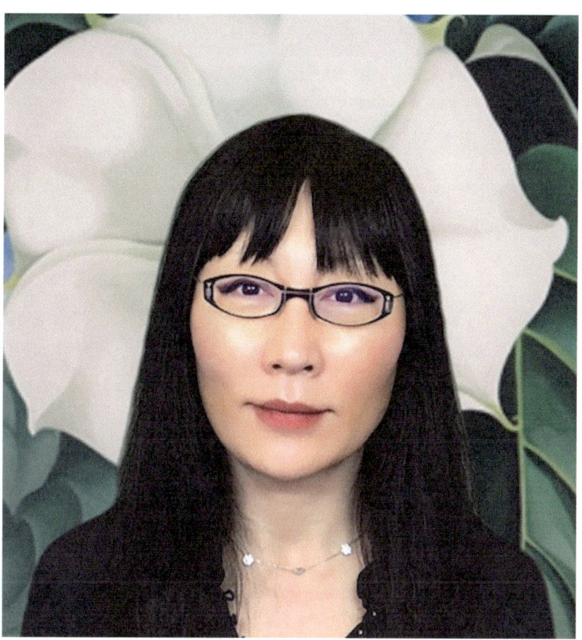

Fig. 26.38 Soonme Cha

Ellen Grant, MD

Ellen Grant (Fig. 26.39) is the Käthe Beutler, MD, Harvard Professor of Pediatrics and Professor of Radiology. She is the Director of Faculty Affairs in Radiology and Director of Research for the Fetal Care and Surgery Center at Boston Children's Hospital (BCH). At BCH, she founded the Fetal Neuroimaging and Developmental Science Center (FNNDSC) to develop tools to better detect and understand fetal and neonatal brain physiology and pathology, now including 15 faculty and raising over $85M in funding. She is a pioneer of neonatal frequency domain near infrared spectroscopy (FDNIRS) combined with diffuse correlation spectroscopy (DCS), the latter of which provides quantitative bedside measures of cerebral blood flow and oxygen consumption. More recently, she has been leading projects that combine artificial intelligence on images and electronic health care records to predict outcomes of neonatal hypoxic-ischemic encephalopathy. Dr. Grant is a Senior Fellow of the ISMRM, received the ASNR Outstanding Contributions in Research Award in 2021, and received the ASPNR Gold Medal Award in 2022.

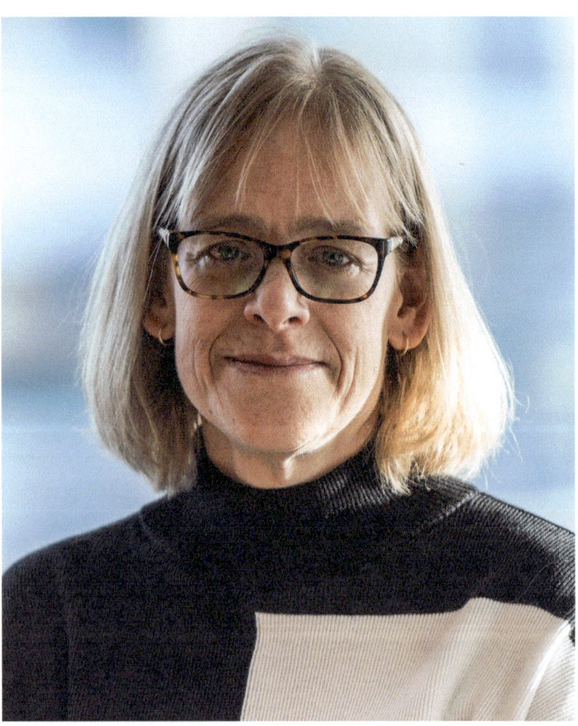

Fig. 26.39 Ellen Grant

Conclusion

In the last 30 years, women Neuroradiologists in North America have made extraordinary strides in the areas of leadership, research, education, clinical innovation, global health, and diversity, equity and inclusion. They have increasingly become presidents of societies, deans, department chairs, vice chairs across multiple domains, and neuroradiology division chiefs. They have increasingly secured grant funding and performed ground-breaking research. They have been more widely recognized for their innovative clinical and education programs, and are at the forefront of global outreach and health equity initiatives. Nevertheless, there is more progress to be made. For example, in 2018, Ahmadi et al. demonstrated that 87.5% of leadership positions within academic neuroradiology in the United States and Canada are held by men [1]. Furthermore, Nguyen et al. showed that for 155 international neurology-related journals, neuroradiology had the largest gender disparity in authorship compared with neurology and neurology-related subspecialties, and the percentage of women authors was significantly lower than the percentage of women in their respective fields [2]. Meltzer et al. showed that although women are receiving more grants and other awards from ASNR, the rates still lag behind the proportion of female applicants [3]. Also, there has never been a female editor in chief of the AJNR. It is imperative that all neuroradiologists continue to support and enhance leadership and career development courses for women, more robust mentorship and sponsorship programs for women, grant support for women, Women in Radiology Committees, and diversity in our Neuroradiology workforce. The amazing women highlighted in this chapter and our supportive male colleagues are paving the way to make this happen.

References

1. Ahmadi M, Khurshid K, Sanelli PC, et al. Influences for gender disparity in academic neuroradiology. AJNR Am J Neuroradiol. 2018;39:18–23. https://doi.org/10.3174/ajnr.A5443.
2. Nguyen AX, Yoffe L, Li A, et al. Gender gap in neurology research authorship (1946–2020). Front Neurol. 2021;12:715428. https://doi.org/10.3389/fneur.2021.715428.
3. Meltzer CC, Sanelli PC, Hepp MB, et al. Women rising to the top: the tipping point for the ASNR. AJNR Am J Neuroradiol. 2019;40:2–4. https://doi.org/10.3174/ajnr.A5893.

Correction to: A World History of Neuroradiology

Daniel Birchall

Correction to:
D. Birchall (ed.), *A World History of Neuroradiology*, https://doi.org/10.1007/978-3-032-16653-1

The original version of the book had been published with errors in Acknowledgments section, Part opener, and Chapters 1, 22, 24, and 25. The errors have been corrected as listed below.

Acknowledgments, Page xi: The name "Karen Lyn" was corrected to "Karen Lyp."

Part II, Women in Neuroradiology, Introduction: A signature was omitted in the original version and has now been added at the end of the matter after the sentence, "With fraternal greetings."

Maria de Fátima Viana Vasco Aragão, MD, PhD Radiologist and Neuroradiologist Recife, Pernambuco, Brazil; Member-at-Large, WFNRS

Chapter 1, Page 22: The year "2026" was corrected to "2030" in the section "2026—The XXIVth SNR—Sapporo—Prof. Kohsuke Kudo and Prof. Minako Azuma."

Chapter 17, Page 185, last paragraph: The name "Thandi Buthelezi" was omitted from the list of SANIS members and has now been added.

Chapter 22, Pages 242-245: The figure references for the following authors were incorrectly assigned and were corrected as follows:

Gopolang Mndebele (Fig. 22.12 → Fig. 22.14)
Thandi Buthelezi (Fig. 22.13 → Fig. 22.12)
Boitumelo Khoza(Fig. 22.14 → Fig. 22.13)

The updated version of this book can be found at
https://doi.org/10.1007/978-3-032-16653-1

D. Birchall (ed.), *A World History of Neuroradiology*,
https://doi.org/10.1007/978-3-032-16653-1_27

Page 238 (Kenya section): The sentence has been corrected to read "dates back to 1967" instead of "dates to 1967."

In the same section, sixth paragraph: "dir. Wangari Maina" has been corrected to "Dr. Wangari Maina."

Chapter 24, Pages 400 and 402: Images of the following authors were missing and have now been added at the appropriate locations:

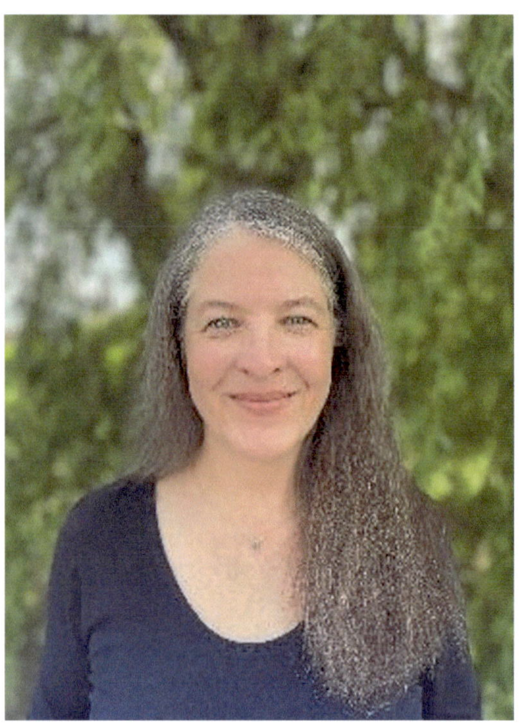

Dr. Isabella Björkman-Burtscher (Page 399)

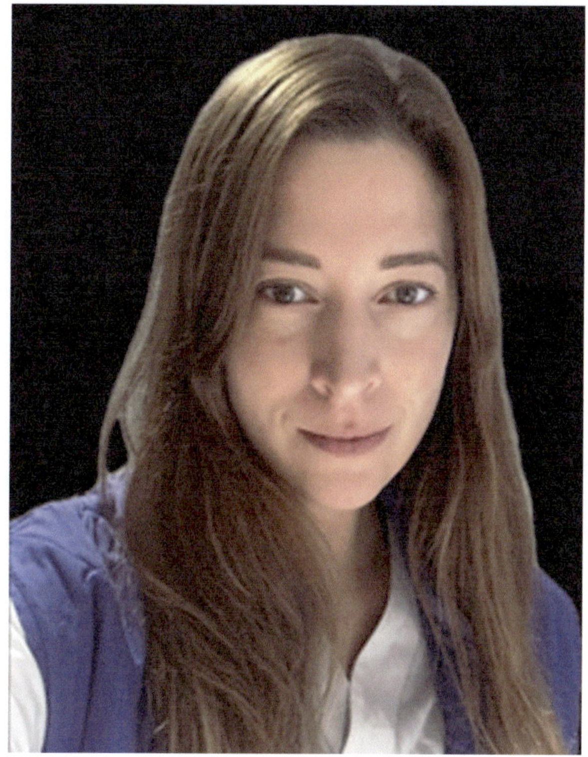

Dr. Anna Falk Delgado (Page 401)

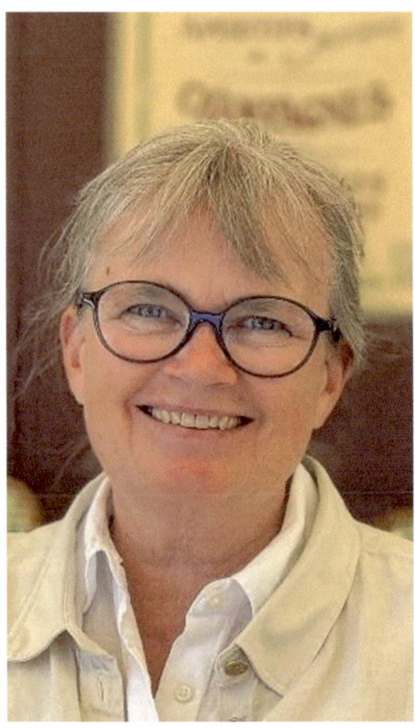

Dr. Birgitta Ramgren (Page 402)

Chapter 25, Page 423: An image of Dr. Fabiane Lorenzoni Sesti has been added to her biography.

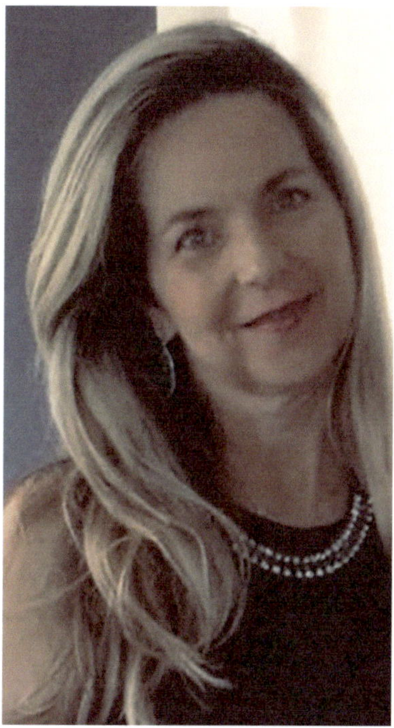

Dr. *Fabiane Lorenzoni Sesti*

Epilogue of the Book

History is the chronicle of past events in human affairs. It encompasses insights into how humans have evolved over time and how past events shape present and future developments. History ranges from local to global contexts and involves exploring various aspects of human experience. We believe that everyone, whether they are professionals or not, should honestly and thoroughly document and take responsibility for recording the paths they have traveled.

Since 1990, the field of neuroradiology has seen significant evolution. The World Federation of Neuroradiological Societies (WFNRS) is committed to publishing a book that highlights many of these developments in neuroradiology over the past three decades. From the moment we began conceptualizing and planning to publish this book, we held the belief that history should belong to everyone, not be the exclusive domain of a few. Therefore, we published this book using an open-source approach and entirely in a digital format, with the hope that people from various fields will make good use of its valuable content. However, we also ask that those who reference the book help by acknowledging the source and citation properly.

We acknowledge the contributions of the Member Societies/Associations/Federations of WFNRS for providing the materials that make this book rich in content. It would be impossible to gather such a wealth of information and data from around the world without the efforts of each individual WFNRS Member. A notable highlight of the book is the section on the "History of Women in Neuroradiology," which owes its realization to the enthusiasm and dedication of Professor Maria de Fátima Aragao. We would also like to express our sincere gratitude to Springer Nature, our publishing partner, for their professional guidance and support throughout the project. We greatly appreciate the administrative assistance provided by Ms. Karen Lyp from the WFNRS Chicago Central Office and Ms. Hui-Yun Chen from the WFNRS Taiwan Office. Finally, special recognition and appreciation go to Professor Daniel Birchall, WFNRS Vice-President and the Book's Editor. His brotherly support and encouragement were key in guiding me through the many challenges involved in bringing this book to fruition.

D. Birchall (ed.), *A World History of Neuroradiology*,
https://doi.org/10.1007/978-3-032-16653-1

Last but not least, this book would not have been possible to publish without the generous support provided by the Memorial Foundation of Mr. Ching-The Hsu (許金德紀念基金會). We appreciate the Medical Scholarship Foundation in Memory of Professor Albert Ly-Young Shen (財團法人沈力揚教授醫學教育獎學紀念基金會) and the Vivian W. Yen Neurological Foundation (財團法人吳舜文神經科學發展基金會) for their full assistance in the process of book publication. We are proud to announce that the book, titled "A World History of Neuroradiology: 1990 to the Present Day," is now published.

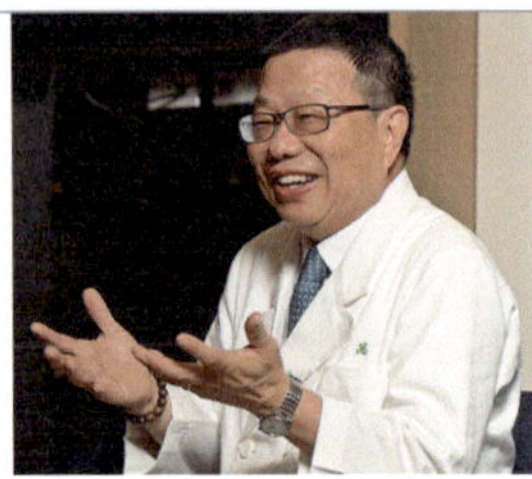

Wan-Yuo, Guo, MD. PhD,
President, WFNRS (2022–2026)
March 2026, China Medical University, Taichung, Taiwan

Index

A

Aboagye, Rosemond N.D., 237
Africa, women in neuroradiology in, 229
  diagnostic neuroradiology, 246, 248, 249
  interventional neuroradiology, 244, 245
  paediatric neuroradiology, 242, 243
  Tanzania, 249–251
  Uganda, 252–254
  Zambia, 257–259
Ahn, Sung Soo, 322
Aida, Noriko, 290
Alkan, Ozlem, 415
Alzheimer's disease (AD), 274, 294
Amemiya, Shiori, 305
American Board of Radiology, 30
American Certificate of Added Qualification (CAQ), 92
American College of Radiology (ACR), 30
American Journal of Neuroradiology (AJNR), 10, 134
American Roentgen Ray Association (ARRS), 437
American Society of Head and Neck Radiology (ASHNR), 139
American Society of Neuroradiology (ASNR), 29, 30, 62, 422, 456–462, 464–466
  ASNR Research Committee, 42, 43
  constitution, evolution of, 38–40
  education/training, 31
    annual meeting, 31, 32
    digital presence and social media, 34
    publications, 33
    standards, guidelines and curriculum development, 34
  executive leadership, 35
  foundation of, 41, 42
  governance
    committee structure, 37, 38
    executive committee, 36, 37
    physician leadership, 36
  International Outreach Program, 186
  policy and procedure manual, 40
  practice/advocacy, 30, 31
  research, 40, 41
  strategic goals and initiatives, 30
American Society of Paediatric Neuroradiology educational scholarship (ASPNR), 259, 476–481
Ames, Romy, 430
Andica, Christina, 283
Ando, Kumiko, 286
Annual Business Meeting (ABM), 93
Annual Meeting, 31, 32
Annual Scientific Meeting (ASM), 63
Anzai, Yoshimi, 466
Anzalone, Nicoletta, 375, 376
APTw imaging, 221
Aragao, Maria de Fátima Viana Vasco, 421
Argentina, neuroradiology in, 434–438
Argentinian Society of Radiology (SAR), 437
Artificial intelligence (AI), 21, 139, 332
ASEAN Oceanian Congress of Radiology, 331
Asian and Oceanian Society of Neuroradiology, 206

D. Birchall (ed.), *The World History of Neuroradiology*,
https://doi.org/10.1007/978-3-032-16653-1

Asian and Oceanian Society of Neuroradiology and Head & Neck Radiology (AOSNHNR), 49, 348
  Asian-Oceanian context, challenges in
    financial viability and secretariat, 58
    local disease patterns and healthcare systems, 58
    working together, 58, 59
  founding of, 49, 50
    1st Congress & XV symposium neuroradiologicum, 50, 51
    2nd Congress, 51
    3rd Congress, 51
    4th Congress, 51
    5th Congress, 52
    6th Congress, 52, 53
    7th Congress, 53
    8th Congress, 53
    9th Congress, 54
    10th Congress, 54
    11th Congress, 54, 55
    12th Congress and XXI symposium neuroradiologicum, 55
    13th Congress, 55
    14th Congress, 56
  future and challenges facing neuroradiology and
    artificial intelligence and technical advances, 57
    information overload, 57
  story of, 56
Asian Oceanian Congress of Neuroradiology (AOCNR), 138, 139, 273
Asia Oceania, neuroradiology in, 265, 266
Asian-Australasian Federation of Interventional and Therapeutic Neuroradiology (AAFITN), 199
Asian-Oceanian Congress of Neuroradiology and Head & Neck Radiology (AOCNHNR), 67, 137, 197
Associazione Italiana di Neuroradiologia (AINR), 117
A*STAR Institute for Human Development and Potential (A*STAR IHDP), 339
Audience Response System, 32
Australasian interventional neuroradiologists, 68
Australia, neuroradiology and neurointervention in, 267–272
Australia and New Zealand Association of Neurologists (ANZAN), 65
Australian and New Zealand Society of Neuroradiology (ANZSNR), 62
  committee of, 62, 64
  current status, 68
  publications, 68, 69
  society presidents, 66–68
  training, 65, 66
Australian medical association (AMA), 66
Australian medical council (AMC), 67
Austrian society of neuroradiology, 71, 72
  academia, 77
  annual meetings, 73, 75
  list of annual meetings, 74–75
  list of honorary members, 73
  list of presidents, 72
  neuroradiology, current situation of, 76
  organization, 72, 73
  training, 76
Azambuja, Néstor, 12, 13
Azuma, Minako, 22–23, 312

B

Badu-Peprah, Augustina, 235
Bae, Yun Jung, 322
Baral, Akriti, 333, 334
Bargalló, Núria, 391
Belgium, 358–360
Bello, Jacquelline A, 461
Benzinger, Tammie L.S., 492
Berner, Silvia, 436
Bertolotti, Mario, 374
Besada, Cristina, 436
Bhargava, Sneh, 285
Bhoopat, Wiyada, 349, 350
Bison, Brigitte, 371
Björkman-Burtscher, Isabella, 399
Bladowska, Joanna, 384
Blaser, Susan, 480
Blood oxygen level-dependent (BOLD) fMRI, 305
Blystad, Ida, 400
Bosnia, neuroradiology, 362–365
Brain death, 12
Brandão, Lara, 426
Braun, Jean-Paul, 72
Brazilian college of radiology (CBR), 425, 427
Brazilian society of diagnostic and therapeutic neuroradiology (SBNRDT), 82, 87
  advancements and collaborations, 87, 88
  COVID-19, period of, 83, 84
  history, 82, 83
  International Symposium of Neuroradiology, 85

Interventional Neuroradiology simulation, 85
interventional neuroradiology, challenges for, 88, 89
Lasjaunias, Pierre, 86, 87
partnership with institutions, 85, 86
simulator-based learning with remote online teaching, 85
Brazilian society of neuroradiology (SBNR), 80–82, 422
Brazil, neuroradiology in, 420–428
British neuroradiology/British society of neuroradiologist (BSNR), 91
1990s, 92, 93
academic subcommittee, 94
BSNR Constitution, 96
2000 onwards, 93, 94
standards subcommittee, 94
TESC, 95
Bull, James William Douglas, 8, 9
Bunnag, Tawan Surawongse, 347
Buthelezi, Thandi, 244

C
Caballo, María Rosario Barrena, 392
Cabrera, María Elizabeth Morón, 430
Cala, Lesley, 270
California Institute for Regenerative Medicine (CIRM), 458
Candy, Sally, 246
Cape Universities Body Imaging Centre (CUBIC), 186
Carpio-O'Donovan, Raquel del, 487
Casares, Katiuzka, 442
Castillo, Mauricio, 21, 22
Catholic University of Rio Grande do Sul (RGS), 422
Cejas, Claudia, 437
Central ventriculography, 13
Centro Hospitalar Universitário de Lisboa Norte, 152
Ceratto, Rosana, 438
Cerebral aneurysm, 149
Cerebral angiography, 63
Cerebral blood flow, 17
Certificate of Added Qualification (CAQ), 92
Cervical spine, 9
Chadrycki, Edla, 421
Charcot-Marie-Tooth disease, 332
Chawalparit, Orasa, 350, 351
Chen, Hung-Chieh, 344
Chen, Ya-Fang, 344
Child-care, 261
Chile, neuroradiology in, 443
China, neuroradiology and neurointervention in, 272–282
Chiro, Giovanni Di, 14
Choi, Hye Young, 315
Choi, Yoon Sung, 325
Chong, Vincent, 336
Churojana, Anchalee, 346
Cila, Aysenur, 413
Clinical Practice Committee (CPC), 30
Cognitive neuroscience, 305
Coimbra Hospital Centre (CHC), 150
College of Radiology Annual Scientific Meetings, 331
Colleges of Medicine of South Africa (CMSA), 248
Colombia, neuroradiology in, 432–434
Committee structure, ASNR, 37, 38
Comparative Effectiveness Research Training (CERT) program, 462
Competency matrix, 82
Competency-based curriculum, 82
Competency-based medical education (CBME), 82
Computed tomography (CT), 15, 61, 143, 144, 216, 288, 376
Conjoint Committee for Recognition of Training in INR (CCINR), 66
CONNECTA BRASIL, 84
Consortium for Advancement of MRI Education and Research in Africa (CAMERA), 262
Constitution, ASNR, 38–40
Consumer price index (CPI), 67
Continuing Medical Education (CME), 33
Corticobasal degeneration (CBD), 295
Costa Rica, neuroradiology in, 434
Course in Diagnostic and Interventional Neuroradiology, 102
COVID-19, 83–85, 118, 138, 337
Craniocervical junction, 9
Croatia, 97, 365–367, 369
Croatian Neuroradiological Congress, 102
Croatian Neuroradiological Society, 98–100, 104, 367
Croatian neuroradiology, 100
Croatian Society of Radiology (CSR), 98, 366
CSNR, 467–468
Current Procedural Terminology Editorial Panel (CPT), 31
Curriculum standardization, 88
Cyprus, 217

D

Da Cunha, Barbara Castellano, 441
Danish Society for Medical Magnetic Resonance (DSMMR), 396
Daoying, Geng, 273
de Lima Petribu, Natacha Calheiros, 428
de Pardal, Maria Luisa Morete, 435
de Siqueira Campos, Christiane Monteiro, 425
de Villiers, Laetitia, 267
Delavelle, Jacqueline, 405
Delgado, Anna Falk, 401
Dementia with grains (DG), 294
Denktaş, Hayrünnisa, 413
des Plantes, Bernard George Ziedses, 6–7
Desmond, Tricia, 271
DGNR, 372
Diagnostic and interventional neuroradiology, 72
Diagnostic neuroradiology
  paediatric neuroradiology, 181
  South Africa, 176–180
Diagnostic Neuroradiology Forum (DNF), 92
Diaz, Gloria Efigenia, 434, 438
Digital subtraction angiography (DSA), 149, 205
Domain Specific Review Board (DSRB), 339
Dominican Republic, neuroradiology in, 446
Dorn, Franziska, 372
Dresdner Neurovascular Centre (DNVC), 374
du Boulay, Edward Philip George Houssemayne, 16
Dutch Society for Neuroradiology (DSNR), 407
Dzefi-Tettey, Klenam, 234

E

East-Saxonian Neurovascular Network (SOS-NET), 374
Education, SSNR, 216
Egypt, women in neuroradiology in, 229–231
Electronic Learning Center, 32
Emergency Clinical Radiology Symposia, 102
Endovascular treatment for stroke (EVAS), 402
Enokizono, Mikako, 306, 307
Entrustable professional activities (EPAs), 82
Epilepsia Chirurgic Unit, 441
Epilepsy, 309
ERANET, 386
Erasmus Course on Magnetic Resonance Imaging (EMRI), 360
Ernemann, Ulrike, 371
Ertl-Wagner, Birgit, 491
Essential Skills in Medical Education (ESME), 340
Ethiopia, neuroradiology in, 232, 233
Eurocentric, 23
European Board of Neuroradiology (EBNR), 402
European Congress of Radiology (ECR), 399
European Course of Head and Neck Radiology (EDiHNNR), 363
European Course of Neuroradiology (ECNR), 217, 360
European Course of Neuroradiology (EDiNR), 363
European Diploma in Interventional Neuroradiology (EDiINR), 363, 402
European Diploma in Neuroradiology (EdiNR), 104, 217, 363, 364, 425, 427
European Society, 216
European Society of Head and Neck Radiology (ESHNR), 139
European Society of Magnetic Resonance Imaging (ESMRMB), 331, 396
European Society of Minimal Invasive Neurological Therapy (ESMINT), 371
European Society of Neuroradiology (ESNR), 62, 139, 144, 248, 360, 375, 398, 402, 415
European Society of Pediatric Oncology (SIOP-E), 370
Executive committee, ASNR, 36, 37

F

Federal Department of Health Australia (DOHA), 64
Federal University of Rio De Janeiro (UFRJ), 426
Fei-Yun Wu, 278
Fellowship of the Royal College of Radiologists (FRCR), 93
Feng, Chen, 277
Feng, Feng, 274
Fetal Neuroimaging and Developmental Science Center (FNNDSC), 494
Figueroa, Jeaneth Bu, 442
Figueroa, Virginia, 442
Fischbein, Nancy, 472
Fischgold, Hermann, 11
Foreign Honorary Members, 129
Foundation of the ASNR (FASNR), 41, 42

French period, 81
Frequency domain near infrared spectroscopy (FDNIRS), 494
Fun, Fan Yoke, 336

G
Garbugino, Silvia, 438
Gbadamosi, Hafisatu, 236
General Medical Council (GMC), 95
Geographic distribution, 88
Germany
  neuroradiology, 370–374
    certification, 109
    organizational structures, 110
    statistics, 107
    stroke treatment, 108
    Young Neuroradiology-Junge Neuroradiologie, 110
Ghana, neuroradiology in, 233, 234, 236–238
Ghana College of Physicians & Surgeons (GCPS), 234
Gibbs, Wende, 485
Gizewski, Elke, 372
Glastonbury, Christine M., 474
Gomyo, Miho, 303
Grant, Ellen, 494
Greitz, Torgny, 15
Gugliemi detachable coil (GDC), 64
Guo, Wan-Yuo, 20, 21

H
Hacettepe University, 413
Hara, Shoko, 313, 314
Hattingen, Elke, 371
Hayashida, Yoshiko, 302
Head and neck radiology, 51, 206
Health Manpower Development Plan (HMDP), 342
Health Professions Council of South Africa (HPCSA), 174
Healthcare reform, 29
Herzegovina, neuroradiology, 362–364
Hewlett, Richard, 177
Highly specialized medicine (HSM), 195
Hilal, Sadek Kamel, 17
Honduras, neuroradiology in, 442
Hospital Departments of Neuroradiology, 118, 119
Hospital Geral of Fortaleza (HGF), 86
Hrvatsko neuroradiološko društvo (HNRD), 101, 102
Hunter, Jill V., 476
Hwee, Tang Phua, 340

I
Idun, Ewurama Andam, 235
Imaging diagnostic service, 423
India
  neuroradiologists in, 285
  women, in neuroradiology in, 302, 314
Indonesia women, in neuroradiology in, 282–284
Instituto Nacional de Ciencias Neurologicas (INCN), 431
Instituto Nacional de Enfermedades Neoplasicas (INEN), 430
International Fellowship programmes, 248
International Outreach, 39
International Outreach Professor Program, 262
The Intervention Register of the German Society for Interventional Radiology (DeGIR), 108
International Society for Magnetic Resonance in Medicine (ISMRM), 263, 273, 276, 337, 398, 399
The International Subarachnoid Aneurysm Trial (ISAT), 93
International Symposium of Neuroradiology, 85
Interventional neuroradiology (INR), 75, 206
  Africa, 244–245
  simulation, 85
Interventional radiology (IR), 255
Ischemic stroke, 108
Israeli, 113
Italian Association of Neuroradiology (AINR), 375
Italian neuroradiology, 115
  academic positions, teaching and research, 119, 120
  congresses and courses, 120
  future, 121, 122
  international relationships, 120
  lost colleagues 1990–2023, 121
  neuroradiologists abroad, 120, 121
Italian Society of Medical and Interventional Radiology (SIRM), 375
Italy, neuroradiology, 374, 375, 377, 378

J
Jacobs, Kathleen, 247
Japan, women, in neuroradiology in, 286–314

Japanese Society of Neuroradiology (JSNR), 127, 312
- Fiftieth Anniversary Commemorative Events, 128
- Foreign Honorary Members, 129
- future prospects, 130
- Kato Prize, 129
- leadership, 127
- legal status, 128
- logo, 130
- membership composition, 127
- official journal, 130
- SNR, 129
- standing committees, 128
- website, 129

Jefić, Svjetlana, 363
Jensen, Mary E., 486
Johnson, Michele H., 483
Joshi, Varsha, 285
Jung, Lyung, 315
Jung, So Lyung, 316

K

Kanchanathiti, Preeya, 349
Kang, Koung Mi, 322
Karlović-Vidaković, Marijana, 362
Kasirye-Mbugua, Napo, 248
Kato Prize, 129
Kennedy, Tabassum, 489
Kenya, neuroradiology in, 238, 239
Khoza, Boitumelo, 245
Kikuta, Junko, 309, 310
Kim, Hyun Jung, 319
Kim, Hyun-Sook, 315
Kim, Jinna, 317
Kitajima, Mika, 301, 302
Korean Board of Radiology, 135
Korean Society of Neuroradiology (KSNR), 132, 314
- Annual Academic Conference and General Assembly, 138
- AOCNR, 139
- logo, 136
- period of birth, 132–134
- period of diversity, 137–140
- period of dynamicity, 135–137
- period of growth, 134, 135
- roster of, 133

Korea, women, in neuroradiology in, 314
- current leaders, 316, 317, 319
- futures, 319, 325
- gradual change, 315
- persistent problems, 327

Korle Bu Teaching Hospital (KBTH), 234, 235
Kudo, Kohsuke, 22, 23
Kumar, Sumeet, 337
Kurihara, Noriko, 297
Kwikima, Ugumba Mussa, 250
Kyoto University, 291

L

Lambart, Lena, 259
Laothamatas, Jiraporn, 346
Larsson, Elna-Marie, 396
Lasjaunias, Pierre, 86–87
Latin America, neuroradiology in, 425
Lee, Eun Ja, 319
Lee, Jeong Hyun, 315, 317
Lee, Young Hen, 317
Leiden University Medical Center (LUMC), 338
Leite, Claudia Costa, 424
Leonardi, Marco, 19, 20, 117
Liauw, Lishya, 338
Lim, Soo Mee, 319
Lim, Tchoyoson, 341
Lima, Alessandra Mertens Brainer, 427
Lin, Chao-Chun, 344
Lindgren, Erik, 7–8
Ling, Chan Ling, 334, 335
Linn, Jennifer, 373
Loevner, Laurie A., 460
Logo, 130
Lohani, Benu Wagle, 333
Lopez, Rosanna Meza, 439
Lui, Yvonne W., 465
Lu, Jie, 276

M

Magnetic resonance imaging (MRI), 14, 21, 22, 61, 143, 144, 360, 376, 386, 426
Magnetic resonance imaging workshop, 176
Mallorca, 217
Malwadde, Elsie Kiguli, 253
Maric, Daliborka, 363
McRae, Donald Lane, 9
Medical Research Council, 176
Medical School in the National University of Singapore, 336
Megret, Marcelle, 404
Meltzer, Carolyn C., 458
Merhemic, Zulejha, 364

Metropolitan Emergency Units in Porto and Lisbon, 153
Mexico, neuroradiology in, 441, 442
Mezue, Phyllis, 241
Michel, Michelle, 470
Microcephaly Epidemic Research Group (MERG), 427
Ministry of Health of the Republic of Croatia, 367
Mndebele, Gopolang, 243
Moon, Won-Jin, 315, 317
Moreno, Thalía, 441
Morimoto, Emiko, 307, 309
Mosier, Kristine, 473
Moyamoya disease, 344
Mulopwe, Juliet, 261
Multidisciplinary case-based reviews, 32
Multidisciplinary interaction, 59
Multislice CT machines, 340
Myelin Oligodendrocyte Glycoprotein Antibody associated Disease (MOGAD), 248

N

Nabawanuka, Eva, 256
Nabbosa, Valeria, 255
Nassanga, Rita, 254
National Board of Medical specialties (NBMS), 333
National Center of Neurology and Psychiatry (NCNP), 292
National Congress, 117, 118
National health care development, 220
National Magnetic Resonance Research Center, 415
National Medical Research Council (NMRC), 339
National Neuroscience Institute (NNI), 337
National Taiwan University College of Medicine, 344
Nepal women, in neuroradiology in, 333, 334
Nepal Radiologists' Association (NRA), 333
Netherlands, neuroradiology, 406–410, 412
Neuroanatomy, 341
Neurofibrillary tangle disease (NFTD), 294
Neurographics, 33
Neuroimaging Professional Committee, 275
Neuro-intervention
  in Australia, 267–270
  South Africa, 182–187
Neuro-IR practice, 183
Neuroradiological Society of Taiwan, 197, 198
  achievements, 198
  Asian-Australasian Federation of Interventional and Therapeutic Neuroradiology, 199
  milestones of, 198, 199
  XXIst SNR, 199, 200
Neuroradiology, 57, 58, 80, 113
  in Africa, 229
    diagnostic neuroradiology, 246, 248, 249
    interventional neuroradiology, 244, 245
    paediatric neuroradiology, 242, 243
    Tanzania, 249–251
    Uganda, 252–254
    Zambia, 257–259
  in Argentina, 434–438
  Asia Oceania, 265, 266
  Australia, 267–272
  in Brazil, 420–428
  Belgium, 358–360
  Bosnia and Herzegovina, 362–365
  in Chile, 443
  China, 272–282
  in Colombia, 432–434
  in Costa Rica, 434
  Croatia, 365–367, 369
  current situation of, 76
  in Dominican Republic, 446
  in Egypt, 229–231
  in Ethiopia, 232, 233
  Germany, 370–374
    certification, 109
    organizational structures, 110
    statistics, 107
    stroke treatment, 108
    Young Neuroradiology-Junge Neuroradiologie, 110
  in Ghana, 233, 234, 236–238
  history of, 97–99, 101, 103, 116, 117
  in Honduras, 442
  India, 285, 302, 314
  Indonesia, women in, 282–284
  in Italy, 374, 375, 377, 378
  in Kenya, 238, 239
  in Latin America, 425
  Japan, women in, 286–314
  Korea, women in, 314
    current leaders, 316, 317, 319
    futures, 319, 325
    gradual change, 315
    persistent problems, 327
  in Mexico, 441, 442
  Nepal, women in, 333, 334

Neuroradiology (*cont.*)
  Netherlands, 406–410, 412
  in Nigeria, 240
  in North America, 452
    ASFNR, 475
    ASHNR, 468–470, 473, 474
    ASNR, 456–466
    ASPNR, 476, 478–480
    ASSR, 481, 482, 484, 485
    CSNR, 467
    diversity, equity and inclusion and global outreach, 455
    education, 455
    functional neuroimaging and artificial intelligence, 454
    head and neck radiology, 453
    health services research, 454
    interventional neuroradiology, 454
    leadership, 452, 453
    luminaries, 487, 490–494
    pediatric neuroradiology, 453
    SNIS, 486
    spine imaging and intervention, 454
  in Paraguay, 439–441
  in Peru, 429–431
  Poland, 378, 379, 381–384
  Portuguese, 147–150, 152, 155, 156
  Singapore, women in, 334–343
  in Somalia, 241
  in South Africa, 174, 175, 241, 242
    diagnostic neuroradiology, 176–180
    early years, 175, 176
    neuro-intervention, 182–187
    paediatric neuroradiology, 181, 182
  Southeast Asia, women in, 327–333
  South Korea, 131, 132
  Spanish
    medicine and radiology, history of, 387
    prominent female, 388, 390–392
    role of women, 387, 388
  subspecialization, 97
  in Sweden, 394, 396–398, 400–403
  Switzerland, 404–406
  Taiwan, women in, 343–345
  Thailand, women in, 345–350, 352, 353
  Turkey, 413
  in Türkiye, 203, 205–207, 210–213
  in Uruguay, 446
  world history of, 143–145
Neuroradiology Consultant in Emergency Medicine Center, 384
Neuroradiology Departments 2023, 119
Neuroradiology Unit, 152
Neuroscience Department at WL-ULS (HEM), 150
Neurosurgery, 13
Neurosurgical Society of Australasia (NSA), 65
NeuTex, 268
Nigeria, neuroradiology in, 240
Nordic Society of Neuroradiology (NSNR), 396
Noriko, Salamon, 299
North America
  neuroradiology, 452
    ASFNR, 475
    ASHNR, 468–470, 473, 474
    ASNR, 456–466
    ASPNR, 476, 478–480
    ASSR, 481, 482, 484, 485
    CSNR, 467
    diversity, equity and inclusion and global outreach, 455
    education, 455
    functional neuroimaging and artificial intelligence, 454
    head and neck radiology, 453
    health services research, 454
    interventional neuroradiology, 454
    leadership, 452, 453
    luminaries, 487, 490–494
    pediatric neuroradiology, 453
    SNIS, 486
    spine imaging and intervention, 454
North America and Neuroimaging Clinics (NIC), 426
Norway, 144
Nshimbi-Makaliki, Sarah, 262

O

O'Donovan, Raquel del Carpio, 429
Oculoplastic X-ray, 335
OECD, 219
Official journal, 130
Ojeda, Adriana, 437
Oleaga, Laura, 390
Olvera, Teresa, 441
Ono, Yuko, 288
Osborn, Anne G., 456, 457
Oslo University Hospital (OUS), 143
Ovalı, Gülgün Yılmaz, 415

P

Palasis, Susan, 478
Paraguay, neuroradiology in, 439–441
Park, Ji Eun, 325
Park, Mina, 325
Park, Sun Won, 315, 319

Parkinson's disease, 274
Patient-centered Ad Hoc Committee, 31
Pazos, Beatriz, 436
Peru, neuroradiology in, 429–431
Phiri, Ruth, 260
Photography Exhibition Competition, 200
Physician leadership, ASNR, 36
Picard, Luc, 18
Poland, neuroradiology, 378, 379, 381–384
Portuguese neuroradiology, 147–150, 152, 155, 156
Post, Judith Donovan, 481
Poussaint, Tina Young, 463
Precision BRAin COnnectivity Profiling of Learning Difficulties for future therapeutic strategy using network-targeted neurostimulation (BRACO-LD), 339
Prince Leopold Institute of Tropical Medicine (ITM), 6
Progressive supranuclear palsy (PSP), 294–295
Public-private partnerships, 187
PURE-Mind, 386

R
Rabadán, Alejandra Teresa, 435
Radiological Sciences Academic Clinical Programme (RADSc ACP), 337, 343
Radiological society of South Africa (RSSA), 175, 249
Radiology, 13, 19
Radiology Academy, 102
Rahmat, Kartini Binti, 331–333
Raininko, Raili, 394
Ramgren, Birgitta, 402
Ramli, Norlisah Mohd, 327–328, 330, 333
Ramos, Ana, 388
Rao, Vijay M., 469
RAPNO (Response Assessment in Pediatric Neuro-Oncology) committee, 370
Reference Centers for Interventional Neuroradiology, 153
Regional Committee for Latin America (RCLA), 422
Remote online teaching, 85
Reneman, L. (Liesbeth), 412
Republic of Croatia, 100
Research, ASNR, 40, 41
Residency Advisory Committee (RAC), 343
Rhyner, Patricia, 457
Ribbeck, Lourdes Simbron, 431
Robson, Caroline, 477
Robust library online, 84
Rodríguez, Aleyda, 432
Rose, Norzaini, 330, 331, 333
Royal Australian and New Zealand College of Radiology (RANZCR), 61
Royal Perth Hospital (RPH), 61
RSNA GLC, 250
Ruggiero, Giovanni, 9, 10

S
Saatci, Isil, 414
Sadato, Akiyo, 291
Sage, Michael R., 18, 19
Salamon, Noriko, 299
Saleem, Sahar, 230
Saleh, Amal, 233
Salvatico, Rosana, 438
SAMRC, 176
Sanelli, Pina, 462
SA society of Neuro-intervention (SANIS), 175
Sato, Noriko, 292
SBNRDT, 421
Schaefer, Pamela W., 459
Schüller, Arthur, 71
Schwartz, Erin Simon, 464
Sesti, Fabiane Lorenzoni, 422
Shah, Lubdha, 484
Shanxi Medical University (SXMU), 275
Shatzkes, Deborah R., 471
Shawa, Jane, 258
Shin, Na-Young, 322
SIG-CONNECTA Neuro, 84
SILAN III Annual Congress, 161
SILAN VI Annual Congress, 162
SILAN IX Annual Congress, 163
SILAN XIII Annual Congress, 164
SILAN XVIII Annual Congress, 165
SILAN XXII Annual Congress, 166
SILAN XXVII Annual Congress, 166
SILAN XXXI Annual Congress, 167
SILAN XXXII Annual Congress, 168
SILAN XXXIII Annual Congress, 169
SILAN Congresses, 153
SILAN-ENERI, 163
SILAN-Garrahan Pediatric Neuroradiology scholarship, 170
SILAN-HUFJD Interventional Neuroradiology program, 158, 170, 171
SILAN-HUGC, 163

SILAN-HUGC Interventional Neuroradiology Scholarship program, 170
SILAN-MCG, 161
SILAN-Oulton Neuroradiology program, 167
SILAN-Vall d'Hebrón Diagnostic Neuroradiology program, 165
SILAN-Zaragoza, 165
Silva, Patricia, 441
Silvera, V. Michelle, 479
Simulator-based learning, 85
Singapore, women, in neuroradiology in, 334–343
SingHealth Duke-NUS Radiological Science Academic Clinical Program, 340
Skåne University Hospital (SUS), 399
Smits, M. (Marion), 410
Smoker, Wendy R. K., 468
SNIS, 486–487
SNR XXIV, 129
Soares, Maria Lúcia, 420
Sociedad Ibero Latino Americana de Neurorradiología Diagnóstica y Terapéutica (SILAN) Society, 157
  establishment of, 158
  founding meeting of, 159
  logo, 158
  nonprofit organization, 159
  past presidents of, 159
  professional society, 160
  SILAN-ENERI, 163
  SILAN-Garrahan Pediatric Neuroradiology scholarship, 170
  SILAN-HUFJD Interventional Neuroradiology program, 170, 171
  SILAN-HUGC, 163
  SILAN-MCG, 161
  SILAN-Oulton Neuroradiology program, 167
  SILAN-Vall d'Hebrón Diagnostic Neuroradiology program, 165
  SILAN-Vall d'Hebrón Neurointerventional program, 167
  SILAN-Zaragoza, 165
Sociedade Brasileira de Neuroradiologia (SBNR), 425
Sociedade Paulista de Radiologia (SPR), 425
Society of British Neurological Surgeons (SBNS), 91
Söderqvist, Åsa Kuntze, 403
Somalia, neuroradiology in, 241
South Africa, neuroradiology in, 174, 175, 241, 242
  diagnostic neuroradiology, 176–180
  early years, 175, 176
  neuro-intervention, 182–187
  paediatric neuroradiology, 181, 182
South African Society of Neurological Imaging (SASNI), 175, 241
Southeast Asia, women, in neuroradiology in, 327–333
South Korea, neuroradiology in, 131, 132
Spanish, neuroradiology
  medicine and radiology, history of, 387
  prominent female, 388, 390–392
  role of women, 387, 388
Spanish Radiological Society (SERAM), 390
Spanish Society of Neurology (SEN), 387
Spanish Society of Neuroradiology (SENR), 387
Špero, Martina, 369
Stenvers, Hendrik W., 407
Stockholm School of Neuroradiology, 215
Sundgren, Maly, 398
Sunkutu-Sichizya, Veronica, 257
Suwanwela, Nitaya, 346–348
Sweden, neuroradiology, 394, 396–398, 400–403
Swedish Cardiopulmonary bioimage study (SCAPIS), 221
Swedish National Board of Health and Welfare, 219
Swedish Society of Medicine (SLS), 217
Swedish Society of Neuroradiology (SSNR), 215–221, 396, 399
Swedish Society of Radiology (SFMR), 217, 399
Swiss Neuro Radiology Institute (SNRI), 371
Swiss neuroradiology
  institutions and Cantons, neuroradiology in, 191–193
  and research, 194, 195
  Swiss Society for Neuroradiology, 189–191
  Swiss title in, 193, 194
Swiss Society for Neuroradiology (SGNR/SSNR), 189–191, 193, 194
Switzerland, neuroradiology, 404–406
Symposium neuroradiologicum (SNR), 3, 4, 129, 139
  bibliographic sources, acknowledgement of, 5
  Ist SNR, 5, 6
  IInd SNR, 6, 7
  IIIrd SNR, 7–9
  IVth SNR, 8–9
  Vth SNR, 9
  VIth SNR, 9, 10
  VIIth SNR, 10, 11
  VIIIth SNR, 11
  IXth SNR, 12

Xth SNR, 12, 13
XIth SNR, 13
XIIth SNR, 14
XIIIth SNR, 15
XIVth SNR, 16
XVth SNR, 16, 17
XVIth SNR, 17
XVIIth SNR, 18
XVIIIth SNR, 18, 19
XIXth SNR, 19, 20
XXth, 20
XXIst SNR, 20, 21
XXIInd SNR, 21, 22
XXIIIrd, 22
XXIVth SNR, 22, 23

T
Taiwan, women, in neuroradiology in, 343–345
Taiwan Neurological Society, 197
Takahashi, Chihiro, 300
Takahashi, Mutsumasa, 16, 17
Tamer, Ines del Valle, 438
Tampieri, Donatella, 467
Tanabe, Jody, 475
Tan, Ai Peng, 339
Tan, Judy, 339
Tanzania, neuroradiology, 249–251
Taveras, Juan Manuel, 10, 11, 435
Thailand, women, in neuroradiology in, 345–350, 352, 353
Thienpondt, Rudolph, 5–6
Ti, Joanna Pearly, 341
Tokumaru, Aya, 293
Tokyo Medical and Dental University (TMDU), 313
Toyoda, Keiko, 296
Training and Education Subcommittee (TESC), 95
Tramontini, Carolina, 433
Transcatheter thrombectomy, 144
Traumatic brain injury (TBI), 328
Turkey, neuroradiology, 413
Turkish neuroradiology, 206
Turkish Society of Neuroradiology (TSNR), 206, 207
Türkiye, neuroradiology in, 203, 205–207, 210–213

U
Uganda, 252–257
Ullevil Hospital University, 349
Ultrasonography, 338
Umino, Maki, 311
United Kingdom Neurointerventional Group (UKNG), 92
Universidad Nacional Mayor de San Marcos (UNMSM), 430
Universidad Peruana Los Andes (UPLA), 430
Universiti Kebangsaan Malaysia (UKM), 330
University Chairs, 118
University Hospital Centre Sestre milosrdnice (UHC), 98
University Hospital of Coimbra (HUC), 150
University of Cape Town (UCT), 175, 242
University of John Hopkins, 415
University of Southern California (USC), 401
University of the Witwatersrand (WITS), 242
University of Zagreb School of Medicine, 369
University Professors, 120
Uppsala University (UU), 401
Uruguay, neuroradiology in, 446
US policymakers, 29
Utomo, Andreani, 283

V
Vagal, Achala, 490
Valk, Jaap, 407
Van Cauter, Sofie, 361
van der Knaap, Marjo S., 407
Vargas, María Isabel, 405
Vernooij, M.W. (Meike), 409
von Einsiedel, Helga Gräfin, 370

W
Waa, Sheila, 239
Wai-Yung, Yu, 343
Wanke, Isabel, 371
Warmuth-Metz, Monika, 370
Watanabe, Alyssa, 482
Wei, Kheok Si, 336
Weldehawariat, Tequam Debebe, 232
Wende, Sigurd, 13
West African College of Surgeons (WACS), 234
WFNRS project, 24, 25, 174
Wiberg, Maria Kristoffersen, 397
Wickbom, Ingmar, 12
Woldenberg, Rona, 488
Wong, Jocelyn, 341
World Federation of Interventional and Therapeutic Neuroradiology (WFITN), 217
World Federation of Neuroradiological Societies (WFNRS), 49, 138, 144, 206, 217, 398, 422

World Live Neurovascular Conference (WLNC, 414
Wu, Hsiu-Mei, 343

X
Xia Shuang, 279

Y
Yan Zhou, 281
Yian, Sitoh Yih, 341
Yongmei Li, 280
Yoo, Roh-Eul, 322
Young Neuroradiology-Junge Neuroradiologie (JUNRAD), 110
Yousry, Tarek, 22
Yunjing Xue, 280

Z
Zambia, 257–259
Zardini, Carolina Servin, 439
Zhang, Bing, 276
Zhang, Minming, 274
Zimny, Anna, 386
Zuccaro, Graciela Noemi, 435

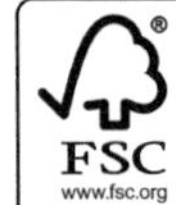

MIX
Papier aus verantwortungsvollen Quellen
Paper from responsible sources
FSC® C105338

If you have any concerns about our products,
you can contact us on
ProductSafety@springernature.com

In case Publisher is established outside the EU,
the EU authorized representative is:
Springer Nature Customer Service Center GmbH
Europaplatz 3, 69115 Heidelberg, Germany

Printed by Libri Plureos GmbH
in Hamburg, Germany